The
5-Minute
Orthopaedic
Consult

ASSOCIATE EDITORS

JAMES F. WENZ, M.D.

ASSISTANT PROFESSOR OF ORTHOPAEDIC SURGERY

CHAIRMAN, DEPARTMENT OF ORTHOPAEDIC SURGERY

JOHNS HOPKINS BAYVIEW MEDICAL CENTER

BALTIMORE MD

FRANK J. FRASSICA, M.D.

PROFESSOR OF ORTHOPAEDICS AND ONCOLOGY

CHAIRMAN, DEPARTMENT OF ORTHOPAEDICS

JOHNS HOPKINS UNIVERSITY

BALTIMORE, MD

The 5-Minute Orthopaedic Consult

EDITOR

PAUL D. SPONSELLER, M.D.

PROFESSOR OF ORTHOPAEDIC SURGERY

HEAD, DIVISION OF PEDIATRIC ORTHOPAEDICS

JOHNS HOPKINS UNIVERSITY

BALTIMORE, MD

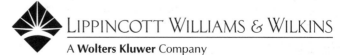

LIPPINCOTT WILLIAMS & WILKINS
A **Wolters Kluwer** Company
Philadelphia · Baltimore · New York · London
Buenos Aires · Hong Kong · Sydney · Tokyo

Acquisitions Editor: Robert Hurley
Production Editor: Steven P. Martin
Manufacturing Manager: Colin J. Warnock
Cover Designer: Christine Jenny
Compositor: The PRD Group
Printer: R.R. Donnelley-Willard

© 2001 by LIPPINCOTT WILLIAMS & WILKINS
530 Walnut Street
Philadelphia, PA 19106 USA
LWW.com

Printed in the USA

Library of Congress Cataloging-in-Publication Data

The 5-minute orthopaedic consult / editor, Paul D. Sponseller; associate
  editors, Frank J. Frassica, James F. Wenz.—1st ed.
      p. cm.
    Includes bibliographical references (p.   ) and index.
    ISBN 0-683-30088-1
    1. Orthopedics—Handbooks, manuals, etc.
    [DNLM: 1. Orthopedics—Handbooks. WE 39 Z999 2000] I. Title:
Five-minute orthopaedic consult. II. Sponseller, Paul D.
III. Frassica, Frank J. IV. Wenz, James F.
RD732.5 .A16 2000
616.7—dc21   98-003652
                                                   CIP

Care has been taken to confirm the accuracy of the information presented and to describe generally accepted practices. However, the authors, editors, and publisher are not responsible for errors or omissions or for any consequences from application of the information in this book and make no warranty, expressed or implied, with respect to the currency, completeness, or accuracy of the contents of the publication. Application of this information in a particular situation remains the professional responsibility of the practitioner.

The authors, editors, and publisher have exerted every effort to ensure that drug selection and dosage set forth in this text are in accordance with current recommendations and practice at the time of publication. However, in view of ongoing research, changes in government regulations, and the constant flow of information relating to drug therapy and drug reactions, the reader is urged to check the package insert for each drug for any change in indications and dosage and for added warnings and precautions. This is particularly important when the recommended agent is a new or infrequently employed drug.

Some drugs and medical devices presented in this publication have Food and Drug Administration (FDA) clearance for limited use in restricted research settings. It is the responsibility of the health care providers to ascertain the FDA status of each drug or device planned for use in their clinical practice.

10 9 8 7 6 5 4 3 2 1

This book is dedicated to the members of the Department of Orthopaedic Surgery at Johns Hopkins University, whose excellence has provided both the motivation and the support for this work. We especially dedicate it to our wives, Amy, Lidia and Deborah, with love and thanks.

Preface

The 5-Minute Orthopaedic Consult is designed to provide easy-to-use, subject-specific information. The organization and indexing make this a reference clinicians can use to help make decisions on the spot while seeing patients in the clinic or in the hospital. The consistent page presentation within each topic enables the user to scan the topic to find specific information, or to gain an overview of the topic within minutes by reading through. We have also included some relevant in-depth information such as etiology and pathogenesis, but in a condensed fashion.

Section I, Orthopaedic Essentials, guides the reader through commonly-performed examinations of the elbow, foot and ankle, hand, hip, knee, neck, shoulder, spine, and wrist and reviews techniques commonly used in orthopaedics; arthrocentesis, arthroscopy, fracture treatment, the Ilizarov method, and splinting. Section II, Specific Conditions, addresses 212 specific conditions from accessory navicular through wrist sprain.

We want this to be a useful reference. Please take a few minutes to leaf through it and get an idea of the scope and organization. We welcome suggestions for future editions. Please feel free to e-mail me at psponse@jhmi.edu.

Acknowledgment

The authors would like to thank Darlene B. Cooke, who helped design the initial concept, and Fran Klass and her staff, who assisted in bringing it to completion. The line drawings were expertly done to fit each topic by Hong Cui MD. Without their help this reference would not have been possible!

Contributing Authors

The following individuals contributed to this book during their residency at the Johns Hopkins University School of Medicine in the Department of Orthopaedics.

NICHOLAS AHN, MD

BRENDON ALBRACHT, DO

URI M. AHN, MD

MELANIE BATTLE KINCHEN, MD

SCOTT BERKENBLIT, MD

BARBARA BUCH, MD

MICHELLE CAMERON, MD

JOHN CARBONE, MD

ANDREW CORDISTA, MD

DAMIEN DOUTÉ, MD

WILLIAM HOBBS, MD

EMMANUEL HOSTIN, MD

MARC HUNGERFORD, MD

CHRISTOPHER HUTCHINS, MD

JOHN HWANG, MD

JAMIL JACOBS-EL, MD

PETER JAY, MD

CLIFF JENG, MD

DAWN LAPORTE, MD

TUNG B. LE, MD

JENNIFER LINDSEY, MD

DAVID LUMSDEN, MD

SAJONG MATHUR, MD

SIMON MEARS, MD

RON SABBAGH, MD

DAVID SOLACOFF, MD

DARYL THOMAS, MD

SEAN TOOMEY, MD

MARC URQUHART, MD

JINSONG WANG, MD

Contents

SECTION I.
Orthopaedic Essentials

Arthrocentesis

 Basics

DESCRIPTION

Aspiration of synovial joints is performed for diagnostic or therapeutic purposes.

CAUSES

Causes of joint effusions include infection, crystalline arthropathies, hemophilia, autoimmune arthropathies, trauma, and pigmented villonodular synovitis.

CPT CODES

- Small joint 20600 (hand, foot)
- Intermediate 20605 (ankle, wrist)
- Large 20610 (shoulder, knee, hip)

 Diagnosis

SIGNS AND SYMPTOMS

Synovial joints are aspirated for myriad reasons, the most common of which include the following:

- Rule out infection.
- Diagnose arthropathies.
- Relieve pain.

Joints with enough fluid to perform arthrocentesis generally have a palpable effusion. Infectious, autoimmune, and crystalline arthropathies are often warm to the touch and may display overlying erythema or cellulitis.

DIFFERENTIAL DIAGNOSIS

- Septic arthritis
- Gout
- Pseudogout
- Autoimmune disorders, such as rheumatoid arthritis or systemic lupus erythematosus
- Trauma
- Hemophilia

PHYSICAL EXAMINATION

An effusion is generally palpable. In infectious and crystalline arthropathies, as well as in trauma, the patient may have difficulty with range of motion of the affected joint. There may be outward signs of trauma or inflammation such as abrasions, erythema, or cellulitis.

LABORATORY TESTS

Joint aspirates should be sent for the following:

- Cell count and differential
- Microscopic examination for crystals
- Culture
- Gram stain
- Special immunologic tests, depending on the purpose of the aspiration

PATHOLOGIC FINDINGS

Crystalline arthropathies demonstrate crystals when specimens are examined with polarized light. Urate crystals appear sharp (needlelike) and display birefringence. The calcium pyrophosphate crystals of pseudogout have blunt ends and are not birefringent. Aspirates from septic arthritis often have cell counts greater than 100,000 with more than 80% to 90% polymorphonuclear cells, and they may have organisms present on Gram staining. Crystalline and inflammatory arthropathies can also have high white cell counts in the range of 50,000/mm^3.

IMAGING PROCEDURES

Radiographs are often helpful to rule out trauma and to evaluate degenerative changes within the joint.

 Management

GENERAL MEASURES

Patients with traumatic effusions should be treated appropriately for their underlying traumatic injury; however, arthrocentesis of the affected joint often makes these patients more comfortable. Patients with septic arthritis require irrigation and débridement of the joint; the type of débridement depends on the joint involved. Appropriate antibiotics should also be administered after all cultures are obtained. Patients with inflammatory and crystalline arthropathies generally respond well to anti-inflammatory medications and should be referred to a rheumatologist for evaluation.

SURGICAL TREATMENT

Sterile skin preparation is required before aspiration. The needle gauge should be large enough to withdraw the viscous joint fluid (usually 20 gauge or larger) (Fig. 1).

COMPLICATIONS

Care should be taken, especially when aspirating a potentially infected joint through cellulitic skin. Cellulitis can initially be thought of as septic arthritis. If the joint is aspirated, care should be taken to do so through uninvolved skin, because the arthrocentesis can infect a previously aseptic joint. The risk of infection in a straightforward aspiration is less than 1 in 10,000.

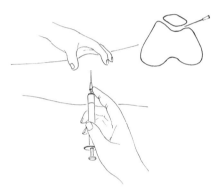

Fig. 1. Arthrocentesis of the knee is most easily done from the lateral side, under the patella.

RECOMMENDED READING

Campbell WC. *Campbell's operative orthopaedics,* vol 1, 9th ed. St. Louis: CV Mosby, 1992:601–617.

Basics

DESCRIPTION

Arthroscopy should be performed after a complete history and physical examination and after appropriate imaging studies have been obtained. Most procedures can be performed on an outpatient basis.

Knee

Indications

Indications include meniscal repair or débridement, meniscal cyst, osteochondral fragment removal, anterior or posterior cruciate tear débridement or reconstruction, synovial biopsy or synovectomy, determination of uncertain origin of instability or pain, and débridement of degenerative joint disease.

Procedure

Two or more portal incisions approximately one-half centimeter in length allow visualization through the arthroscope and instrument placement through another portal. The articular cartilage can be visualized in the three compartments of the knee (patellofemoral, medial, and lateral). The medial and lateral menisci, as well as the anterior cruciate ligament, can be visualized and probed to assess stability and integrity. Meniscal tears can often be treated definitively through the arthroscopic portals with débridement. Anterior cruciate ligament tears can also be reconstructed with arthroscopic assistance. The arthroscopic procedure can usually be performed on an outpatient basis.

Rehabilitation

Postoperatively, most patients can resume partial or full weight bearing with crutch assistance. The rehabilitation period after arthroscopy varies, depending on the type of procedure performed. Many patients who have undergone arthroscopy have some physical therapy for strengthening of the quadriceps and hamstrings; the duration and method of rehabilitation are specific to the injury.

Shoulder

Indications

Indications include treatment of instability, biopsy, removal of loose bodies, treatment of impingement, rotator cuff repair, and management of osteochondral lesions.

Procedure

Involves two or more half-centimeter portals. The articular cartilage of the glenoid and humeral head can be visualized for any pathologic process (e.g., osteoarthritis, osteochondral fragments). The soft tissue stabilizers of the shoulder can also be assessed: inferior glenohumeral ligament complex, middle glenohumeral ligament complex, and superior glenohumeral ligament complex. The integrity of the labrum can be determined arthroscopically as well. The diagnostic part of the procedure involves visualizing the subacromial space and rotator cuff for causes of impingement. Definitive procedures that can be performed arthroscopically include soft tissue stabilization procedures for instability of recurrent dislocations (e.g., Bankart's), acromioplasty, and rotator cuff repair.

Rehabilitation

Physical therapy is a necessary modality for anyone who has undergone shoulder arthroscopy. In general, the emphasis is on regaining motion and strengthening the shoulder girdle muscles and dynamic stabilizers of the shoulder. The duration and mode of rehabilitation vary with the type of injury.

Hip

Indications

Indications are synovial biopsy or synovectomy, loose body removal, and treatment of labral tears.

Ankle

Indications

Indications are synovial biopsy or synovectomy, loose body removal, bone spur removal, osteochondral fragment removal, drilling, and stabilization.

Elbow

Indications

Indications are synovial biopsy or synovectomy, loose body removal, and débridement of cartilage lesions.

Wrist

Indications

These include synovial biopsy or synovectomy, loose body removal, and diagnosis or débridement of triangular fibrocartilage complex injuries.

Elbow Anatomy and Examination

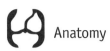 Anatomy

DESCRIPTION

The elbow joint is made up of two major articulations: the ulnohumeral joint and the humeroradial joint. In some ways, the elbow is similar to a hinged joint, with a range of motion restricted to extension and flexion (135 degrees). The triceps muscle extends the elbow joint, whereas the biceps and brachialis muscles flex the joint. The carrying angle of the elbow joint is approximately 7 degrees of valgus (away from the body) and allows the hand to be away from the body when the elbow is extended.

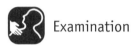 Examination

PHYSICAL EXAMINATION

History

A thorough history of the mechanism of injury (e.g., whether the patient fell onto an outstretched hand) can help to guide and focus the physical examination of the upper extremity.

Cervical Spine

The physical examination is begun by evaluating the cervical spine and shoulder (proximally) and the neurovascular status of the wrist and hand (distally). This includes range and palpation of the cervical spine, shoulders, wrists, and hands. Only then should one proceed with a focused elbow examination.

Upper Extremities

The patient should have both upper extremities from the shoulder girdle to the hand fully exposed for inspection and side-to-side comparison.

Inspection

- The elbow should be inspected for any asymmetry, such as alignment (carrying angle).
- Ecchymosis and edema should raise the suspicion of a fracture, dislocation, or ligamentous injury.
- Next the patient is asked to flex and extend both elbows actively, to compare the range of motion to the contralateral, uninjured side.
- Then the patient's ability to pronate and supinate the elbow fully is assessed.
- Elbow effusion (fluid in the joint) can be detected by palpating the elbow laterally in the center of the anatomic triangle formed by the lateral epicondyle, the radial head, and the tip of the olecranon.

Palpation

- Bony landmarks help to narrow the differential diagnosis.
- Laterally, bony landmarks are the lateral epicondyle and the radial head. The lateral epicondyle is the site of origin of the wrist and digit extensors and lateral collateral ligament complex.
- Medially, the medial epicondyle is easily palpated. This is the attachment of the medial collateral ligament complex, wrist flexor muscles, and a forearm pronator.
- The cubital tunnel is immediately posterior to the medial epicondyle. It is the groove containing the ulnar nerve as it crosses the elbow.
- Anteriorly, the tendon of the biceps can be easily palpated.
- Posteriorly, the olecranon bursa (a potential space) lies subcutaneously over the bony prominence of the olecranon.
- The triceps tendon and its attachment to the olecranon can be palpated.

Special Tests

"Tennis Elbow" Pain

- This pain can be elicited by palpating the lateral epicondyle, and it can be exacerbated by having the patient extend the wrist during palpation.
- The patient typically gives a history of an overuse activity.

Medial (Ulnar) Collateral Ligament Injury

- This injury is characterized by medial elbow tenderness and swelling after a fall onto an outstretched hand.

Biceps Tendon Rupture

- Rupture of the biceps tendon from its insertion on the bicipital tuberosity causes anterior swelling with or without ecchymosis.
- The muscle retracts proximally to cause a prominent, fusiform asymmetry in the midmuscle belly.
- The patient exhibits pain and weakness with resisted supination of the forearm.

Olecranon Bursitis

- This condition presents with a fluctuant subcutaneous area with or without erythema or tenderness over the tip of the olecranon.

"Nursemaid's Elbows"

- These injuries occur commonly in young children who have sustained a traction or pulling force to the arm.

Pediatric Elbow Fractures

- These fractures are common.
- A high level of suspicion of fracture is warranted in any child with painful motion and swelling of the elbow.
- With these clinical signs (despite normal-appearing radiographs), the child's elbow should be immobilized in a posterior splint and sling, with orthopaedic follow-up within the week.

IMAGING PROCEDURES

- Anteroposterior and lateral radiographs of the elbow are standard.
- An anterior "sail sign" on a lateral radiograph may be normal.
- A posterior "fat pad sign" on the lateral radiograph usually indicates intraarticular injury or fracture.
- The varied appearance of the ossification centers and physes in pediatric elbows make comparison views of the contralateral, uninjured elbow beneficial.

RECOMMENDED READING

Morrey BF. Anatomy of the elbow joint. In: Morrey BF, ed. *The elbow and its disorders,* 2nd ed. Philadelphia: WB Saunders, 1993:16–52.

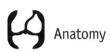 ## Anatomy

DESCRIPTION

The major functions of the foot and ankle are to allow even stress distribution between the foot and the lower extremity during walking and running. For adequate function, the foot must be plantigrade (i.e., rest evenly flat on the ground) and painless.

Functionally, the muscles and tendons can be divided into four groups: dorsiflexors, plantar flexors, invertors, and evertors.

The extensor tendons dorsiflex the ankle and toes. These tendons (anterior tibialis, extensor digitorum longus, and extensor hallucis longus) are easily palpable as they cross the ankle and can be cut by glass or other sharp objects.

The evertors (peroneus longus and brevis) lie on the lateral aspect of the leg, and their tendons run behind the lateral malleolus.

The plantar flexors and invertors all travel behind the ankle. The posterior tibial tendon is the main invertor and is prone to tenosynovitis and rupture in the adult, a condition leading to acquired flatfoot. Toe flexors (flexor digitorum longus and flexor hallucis longus) are not palpable at the ankle, and their function can be tested by checking passive and active toe flexion.

The bones of the foot and ankle are easily palpable (Fig. 1).

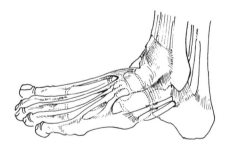

Fig. 1. The dorsal aspect of the ankle contains the extensor tendons (long and short) and the peronei, each constrained by separate retinacula.

Examination

PHYSICAL EXAMINATION

- Always address neurovascular status:

—Palpate the dorsalis pedis pulse at the front of the middle of the ankle and the posterior tibial pulse behind the medial malleolus.

- Perform a motor examination:

—Assess foot and toe dorsiflexion.
—Assess foot and toe flexion.
—Assess foot inversion and eversion.

- These tests confirm neurologic motor integrity to the foot.
- Sensation to light touch should also be intact along:

—The foot dorsum (superficial peroneal nerve)
—The first dorsal web space (deep peroneal nerve)
—The medial aspect (saphenous nerve)
—The lateral aspect (sural nerve)

- Evaluate motion of the affected foot:

—Check ankle plantar flexion and dorsiflexion and inversion and eversion of the hind foot to assess subtalar motion (allows for walking on uneven surfaces).
—Distally assess Chopart's joint (includes the calcaneocuboid and talonavicular joints) with midfoot abduction and adduction.
—Assess Lisfranc's joint with palpation and motion of the joints between the metatarsal bases and the tarsal bones.
—Perform metatarsal motion and palpation.
—Always compare motion with that of the other foot.

- Examine the plantar fascia:

—Palpate the plantar fascia, originating at the heel base.
—This may help the clinician to identify plantar fasciitis, especially if there is tenderness accentuated with the toes dorsiflexed.

- Examine the medial malleolus:

—Tenderness behind the medial malleolus may reveal tarsal tunnel syndrome, posterior tibial tendinitis, or flexor hallucis longus tenosynovitis.

- Examine the lateral malleolus:

—Tenderness behind the lateral malleolus may indicate a peroneal tendon disorder, such as tendon subluxation, impingement, or tear.
—Tenderness directly below the lateral malleolus indicates a calcaneofibular ligament injury.
—The anterior drawer test (an attempt to sublux the talus from the tibiotalar joint anteriorly) with the ankle dorsiflexed can identify a complete tear of this structure.

- Examine the anterior talofibular ligament:

—This is the most commonly injured ankle ligament.
—Injury causes tenderness just anterior to the lateral malleolus.
—The anterior drawer test with the ankle in plantar flexion can demonstrate a complete tear.

IMAGING PROCEDURES

Radiography

Radiographs should be taken with patient in the standing position. This view demonstrates bony relationships in the physiologic state and is much more likely to reveal foot disorders than a nonstanding view.

Computed Tomography

This technique is helpful to identify and delineate occult fractures, especially of the talus, navicular, and calcaneus.

Magnetic Resonance Imaging

This imaging technique may help to demonstrate tendon ruptures and soft tissue lesions.

RECOMMENDED READING

Mann RA. Principles of examination of the foot and ankle. In: Mann RA, Coughlin MJ, eds. *Surgery of the foot and ankle,* 6th ed. St. Louis: CV Mosby, 1993:45–60.

Fracture Treatment

 Basics

DESCRIPTION

General treatment guidelines exist for treating fractures.

CLASSIFICATION

Nondisplaced

• Single or both cortices are involved, but the bone has not moved. This fracture can be difficult to detect.
• Radiolucent line: This is the so-called "hairline fracture."

Displaced

• Angulation: This is described in many ways. A clear way to describe this deformity is to state the direction of the apex of the fracture, such as "angulated fracture apex anterior." Another method is to state the type of deformity, such as "varus angulation."
• Shortening: This is sometimes subtle. Look for overlaps on the radiograph.
• Rotation: Compare to the opposite extremity. Often easier to detect clinically, it can be difficult to assess radiographically. With metacarpal or digit fractures, check the flexion arcade by having the patient make a fist.
• Translation: This is most commonly described by the location of the distal fragment, that is, medially displaced.

Open Versus Closed

This is one of the most important determinations to make when evaluating a patient with a fracture. Any wound anywhere on a limb with a fracture must be suspect. If the wound communicates with bone and one believes that there could be a communication with the fracture site, this must be considered an open fracture. Patients with open fractures must go to the operating room within 6 to 8 hours to decrease the risk of infection. Patients should be given an antibiotic with good gram-positive coverage (often cefazolin, 1 g in adults and 25 mg/kg in children) and tetanus prophylaxis. For patients with grade II fractures (see later), an aminoglycoside should also be given. For patients with fractures that occurred in a farm environment, with vascular compromise, or with extensive soft tissue crush, 4 to 5 million units of aqueous penicillin G every 4 to 6 hours should be added (first-generation cephalosporin plus an aminoglycoside plus penicillin). Although no data support it, covering the wound with an antiseptic-soaked (povidone-iodine [Betadine]) sterile dressing until the patient is in the operating room is believed to decrease bacterial colonization. The patient must be given nothing by mouth, and it is important to document the last time the patient ate or drank anything.

A useful classification of open fractures is the modified classification described by Gustilo and Anderson. (It was actually described for tibia fractures, although most clinicians have now generalized it to all open fractures.)

I. Low energy, laceration less than 1 cm
II. Moderate energy, greater than 1 cm and usually less than 10 cm
III. High energy, more than 10 cm
IIIA. Adequate soft tissue coverage (muscle flap not necessary)
IIIB. Massive soft tissue destruction, bony exposure (muscle flap necessary)
IIIC. Fractures associated with a vascular injury

Fracture Sites

• Diaphysis: The shaft is mostly hard cortical bone. It is also often described by relative anatomic level—proximal third, middle third, and distal third.
• Metaphysis: This is composed of spongy cancellous bone.
• Intraarticular: This occurs within a joint, with low tolerance for any incongruence (also referred to as "step-off").
• Physis: See later.
• Epiphysis: See later.

Fracture Pattern

• Transverse: The fracture is straight across the bone.
• Oblique: The fracture is oblique across the bone.
• Spiral: The fracture is spiraling around the bone.
• Comminuted: Fragments are present at the fracture site.
• Segmental: The same bone is fractured in two places, so there is a "floating segment of bone."
• Impacted
• Avulsion: The size of the fragment and the amount of displacement help to guide treatment.
• Compression
• Pathologic: The fracture occurs through some other process in bone, such as a tumor (benign or malignant) or a metabolic process. One must have a high index of suspicion when the mechanism appears mild compared with the injury sustained (e.g., humerus fracture while throwing a ball or femur fracture while stepping off a curb).

Special in Children

• Greenstick: The cortex and periosteum on the concave side are intact, whereas the cortex and, often, the periosteum on the convex side are fractured.
• Buckle (torus fracture): This metaphyseal compression injury is relatively stable and is splinted for comfort.
• Growth plate injuries: The growth plate is called the physis; the articular side of the bone relative to the growth plate is called the epiphysis; the other side is the metaphysis.

Salter Classification

I. Transverse fractures through the physis
II. Through the physis with a metaphyseal fragment
III. Fractures through the physis and the epiphysis: intraarticular
IV. Fractures through the epiphysis, physis, and metaphysis: intraarticular
V. Crush injury of the physis
VI. Injury to the perichondral ring (not part of the original classification)

The clinician must suspect child abuse in cases of multiple bruises and fractures of different ages, as well as when the reported mechanism of injury does not account for the injury observed or when the reported mechanism keeps changing or is reported differently by different people. The bones most commonly fractured are the humerus, tibia, and femur, in that order. The clinician must involve social work and the pediatrician.

ICD-9-CM 829.0 Fracture

Management

GENERAL MEASURES

Ice, elevation, and immobilization should begin as soon as the patient is encountered in the emergency department, even before and during the evaluation.

Immobilization

Immediate and definitive immobilization protects soft tissue and allows soft tissue and bone to heal. Types are as follows:

• Splint: Options include sugar tong, U splint, ulnar or radial gutter, thumb spica, and anterior, posterior, medial, and lateral splints. They can be used for immediate treatment during evaluation, as well as for early definitive care. Actually, splinting is preferred for early definitive treatment with closed therapy because of a lower risk of compartment syndrome and soft tissue injury than with a circularized cast.
• Cast: Types include long arm, short arm, thumb spica, long leg, short leg, weight-bearing (walking), or non–weight-bearing, and patella weight-bearing short leg. Casts are the current standard for closed treatment of fractures. They are often not placed in the acute setting because of the theoretic risk of compartment syndrome. Casts can be univalved or bivalved to reduce the risk of compartment syndrome. They must be molded with three-point fixation to maintain fracture reduction.
• Functional bracing: This approach has been successful in the humerus.
• Internal fixation: This involves operative treatment.
• Plates and screws: These devices allow for anatomic reduction, more rigid fixation, reduction of joint surfaces, and early motion.
• Intramedullary rods: These devices can allow for anatomic reduction, more rigid fixation, and earlier motion and weight bearing.
• External fixation: This approach is used in situations of tenuous blood supply, marked soft tissue injury, or gross contamination, as well as in comminuted distal radius fractures.

COMPLICATIONS

Bone-Healing Abnormalities

• Delayed union: Healing has not occurred in 3 to 4 months (slow but steady progress).
• Nonunion: Healing has not occurred in 6 months (classified as hypertrophic or atrophic).
• The foregoing complications can be caused by too much or too little motion, inadequate fixation, soft tissue interposition, space between fragments, infection, or poor blood supply. These time allotments are arbitrary.
• Treatment can include electric stimulation, surgical débridement, surgical removal of interposing tissue, bone grafting, conversion to more or less rigid fixation, revision to reamed intramedullary nail, and use of osteogenic materials at the fracture site.
• Malunion: This term refers to healing with a malalignment.
• Osteonecrosis (avascular necrosis): This condition occurs secondary to the disruption of the blood supply to the bone. It is more common with intraarticular fractures and is most commonly seen with fractures of the femoral neck, femoral head, femoral condyles, proximal scaphoid, proximal humerus, and talar neck.

Infection

See Osteomyelitis.

Soft Tissue Disorders

• Arterial injury: This is rare, but consequences are severe. One must carefully assess this possibility during the physical examination and must maintain a high index of suspicion.
• Compartment syndrome: See the specific chapters on this syndrome.
• Nerve injuries: These are rare but are more common than arterial injuries. Most are neuropraxias, and about 70% resolve over time. More common injuries are as follows:

—Fracture and fracture-dislocation of the cervical, thoracic, and lumbar spine: cauda equina or spinal cord injury
—Shoulder fracture or dislocation: axillary nerve
—Humerus: radial nerve
—Medial epicondyle fracture: ulnar nerve
—Radial head or Monteggia's fracture: posterior interosseous nerve
—Hip dislocations, acetabular fractures: sciatic nerve
—Lateral knee injuries: common peroneal nerve

Pulmonary Disorders

• Adult respiratory distress syndrome
• Fat emboli syndrome
• Pulmonary embolism

Gastrointestinal Disorders

• Related to the trauma (e.g., spleen injury)
• Stress ulcers in the intensive care setting
• Cast syndrome: after body or hip spica casting, compression of the second portion of the duodenum by the superior mesenteric artery
• Reflex sympathetic dystrophy: see specific chapter

RECOMMENDED READING

Browner BD, Jupiter JB, Levine AM, et al. *Skeletal trauma*, vol 2. Philadelphia: WB Saunders, 1992.

Heckman JD. Clinical symposia—fractures: emergency care and complications. *Clin Symp* 1991;43,2–32.

Rockwood CA, Wilkins KE, Beaty JH, eds. *Fractures in children*, 4th ed. Philadelphia: Lippincott–Raven, 1996:3–18.

Hand Anatomy and Examination

 Anatomy

DESCRIPTION

The hand is a unique organ that allows humans to work and to create. The hand can be conveniently divided into the volar and dorsal parts. The volar portion of the hand contains the major digital nerves, the flexor tendons, and the muscles that allow us to move our fingers. The bony architecture is complex, with the distal surface of the radius making up the major portion of the wrist, eight carpal bones and then five metacarpals, three phalanges for each of the fingers, and a proximal and distal phalanx for the thumb.

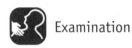 Examination

PHYSICAL EXAMINATION

General Considerations

• Examination of the hand is extremely complex.
• It is essential to understanding the anatomy and biomechanics of the hand.
• An examiner should have his or her own system of examining the key components of hand anatomy and function.

EXAMPLE OF HAND EXAMINATION

Check Vascular Status

• Palpate the radial and ulnar arteries; use a Doppler examination as needed.
• Digital arteries can be examined using a Doppler technique.
• Check the capillary refill in each finger (should be less than 2 seconds).
• Some hand surgeons examine individual digits by measuring the temperature of fingers and by placing a pulse oximeter and measuring oxygen saturation.
• Perform the Allen test (to check the competence of the palmar arch).

—Press firmly on both radial and ulnar arteries and have the patient open and close his or her hand actively several times.
—Then, take the pressure off the ulnar artery and see whether blood returns to the hand.

Nerve Innervation

Check Median Nerve

• Examine the sensation on the volar tip of the thumb.
• Perform a two-point examination (normal: less than 5 mm).
• Ask the patient to appose the thumb to the little finger to test the motor function of the median nerve.

Check Ulnar Nerve

• Examine the sensation on the volar tip of the little finger.
• Ask the patient to cross his or her fingers (the motor branches of the ulnar nerve innervate the intrinsic muscles of the hand) to test the motor function of the ulnar nerve.

Check Radial Nerve

• The radial nerve has no motor branch in the hand.
• The sensation of the radial nerve is tested on the first web space of the dorsal aspect of the hand.

Check Bones, Tendons, and Ligaments

• Each bone is palpated to rule out a fracture.
• Swelling can be variable.

Range of Motion (ROM)

• Check each joint for active and passive ROM:
• Normal ROM in the interphalangeal joint of the thumb: 0 to 80 degrees
• Normal ROM in the metacarpophalangeal joint of the thumb: 0 to 50 degrees
• Normal ROM in distal interphalangeal and metacarpophalangeal joints of the fingers: 0 to 90 degrees
• Normal ROM in the proximal interphalangeal joint of the fingers: 0 to 100 degrees
• Normal ROM of the wrist: 80 degrees of flexion and 70 degrees of extension

Special Tests

Tinel's Sign

• Percussion over the median nerve at the wrist produces numbness, tingling, and pain in the thumb and the index and middle fingers.
• Test for carpal tunnel syndrome.

Phalen's Test

• Flexion of the wrist completely for 1 minute produces numbness, tingling, and pain in the hand.
• Test for carpal tunnel syndrome.

Aspiration of the Wrist Joint (Two Approaches)

• Dorsal approach: Insert a needle between the third compartment (extensor pollicis longus) and the fourth compartment (extensor digitorum communis and extensor indicis proprius).
• Palpate Lister's tubercle (bony prominence in distal radius) and introduce the needle just distal to it; flexing the wrist facilitates entry.

Finkelstein's Test

• Passive hyperflexion of thumb metacarpophalangeal and interphalangeal joints (thumb in fist) with ulnar deviation of wrist causes pain over abductor pollicis longus and extensor pollicis brevis.
• Test for de Quervain's tenosynovitis.

Grind Test

• Hold the proximal phalanx and the metacarpophalangeal joint and forcefully push against the trapeziometacarpal joint.
• Pain during this maneuver is consistent with arthritis in the trapeziometacarpal joint.

IMAGING PROCEDURES

Anteroposterior and lateral radiographs should be obtained as the first step in imaging.

Anatomy

DESCRIPTION OF BONY ANATOMY

Pelvis

• The pelvis is composed of three bones on each side that form a normal hemipelvis:

—Ischium, which forms the main support during sitting
—Pubis (anterior portion)
—Ilium (main wing)

• Acetabulum

—The bones of the pelvis are joined together at the acetabulum.
—It is the articulation of the femoral head.

• The pelvis has numerous growth lines in the immature patient, especially the triradiate cartilage of the acetabulum and the apophysis of the ilium.
• Apophysis

—It is the cartilage cap that provides growth to the ilium.
—In preadolescence and adolescence as it matures, the growth cartilage of the ilium ossifies and provides a sign of advancing maturity.

Femoral Head

• The femoral head should be perfectly spheric on the anteroposterior and lateral radiographs (Fig. 1).
• The proximal femur is composed of the femoral head, the greater and lesser trochanters, and the intertrochanteric area (Fig. 2).
• Fovea

—It is a small indentation medially where the ligament inserts.

• Greater trochanter

—It is the site for insertion of the abductor muscles, gluteus medius, and gluteus minimus.
—Its tip should be at the same level as the femoral head.

• Lesser trochanter

—It is the small prominence posteromedial and distal to the femoral neck.
—This is the attachment of the iliopsoas muscle, the major hip flexor.

• Growth plate of the femoral head

—It usually remains open until approximately 13 years of age in girls and 14 to 15 years in boys. Before this, forces on the growth plate may cause displacement, especially in the heavy child or as a result of major trauma: the slipped capital femoral epiphysis.
—Loss of sphericity of the femoral head is most often due to avascular necrosis or a degenerative cyst.
—Loss of the joint space around the femoral head is a sign of arthritic change or chondrolysis.

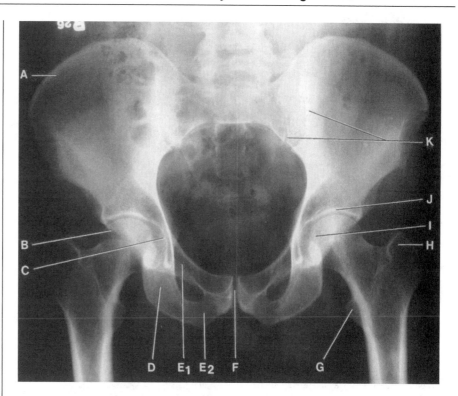

Fig. 1. Anteroposterior radiograph of the pelvis and hips. Important points of bony anatomy are noted: *A*, italic crest; *B*, posterior acetabular margin; *C*, medial acetabular wall; *D*, ischium; *E*, pubis; *E1*, superior ramus; *E2*, inferior ramus; *F*, symphysis pubis; *G*, lesser trochanter; *H*, greater trochanter; *I*, fovea of the femoral head; *J*, acetabular dome; *K*, sacroiliac joint. (From Steinberg GG, Akins CM, Baran DT. *Orthopaedics in primary care*, 3rd ed. Philadelphia: Lippincott Williams & Wilkins, 1999, with permission.)

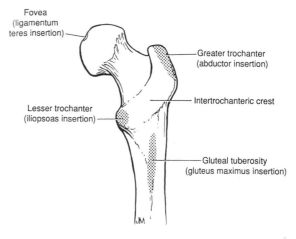

Fig. 2. Proximal femur (posterior view). (From Steinberg GG, Akins CM, Baran DT. *Orthopaedics in primary care*, 3rd ed. Philadelphia: Lippincott Williams & Wilkins, 1999, with permission.)

Hip Anatomy and Examination

DESCRIPTION OF SOFT TISSUE ANATOMY

- Major muscles that propel the hip:

—The flexors: iliopsoas and rectus
—The abductors: gluteus medius and gluteus minimis, which insert on the greater trochanter
—The extensors: gluteus maximus and hamstrings
—The adductors: medially

- Structural abnormalities of the hip and damage to the muscles and nerves often result in a limp.

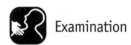 Examination

PHYSICAL EXAMINATION

Standing Examination

Observation of Patient Walking

- Ideally do this before he or she knows about being observed.
- Look for any asymmetry of stride lengths between the two sides.
- From the side, observe the lumbar spine and pelvis for excessive motion, which may occur if the hip is stiff.
- From the front, observe for any dropping of the pelvis on one side, which may indicate a hip disorder.

Trendelenburg's Sign

- The shoulders lean over to the side of the stance.
- This is a sign of hip muscle weakness or hip guarding.

Trendelenburg's Test (Confirms Abductor Weakness)

- Have the patient stand on one leg alone first, then the other.
- Look for any dropping of the opposite hemipelvis or tilting of the shoulders over toward the side of the stance (compensatory mechanisms for weak abductors or painful hips).
- Be aware that pain from within the hip joint is often referred to the groin or to the lower thigh.
- This latter phenomenon is especially common in children and adolescents, whose complaints are often mistaken for knee disorders.

Supine Examination

- Ask the patient to lie supine.
- Look for symmetric positioning of the legs:

—Is one leg more externally rotated or more adducted than the other (from fracture, slipped epiphysis, or contracture)?
—Is one leg shorter than the other (from a prior bony disorder)?

- Measure the leg lengths:

—Use a tape measure.
—Measure between the inferior edge of the anterior superior iliac spine and the inferior edge of the medial malleolus.

- Check the range of motion: roll the hip in extension from side to side:

—Is there is any guarding or spasm?
—If it does not roll far, this is an indication of stiffness in the joint.

- Quantify rotation:

—Flex the hip and knee up to 90 degrees and check the following:
    —Internal rotation (normal, 15 to 45 degrees)
    —External rotation (normal, 40 to 65 degrees)
    —The abduction (normal, 35 to 70 degrees)

—Check the range of abduction.
    —Measure this by the ability to move the knee of the flexed hip sideways toward the examination table.
    —Do not allow the patient's pelvis to move while doing this test because it may give a false impression of increased motion.

—Internal rotation and abduction are the motions usually lost first in hip disorders.

- Palpate the trochanteric bursa as a site for pain:

—This is a thin layer of smooth tissue over the prominence of the greater trochanter and under the fascia lata. It is formed because the fascia lata is so tight that it acts as a pressure point against the trochanter and the femur.

- Perform Thomas' test (hip flexion contracture):

—This is measured while the patient lies supine.
—The opposite leg is brought up to full flexion and is held there, to lock the pelvis. The limb in question is then extended down as far as possible. The lack of extension is measured as a flexion contracture.
—(In the standing position, flexion contracture can be masked when a patient increases lumbar lordosis to bring the hips down straight.)

RECOMMENDED READING

Moore K, Dalley AF II. *Clinically oriented anatomy*, 4th ed. Philadelphia: Lippincott Williams & Wilkins, 1999:506–514.

Basics

DESCRIPTION

The Ilizarov method refers to use of a versatile external fixator to produce gradual changes in the length and alignment of an extremity. The fixator consists of circular rings attached to bone with wires. These rings are distracted (spread apart) by threaded rods. Each fixator is custom assembled for the given patient and indication. The method was developed in Kurgan, Russia, by G.I. Ilizarov, as a means of slowly and completely correcting many congenital and acquired abnormalities. The process of forming new bone by slow, gentle stretching is called distraction osteogenesis. Although other fixators are available to accomplish these effects, the system that Ilizarov initiated is probably the most versatile. Nevertheless, the principles described here are general and apply not to the device, but rather to the concept and procedure.

The Ilizarov method is applicable to all extremities. However, it is used most commonly in the lower extremities because alignment is more critical in these than in the upper extremities. The ideal age for performing the Ilizarov method is in the preteen and teen years. At this time, the skeleton is almost finished growing, so its final shape can be determined, yet the potential for healing and remodeling is that of a child. In addition, the patient has the maturity to undergo an arduous treatment process. Bone healing, however, is slower with advancing age.

For certain indications, this procedure can be performed in younger patients (with severe congenital abnormalities) or in adults (with nonunions and acquired deformities).

SYNONYM

Limb lengthening

CLASSIFICATION

The types of procedures performed using the Ilizarov method are as follows:

- Extremity lengthening
- Angular correction
- Repair of nonunion
- Restoration of lost bone
- Correction of contracture
- Fracture treatment

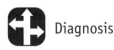

Diagnosis

PHYSICAL EXAMINATION

The patient should be checked for pin tract problems, nerve function, and joint range of motion at each visit.

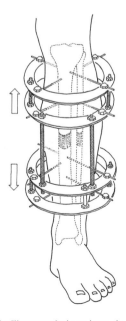

Management

SURGICAL TREATMENT

The surgery is done with the patient under general anesthesia, and the elongation of the bone is performed later. The external fixator frame is assembled on the patient's limb according to its shape and the goal of treatment. Several pins or rings are needed above and below the site of bone correction. Threaded distraction rods are positioned to provide the needed correction over time (Fig. 1). Then the osteotomy is done, once the bone is stabilized. This should be done through a small incision, and the surgeon should try to disrupt as little of the blood supply as possible. Often, the fixator is extended to the adjacent bone for stability. The correction is usually not done while the patient is under anesthesia, unless the correction is minor. Usually, no distraction or lengthening is done at the time of the surgery. Distraction is started at 7 to 10 days later, about the time the healing callus is first seen radiographically. Distraction is continued at a rate of 1 mm per day, usually divided into at least four segments so the tissues are not stretched too suddenly. In this way, the callus is slowly stretched outward. This is termed "distraction osteogenesis." Once the desired length is achieved, the new bone is allowed to strengthen. This occurs with time and weight bearing. The fixator is removed when the bone appears strong enough. The total time spent in the fixator can be estimated by the "lengthening index," which is the time (per centimeter of length gained) needed for the process of lengthening and consolidation. It averages 1 to 1.6 months per centimeter.

Fig. 1. The Ilizarov method may be used to lengthen a limb. Bone regenerates to fill in the gap.

Other fixators may be used instead of the Ilizarov fixator, which tends to be bulky. If complex rotation and angular correction are not needed, fixators with pins in a straight line may be used. Many different models are currently available.

PHYSICAL THERAPY

Patients may benefit from the following:

- Teaching appropriate weight bearing
- Maintaining joint range of motion
- Strengthening
- Teaching transfers
- Monitoring the correction process on a daily basis

MEDICAL TREATMENT

Nonsteroidal antiinflammatory agents should not be taken for a long period because they may suppress bone healing.

PATIENT EDUCATION

Patients should be told of the duration of treatment, which usually runs many months. They should be helped to make arrangements for school or work and for extensive care after the procedure. Admission to a rehabilitation hospital is sometimes indicated. Patients should be assessed to determine whether they have the level of maturity needed for the treatment. Patients may be allowed to bear weight and to swim with the device, if the surgeon allows.

MONITORING

Patients need to be seen periodically during the procedure to monitor the correction process and to check on the status of the pin sites. Radiographs are usually necessary.

COMPLICATIONS

- Nonunion
- Joint stiffness or subluxation
- Fracture
- Nerve injury

PROGNOSIS

The results are largely good because the frame is smaller and more predictable. An 80% to 90% success rate may be expected, although the time for healing is often prolonged.

RECOMMENDED READING

Paley D. Current techniques of limb lengthening. *J Pediatr Orthop* 1988;8:733–792.

Knee Anatomy and Examination

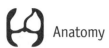 Anatomy

DESCRIPTION

The knee joint is complex and is composed of two major articulations with three compartments: patellofemoral, medial femorotibial (medial compartment), and lateral femorotibial (lateral compartment). The patella, the largest sesamoid bone in the body, helps to center the action of the quadriceps muscles while it increases the lever arm. The quadriceps tendon attaches the four quadriceps muscles to the patella, and the patellar tendon connects the patella and the tibia. The four quadriceps muscles extend the knee powerfully through their contraction and attachment by the quadriceps tendon. The four hamstring muscles (biceps femoris, semimembranosus, semitendinosus, and gracilis) flex the knee. The medial and lateral menisci are composed of fibrocartilage and distribute force between the femoral and tibial condyles. Four major ligaments guide motion of the joint: the two central ligaments are the anterior cruciate ligament (ACL) and the posterior cruciate ligament (PCL), and the two outside ligaments are the medial and lateral collateral ligaments. The proximal portion of the fibula (called the head) can be felt just distal to the lateral joint, and it articulates with the tibia through a small head (Fig. 1).

 Examination

HISTORY

Pain

- Acute onset

—ACL: cutting maneuvers associated with a "pop"
—PCL tear: dashboard injuries
—Meniscus: twisting injuries with moderate edema and later locking and clicking of knee

- Chronic: degenerative joint disease, gout, pseudogout
- Specific location

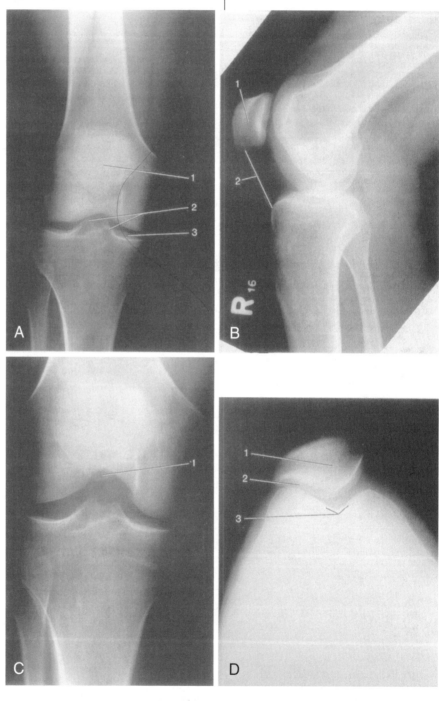

Fig. 1. Radiographic views of the normal knee. **A:** Anteroposterior view: *1*, patella; *2*, tibial spines; *3*, medial joint space. **B:** Lateral view: *1*, patella; *2*, patellar ligament. **C:** Notch view: *1*, intercondylar notch. **D:** Skyline patellar view: *1*, Patella: *2*, Patellofemoral joint: *3*, trochear groove. (From Steinberg GG, Akins CM, Baran DT. *Orthopaedics in primary care*, 3rd ed. Philadelphia: Lippincott Williams & Wilkins, 1999, with permission).

- Specific activities causing pain (e.g., pain with climbing stairs and on rising from sitting may be patellofemoral)

Swelling

- Posttraumatic

—Immediate: fracture versus ligament tear
—Delayed: meniscal versus chondral tear

- Chronic: degenerative joint disease, gout, pseudogout
- Associated with erythema, fever, increased white blood cell count and erythrocyte sedimentation rate, and severe pain
- Range of motion: think infection

Mechanical Factors

- Locking: meniscal tear versus loose body
- Giving way: ACL, knee felt to "shift," meniscal tears, patellar dislocation, or subluxation
- Grinding: specific location (medial, lateral, patellofemoral)

Neurologic Conditions

- Weakness or numbness
- Back pain
- Groin pain or with range of motion of hip (hip pain can be referred to the knee)

Associated Conditions

- Rheumatologic disorders

PHYSICAL EXAMINATION

General Considerations

- The patient must undress or wear shorts.
- Most maneuvers must be done with the patient relaxed and avoiding contraction of muscles.

Standing

- Alignment (normal adult is 7 degree valgus angle)
- Varus: foot toward the midline
- Valgus: foot away from the midline
- Muscle mass: possible atrophy

Gait

- Antalgic: This gait has short strides and short length of time in the stance phase on the affected leg (often an indication of pain in affected leg).
- Trendelenburg's: The contralateral pelvis tips toward the floor or the upper body tilts toward the affected side when standing on the affected leg (an indication of weak hip abductors).
- Medial or lateral thrust: Tibial translation and angular displacement during stance phase (of affected knee) may indicate a posterolateral or posteromedial injury.
- Squatting: Patients with a meniscal tear often have symptoms during squatting.

Sitting

- Active leg extension

—Inability to extend the leg actively; a possible indication of extensor mechanism rupture

- Patella position

—"Grasshopper patella": patella pointing upward and outward
—Patella alta: patella facing upward rather than straight

- Patellar tracking with range of motion

—Terminal J sign: patella deviating laterally when moving into terminal extension

- Palpation for crepitance

Supine (Knee Extended Unless Otherwise Noted)

Back and Neurologic Examination

- Straight leg raises, sensation, reflexes

Hip Examination

- Especially internal rotation (hip disorders often referred as pain to the knee)

Observation

- Signs of erythema or effusion

Palpation

- Warmth
- Pain to palpation: note specific location

Effusion

- Blot test: Press the patella against the femoral groove. If a large effusion is present, the fluid is first forced out of the groove and then the patella rebounds as fluid flows back.
- Milk test: Milk the fluid from the lateral side of the knee and the suprapatellar pouch to the medial side of the knee with several strokes of the examiner's hand. Next quickly tap the medial joint (just dorsal to the patella) with two fingers and look for a fluid wave on the lateral knee.
- Milk test II: Milk the fluid from the medial side of the knee into the suprapatellar pouch with several strokes of the examiner's hand. Next blot the suprapatellar pouch with the examiner's hand (palm and fingers across the entire pouch) and look for a fluid wave on the medial side of the knee.

Patellar Assessment

- Q angle: This is the angle of the anterior superior iliac spine, patella, and tibial tubercle. (The normal limit is less than 15 degrees; an increased angle may lead to dislocations or subluxations.)
- Palpation: In the medial and lateral articular facets of the patella, one should assess for pain.
- Passive mobility should be assessed.

—Medial and lateral glide test (knee flexed 30 degrees): This test determines the number of quadrants the patella will move over the trochlear groove and tests the integrity of medial and lateral restraints.
—Tilt test: This evaluates the number of degrees the patella will passively elevate; less than 0 degrees of lateral elevation may indicate tightness of the lateral retinaculum.

- Apprehension test: In patients with subluxation of the patella, pressing the patella laterally causes the patient's face to show distress and apprehension as the patella subluxes.
- Grind test: Press the patella distally against the trochlear groove, then have the patient contract the quadriceps while palpating for crepitance. Patients with patellofemoral disease often have a roughened surface causing a grind, and this maneuver often causes pain in this condition.

Range of Motion

- Normal is an angle 3 to 5 degrees of hyperextension to 135 degrees of flexion.

Palpating the Knee at 90 Degrees of Flexion

- Palpate the extensor mechanism.

—Patellar tendon and its insertion on the tibial tuberosity
—Quadriceps tendon

- Palpate the medial structures.

—Joint line: pain is possible indication of medial meniscal tear
—Medial collateral ligament
—Pes anserinus (insertion on proximal tibia of the semitendinosus, gracilis, and sartorius tendons): pain is possible indication of bursitis or tendinitis
—Saphenous nerve: pain is possibly elicited by tapping of nerve

- Palpate the lateral structures.

—Placement of foot across the opposite knee to place the lateral structures on stretch
—Joint line: pain is a possible indication of a lateral meniscal tear
—Lateral collateral ligament: iliotibial band
  —Insertion onto "Gerdy's tubercle": proximal, anterior lateral tibia
  —Pain is a possible indication of tendinitis or bursitis

Knee Anatomy and Examination

Stability Examinations

- Lachman's test (Fig. 2)

—This is the most sensitive test for ACL integrity (80% in acute tears, 98% in chronic tears).
—With the patient's knee relaxed, flex the knee 30 degrees and hold one hand on the distal thigh and a second hand on the proximal lower leg. The tibia is then translated anteriorly.
—Assess the following:
   —Quality of end point (solid, firm end point versus indeterminate or soft end point)
   —Amount of translation
      —Normal limit: 1+ = 0 to 5 mm of translation
      —2+ = 5 to 10 mm of translation
      —3+ = more than 10 mm of translation
      —Abnormal: 3-mm difference to the contralateral knee

- Anterior and posterior drawer test

—Increased posterior translation or posterior starting point (sag sign) is the most sensitive test for detecting an isolated PCL injury.
—Increased anterior drawer is less sensitive than Lachman's test in ACL injuries (30% to 50% in acute tears).
—Place knees at 90 degrees of flexion and neutral rotation and stabilize the patient's feet by sitting on them. Place both hands around the proximal lower leg and attempt to translate the tibia anteriorly and posteriorly on the femur.
—Note the starting point of tibia relative to the femur: normal knees have the lip of the tibial plateau anterior to the femoral condyles by about 1 cm (N1 = 10 mm, 1+ = 5 mm, 2+ = 0 mm [flush], 3+ = more than −5 mm).
—Grade translation is like that in Lachman's test.
—Also look for the tendency of the tibia to spin in a posterolateral, posteromedial or anteromedial direction; with the posterior drawer test, posterior movement of lateral tibia on the femur but no movement of the medial tibia indicates a posterior lateral corner instability.

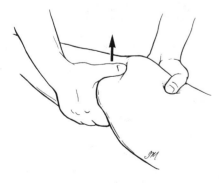

Fig. 2. Lachman's test. The knee is flexed 20 degrees. The proximal tibia is grasped and moved forward while the femur is held with the other hand. (Adapted from Torg JS, Conrad W, Kalen V. Clinical diagnosis of anterior cruciate ligament instability in the athlete. *Am J Sports Med* 1976;4:84–92, with permission.)

—Drawer test with the tibia in external rotation
   —This test assesses the posterior lateral corner instability.
   —If the PCL is out but the posterior lateral corner is intact, there is less translation than in a posterior drawer test in neutral rotation.
—Drawer test with tibia in internal rotation
   —This test assesses the posterior medial corner.
   —If the PCL is out but the posterior medial corner is intact, there is less translation than in a posterior drawer test in neutral rotation.

- Varus and valgus stability tests

—One of the examiner's hands is held at the patient's knee and the other hand is held at the ankle while the knee is stressed in the coronal plane.
—Assessment:
   —Grade 1: 0 to 5 mm opening—minimal tear
   —Grade 2: 5 to 10 mm opening and firm end point—moderate tear
   —Grade 3: greater than 10 mm opening and minimal end point—complete tear
—At 30 degrees of flexion:
   —Specific for medial and lateral collateral ligament tears
—At full extension:
   —Palpate the joint to make sure any laxity is not actually pseudolaxity (fracture reduction or arthritic bone loss).
   —Valgus laxity signifies an injury to the medial collateral ligament, the posteromedial capsule, the PCL, and possibly the ACL.
   —Varus laxity signifies an injury to the lateral collateral ligament, the posterolateral capsule, and the PCL.

Additional Ligament Tests

- ACL

—Attempt to show anterior tibial subluxation and reduction.
—Perform a pivot shift.
—Flex the hip to the abdomen, with mild knee valgus, flex and extend the knee.
—If the ACL is out, the tibia will go from the subluxed position in extension to a reduced position in flexion (tibia moves posterior in relation to the femoral condyles).

- PCL

—Attempt to show posterior tibial subluxation and reduction.
—Perform the quadriceps active test.
—The knee is placed as in the drawer tests, and the patient attempts to extend the knee.
—If the PCL is out, the tibia will sag posteriorly at the start, but when extension is attempted, the tibia is reduced (moves anterior in relation to the femoral condyles).

- Isolated posterior lateral corner

—Perform prone rotation at 30 and 90 degrees.
—If an isolated PLC tear is present, there will be increased external rotation at 30 degrees.

- Posterior lateral corner and PCL

—Hyperextension recurvatum: The patient is supine and the examiner lifts the patient's toes.
—If both are out, the knee will move into hyperextension and varus.

Meniscal Examinations

- Pain to palpation along the joint line
- Pain along the joint line with full flexion
- Maneuvers to elicit pain or a click (torn meniscus catching in the joint)

—McMurry's test: varus and valgus stress and tibial rotation as the knee is extended from full flexion to extension (Fig. 3)
—Steinman's test: quick tibial rotation with the knee in flexion
—Appley's test: prone flexion and rotation of the knee

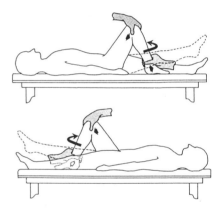

Fig. 3. McMurry's test for meniscus tear is positive if pain is reproduced along the medial or lateral joint line. (From Steinberg GG, Akins CM, Baran DT. *Orthopaedics in primary care*, 3rd ed. Philadelphia: Lippincott Williams & Wilkins, 1999, with permission).

RECOMMENDED READING

Hoppenfeld S. *Physical examination of the spine and extremities.* Norwalk, CT: Appleton & Lange, 1976:171–196.

Miller MD, Cooper DE, Warner JJ, *Review of sports medicine and arthroscopy.* Philadelphia: WB Saunders, 1995:8–13.

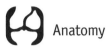 Anatomy

DESCRIPTION

- Soft tissues of the neck
- Vascular structures of the neck
- Neurologic structures of the neck
- Cervical spine

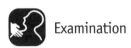 Examination

Examination of the neck starts there and is done only after a complete neurologic examination. It includes local examination of the neck, including the bony and soft tissues of the neck itself, as well as the structures that traverse the neck to go to the other parts of the body.

NEUROLOGIC EXAMINATION

A careful neurologic examination is performed.

Motor Examination

- Deltoids—shoulder abduction
- Biceps—arm flexion
- Triceps—arm extension
- Wrist extensors—wrist
- Wrist flexors—wrist
- Finger extension
- Finger flexion

Deep Tendon Reflexes

- Biceps
- Triceps
- Brachioradialis

Sensation

- Ulnar nerves
- Median nerves

PHYSICAL EXAMINATION

Inspection

- Attitude and posture of the head
- Posture of the body
- Gait
- Scars on the neck

Bony Palpation: Anterior

- Hyoid bone: C-3 vertebral body
- Tip of thyroid cartilage: C-4 vertebral body
- First cricoid ring: C-6 vertebral body
- Carotid tubercle: C-6 transverse process (The two carotid tubercles of the C-6 vertebra should be palpated separately, because simultaneous palpation can restrict the flow of both carotid arteries.)

Bony Palpation: Posterior

- Occiput
- Inion: This is the lower, most palpable part of the occiput.
- Spinous processes of the cervical spine: C-7 and T-1 are the most prominent. (All the spinous processes are aligned in one line, and any shift may be due to a unilateral facet dislocation. C3-5 may be bifid.)
- Facet joints: About 1 inch lateral to the spinous processes, the most common joint involved in osteoarthritis is C5-6.

Soft Tissue Palpation: Anterior

- Sternocleidomastoid
- Lymph nodes
- Thyroid gland
- Carotid pulse
- Palpation for a cervical rib in the supraclavicular region

Soft Tissue Palpation: Posterior

- Trapezius
- Greater occipital nerves
- Ligamentum nuchae: inion to C-7 spinous process

Range of Motion

- Flexion and extension: 50% occurs between the occiput and C-1, and the rest is distributed among C-2 to C-7; slightly greater motion occurs at the C5-6 level.
- Rotation: 50% occurs between C-1 and C-2, and the rest is evenly distributed in the remainder of the cervical spine.
- Lateral bending: This is evenly spread throughout the cervical spine and is usually not a pure movement but rather functions in conjunction with rotation.

IMAGING PROCEDURES

Radiographs

- Anteroposterior and lateral views are used to screen for most conditions.
- Oblique views are used to detect facet dislocation and subluxation.
- The open-mouth view is used to detect odontoid fractures (patients with neck pain who have struck their heads).

Magnetic Resonance Imaging

- This method is used to detect and define disc herniation.

Computed Tomography

- This technique is used to define the anatomy of cervical spinal structures.

Shoulder Anatomy and Examination

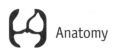 Anatomy

DESCRIPTION

The shoulder is a suspensory structure composed of three bones:

- Scapula
- Clavicle
- Humerus

Scapula

- This triangular bone has an anterior projection called the coracoid process.
- Its acromial process articulates with the clavicle, and the glenoid process articulates with the humeral head.

Clavicle

- This bone acts as an anterior strut.
- It articulates with the scapula and the sternum.

Glenohumeral Joint

- This joint, together with the scapulothoracic joint, allows range of motion of the upper arm.

Shoulder Joint

- This has greater range of motion than any other joint in the body.
- This range is possible because only 30% of the humeral head articulates with the glenoid at any given time.
- The shoulder joint has little inherent bony stability.
- It relies on the strong glenohumeral ligaments that form the joint capsule and the many muscles that cross the joint to provide stability.

Muscles of the Shoulder

Deltoid

- This is the most superficial muscle.
- It abducts the arm; it originates on the acromioclavicular arch and inserts on the lateral humerus.
- Deep to the deltoid is the rotator cuff, which is composed of four muscles:

—Subscapularis (internal rotator)
—Supraspinatus (external rotator)
—Infraspinatus (external rotator)
—Teres minor (external rotator)
—(These muscles stabilize the humeral head in the glenoid and primarily internally and externally rotate the humerus.)

Coracobrachialis and Biceps

- They cross the shoulder joint and help the forward flex of the upper arm.
- The tendon of the short head of the biceps passes through the joint capsule and can be involved with intraarticular disease.

Pectoralis Major and Minor

- These muscles originate from the chest wall to insert on the medial humerus and function to adduct the arm.

Nerves

- The brachial plexus passes through the axilla and innervates the shoulder muscles, skin, and the arm and hand distally. Its many branches originate in the neck from C-5 to T-1 and divide.
- The axillary nerve wraps around the proximal humerus and innervates the deltoid. It can be injured by proximal humerus fractures or dislocations.
- The musculocutaneus nerve innervates the biceps and coracobrachialis before continuing distally as a sensory nerve.
- The radial, median, and ulnar nerves all branch out from the axilla and innervate the forearm and hand distally.

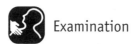 Examination

PHYSICAL EXAMINATION

Inspection

- This should include the scapula, clavicle, and musculature of the back and chest.
- An elevated clavicle may be the result of a prior acromioclavicular subluxation.
- A winged scapula or malunited fracture may be detected.
- Swelling may indicate trauma or inflammatory arthritis.

Palpation

- This should include the clavicle, all four joints, the acromion, shoulder capsule and biceps tendons.
- The insertions of the rotator cuff on the greater and lesser tuberosities should be palpated.

Range of Motion and Strength

- Forward flexion, extension, and internal external rotation should be measured.
- Internal rotation can be assessed by asking the patient to put his or her hand as high up behind the back as possible. The spinal level obtained can then be recorded as the measure of internal rotation.
- The contribution of the scapula should be noted because patients supplement glenohumeral motion with motion of the scapula.
- Failure of abduction above the shoulder level may indicate rotator cuff disease.

Neurovascular Examination

- This should include the axial nerve, which innervates the deltoid and the lateral skin of the shoulder, and the entire brachial plexus both proximally and distally.
- Biceps and triceps reflexes should be elicited.

Special Tests

Glenohumeral translation with the scapula stabilized by the examiner's hand may reveal anterior or posterior shoulder instability; this maneuver may cause the patient apprehension or a feeling of impending dislocation, a finding indicative of instability.

Sulcus Sign

- Inferior traction on the elbow may reveal a "sulcus sign" beneath the acromion that indicates instability.

Impingement Sign of Neer

- This involves elevation of the arm and forces the proximal humerus against the inferior glenoid.
- This may indicate acromial impingement syndrome.
- The impingement test is positive if symptoms are relieved by an injection of local anesthetic into the acromioclavicular joint.
- Active supination of the forearm against resistance may cause pain in the bicipital groove of the proximal humerus that is typical of bicipital tendinitis.

IMAGING PROCEDURES

- Radiographs of the shoulder should include anteroposterior, lateral, and axillary views.
- A scapular Y view may also help to assess congruence of the glenohumeral joint.

RECOMMENDED READING

Moore K, Dalley AF II. *Clinically oriented anatomy*, 4th ed. Philadelphia: Lippincott Williams & Wilkins, 1999:676–719.

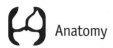 Anatomy

DESCRIPTION

The spine is a complex composite of bony elements, articulations, ligaments, muscles, spinal cord, and peripheral nerves. The bony spine is conveniently and arbitrarily divided into anterior, middle, and posterior columns. When two or more of these columns are disrupted, the spine is considered unstable and must be surgically stabilized with internal fixation. The anterior column consists of the anterior portion of the vertebral body and the anterior longitudinal ligament.

The middle column is composed of the middle of the vertebral body and the posterior longitudinal ligament. The posterior column consists of the lamina, facet joints, and spinous processes. The spinal cord is protected by the vertebral body, lamina, and the spinous process.

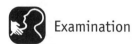 Examination

PHYSICAL EXAMINATION

Exposure

• The patient undresses and puts on a hospital gown.

Gait

• Look for an antalgic (painful) gait.
• Look for muscle weakness.
• Look for signs of hip or knee problems.
• Look for Trendelenburg's sign (abductor weakness with an ipsilateral pelvic tilt when the leg is lifted off the ground).

Inspection

• Examine the patient from the side and from behind.
• Check the patient's posture and view the spine from behind the patient to check for curvature of the thoracic or lumbar spine.
• Structural scoliosis is characterized by a fixed curve, with no change with flexion or recumbency.
• Sciatic scoliosis is characterized by a more diffuse curve; on forward flexion, the curve worsens; flexion is more limited, and it disappears with recumbency.
• In spondylolisthesis, note the skin crease changes at the junction of the lumbar spine and the sacrum.
• In neurofibromatosis, note the café-au-lait spots and masses.

Spine Range of Motion

• The patient's hands should be extended toward the floor.
• While standing:

—Spine forward flexion
—Spine forward extension
—Lateral flexion
—Rotation: palpation of spinous process separation

• Root irritation from disc herniation

—Deviation to painful side with spine flexion

• Ankylosing spondylitis

—Whole spine is rigid.
—Have patient rise up and down on his or her toes repeatedly: tests gastrocnemius soleus (S-1 nerve root).
—Have patient walk on his or her heels: tests L-5 nerve root.

Sitting Tests

Reflexes

REFLEX	NERVE ROOT
Knee	L3-4
Ankle	S-1
Biceps	C-5
Triceps	C-7
Brachioradialis	C-6

Flip Test

Straight leg raising is tested with the patient in the sitting position to check for malingering.

Supine Tests

Strength Testing

This systematically examines nerve roots.

MUSCLE GROUP	ACTION	NERVE ROOT
Iliopsoas	Hip flexion	L1-2
Quadriceps	Knee extension	L3-4
Tibialis anterior	Foot dorsiflexion	L-4
Extensor hallucis longus	Big toe extension	L-5
Gastrocnemius	Foot plantar flexion	S-1
Flexor hallucis longus	Big toe flexion	S-1
Deltoid, biceps	Arm abduction, elbow flexion	C-5
Extensor carpi radialis longus and brevis	Wrist extension	C-6
Wrist flexors, finger extensors, triceps	Elbow and finger extension, wrist flexion	C-7
Interossei,	Finger flexion, hand intrinsics	C-8

Muscle Strength Grading

5: Normal strength
4: Movement against gravity, weakness with resistance
3: Marked weakness against resistance
2: Some muscle or tendon movement with gravity eliminated
1: Flicker of tendon unit
0: No movement

Spine Anatomy and Examination

Sensory Levels

Pinprick testing is used to compare sensibility on the upper and lower extremities.

NERVE ROOT	AREA OF SKIN INNERVATION
L-1	Groin
L-2	Lateral thigh
L-3	Knee cap region
L-4	Anteromedial shin
L-5	Dorsum of foot, anterior aspect lower leg
S-1	Sole and outer border of foot
C-5	Lateral arm
C-6	Lateral forearm, thumb, index and half middle fingers
C-7	Middle finger
C-8	Medial forearm, ring and small fingers
T-1	Medial arm

Vibration sensibility and temperature sense are tested as well.

Nerve Root Tension Tests

Straight Leg Raising with Knee Extended

• The patient is supine with the foot relaxed.
• Raise the leg slowly: this reproduces the sciatic-type radicular leg pain that is relieved when the knee is bent and is exacerbated by foot dorsiflexion.

Unaffected Leg Raising

• Pain is felt in the affected extremity.
• This finding suggests disc herniation axillary or medial to the root.

Femoral Nerve Stretch Test

• The patient is lying face down, and the hip is extended with the knee slightly flexed.
• Pain radiating down the front of the thigh indicates L3-4 nerve root irritation.

Patrick's Test

• Test the sacroiliac joint by abducting and extending the hip, to reproduce sacroiliac joint pain.

Rectal Examination

• This is a "must-do" examination.
• Check for the following:

—Tone
—Volition
—Anal wink (stroke perianal skin, feel anal sphincter contraction around finger)
—Bulbocavernosus maneuver (signals end of "spinal shock": pull on Foley catheter in urethra or pull on glans penis, feel anal wink)
—Perianal sensation: S-2, S-3, S-4 (if sensation is absent, a mass lesion such as a disc or tumor may be pressing on the nerve roots)

Upper Motor Neuron Disorders

Hoffman's Sign

• Nip the nail of the patient's middle finger.
• A positive reaction produces flexion of the terminal phalanx of the thumb and of the second and third phalanx of another finger.

Babinski's Sign

• Stroke the plantar lateral foot.
• If the sign is positive, the big toe will extend upward.

Waddell Signs

If three of the following five signs are positive, the patient is malingering:

• Nonanatomic superficial tenderness
• Simulation tests (pain with axial loading or rotation of the spine)
• Flip test
• Nonanatomic weakness and sensory findings
• Overreaction: "cogwheeling" or jerky muscle relaxation

IMAGING PROCEDURES

• Imaging confirms or supports the diagnosis of disorders suspected from the history and physical examination.
• The radiograph should demonstrate normal alignment of the vertebrae, the presence of bony landmarks, and maintenance of the disc spaces (Fig. 1).

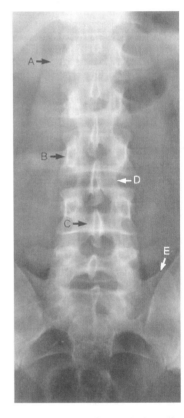

Fig. 1. Roentgenogram of normal lumbosacral spine. **A:** Transverse process. **B:** Pedicle. **C:** Posterior spinous process. **D:** Lamina. **E:** Sacrum. (From Steinberg GG, Akins CM, Baran DT. *Orthopaedics in primary care,* 3rd ed. Philadelphia: Lippincott Williams & Wilkins, 1999, with permission).

RECOMMENDED READING

Orthopaedic neurology: a diagnostic guide to neurologic levels. Philadelphia: JB Lippincott, 1977:80–106.

Basics

DESCRIPTION

When a patient is discovered to have a fracture, the physician should do the following:

• Assess and stabilize vital systems.
• Evaluate and document the neurovascular status of the limb with the fracture.
• Determine whether the fracture is open or closed.
• Splint the fracture.

—This is often done in the field or at the site of the accident by emergency medical technicians. Adequate splinting has the following advantages:

—1. It provides immobilization, which relieves pain.
—2. It prevents further soft tissue injury and keeps closed fractures from becoming open fractures.
—3. It may lower the incidence of clinical fat embolism and shock.

TYPES OF SPLINTS

Almost anything rigid can be used as a splint in the field, such as sticks, slats of wood, a pillow, or rigid cardboard. Most emergency equipment includes the splints described in the following paragraphs.

Thomas Splints

This type of splint is used for femoral shaft fractures and sometimes for knee injuries. One should use a half-ring or full-ring splint that measures 2 inches more than the circumference of the proximal thigh. If a half-ring splint is used, a strap is placed anteriorly. The ring engages the ischial tuberosity for countertraction, and traction is applied to the end of the splint with an ankle hitch. This temporary splint should not be left on for longer than 2 hours, because the ankle hitch places significant pressure on the skin and may cause skin necrosis.

Inflatable Splints

Inflatable splints consist of a double-walled polyvinyl jacket with a zip fastener placed around the injured limb. The splint is inflated by blowing air into the mouth tube. A mechanical pump can produce circulatory embarrassment and should be avoided. The pressure from inflation is believed to be transmitted directly into the soft tissue compartments, and therefore, one must be careful to monitor for compartment syndrome. In addition, inflatable splints should not be applied over clothing, because folds can cause high-pressure points and blistering. Skin maceration may occur if air splints are used for any extended period.

Structural Aluminum Malleable Splints

These splints are made of a strip of soft aluminum, coated with polyethylene foam. They are cut into strips, weigh little, and take up little room. When folded longitudinally, these floppy, malleable strips change to rigid members. They are self-padded, can be trimmed to size by scissors, conform to any contour, and are radiolucent.

Sugar Tong Splints

Sugar tong splints may be used for wrist, elbow, or forearm fractures. The arm is well padded from the metacarpophalangeal (MCP) joints to above the elbow with Webril or Softroll, with higher padding or ¼-inch felt applied over bony prominences. The padding may also be placed directly onto the plaster slabs and applied as a single unit. Plaster is measured to span from the MCP joints in the volar direction to and around the elbow and back to the MCP joints dorsally. Eight to 12 layers (3 or 4 width inch) plaster are measured, and these are laid on top of each other and are dipped in water. The bandages are sufficiently soaked when the bubbling stops. (They can be left in the water up to 4 minutes without lowering the strength of the splint.) The operator places the splint on the patient's arm, with adequate padding between the arm and the plaster, so it spans from the MCP joints in the volar direction, around the elbow, which is flexed at 90 degrees, to the MCP joints dorsally. The wrist should be held in the neutral position, and the elbow should be flexed at 90 degrees. The plaster is secured with elastic (Ace) wraps. Three points of force are produced by the operator, who molds the splint firmly against the proximal and distal portions of the extremity (two of the points) and locates the third point directly opposite the apex of the fracture. The position is held until the splint becomes hard. The limb is supported in a sling.

Ankle Splints

Ankle splints consist of two components, a posterior slab and a U that runs from medial to lateral. This splint may be used for distal tibia, fibula, or tibia and fibula fractures, ankle sprains, or Achilles tendon tears, and the posterior slab alone may be used for metatarsal fractures. If the patient's condition allows, the position most conducive for applying this splint is prone, with the affected limb flexed off the bed at the knee. This position makes it easier for a single person to apply this splint and to hold the patient's foot and ankle in the neutral position. The leg should be well padded with Webril or Softroll from the toes to just below the knee. Attention and extra padding should be given to the medial and lateral malleolus.

Four, 5, or 6 inch width plaster are measured from 2 inches below the popliteal space to 2 inches beyond the toes. Ten to 12 sheets are then measured. Then a U is measured from the medial aspect of the knee under the foot and up to the lateral side of the knee, using 3- or 4-inch plaster, and, again, 10 to 12 sheets are measured. The posterior slab is applied, and the distal aspect is folded back to make a reinforcing toe plate. The U slab is then applied, and the splint is secured with elastic wraps. The ankle is held in the neutral position with the ankle at 90 degrees until the splint hardens.

Posterior Elbow Splints

A posterior elbow splint may be used for supracondylar humerus fractures, elbow sprains, radial head fractures, or elbow strains. The arm is well padded from its distal portion to the wrist all the way up the arm. Four or 5 inch plaster are measured from 2 to 3 inches from the axilla to the base of the fifth metacarpal. Ten to 12 sheets are measured and are placed together. The splint is applied to the patient from 2 to 3 inches distal to the axilla over the elbow and along the ulnar aspect of the forearm to the base of the fifth metacarpal. Before wrapping the elbow, the operator should overlap the corners of the splint to make a dart and should be careful not to cause a pressure point. The arm is positioned with the wrist in the neutral position and the elbow flexed at 90 degrees. The position may be further secured with a separate slab of plaster extending from the ulnar aspect of the forearm to above the elbow. The splint is secured with elastic bandages, and the position is held until the splint is hard. The arm is then supported in a sling.

Metacarpal Splints

A boxer's fracture is a fracture of the distal fifth metacarpal and is a common injury. The "boxer splint" can also be used for fourth metacarpal fractures. Adequate padding is applied and 4 inch plaster are measured from the tip of the fifth finger to 2 inches from the antecubital fossa. A gauze pad is placed between the fourth and fifth fingers. The splint is applied to the ulnar side of the hand, to create a "gutter." The patient's wrist is positioned at 25 to 30 degrees of extension, and the MCP joint is positioned at 90 degrees of flexion. The operator should secure the splint with an elastic wrap and hold the MCP joint at 90 degrees until the splint is hard.

Wrist Anatomy and Examination

- The lunate, capitate, and base of the third metacarpal are in line with each other and are covered by the extensor carpi radialis brevis tendon, which inserts into the base of the third metacarpal.
- Ulnar styloid process

—It can be palpated at the distal aspect of the ulna medially and posteriorly.
—The extensor carpi ulnaris tendon runs through a groove on the distal tip of the ulnar styloid process.

- Triquetrum

—It lies just distal to the ulnar styloid process.

- Pisiform

—It is a small sesamoid bone, which lies anterolateral to the triquetrum and is formed within the flexor carpi ulnaris tendon.

- Hook of the hamate

—It is located slightly dorsal and radial to the pisiform.
—The hook forms the lateral (radial) border of the tunnel of Guyon, which encompasses the ulnar nerve and artery; the medial border of the tunnel of Guyon is the pisiform bone.

Palpation of Soft Tissues

- Finkelstein's test

—This test evaluates specifically for stenosing tenosynovitis of the tendons in tunnel I.
—The patient is instructed to make a fist with the thumb tucked inside the other fingers.
—Then the examiner stabilizes the patient's forearm with one hand and deviates the patient's wrist in an ulnar direction with the other hand.
—If the patient feels a sharp pain in the tunnel region, this strongly supports a diagnosis of stenosing tenosynovitis.

- Volar wrist

—Palmaris longus
  —It bisects the anterior aspect of the wrist, and its distal end is also the anterior surface of the carpal tunnel.
  —To palpate palmaris longus, have the patient flex the wrist and touch the tips of the thumb and small finger together in apposition; the palmaris longus becomes prominent along the midline of the anterior aspect of the wrist.

—Carpal tunnel
  —It lies deep to the palmaris longus and is defined proximally by the pisiform and the tubercle of the scaphoid and distally by the hook of the hamate and the tubercle of the trapezium.
  —The transverse carpal ligament, a portion of the volar carpal ligament, runs between these bony prominences and forms a fibrous sheath that contains the carpal tunnel anteriorly within a fibroosseous tunnel.
  —Posteriorly, the tunnel is bordered by the carpal bones.
  —The tunnel transports the median nerve and the finger flexor tendons from the forearm to the hand.
  —Clinical significance: compression of the median nerve (carpal tunnel syndrome) can restrict motor function as well as sensation along the median nerve distribution of the hand. Patients note discomfort over the wrist and numbness of the thumb and the index and middle fingers. Patients often have paresthesias at night.
  —To support a diagnosis of carpal tunnel syndrome, one can reproduce pain in the median nerve distribution by tapping over the volar carpal ligament (Tinel's sign.) Flexing the patient's wrist to its maximal degree and holding for at least 1 minute (Phalen's test) may also reproduce the patient's symptoms.

—Flexor carpi radialis
  —Flexor carpi radialis tendinitis can cause pain over the flexor aspect of the wrist.
  —On examination, pain is noted with palpation over the flexor carpi radialis tunnel (from 3 cm proximal to the wrist to the main insertion of the flexor carpi radialis on the base of the second metacarpal).
  —Examination also usually demonstrates increased pain with resisted wrist flexion and resisted radial deviation of the wrist.

- Vascular anatomy

—The radial artery can be palpated just radial to the flexor carpi radialis tendon.
—The pulse of the ulnar artery may be palpated proximal to the pisiform bone just before it crosses the wrist on the anterior aspect of the ulna. Most patients have both arteries, with the ulnar artery usually providing the dominant blood supply.

Range of Motion

Active range of motion should be assessed using bilateral comparison to evaluate the patient's restrictions. Evaluate the following:

- Flexion (normal is usually 70 to 80 degrees)
- Extension (normal is usually 70 to 80 degrees)
- Radial deviation (normal is up to approximately 20 degrees)
- Ulnar deviation (normal is up to approximately 30 degrees)
- Supination (normal is 90 degrees)
- Pronation (normal is 90 degrees)

Neurologic Examination

This examination focuses on muscular assessment and sensation testing.

Motor Testing

- Wrist extension (C-6)
- Flexion (C-7)
- Supination (C-5, C-6)
- Pronation (C-6, C-8, T-1)

Sensation Testing

Sensation on the volar and dorsal aspects of the wrist should be tested and compared with that of the contralateral wrist.

Peripheral Nerve Innervation

Peripheral nerve innervation is best assessed by testing sensation in the median, ulnar, and radial nerve distributions in the hand.

Symptoms

Symptoms can be referred to the wrist from the elbow, shoulder, and the cervical spine, and causes include the following:

- Herniated cervical discs
- Osteoarthritis
- Brachial plexus outlet syndromes
- Elbow and shoulder entrapment syndromes

RECOMMENDED READING

American Society for Surgery of the Hand. *The hand: examination and diagnosis*. New York: Churchill Livingstone, 1990:15–25, 47–56.

Hoppenfeld S. *Physical examination of the spine and extremities*. Norwalk, CT: Appleton & Lange, 1976:59–104.

Watson HK, Weinzweig J. Physical examination of the wrist. *Hand Clin* 1997;1:17–34.

SECTION II.
Specific Conditions

Accessory Navicular

 Basics

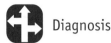 Diagnosis

Management

DESCRIPTION

This anatomic variant consists of an ossicle medial to the navicular of both feet.

Synonyms

- Os tibiale
- External prehallux

Incidence

- In normal feet, a 10% incidence; 89% of cases are bilateral
- Most commonly symptomatic in second decade of life
- Usually affects teens and young adults
- More frequent in girls

CAUSES

This ossicle is a variant of normal. It may cause problems by its prominence or by diminishing the pull of the posterior tibial tendon, which normally inserts in that region.

ICD-9-CM

755.56 Accessory Navicular
734 Pes planus

SIGNS AND SYMPTOMS

Pain may begin after wearing of ill-fitting shoes or after trauma to the foot. Pain is characterized as follows:

- Pain and tenderness along the medial aspect of the foot in the region of the accessory navicular
- Pain with motion of the posterior tibial tendon when the patient attempts to rise on tiptoes
- Often increased prominence over the medial end of the navicular

DIFFERENTIAL DIAGNOSIS

- Navicular fracture, acute fracture of the first or second metatarsal
- Posterior tibial tendinitis
- Stress fracture of navicular
- On plain radiograph, accessory navicular possibly resembling a calcaneal fracture

PHYSICAL EXAMINATION

- The tenderness is localized to the medial pole of the navicular. This may be localized by abducting and adducting the foot and feeling it move along the head of the navicular. Some degree of prominence in this area is normal, however.
- Look for hard material on the arch of the shoe, which may exacerbate symptoms.

PATHOLOGIC FINDINGS

This is a separate osteocartilagenous fragment located in the place of the normal medial pole of the navicular. The posterior tibial tendon sends a slip to insert on this bone.

IMAGING PROCEDURES

Obtain routine anteroposterior and lateral radiographs of the foot. The injury is best seen on a reverse oblique view. Smooth margins with well-formed cortex differentiate this from a fracture. Bone scan may be needed if a navicular stress fracture is suspected in the differential diagnosis. A bone scan may have increased activity over an accessory navicular if the condition is symptomatic.

GENERAL MEASURES

The patient should decrease activity to tolerance, and antiinflammatory medication and use of a softer, wider shoe are recommended. Mild symptoms may only require a decrease in activity. If a flatfoot is present, a felt arch support may be useful. Short leg walking casts may be used for 3 to 6 weeks for persistent symptoms. If pain is acute, these measures may be combined with injection into the bursa on the surface of the accessory navicular, which may be swollen.

MEDICAL TREATMENT

There is no proof that one nonsteroidal agent is superior to another.

PATIENT EDUCATION

Instruct patients on the benign nature of the condition. If the condition is to medial pressure from the shoe, suggest a wider, softer shoe. Recommend rest from sports with more gradual return when symptoms subside.

MONITORING

Patients may be counseled to follow-up as needed.

COMPLICATIONS

Complications include callus formation and recurrence of symptoms with continued activity.

RECOMMENDED READING

Coughlin MJ. Sesamoids and accessory bones of the foot. In: Mann RA, Coughlin MJ, eds. *Surgery of the foot and ankle*, 6th ed. St. Louis: CV Mosby, 1993:499–539.

Basics

DESCRIPTION

An Achilles tendon rupture is a disruption of the Achilles tendon, usually at 2 to 6 cm proximal to its insertion in the calcaneus (Fig. 1). It commonly occurs in patients between 30 and 50 years of age, and it affects men and women equally.

CAUSES

Achilles tendon rupture is caused by sports activities that require rapid push-off, trauma, chronic Achilles tendinitis, or a partial tear that is not properly treated.

RISK FACTORS

It has been suggested that increased vascularity of the tendon during active years and a subsequent relative decrease in perfusion to the tendon during an inactive period lead to the degenerative changes found in the ruptured tendon.

CLASSIFICATION

- Acute versus chronic
- Complete versus incomplete

ASSOCIATED CONDITIONS

- Achilles peritendinitis
- Tendinosis

ICD-9-CM

727.67 Nontraumatic
845.09 Traumatic

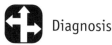 Diagnosis

SIGNS AND SYMPTOMS

Usually, a sudden snap in the back of the ankle is felt on forced plantar flexion of the foot. Pain may be severe. Local pain, swelling with a palpable gap along the Achilles tendon near its insertion site, and decreased active plantar flexion strength all strongly suggest the diagnosis.

DIFFERENTIAL DIAGNOSIS

- Posterior heel bursitis
- Achilles peritendinitis
- Partial Achilles tendon tear

PHYSICAL EXAMINATION

- Examine the back of the ankle for pain and swelling. Patients may still be able to plantar flex the ankle despite a rupture of the Achilles tendon by using the other muscles of the ankle and foot.
- Thompson's test is performed by strongly squeezing the muscular section of the calf and noting whether the heel moves upward . It is useful in this situation to detect continuity of the Achilles tendon.

LABORATORY TESTS

Obtain preoperative laboratory tests only if surgery is planned.

PATHOLOGIC FINDINGS

- Features are inconsistent.
- Findings range from normal tendon to degenerative or chronic inflammatory changes in patients with a previous history of Achilles peritendinitis.

IMAGING PROCEDURES

- Plain films are used to evaluate bony structure.
- Computed tomography is needed to rule out avulsion of the Achilles tendon insertion into the calcaneus with bony separation. Preexisting ankle joint arthritis must also be excluded.
- Magnetic resonance imaging is preferred because of its superior soft tissue resolution. It is also useful to distinguish complete rupture from peritendinitis, tendinosis, and incomplete rupture.

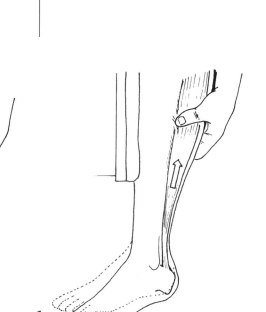

Fig. 1. Achilles tendon rupture is an irregular tear in the midsubstance.

Achilles Tendon Rupture

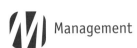 Management

GENERAL MEASURES

Management is controversial and can be operative or nonoperative. Nonoperative therapy in general requires the patient to be in a short leg cast with the foot in maximal equinus for 4 weeks, followed by several short leg casts with the affected foot gradually brought into neutral position.

SURGICAL TREATMENT

Primary tendon repairs are associated with normal surgical risks. Wound infection, if it occurs, may be particularly bothersome because the incision is just under the heel of the shoe. Management must be individualized. Most authors advocate surgical treatment for Achilles tendon rupture in a young, athletic patient without medical problems. However, cast treatment alone works almost as well, and this continues to be a controversial subject.

Direct end-to-end anastomosis is recommended for acute ruptures. For neglected or previously misdiagnosed injuries, excessive scarring or contracture makes end-to-end repair difficult. Various methods including a V-Y lengthening technique, tendon transfers, tendon grafts, or the use of synthetic materials have all been described.

PHYSICAL THERAPY

After casting, physical therapy begins with gentle active dorsiflexion and plantar flexion. After a few weeks, the patient is then advanced to Achilles tendon stretching exercises and progressive resistance exercises to restore calf muscle strength.

PATIENT EDUCATION

The patient should be actively involved in the decision-making process, with a clear understanding of the risks and benefits of surgical and nonsurgical treatments.

Prevention

Proper warm-up exercises are warranted before participation in sporting events.

MONITORING

Postoperatively, the affected leg is placed in a short leg cast with the knee flexed and the foot in maximum plantar flexion for 2 to 3 weeks. During the next 4 to 6 weeks, a short leg cast is placed with the foot in about 10 degrees of equinus. Partial weight bearing with crutches can begin after about 6 weeks of casting. After the cast is discontinued, the foot is then brought into neutral position with a brace.

COMPLICATIONS

Common surgical complications, aside from the risks associated with anesthesia, include the following:

- Deep infection (0.2%)
- Superficial infection (1.3%)
- Suture granuloma (0.5%)
- Skin necrosis (0.4%)
- Chronic fistula (0.3%)
- Disturbance of sensibility (1.9%)
- Longer hospitalization time

The advantages of surgical repair include the following (Cetti):

- Less time spent in cast (6.7 versus 8.3 weeks)
- Slightly stronger plantar flexion strength (87 versus 78%)
- Lower incidence of recurrent rupture (1.4 versus 13.4%)

PROGNOSIS

For acute injuries, 57% of operative patients return to their preinjury level of sporting activity as compared with 29% in the nonoperative group. The rate of rupture recurrence is discussed the previous section. In general, for uncomplicated Achilles tendon rupture, most patients can expect to return to their daily routines with minimal problems.

RECOMMENDED READING

Cetti R, Christensen SE, Ejsted R, et al. Operative versus nonoperative treatment of Achilles tendon rupture. *Am J Sports Med* 1993;21:791.

Elstron J, Pankovich AM. Muscle and tendon surgery of the leg. In: C. McCollister Evarts, ed. *Evarts surgery of the musculoskeletal system,* vol 4, 3rd ed. New York: Churchill Livingstone, 1990:3915–3962.

Plattner P, Mann RO. Miscellaneous conditions of the foot. In: Mann RO, ed. *Surgery of the foot and ankle,* vol 2. St. Louis: CV Mosby, 1993:810–816.

Basics

DESCRIPTION

This condition is a chronic, painful inflammation of the Achilles tendon and its sheath, the fibrous terminal attachment of the gastrocnemius and soleus muscles into the calcaneus, and associated structures. It is also known as Achilles or calcaneal paratenonitis.

INCIDENCE

- This common overuse injury is seen particularly among recreational and competitive athletes and occurs in 6% to 11% of runners.
- It affects active persons 15 to 45 years old.
- It is extremely prevalent in the high school and college track circuit.
- It is found in middle- to long-distance runners (800 m to marathon)
- It is more common in active middle-aged individuals.
- The male-to-female predominance roughly parallels that of participation in athletic activities.

CAUSES

This overuse injury of the affected leg is often due to the following conditions:

- Rough terrain or uneven surfaces
- Improper shoe wear (10%)
- Adverse weather conditions (ice, snow, cold)
- Biomechanical abnormalities of the lower extremity, from lumbar spine to foot (up to 35% to 55%)
- Training errors (75%): sudden increase in training regimen (mileage)
- Chronically inappropriate short or absent warm-up and stretching period

RISK FACTORS

- Microvascular disease: diabetes, lupus, rheumatoid disease, endarteritis
- Hemodialysis or peritoneal dialysis: renal disease
- Connective tissue disease

CLASSIFICATION

- Insertional versus noninsertional
- Paratenonitis: paratenon inflammation
- Paratenonitis with tendinosis: intrasubstance degeneration with paratenon inflammation
- Tendinosis: intrasubstance degeneration secondary to atrophy
- Terminal condition after long-term symptoms, often at this point asymptomatic

ASSOCIATED CONDITIONS

Achilles tendon rupture

ICD-9-CM

726.71 Achilles tendinitis

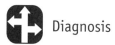

Diagnosis

SIGNS AND SYMPTOMS

- A gradual increase in painful swelling and warmth occurs at any point along the tendon substance, from the musculotendinous junction to the bony insertion (os calcis).
- Most pain is 3 to 5 cm proximal to the insertion onto the calcaneus.
- Microtrauma such as continued running, or even gross trauma such as a single leap (in jumpers), exacerbates the symptoms.
- Pain is somewhat relieved by unloading (rest).

DIFFERENTIAL DIAGNOSIS

- Precalcaneal bursitis
- Retrocalcaneal bursitis
- Peroneal tendinitis or rupture
- Posterior tibialis tendinitis or rupture
- Achilles tendon rupture, partial or complete: may represent terminal stage
- Inflamatory Arthritis (Reath's Syndrome)

PHYSICAL EXAMINATION

A full lower extremity history should be obtained. The examiner should check for pain on dorsiflexion of the ankle. Placing both fingers around the tendon localizes the pain. In severe cases, the tendon sheath may be swollen and crepitant with ankle motion (Figs. 1 and 2).

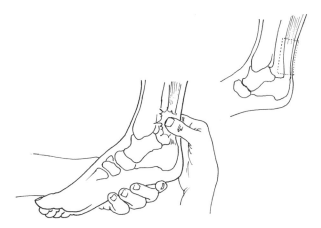

Fig. 1. The area of tenderness in Achilles tendinitis is above the heel, over a broad area.

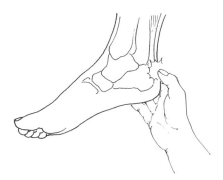

Fig. 2. Retrocalcaneal bursitis produces pain in the back of the heel, at the insertion of the Achilles tendon.

Achilles Tendinitis

- Use Thompson's test to rule out tendon rupture.
- Note any intrinsic foot, ankle, or leg deformities: pes cavus, leg length discrepancy, scoliosis, equinus deformity, residual clubfoot.

LABORATORY TESTS

Usually none are indicated. Serum chemistry study with glucose is recommended if one of the foregoing systemic conditions is suspected, if diabetes needs to be ruled out, or if an overuse history is not present. Evaluation for inflamatory arthritis if clinically indicated.

PATHOLOGIC FINDINGS

Chronic inflammatory changes are noted in the sheath.

IMAGING PROCEDURES

Magnetic resonance imaging is indicated if the clinical picture suggests tendinosis.

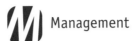 Management

GENERAL MEASURES

Nonsteroidal medications, ice, rest, footwear modification, and orthotic correction of the foot and leg abnormality are used. Retrocalcaneal bursa injection may also help to relieve symptoms and inflammation. For patients who are not responsive to the foregoing treatments, a trial of cast immobilization with weight bearing is appropriate.

SURGICAL TREATMENT

Treatment involves removal or release of the paratenon through a straight medial incision. This method is reserved for the fewer than 25% of patients in whom 3 to 12 months of conservative management has failed. Seventy percent to 90% respond favorably, with a return to activity after a further period of rest. Patients with previous surgical failures respond well to repeat surgery. If intratendinous débridement is performed, it may require augmentation or local tendon transfer.

PHYSICAL THERAPY

Ultrasound therapy (during proliferative phase healing), phonophoresis, iontophoresis, and short-term heel wedge use (to unload tendon unit) are used. Eventually, flexibility, strengthening, and conditioning through eccentric exercise gain maximal benefit.

MEDICAL TREATMENT

- Nonsteroidal antiinflammatory drugs
- Analgesics

PATIENT EDUCATION

- Adequate pretraining stretching and warm-up
- Proper shoe wear and terrain adjustment, with avoidance of steep hills and stairs

MONITORING

Routine follow-up is indicated until the symptoms are resolved.

COMPLICATIONS

Tendon degeneration and eventual rupture with loss of function, particularly with a high rate of surgical failure, are possible.

PROGNOSIS

The prognosis is good; however, recovery can be prolonged.

RECOMMENDED READING

Clain MR, Baxter DE. Achilles tendinitis. *Foot Ankle* 1992;13:482–487.

Griffin LY. *Orthopaedic knowledge update: sports medicine*. Rosemont, IL: American Academy of Orthopaedic Surgeons, 1994.

Kasser JR, ed. *Orthopaedic knowledge update 5*. Rosemont, IL: American Academy of Orthopaedic Surgeons, 1996:225–298.

Lutter LD, Mizel MS, Pfeffer GB. *Orthopaedic knowledge update: foot and ankle*. Rosemont, IL: American Academy of Orthopaedic Surgeons, 1994:270–273.

Basics

DESCRIPTION

Achondroplasia is the most common skeletal dysplasia, by a significant margin. It is characterized by patient height less than 4½ feet, with the greatest shortening of the proximal humerus and femur. There may be hypoplasia of the midface and frontal bossing (Fig. 1). Arthritis is rarely seen, but spinal stenosis is the most serious possible complication. Achondroplasia affects the skeletal and neurologic systems. Its features are immediately evident at birth, but life expectancy is not significantly altered in the heterozygote. The incidence of spinal stenosis and degenerative disc disease increases with age. It affects males and females equally.

• Skeleton: ligamentous laxity, undergrowth of growth plates
• Neurologic: stenosis of the foramen magnum in infancy or the lumbar spine near maturity

INCIDENCE

1 per 15,000 population

GENETICS

• Autosomal dominant
• Acquired by most patients (70%) as a new mutation
• Homozygous cases (with two affected parents) usually fatal in infancy

CAUSES

Achondroplasia results from a defect in the fibroblast growth factor receptor protein. The reason for spontaneous mutations is unclear, but the pathologic process begins *in utero*; the epiphyseal cartilage plate growth is slowed and disordered, with a resulting decrease in longitudinal growth.

RISK FACTORS

• Parental age greater than 37 years
• Achondroplastic parent

CLASSIFICATION

Skeletal dysplasia: rhizomelic short stature

ASSOCIATED CONDITIONS

• Hydrocephalus
• Obesity

ICD-9-CM

756.4 Achondroplasia
259.4 Dwarfism
724.00 (general) Spinal stenosis

 Diagnosis

SIGNS AND SYMPTOMS

The characteristic signs of achondroplasia–disproportionate short stature, long trunk, and rhizomelic shortening of the limbs are evident at birth (Fig. 2). The head is both relatively and absolutely large, with a prominent forehead, parietal bossing, and flattening of the occiput. Varying degrees of midfacial hypoplasia occur. Initially, the legs appear straight, but genu varum develops with ambulation. The hands and feet appear large, but the digits are short, broad, and stubby (Fig. 3). Elbow extension is restricted but of little functional significance. Excessive lumbar lordosis and posterior

pelvic tilt are seen, as well as a waddling gait. Stenosis of the lumbar spine, prolapse of the intervertebral discs, osteophytes, and deformed vertebral bodies may compress the spinal cord and nerve roots. Adult height ranges from 42 to 56 inches.

DIFFERENTIAL DIAGNOSIS

• Pseudoachondroplasia: normal facial appearance; irregular epiphyses of hips and knees
• Hypochondroplasia: height usually over 54 inches; no spinal stenosis

PHYSICAL EXAMINATION

• Head: frontal bossing; midface hypoplasia
• Spine: exaggerated lumbar lordosis; possible thoracolumbar kyphosis
• Extremities: short, especially proximally in humerus, femur; muscular appearance
• Elbow with possible flexion contracture; radial head sometimes dislocated
• Space between long and ring fingers giving appearance of "trident" hand
• Bowed (varus) knees common; varus-valgus laxity and hyperextension in childhood
• Lumbar stenosis in adults possibly producing motor weakness in ankles
• Cervical or thoracic stenosis possibly causing hyperreflexia

LABORATORY TESTS

This condition has no characteristic laboratory findings.

PATHOLOGIC FINDINGS

• Seventy percent to 80% of cases result from spontaneous mutations. Growth plates show decreased cellular organization and activity. The result is a defect in endochondral osteogenesis.
• Bones and other tissues are otherwise normal.
• Epiphyseal plates are of normal width; microscopically, the normal, orderly arrangement of cartilage cells into columns is defective.
• Membranous bone formation, which accounts for circumferential growth of the shafts of the long bones, proceeds normally.
• Changes can be recognized radiographically as early as at 3 months' gestation.

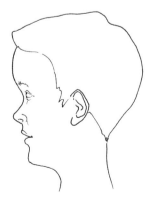

Fig. 1. Frontal bossing and midface hypoplasia are seen in achondroplasia.

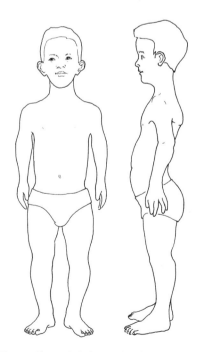

Fig. 2. Characteristic features in achondroplasia include rhizomelic shortening (thighs and upper arms most markedly shortened) and increased lumbar lordosis.

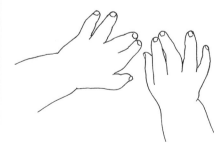

Fig. 3. A characteristic separation between the third and fourth fingers leads to the "trident hand" of achondroplasia.

Achondroplasia

SPECIAL TESTS

- Sleep studies are possibly indicated for infants with developmental delay.
- Routine chromosomal testing is not indicated.

IMAGING PROCEDURES

Radiographs

- Skull: A shortened skull base, a large cranium with prominent frontal and occipital areas, and superimposition of the sphenooccipital synchondrosis over the mastoid are seen. The angle of the base of the skull is 85 to 120 degrees (normal, 10 to 145 degrees), and the foramen magnum is small.
- Lumbar spine: Decreased interpedicular distance, spinal stenosis, and posterior scalloping of the vertebral bodies are noted. Dorsolumbar kyphosis, commonly seen in infancy, disappears with ambulation and is replaced by an exaggerated lumbar lordosis.
- Pelvis: This is short and broad with relatively wide, nonflaring iliac wings, small and deep greater sciatic notches, and horizontal superior margins of the acetabulum.

Magnetic Resonance Imaging

Magnetic resonance imaging studies of the head and neck should be obtained if developmental delay persists.

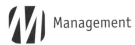 Management

GENERAL MEASURES

No effective treatment is known. Osteotomy is occasionally required to correct specific deformities of the limbs. In adults, low back pain may require symptomatic measures. Neurologic complications including hydrocephalus, nerve root compression, spinal stenosis, and paraplegia may necessitate surgical treatment.

- Foramen magnum decompression is performed for severe infantile stenosis.
- Thoracolumbar kyphosis is followed and patients are treated with a brace if the condition persists beyond the age of 2 to 3 years.
- Laminectomy is indicated for significant spinal stenosis.
- Restriction from sports is not generally necessary.
- Custom chairs and automobile hand controls are helpful.
- Close follow-up for any signs of neurologic compromise is important.
- Children with achondroplasia should not be evaluated against normal developmental milestones but rather against standards developed for children with the condition.
- Motor skills are often delayed because of the physical difficulties posed by short limbs and hypotonia.
- Cognitive skills are usually attained at the expected ages.

SURGICAL TREATMENT

- Tibial valgus-derotation osteotomy: This is usually indicated for persistent varus and torsion of knees. Some surgeons prefer early fibular shortening.
- Spinal fusion: This is indicated for significant kyphosis of more than 40 degrees that fails to respond to bracing.
- Laminectomy: If this is indicated for spinal stenosis, it should be extensive. Usually, the entire lumbar spine, and sometimes the lower thoracic spine, is decompressed. Kyphosis may need to be fused at same time if it is severe or if the patient is young.
- Limb lengthening: This may produce significant gains in height, owing to lax musculature. It may also improve lumbar lordosis and stenosis by stretching hamstrings. Usually, however, bilateral lengthening of the femur, tibia, and humerus is necessary, a treatment lasting several years.
- Foramen magnum decompression: This should be done by an experienced neurosurgeon, only after multidisciplinary consultation.

PHYSICAL THERAPY

Physical therapy is not generally indicated aside from postoperative rehabilitation or cases of severe developmental delay.

PATIENT EDUCATION

- Genetic counseling
- Weight control, which is often a problem and is helped by exercise
- Early detection of spinal stenosis
- Vocational counseling, if needed
- Usually no restriction on activity unless spinal stenosis occurs
- Dwarf Amateur Athletic Association: a competitive forum

MONITORING

Periodic examinations of extremity strength and bladder control are warranted.

COMPLICATIONS

- Spinal stenosis
- Nerve root compression

PROGNOSIS

- Prognosis is good, except for spinal stenosis.
- Visceral involvement is absent.
- The homozygous form usually results in death in a few weeks to months.
- Heterozygous individuals have a normal life span.
- Intelligence is normal.
- Patients are usually independent in daily life.

RECOMMENDED READING

Aryanpur J, Hurko O, Francomano C. Craniocervical decompression for cervicomedullary compression in pediatric patients with achondroplasia. *J Neurosurg* 1990;73:375–382.

Bell DF. Use of the Ilizarov technique in the correction of limb deformities associated with skeletal dysplasia. *J Pediatr Orthop* 1992;12:283–290.

Brashear HR, Raney RB. *Handbook of orthopaedic surgery*, 10th ed. St. Louis, CV Mosby, 1986:61–62.

Netter FH. *Musculoskeletal system*, vol 8. In: Freyberg RH, Hensinger RN, eds. *The Ciba collection of medical illustrations*. Summit, NJ: Ciba-Geigy, 1991:6–8.

Nicoletti B, Kopits SE, Ascani E, et al. *Human achondroplasia*. New York: Plenum Press, 1986:3–462.

Basics

DESCRIPTION

Disruption of the ligaments by which the clavicle helps to suspend the scapula results in increased prominence of the clavicle. The function of the shoulder is not usually seriously impaired once the discomfort of the acute injury subsides.

INCIDENCE

- Varies with activity levels
- Common in athletes participating in football, wrestling, and lacrosse
- Most common in the 16- to 30-year age group
- Rare in skeletally immature individuals
- More common in males because of sports preferences

CLASSIFICATION

- Grade I: Strain of the ligaments occurs but no real displacement. The prognosis is excellent.
- Grade II: A tear of the acromioclavicular ligaments is present but no disruption of the stronger coracoclavicular ligaments. The clavicle is mildly displaced upward.
- Grade III: There is disruption of all ligaments with full dislocation, but it usually does well with time.
- Grade IV: This is the same as grade III but with more disruption of associated muscle (deltoid and trapezius) causing the clavicle to be extremely prominent (Fig. 1).

CAUSES

A fall or blow on the very tip of the shoulder (acromion) causes the scapula to be pushed down from the clavicle and damages the suspensory ligaments.

RISK FACTORS

- Contact sports
- Fall on point of elbow, with fall not broken by arm

ASSOCIATED CONDITIONS

- Shoulder arthritis
- Impingement syndrome

ICD-9-CM

831.04 Acromioclavicular dislocation

 Diagnosis

SIGNS AND SYMPTOMS

- Prominence on the "point" of the shoulder (clavicle)
- Scapula appearing to sag temporarily
- Tenderness in the area of lateral clavicle
- Shoulder movement in all directions painful
- Symptoms usually subsiding over 4 to 8 weeks and rarely recurrent
- A persistent ache with activity in a few patients

DIFFERENTIAL DIAGNOSIS

This includes clavicle fracture, in which tenderness is usually located more medially, and there is more swelling. A variant of this problem is the epiphyseal separation of the clavicle.

PHYSICAL EXAMINATION

Palpate for tenderness over the coracoclavicular ligaments and the acromioclavicular areas. Palpate the rest of the clavicle and the humerus for fracture. Ask the patient to actively abduct the shoulder and look for at least some muscle contraction in the rotator cuff.

PATHOLOGIC FINDINGS

Disruption in the acromioclavicular ligaments and coracoclavicular ligaments is seen, depending on the grade of injury.

IMAGING PROCEDURES

An anteroposterior radiograph of both shoulders allows comparison between the injured and uninjured sides. The distance between the coracoid and the clavicle may be compared. In grade I and II injury, the two sides are equal, but by adding weights to the hand, the distance may increase in grade II. In grade III, the distance is increased even without weights.

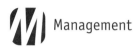 Management

GENERAL MEASURES

Nonsteroidal antiinflammatory drugs or narcotic analgesics are given for the acute injury. A sling should be worn when the patient is up. Braces to reduce the joint (i.e., Kenny-Howard brace) are no longer widely used because of the risk of pressure sores and because of good results with only a simple sling. For patients with grade IV injuries, surgery may be indicated.
Gentle range of motion, then active use of the shoulder may be allowed as symptoms permit. Return to sports should be delayed at least for 6 weeks for patients with grades II to IV injuries.

SURGICAL TREATMENT

If surgery is indicated, the joint may be held in reduction with a screw or with ligament reconstruction.

PHYSICAL THERAPY

This is indicated in severe cases. The therapist should work first on motion, then on strength. Home exercises should also be taught.

MEDICAL TREATMENT

An analgesic of choice is given for 2 to 4 weeks.

MONITORING

Focus on the patient's function. The radiographic appearance of the joint does not correlate with function, so routine follow-up radiographs are not typically needed.

COMPLICATIONS

Mild pain may persist, exacerbated by activity. In rare cases, painful arthrosis may occur.

PROGNOSIS

Most patients may return to their usual activities in several months. A few require reconstructive surgery, owing to persistent pain in the acromioclavicular joint.

RECOMMENDED READING

Rockwood CA. Fractures and dislocations of the shoulder. In: Rockwood CA, Green DP, Bucholz RW, et al. *Rockwood and Green's fractures in adults*, 4th ed. Philadelphia: Lippincott–Raven, 1996:1341–1361.

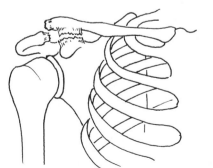

Fig. 1. Acromioclavicular dislocation occurs if there is a tear in the coracoclavicular and acromioclavicular ligaments.

Aneurysmal Bone Cyst

Basics

DESCRIPTION

An aneurysmal bone cyst (ABC) is a lesion of bone that can be locally aggressive and can cause a bone to "balloon" as a result of aneurysmal cystic expansion. It most commonly occurs at the proximal ends of long bones.

INCIDENCE

- It is rare.
- It can occur in any decade of adult life, but nearly 80% of all ABCs occur in the second decade.
- The male-to-female ratio is 1 to 1.3.

CAUSES

There are no known causes of ABCs. However, nearly half of all ABCs are seen to occur in conjunction with another benign tumor and may represent a breakdown in the body's reaction to the other tumor.

RISK FACTORS

There are no known risk factors for ABCs.

CLASSIFICATION

Musculoskeletal tumors have been classified by Enneking based on histologic features as benign (G0), low grade (G1), or high grade (G2). Enneking has further divided benign lesions based on their biologic activity as latent, active (growing within bone), or aggressive (invading surrounding tissues). In general, ABCs are considered benign active lesions.

ASSOCIATED CONDITIONS

None exist, unless the ABC is arising from another tumor.

ICD-9-CM

213.9 Aneurysmal bone cyst

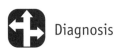

Diagnosis

SIGNS AND SYMPTOMS

- Pain is most common symptom; it is usually mild and intermittent.
- The involved area may swell, and this will tend to increase until the lesion is treated.
- The second most common site for an ABC is the vertebral column, and the lesion may cause signs and symptoms of spinal cord compression (leg weakness, bowel or bladder dysfunction).

DIFFERENTIAL DIAGNOSIS

Depending on the location of the tumor, there can be a widely varying differential diagnosis based on symptoms. Based on radiographs, the differential diagnosis includes the following:

- Unicameral bone cyst
- Giant cell tumor
- Osteosarcoma (telangiectatic type)
- Osteoblastoma
- Fibrous dysplasia

Based on histologic features, the differential diagnosis includes the following:

- Giant cell tumor
- Giant cell reparative granuloma
- Simple bone cyst
- Telangiectatic osteosarcoma

PHYSICAL EXAMINATION

- Check the affected area for tenderness to palpation and the presence of swelling.
- Quantify range of motion to follow the progress of the lesion.

PATHOLOGIC FINDINGS

An ABC appears to be hemorrhagic and consists of a combination of "fleshy" tissue and unclotted blood. The soft tissue is often brown because of hemosiderin deposition. Normally, at the periphery of the lesion is an eggshell-like layer of periosteal bone around the lesion. Microscopically, there appear to be cavernous spaces filled with blood. The walls of the spaces contain fibroblastic cells, multinucleated giant cells, and strands of bone.

IMAGING PROCEDURES

Radiography

Plain radiographs show a "ballooned" expansion of the affected bone. No matrix mineralization is present in the lesion. Lesions are most commonly seen in the metaphyseal regions of the femur and tibia, as well as in the posterior elements of the vertebra. One can often see a sclerotic rim or a fine shell of periosteal bone surrounding the lesion.

Computed Tomography

Computed tomography scans can be used to assess lesions of the pelvis or vertebral column more precisely. This method often allows the physician to assess carefully the presence of the periosteal rim of bone around a lesion. A fluid level can often be seen in a lesion.

Magnetic Resonance Imaging

These scans have allowed more accurate assessment of the extent of an ABC and allow one to look for soft tissue invasion by the lesion that points away from an ABC. On T_2-weighted images, the lesions have high signal levels, and one can often see layering in the blood.

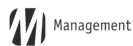

Management

GENERAL MEASURES

After appropriate evaluation of the lesion with radiologic studies, a diagnostic open biopsy may be performed, followed by excision, curet-
tage, and bone grafting. Once the bony defect is healed, patients return to normal function. Metastatic lesions are extremely rare. Lesions can recur locally; however, with the use of topical chemical or cryocauterization of the walls of the ABC, lesions recur less than 15–25% of the time.

Most patients need to limit weight-bearing activity with the involved region while bony healing occurs. Once the bone has healed, there need not be any limitation on activity.

SURGICAL TREATMENT

Treatment of ABCs involves excision, curettage, chemical cauterization of the cyst walls, and bone grafting. If the ABC is in an expendable bone (rib or fibula), resection of the lesion with a local margin is preferred. Radiation therapy should not be performed because of the potential of malignant transformation in the lesion.

PHYSICAL THERAPY

Physical therapy may be needed to regain joint motion or to assist in gait training after surgery.

PATIENT EDUCATION

Patients must be educated to look for signs and symptoms of local recurrence of the tumor that include onset of pain or localized swelling in the area of a prior lesion.

MONITORING

After surgical treatment, regular follow-up is required for several years to evaluate bony healing and to look for local recurrence of the tumor.

COMPLICATIONS

Complications of surgical treatment vary greatly; however, the most common problem after appropriate treatment is local recurrence of the tumor. Other surgical complications such as infection and neurologic or vascular injury occur with a low frequency.

PROGNOSIS

With modern treatment, 95% of patients can be expected to be cured of ABCs. An ABC should not be expected to metastasize unless rare malignant transformation occurs. If a patient does have a local recurrence, repeat surgical excision can be performed.

RECOMMENDED READING

Bruckner JD, Conrad EU III. Musculoskeletal neoplasms. In: Kasser JR, ed. *Orthopaedic knowledge update 5.* Rosemont, IL: American Academy of Orthopaedic Surgeons, 1996:133–148.

Wold LE, McLeod RA, Sims FH, et al. Aneurysmal bone cyst. In: Wold LE, ed. *Atlas of orthopedic pathology.* Philadelphia: WB Saunders, 1990:232–237.

Basics

DESCRIPTION

Osteoarthritis of the ankle joint is rare, except after traumatic injury. It usually develops within 9 months of a traumatic episode and often presents with pain and loss of motion. It occurs in patients older than 50 years.

GENETICS

No predisposition exists. However, patients with rheumatoid arthritis have a high (up to 90%), incidence of foot problems, including ankle arthritis.

INCIDENCE

It is uncommon, although it is more common after injuries that disrupt the joint space.

CAUSES

- Trauma to the ankle joint
- Obesity
- Ankle malalignment or loss of muscle control

RISK FACTOR

- Ankle trauma

CLASSIFICATION

In patients with rheumatoid arthritis, joint involvement may be staged as follows:

- No bony deformity
- Minimal erosive changes
- Soft tissue change and bony erosion
- Articular cartilage destruction

ICD-9-CM

716.97 Arthropathy, ankle not otherwise specified

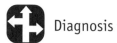 Diagnosis

SIGNS AND SYMPTOMS

- Pain
- Impaired joint function
- Decreased range of motion

DIFFERENTIAL DIAGNOSIS

- Osteochondritis dissecans
- Posterior tibial tendinitis
- Subtalar joint arthritis

PHYSICAL EXAMINATION

- Decreased range of motion, swelling, and tenderness along the joint surface are noted.
- The range of ankle dorsiflexion and plantar flexion should be quantified.
- The gait should be observed with patient's shoes off.
- Strength of ankle muscles should be tested, and pulses of the foot should be checked.

IMAGING PROCEDURES

Plain anteroposterior, lateral, and mortise views of the ankle are sufficient to establish the diagnosis. Osteophytes, a narrowed joint space, cysts, and subchondral sclerosis are characteristic findings of plain films.

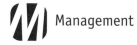 Management

GENERAL MEASURES

Initial treatment should be nonoperative. Decreased activity, nonsteroidal antiinflammatory drugs, and a well-cushioned shoe with a heel lift may be adequate treatment. Use of a rocker-bottom shoe may decrease pain associated with ankle arthritis. If nonoperative treatment is not effective after 3 to 4 months, the patient may be counseled about surgery. Decreased activity for the affected ankle may help to alleviate the symptoms.

SURGICAL TREATMENT

The treatment of choice for posttraumatic or inflammatory arthritis of the ankle is an ankle fusion. This controls the pain at the expense of range of motion. Usually, patients tolerate the loss of ankle motion well, and function is improved. Total ankle arthroplasty has not been proven effective reliably. Subtalar motion should be maintained. Fusion of the ankle requires removal of the remaining articular cartilage between the talus and the tibial plafond. Typically, the bones are then fixed with screws and possibly with plates. The patient is placed in a cast and is kept non–weight bearing until solid fusion has occurred.

PHYSICAL THERAPY

This is not typically helpful.

MEDICAL TREATMENT

- Decreased activity
- Cushioned shoe (with heel lift, if needed)
- Rocker-bottom shoe
- Medications

—Nonsteroidal antiinflammatory drugs
—Analgesics

PATIENT EDUCATION

The patient should be taught about the distinction between the ankle joint, which allows dorsiflexion and plantar flexion, and the subtalar joint, which allows inversion and eversion. The various options for treatment including analgesics, orthotics, and surgery should be mentioned so patients may self-select their treatment. The patient should be instructed that this problem may not improve and that the affected ankle will most likely will never be the same as the opposite joint.

PREVENTION

Treatment of ankle fractures, when indicated, to obtain anatomic alignment of the talus and ankle mortise with open reduction and internal fixation will decrease the likelihood of posttraumatic arthritis, although arthritis may still follow if there has been significant cartilage damage. Weight reduction helps to reduce symptoms.

MONITORING

The patient should be seen at appropriate intervals to monitor symptoms and range of motion and to discuss treatment options.

COMPLICATIONS

Although fusion is usually successful, it may result in transfer of stress to the subtalar joint or midfoot, with occasional symptoms in either of these areas.

PROGNOSIS

Prognosis is fair. Many patients with significant arthritis ultimately need surgical fusion to control pain.

RECOMMENDED READING

Trafton PG, Bray TJ, Simpson LA. Fractures and soft tissue injuries of the ankle. In: Brown B, Jupiter J, Levine, AM, et al. *Skeletal trauma,* 2nd ed. Philadelphia: WB Saunders, 1992:1871–1957.

Ankle Fracture

 Basics

DESCRIPTION

Fractures of the distal end of the fibula and tibia are referred to as ankle fractures. These usually result from twisting of the body around a planted foot or a misstep that results in overstressing the ankle joint. Severe fractures may result in dislocation of the ankle.

INCIDENCE

- These fractures are common.
- Fractures in children typically involve the growth plate.
- Fractures in adolescents can have special patterns because of the partial closure of the growth plates.

CAUSES

- Most often, these fractures result from acute trauma caused by a fall, misstep, or sports injury.
- They are rarely caused by a pathologic lesion.

RISK FACTORS

Osteoporosis can increase the risk of ankle fracture.

CLASSIFICATION

Two fracture classification systems are currently used.

Lauge-Hansen System

The Lauge-Hansen system is based on the position of the foot at the time of injury and the force applied to it. The first word in the classification refers to position and the second is the force applied. The four main types are supination-external rotation, supination-adduction, pronation-external rotation, and pronation-abduction.

Weber or AO System

The Weber or AO classification is simpler and relies on the level of the fibular fracture. A is below the ankle joint line, B is at the joint line, and C is above the joint line. *Tibial plafond* or *pilon* fracture is a comminuted fracture of the distal end of the tibia that is caused by high-energy trauma.

ASSOCIATED CONDITIONS

- Ankle sprain
- Posterior tibial tendon sprain

ICD-9-CM

824.9 Fracture, ankle

 Diagnosis

SIGNS AND SYMPTOMS

- Pain in the ankle and failure to bear weight are noted.
- Deformity may be present with a fracture-dislocation.
- Swelling and ecchymosis are common.

DIFFERENTIAL DIAGNOSIS

- Ligamentous injury (sprain) resulting from acute trauma and not evident on a radiograph
- Stress fractures of the distal fibula
- Osteochondritis dissecans
- Metatarsal fracture

PHYSICAL EXAMINATION

- Palpate the affected area and inspect for any breaks in the skin or tenting.
- Assess the dorsalis pedis and posterior tibial pulse and all nerves to the foot.
- Check compartments for compartment syndrome.

LABORATORY TESTS

- Generally, testing is only for preoperative evaluations.
- Patients with severely comminuted fractures may benefit from a preoperative computed tomography scan to evaluate the fracture pattern and the joint surfaces.

IMAGING PROCEDURES

Although there is a tendency to obtain radiographs of the ankle of any patient who complains of pain and swelling, limiting radiography to those ankles with specific indications may reduce radiograph usage by 50% without missing any significant fractures. These indications are gross deformity, instability of the ankle, crepitus, localized bone tenderness, swelling, and inability to bear weight.
In general, three radiographs of the ankle are obtained: an anteroposterior view, a lateral view, and 15-degree internally rotated oblique view called a mortise view. A good case has also been made for obtaining only lateral and mortise views, because the anteroposterior view has not been found to add significant information.
Stress views may also be helpful in evaluating ligamentous injuries, but obtaining them can be painful in an acute setting.

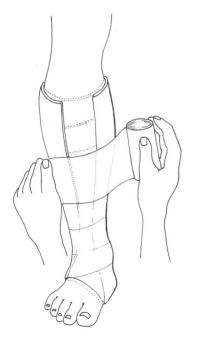

Management

GENERAL MEASURES

Pain medication and elevation should be prescribed. All ankle fractures should be splinted or casted in a neutral position acutely (Fig. 1). Isolated fibular fractures or undisplaced fractures of the medial malleolus may be treated in a cast. Congruity of the ankle joint is thought to be important to reduce the incidence of posttraumatic arthritis. If radiographs reveal widening of the joint, operative treatment is usually indicated. Dislocations should be reduced with adequate sedation as soon as possible.

Patients with open fractures should be taken to the operating room for irrigation, débridement, and fixation within 6 to 8 hours of the injury. Patients should be kept non-weight bearing on the affected side until pain has subsided and there are some signs of fracture healing on follow-up radiographs. Early weight bearing and range of motion are important to prevent stiffness.

SURGICAL TREATMENT

• The fibular fracture is usually plated through a lateral incision.
• Medial malleolar fractures are fixed with compression screws placed in a retrograde fashion.
• Open fractures or comminuted pilon fractures may require an external fixator with or without internal fixation.

PHYSICAL THERAPY

Range of motion of the metatarsophalangeal joints and, later, range of motion of the ankle and midfoot are important to prevent contractures and to reduce scarring of soft tissues.

MEDICAL TREATMENT

Treatment consists of analgesics.

PATIENT EDUCATION

Patients should be aware of the potential for posttraumatic arthritis later in life.

PREVENTION

• Proper shoe wear
• Avoidance of irregular walking and running surfaces

MONITORING

Radiographs should be taken every 2 to 6 weeks, depending on the fracture pattern and signs of healing.

COMPLICATIONS

• With severe fractures, blisters may occur and may compromise skin integrity.
• Open fractures may become infected and may require irrigation and débridement.
• Nonunion of ankle fractures may occur, and these patients often need revision surgery.
• Malunion may also occur and sometimes requires corrective osteotomy.
• Elderly patients may have osteoporotic bone, which makes surgery more difficult.
• Elderly patients are also at higher risk for skin or wound breakdown.

PROGNOSIS

Most ankle fractures heal without incident, and the patient is able to return to normal activities.

RECOMMENDED READING

Rockwood CA, Green DP, Heckman JD. *Rockwood and Green's fractures in adults,* 4th ed. Philadelphia: JB Lippincott, 1996:2267–2405.

Fig. 1. Ankle fractures or other injuries may be splinted by a "sugar tong" method employing a layer of padding, fiberglass, or plaster and an elastic (Ace) bandage.

Ankle Osteochondritis Dissecans

 Basics

DESCRIPTION

This lesion is a common cause of ankle pain. It is an osteochondral fracture from the talar dome that affects the articular surface of the talus as it articulates with the tibia. Medial lesions tend to be situated in a posterior area, whereas lateral lesions are usually situated more anteriorly. Patients complain of ankle pain, usually with a history of trauma. Intermittent swelling and grinding in the ankle are common associated symptoms. Radiographs may or may not demonstrate the lesion. Computed tomography or magnetic resonance imaging scans are necessary to define the anatomic features and to detect occult lesions.

Treatment in the acute phase includes conservative therapy, such as casting and reduced weight bearing. Failure to respond to this treatment, or a lesion that includes a displaced fragment, warrants surgery.

GENETICS

- Patients may give a history of affected family members.
- This is most common in adolescents and young adults.

INCIDENCE

Ankle osteochondritis dissecans is found in about 1% to 5% of patients with complaints of recurrent ankle pain or sprains. There is no sex predilection.

CAUSES

- All lateral lesions are believed to be caused by trauma.
- Medial lesions may be caused by trauma or avascular necrosis.

RISK FACTORS

- History of trauma
- Lax ankle joint
- Family history
- History of contralateral osteochondritis dissecans

CLASSIFICATION

- Stage I: subchondral compression
- Stage II: incomplete osteochondral fracture
- Stage III: complete nondisplaced osteochondral fracture
- Stage IV: displaced fragment

ASSOCIATED CONDITIONS

This condition is increased in patients with high activity levels and those taking steroids.

ICD-9-CM

732.7 Osteochondritis dissecans

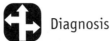 Diagnosis

SIGNS AND SYMPTOMS

- Ankle pain
- Acute swelling
- Chronic intermittent swelling
- Ankle grinding
- Ankle instability

DIFFERENTIAL DIAGNOSIS

- Ankle sprain
- Subluxing peroneal tendon
- Fibular or medial malleolar fracture
- Synovitis

PHYSICAL EXAMINATION

The patient should be checked for bony tenderness over the area of the lesion, and for ankle effusion.

PATHOLOGIC FINDINGS

The fragment is a wedge-shaped ossicle of hardened bone, covered by cartilage and attached to the talus by fibrous tissue.

IMAGING PROCEDURES

In an acute situation, anteroposterior, lateral, and mortise radiographs should be obtained to visualize the lesion. If the lesion cannot be seen radiographically, a bone scan or magnetic resonance imaging may identify the lesion before it is radiographically apparent.

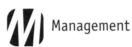 Management

GENERAL MEASURES

Conservative therapy in the acute phase includes casting and reduced weight bearing for 4 to 6 weeks. Failure to respond to such therapy or the presence of a displaced fragment may require surgical intervention.

SURGICAL TREATMENT

The following procedures can be performed arthroscopically or through an arthrotomy:

- Internal fixation of the fragment
- Drilling of the fragment (an attempt to increase the vascularity to the fragment)
- Excision of the fragment
- Fixation of the fragment with bone grafting

PHYSICAL THERAPY

Patients should be partially weight bearing or non–weight bearing during attempts to heal the fragment. It is helpful to teach partial weight bearing and range of motion.

MEDICAL TREATMENT

- Rest
- Activity restriction
- Immobilization of the joint
- Medications (nonsteroidal antiinflammatory drugs may impair bone healing and are not useful during the first 8 to 12 weeks of treatment)

PATIENT EDUCATION

Patients should be warned that healing is slow because of the decreased blood supply and high stress. Alternative activities and exercises should be recommended.

PREVENTION

There is no sure way to prevent this condition.

MONITORING

The patient should be seen periodically as symptoms dictate, for advice on activities.

COMPLICATIONS

- Nonunion
- Displacement of the fragment
- Arthrosis
- Continued pain

PROGNOSIS

Many patients develop progressive pain and stiffness.

RECOMMENDED READING

Coughlin MJ, Mann RA. *Surgery of the foot and ankle*. St. Louis: Mosby—Year Book, 1999:1568–1569.

Lutter LD, Mizel MS, Pfeffer GB. *Orthopaedic knowledge update: foot and ankle*. Rosemont, IL: American Academy of Orthopaedic Surgeons, 1994:311.

Basics

DESCRIPTION

Ankle pain is a complaint that should be approached with a full understanding of ankle anatomy, a proper history, and a thorough physical examination. The ankle joint includes three bones: the talus, the distal tibia, and the distal fibula. Pain about the ankle after trauma warrants an examination of the anatomic structures around the ankle to determine whether a soft tissue or bony injury has occurred. In an elderly person, persistent, chronic ankle pain without a history of specific trauma that increases with weight bearing and decreases with rest and nonsteroidal medications may indicate osteoarthritis. Pain in the ankle associated with other joint pain and characteristic deformities may warrant a rheumatologic evaluation to rule out rheumatoid or other inflammatory arthritides. Severe ankle pain with range of motion in an individual with a history of penetrating trauma, intravenous drug abuse, or an immunocompromised state may signify a septic joint that requires surgery. Ankle pain may even be due to an ulcer in a patient with diabetes who is prone to foot problems. Ankle pain with significant swelling, a history of great toe metatarsophalangeal joint redness, and swelling suggests gout. Although most patients who have ankle pain may have a simple sprain or fracture, the problem may indicate a systemic disorder. Ankle pain involves the following:

- Bones: tibiotalar joint, distal fibula, distal tibia, talus
- Lateral ligaments: anterior talofibular ligament and calcaneofibular ligament
- Medial ligaments: superficial and deep deltoid ligaments
- Ligaments between the tibia and fibula: anterior tibiofibular ligament
- Interosseous membrane

INCIDENCE

- Extremely common
- More common with increasing age
- Equal in both sexes

CLASSIFICATION

- Traumatic
- Degenerative
- Inflammatory
- Infectious

ASSOCIATED CONDITIONS

- Rheumatoid arthritis
- Gout
- Active lifestyle

ICD-9-CM

719.47 Ankle joint pain

 Diagnosis

SIGNS AND SYMPTOMS

Ankle pain that is well localized after a traumatic episode may represent an ankle sprain or a fracture. Pain without a history of trauma but with significant joint swelling, warmth, and extreme pain with passive motion could indicate a septic joint or a gouty attack. The physician should attempt to elicit a history of factors that cause or exacerbate the pain (e.g., duration, location, and severity of traumatic episode, or the presence of swelling in any other joints). The location of the pain may help to focus the examination on the ankle joint itself or on the subtalar joint, tendons, or the heel.

DIFFERENTIAL DIAGNOSIS

- Ankle sprain
- Ankle fracture
- Rheumatoid arthritis
- Septic joint
- Gouty attack
- Osteochondritis dissecans of the talar dome
- Subluxating peroneal tendons
- Peripheral vascular disease
- Bone tumor of the associated bones about the ankle joint
- Pigmented villonodular synovitis
- Tarsal coalition

PHYSICAL EXAMINATION

Palpate the anterior talofibular ligament, calcaneofibular ligament, and the deltoid ligament, as well as the medial and lateral malleoli for well-localized tenderness. Palpate the joint line anteriorly for capsule tenderness. Perform a study of active and passive motion of the ankle and a comparison of the results with the pain-free contralateral ankle. Examine the skin about the ankle. Is the ankle joint swollen and hot? Examine the neurovascular status of the foot. Determine its ability to bear weight, and observe the patient's gait.

Ankle Pain

LABORATORY TESTS

Order serum laboratory tests based on the level of suspicion for specific clinical entities:

• Septic arthritis: complete blood count with differential erythrocyte sedimentation rate
• Rheumatoid arthritis or other inflammatory arthritis: rheumatoid screen, rheumatoid factor, antinuclear antibody
• Gout: serum uric acid level

Arthrocentesis is often the best and only method to establish a definitive diagnosis. In the case of septic arthritis, findings include positive culture, most commonly *Staphylococcus aureus*. In the case of gout, findings include urate crystals.

IMAGING PROCEDURES

Usually plain films—anteroposterior, lateral, and mortise views—are sufficient. An oblique radiograph of the foot may be indicated to rule out calcaneonavicular coalition. Magnetic resonance imaging may be necessary to detect occult processes, such as tumors and stress fractures, and synovial proliferate diseases, such as pigmented villonodular synovitis, synovial chondromatosis, or synovitis. Computed tomography can help to define fracture fragments and intraarticular step-offs in plafond fractures (distal tibial intraarticular fractures). Computed tomography of the subtalar joint may be indicated to rule out coalition.

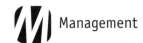 Management

GENERAL MEASURES

Ankle sprains can be treated with rest, ice, compressive dressing (elastic [Ace] wrap), and elevation (RICE) and gradual weight bearing as tolerated. A patient with a nondisplaced distal fibular fracture without medial tenderness, medial space widening, or a medial malleolar fracture can be treated with a short leg walking cast and follow-up with an orthopaedist. Tibial intraarticular fractures, medial malleolar fractures, open fractures, and open fracture-dislocations warrant an orthopaedic consultation. Hot, swollen, erythematous ankles may warrant an arthrocentesis to rule out a gouty attack or a septic joint.

With ankle sprains, nondisplaced distal fibular fractures that are nontender medially and without medial space widening, or a medial malleolar fracture, the patient should gradually begin to bear weight as tolerated. Non–weight-bearing activity is appropriate in patients with a surgically treated fracture.

SURGICAL TREATMENT

Most ankle fractures that warrant surgery can be treated with open reduction and internal fixation with plates and screws. Certain fractures, such as distal tibial intraarticular fractures and open fractures, may require special fixation devices.

PHYSICAL THERAPY

This may be indicated in certain cases once diagnosis and specific treatments are performed.

MEDICAL TREATMENT

• Nonsteroidal antiinflammatory drugs are usually sufficient for sprains and certain fractures.
• Gouty attacks may require indomethacin, colchicine, or allopurinol.
• Septic joints require antibiotic medications.

MONITORING

Careful short-term follow-up is necessary to check range of motion and to prevent contractures.

COMPLICATIONS

Many of the causes of ankle pain may lead to progressive pain and stiffness.

PROGNOSIS

Most causes of ankle pain can be identified and treated with good to excellent results.

RECOMMENDED READING

Lutter LD, Mizel MS, Pfeffer GB. *Orthopaedic knowledge update: foot and ankle*. Rosemont, IL: American Academy of Orthopaedic Surgeons, 1994:241–253.

Basics

DESCRIPTION

Sprains of the lateral ligaments about the ankle are the most common injury in sports and dance and occur commonly in the general population. This injury is most commonly an attenuation, partial tear, or complete rupture of the anterior talofibular ligament. More severe injuries include the calcaneofibular ligament. Patients experience this injury from an inversion mechanism. The clinical presentation includes pain and swelling on the lateral aspect of the ankle. A radiograph should be obtained acutely to rule out a fracture. Most injuries resolve with rest, ice, compression, and elevation (RICE) in the acute phase. Surgery is not necessary unless one is dealing with a high-performance athlete, a child with recurrent ankle sprains, or a patient with chronic ankle instability.

GENETICS

Children 12 to 16 years of age who have frequent ankle sprains may have a tarsal coalition (an autosomal dominant congenital fusion of the calcaneonavicular or talocalcaneal joint).

INCIDENCE

Every day in the Unitd States, 23,000 of these injuries occur.

CAUSES

The injury results from inversion of the foot when weight is placed on the ankle.

RISK FACTORS

- Athletes
- Dancers
- Children with congenital tarsal fusions

CLASSIFICATION

- Grade 1: partial tearing of the ligaments
- Grade 2: partial to complete tear of the anterior talofibular ligament, partial tear of the calcaneofibular ligament
- Grade 3: complete rupture of the anterior talofibular ligament and calcaneofibular ligament

ICD-9-CM

845.0 Ankle sprain

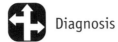 ## Diagnosis

SIGNS AND SYMPTOMS

Patients have pain, tenderness, and swelling over the lateral aspect of the ankle.

DIFFERENTIAL DIAGNOSIS

- Fibular fracture
- Osteochondral fracture of the talar dome
- Peroneal tendon subluxation
- Congenital tarsal fusion
- Talar fracture
- Calcaneal fracture
- Subtalar subluxation

PHYSICAL EXAMINATION

Tenderness and swelling are noted along the lateral aspect of the ankle inferior and anterior to the tip of the lateral malleolus. Instability may be examined with an anterior drawer test of the ankle: holding the distal tibia firmly with one hand, try to displace the hind foot (with the other hand around the heel) anteriorly with the ankle in a neutral position and in plantar flexion. Compare these displacements with those of the other, uninjured ankle.

IMAGING PROCEDURES

Anteroposteriorly, lateral and mortise radiographic views of the ankle are obtained. Computed tomography is indicated if tarsal coalition is suspected.

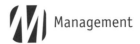 ## Management

GENERAL MEASURES

- RICE and partial weight bearing are indicated as tolerated with crutches in the acute phase (first week).
- Nonsteroidal antiinflammatory medication may help with pain.
- Gentle active range of motion as tolerated is advised.
- Consider a long-term strengthening program in physical therapy if symptoms continue.

SURGICAL TREATMENT

Surgery is indicated only in patients with recurrent instability. In this case, reconstruction of the lateral ankle ligaments with part of the peroneus brevis tendon is usually successful.

PHYSICAL THERAPY

Range of motion, strengthening exercises, and proprioceptive training are indicated.

MEDICAL TREATMENT

Antiinflammatory drugs and analgesics can be used for severe sprains; however, they generally are not necessary.

PATIENT EDUCATION

An appropriate return to activity plan should be determined as indicated by the severity of the ankle sprain.

PREVENTION

Proprioceptive training has been shown to decrease recurrent sprains.

MONITORING

Patients should show full strength and range of motion before returning to sports.

COMPLICATIONS

- Osteochondritis dissecans
- Recurrent sprains

PROGNOSIS

It depends on severity, but most patients have an excellent prognosis.

RECOMMENDED READING

Clanton TO, Schon LC. Athletic injuries to the soft tissues of the foot and ankle. In: Mann RA, Coughlin MJ, eds. *Surgery of the foot and ankle,* 6th ed. St. Louis: CV Mosby, 1993:1121–1150.

Ankylosing Spondylitis

 ## Basics

DESCRIPTION

Ankylosing spondylitis is a seronegative spondyloarthropathy characterized by ossification of the ligaments of the spine, as well as those of the hips and shoulders. This inflammatory arthritis begins in the young adult and affects the ligaments of the spine, sacroiliac joints, hips, and shoulders.

SYNONYM

Marie-Strumpell arthritis

GENETICS

This condition is associated with the HLA-B27 antigen.

INCIDENCE

• Ten percent to 20% of people who are positive for HLA-B27 will develop ankylosing spondylitis or another seronegative spondyloarthropathy.
• It usually begins between the ages of 20 and 40 years and is progressive.
• The male-to-female ratio is 10:1.

CAUSES

There is inflammation of the cartilaginous attachment of the tendon or ligament to bone. The cause of this inflammation is unknown, but a suggestion has been made that bacterial antigens such as *Klebsiella* may be involved.

RISK FACTORS

• HLA-B27
• Family history
• Poorer prognosis for younger patients
• Age less than 40 years

ASSOCIATED CONDITIONS

• Plantar fasciitis
• Achilles tendinitis
• Inflammatory uveitis
• Aortic insufficiency, cardiomegaly, and conduction defects

ICD-9-CM

720.0 Ankylosing spondylitis

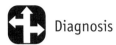 ## Diagnosis

SIGNS AND SYMPTOMS

The diagnosis of ankylosing spondylitis is clinical, based on the following:

• Typical pain pattern
• Duration longer than 3 months
• Age less than 40 years
• No evidence of Reiter's syndrome, psoriasis, or bowel disease
• Commonly, insidious onset of stiffness without pain, malaise, and susceptibility to fatigue

Pain first appears in the hips, buttocks, or lumbosacral region. The pain is worst in the morning and improves with exercise. Tenderness over the sacroiliac joints is usually present. Decreased spinal mobility, diminished chest expansion, kyphosis, and flattening of the lumbar spine develop as the disease progresses. Patients may develop a marked forward lean, which may be severely deforming (Figs. 1 and 2). The upper extremities are rarely involved.

DIFFERENTIAL DIAGNOSIS

• Reiter's syndrome (nongonococcal urethritis and arthritis)
• Psoriatic arthritis
• Intestinal arthropathy (associated with Crohn's disease and ulcerative colitis)

PHYSICAL EXAMINATION

Patients may have no or only subtle physical findings. Reduced motion of the cervical or lumbar spine may be present. Reduced chest expansion (less than 2.5 cm on deep inspiration) is an early finding.

LABORATORY TESTS

• Erythrocyte sedimentation rate (elevated in 80%)
• Rheumatoid factor
• Tissue typing for HLA antigens (90% positive for HLA-B27). (The HLA-B27 antigen test is positive in about 5% of healthy persons. It should not be used as a general screening test but is useful in young patients with chronic back pain.)

PATHOLOGIC FINDINGS

Initial pathologic changes resemble those of rheumatoid arthritis and proceed gradually to extensive bony ankylosis. Progressive ossification occurs in the capsular and other intervertebral ligaments and fuses the lower, and often the entire spine, which may fuse in a kyphotic position. The costovertebral joints may become ankylosed. The vertebral bodies tend to become osteoporotic.

IMAGING PROCEDURES

There are no pathognomonic tests for ankylosing spondylitis. Radiographic changes may not appear until months after symptoms. The earliest changes are increased bone density at the sacroiliac joints. As the disease progresses, smaller erosions and narrowing appear in the facet joints. Later changes include obliteration of the sacroiliac joint and facet joint spaces and ossification of the longitudinal ligaments and the periphery of the annulus fibrosus (disc), giving the "bamboo spine" appearance.

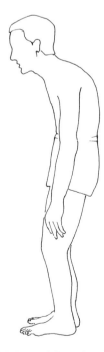

Fig. 1. Ankylosing spondylitis produces kyphosis of the entire spine and flexion contractures of the joints.

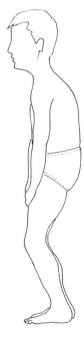

Fig. 2. The patient with ankylosing spondylitis must flex at the knee to look upward.

Management

GENERAL MEASURES

General measures include extension exercises, following a well-balanced diet, and pain control with aspirin or other antiinflammatory medications.

Prevention of deformity is a major focus in this disease process. A firm mattress or bed board and prophylactic bracing should be used to prevent kyphosis. Hyperextension exercises should also be prescribed. In later stages of the disease, if a kyphosis that prevents the patient from looking ahead develops, spinal osteotomy and stabilization may become necessary. Total hip arthroplasty may also be necessary for treatment of intractable hip pain.

SURGICAL TREATMENT

Spinal osteotomy consists of removing wedges of the abnormally ossified bone at the site of maximal deformity. Straightening the spine and holding it in place with rods until fusion occurs may be done in the cervical, thoracic, or lumbar areas.

PHYSICAL THERAPY

Hyperextension exercises are helpful in preventing kyphosis.

MEDICAL TREATMENT

Nonsteroidal drugs should be used to control symptoms. The selection is empiric, although indomethacin is considered to be the drug of choice overall.

PATIENT EDUCATION

Activity should not be prohibited, but patients should be told about the increased risk and danger of spine fracture and should avoid situations placing them at risk for this injury. Patients should avoid contact sports and other activities such as skydiving and bungee jumping. Patients should be given a handout describing proper sleeping posture, as well as extension exercises. The Arthritis Foundation has patient literature and newsletters (404-872-7100).

PREVENTION

- Patients should be discouraged from smoking.
- Patients should be counseled about a 10% to 20% risk of transmitting their disease to their children.

MONITORING

Patients should be seen on a routine basis (every 6 months) to monitor posture, to reinforce the importance of exercises, and to adjust analgesics. They should be monitored for uveitis as well as for development of cardiac and pulmonary problems.

COMPLICATIONS

Spinal fractures may happen with minimal trauma because the ossified spine is brittle and has no "give." Anteroposterior, lateral, and oblique radiographs should be studied carefully because small fracture lines may be difficult to detect. Computed tomography scans with three-dimensional reconstructions are sensitive in detecting fractures. Magnetic resonance imaging can be used to detect epidural hematomas. Spinal fractures should be urgently braced or internally fixed, because paralysis may ensue. Uveitis develops in 25% of patients and may require topical steroids.

PROGNOSIS

Patients with early onset of disease, as well as inflammation of peripheral joints, have a worse prognosis. There is no cure for this disorder, but with aggressive preventive measures, much of the disability associated with it can be prevented.

RECOMMENDED READING

Brashear HR, Raney RB. *Handbook of orthopaedic surgery*, 10th ed. St. Louis: CV Mosby, 1986:150–153.

Clark CR, Bonfilgio M. *Orthopaedics*. New York: Churchill Livingstone, 1994:290.

Anterior Cruciate Ligament Injury

 Basics

DESCRIPTION

The anterior cruciate ligament (ACL) is one of the primary stabilizers of the knee joint, the largest joint in the body. It prevents anterior translation of the tibia on the femur. ACL injuries occur predominantly from noncontact decelerations such as stopping suddenly, pivoting, or landing after jumping. ACL injuries run the gamut from mild sprains, with no resultant functional abnormalities, to complete ruptures. In the pediatric patient, injury to the ACL most often occurs at the ligament-bone interface, whereas in the adult, rupture of the midsubstance of the ligament is more common.

SYNONYMS

In the immature patient, a tibial spine fracture is the equivalent injury.

INCIDENCE

- 100,000 ACL injuries occur in the United States annually.
- They are common in young, active adults.
- They can occur in skeletally immature children and in middle-aged athletes.

SIGNS AND SYMPTOMS

Acute Symptoms

- Pain and swelling
- In approximately half of patients, a "pop" or a tearing sensation at the time of injury

Chronic Symptoms

- Pain, swelling, instability

CAUSES

- Sudden decelerating injuries
- Impacts to the knee with the foot planted

RISK FACTORS

- Female athletes
- Small femoral intercondylar notch

CLASSIFICATION

Partial Tears

These are difficult to differentiate from complete tears on a clinical examination. An arthroscopic examination reveals that some portion of the ACL is intact. Because of plastic deformation, however, the ligament is dysfunctional, resulting in instability.

Complete Tears

Obvious complete rupture of ACL is identified arthroscopically or on magnetic resonance imaging. Avulsion fractures of the ACL tibial insertion, in which a fragment of bone is identified on a radiograph, may be repaired primarily.

ASSOCIATED CONDITIONS

- Meniscal tear
- Collateral ligament injury
- "Bone bruise"
- Articular cartilage injury

ICD-9-CM

717.83 Anterior cruciate ligament

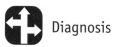 Diagnosis

DIFFERENTIAL DIAGNOSIS

- Osteochondral fracture
- Tibial plateau fracture
- Meniscal injury: prevalence of meniscal injury with coexistent ACL injury ranging from 6% to 100%
- Cartilage injury
- Medial or lateral collateral ligament injury
- Posterior cruciate ligament injury

PHYSICAL EXAMINATION

Often, tense joint effusion is seen. Marked restriction in movement occurs secondary to pain and spasm. Lachman's test and the anterior drawer test are positive. The condition is chronic, not acute. Most of the acute symptoms and signs resolve in approximately 10 days' time. Performance of many of the tests to assess for knee stability (e.g., pivot shift, anterior drawer) is difficult in the acute period because muscle spasm and guarding prevent isolated assessment of the ligamentous structures.

LABORATORY TESTS

Knee aspiration reveals sanguineous fluid. The presence of fat in the aspirate helps to differentiate ACL injury from intraarticular fracture.

PATHOLOGIC FINDINGS

The collagen fibers are usually totally disrupted (mop ends).

IMAGING PROCEDURES

Anteroposterior, lateral, and intercondylar notch views of the knee to rule out fracture. Magnetic resonance imaging is useful for diagnosing ACL injuries as well as for assessing damage to menisci.

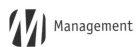 Management

GENERAL MEASURES

In the acute setting, diagnosis of an ACL injury is often difficult to differentiate from other ligamentous and meniscal injuries in the absence of a magnetic resonance imaging scan. Once the immediate pain and spasm have resolved (usually in about 10 days' time), physical examination directed toward assessing for ACL insufficiency and knee instability is much more informative. Therefore, in the acute period, care is directed toward comfort:

• The patient is placed in a knee immobilizer.
• The patient bears weight as tolerated.
• The patient is placed on crutches.
• Ice, elevation, and analgesics are prescribed.
• Gentle range of motion exercises are commenced once comfort allows.
• Isometric quadriceps strengthening exercises are begun as soon as tolerated to prevent quadriceps atrophy.
• Follow-up is arranged for 10 to 14 days after the injury, by which time the pain and swelling should have subsided.

Management of the diagnosed ACL-deficient knee continues to evolve and depends on the symptoms patients experience and their activity demands. For those desiring a return to athletics involving pivoting-type movements or in those patients in whom relatively trivial activities result in knee instability, ACL reconstruction is warranted.

Rehabilitation and functional bracing are beginning to fall out of favor in the younger patient population because of increasing concern that even occasional episodes of instability can result in significant damage to the articular surfaces and the menisci.

SURGICAL TREATMENT

ACL repair involves placement of a graft (most often patellar bone, tendon bone, or hamstring tendons) in place of the preexisting ligament. Concurrent meniscal damage may be repaired at this time as well.

PHYSICAL THERAPY

In both the reconstructed and the nonreconstructed knee, therapy involves hamstring and quadriceps strengthening exercises as well as range-of-motion exercises of the knee.

MEDICAL TREATMENT

• Medications (for use in the acute period)

—Nonsteroidal antiinflammatory drugs
—Acetaminophen
—Mild narcotic analgesics

PATIENT EDUCATION

More than 90% of patients have a stable knee after ACL reconstruction. Patients who have had a "patellar tendon" reconstruction often have anterior knee pain (mild). Most patients do not return to their previous level of activity if they were high-performance athletes, but most patients can return to sports.

PREVENTION

Athletic braces alone do not prevent ACL tears. The key to prevention is proper conditioning. Injury often occurs in recreational athletes when they are tired.

MONITORING

Patients are followed carefully at 4- to 6-week intervals after ACL reconstruction to ensure that they regain their range of motion and rebuild their quadriceps and hamstring muscles. Patients who have not undergone reconstruction are followed closely to check for "giving way" symptoms, which often lead to meniscal and cartilage injuries.

COMPLICATIONS

After surgery, the following complications may occur, fortunately infrequently:

• Arthrofibrosis
• Reflex sympathetic dystrophy
• Anterior knee pain
• Deep venous thrombosis
• Patellar fracture
• Patellar tendon rupture

PROGNOSIS

In the unstable knee, meniscal tears, cartilage damage, and ultimately degenerative arthritic changes may ensue. Patients have an excellent prognosis after ACL reconstruction.

RECOMMENDED READING

Larson RL, Taillon M. Anterior cruciate ligament insufficiency: principles of treatment. *J Am Acad Orthop Surg* 1994;2:26–35.

Johnson RJ, Beynnon BD, Nichols LB, et al. The treatment of injuries of the anterior cruciate ligament. *J Bone Joint Surg Am* 1992;74:140–151.

Back Pain

 Basics

DESCRIPTION

Low back pain is the most common musculoskel-etal condition. Back pain, affecting the bones, joints and ligaments, and muscles of the back, occurs primarily in adults but may also occur in children and adolescents. Back pain has many causes, and the clinician must carefully evaluate each patient to determine the nature of the pain.

SYNONYMS

- Backache
- Low back pain

GENETICS

No genetic predispositions are known.

INCIDENCE

Low back pain is extremely common in adults. Children and adolescents with scoliosis may have mild pain. Significant back pain in children should alert the clinician to look for a potentially serious problem such as a tumor or infection.

Age

- Adults: common
- Children: uncommon

Sex

Back pain is more common in men because they generally do more manual labor and are often injured in motor vehicle and industrial accidents.

CAUSES

Traumatic

- Fractures
- Fracture-dislocations
- Herniated discs
- Ligament tears

Atraumatic

- Degenerative disc disease
- Inflammatory arthritis
- Osteoporosis
- Spondylolysis and spondylolisthesis
- Neoplasms

RISK FACTORS

- Obesity
- Smoking
- Manual labor
- Accidents

CLASSIFICATION

Classification is broadly into traumatic and atraumatic conditions.

ASSOCIATED CONDITIONS

- Ankylosing spondylitis
- Rheumatoid arthritis

ICD-9-CM

847.9 Back Sprain

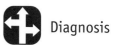 Diagnosis

SIGNS AND SYMPTOMS

Symptoms

- Low back discomfort
- Stiffness
- Numbness

Signs

- Paravertebral muscle spasm
- Motor weakness
- Loss of deep tendon reflexes
- Loss of sensation
- Clonus
- Positive Babinski's sign (upgoing great toe)

DIFFERENTIAL DIAGNOSIS

The differential diagnosis is long and can be broadly outlined according to the age of the patient and whether there was a traumatic event.

Adults

Traumatic

- Herniated discs
- Compression fractures
- Fracture-dislocations
- Spondylolysis (traumatic)

Atraumatic

- Degenerative disc disease
- Spinal stenosis
- Inflammatory arthritis: rheumatoid arthritis, ankylosing spondylitis
- Spondylolysis and spondylolisthesis
- Ligament strains
- Neoplasms: metastatic bone disease, multiple myeloma

Children

Traumatic

- Herniated disc
- Fracture

Atraumatic

- Scoliosis
- Disc space infection
- Vertebral osteomyelitis
- Neoplasms

PHYSICAL EXAMINATION

• Range of motion, detection of local tenderness, and a careful neurologic examination should be performed.
• Flexion, extension, and rotation of the lumbosacral spine should be noted. Pain with extension is common in patients with facet joint arthritis.
• Paravertebral muscle spasms and percussion tenderness should be elicited.
• Neurologic examination is crucial. Specifically, the following should be evaluated:

—Motor testing
—Deep tendon reflexes
—Sensation

LABORATORY TESTS

There are no specific laboratory tests. If one suspects infection, a complete blood count and erythrocyte sedimentation rate should be performed. These determinations are also useful in the older patient as a screening test for multiple myeloma. In young patients with significant stiffness, a serum HLA-B27 test can be used to look for ankylosing spondylitis.

PATHOLOGIC FINDINGS

No pathologic findings are applicable.

IMAGING PROCEDURES

Anteroposterior and lateral radiographs are the first imaging tests to be performed. They are not always necessary in patients who have their first episode of back pain, especially if it is caused by minor trauma (such as lifting). If the back pain persists for more than 6 weeks, radiographs should be done.
Computed tomography and magnetic resonance imaging scans are useful to detect and localize structural abnormalities precisely. These methods can be used singly or in combination:

• Computed tomography is useful to detect bone abnormalities such as fractures or osteoid osteomas.
• Magnetic resonance imaging is useful to detect marrow abnormalities or soft tissue processes such as metastatic bone disease.

Management

GENERAL MEASURES

Most patients with low back pain can be treated conservatively (nonoperatively) with rest, antiinflammatory medications, and physical therapy to improve aerobic conditioning. Prolonged bed rest is not beneficial.
During the initial period of severe spasm and pain (usually 2 to 7 days), patients may have restricted mobility. If plain radiographs are normal, patients should be progressively mobilized with physical therapy and aerobic conditioning.

SURGICAL TREATMENT

The many different operative procedures for back pain are based on the nature of the individual's problem. Common to all procedures are several principles:

• Decompression of any nerve root or spinal cord compression
• Removal of any arthritic joints
• Fusion to achieve a stable spine

Instrumentation has become important to achieve fusion in a reliable manner. There are many different instrumentation systems including pedicle screws, plates, and rods.

PHYSICAL THERAPY

Physical therapy is a key component. Patients are instructed in back exercises to improve posture and strength and aerobic conditioning, and they are taught the proper way to lift things and care for their back. In addition, patients who are injured on the job go through a work-hardening program.

MEDICAL TREATMENT

Nonsteroidal antiinflammatory agents are the drugs of choice to decrease inflammation. They are generally prescribed for an initial 4 to 6 weeks. If the pain has resolved at that time, the medication is discontinued. Muscle relaxants do not have a major role, although they can be very helpful in patients with severe spasm and anxiety. They are best used for short-term pain relief rather than for long-term use.

PATIENT EDUCATION

Education is important so patients understand their condition and the ways to prevent recurrent injuries.

PREVENTION

Prevention is best accomplished through the use of specific back exercises, avoidance of exacerbating activities, and aerobic conditioning.

MONITORING

Patients are followed at 4- to 6-week intervals until the pain subsides. With rest, activity modification, and nonsteroidal pain medications, patients should show progressive improvement. If they do not, one should suspect a structural problem.
Technetium bone scans, computed tomography scans, and magnetic resonance imaging scans can be used to detect pathologic processes.

COMPLICATIONS

Many different surgical complications can occur, including infection, neurologic injury, pseudarthrosis (nonunion), loss of fixation, and chronic unexplained pain.
Cauda equina syndrome is a devastating complication that occurs when an offending agent causes nerve root compression of the cauda equina. If the compression proceeds unchecked, permanent neurologic loss ensues and results in paralysis of the lower extremities and loss of bladder and bowel function.

PROGNOSIS

The prognosis is good (not always excellent) in patients who do not have major structural abnormalities. When major fusions have been performed, patients can return to most activities; however, they do not generally tolerate heavy work or repetitive loading of the back.

RECOMMENDED READING

Johns Hopkins Health, Johns Hopkins University. *Back pain: what you need to know*. Ottenheimer Publishers, 1998:21–49.

White AA. *Your aching back: a doctor's guide to relief*. New York: Simon and Schuster, 1990:129–140.

Bite to the Hand

 Basics

DESCRIPTION

Hand bites are serious injuries that, if not managed correctly, may result in significant morbidity to the hand. Two mechanisms of injury exist: the first is a direct bite to the hand, such as a dog bite. The more common mechanism is a "clenched fist" injury, which occurs over the metacarpophalangeal joint (the knuckle) when a fist strikes an opponent's mouth. This seemingly benign injury is, in fact, treacherous and is unfortunately common. A tooth may lacerate the extensor tendon, the joint capsule, or the joint itself. As the digit is straightened, the underlying wound is obscured by normal soft tissue.

SYNONYMS

- Clenched fist injury
- Dog or cat bite

INCIDENCE

- Common

CAUSES

- Fist fights
- Dog or cat exposure

RISK FACTORS

- Alcohol abuse
- Fighting

CLASSIFICATION

- MINOR—small puncture wound
- MAJOR—large lacerations and soft tissue damage (2-5 cm, exposed bone or cartilage, tendon rupture)

ASSOCIATED CONDITIONS

- Fractures

ICD-9-CM

882.1 Wound hand complicated

 Diagnosis

SIGNS AND SYMPTOMS

Signs

- Puncture or laceration to hand is present.
- Associated swelling and erythema may be present.
- Cellulitis and lymphangitis are present if there is an infection.
- If a tendon has been lacerated, the patient may experience difficulty with finger extension.

Symptoms

- Decreased hand function, such as difficulty with grasping or moving an individual digit
- Pain

DIFFERENTIAL DIAGNOSIS

Any puncture wound over the metacarpophalangeal joints must be regarded with great suspicion and treated as a clenched fist–type bite injury. Many combatants are embarrassed or hesitant to admit injury to this region and consequently present late for evaluation and treatment.

PHYSICAL EXAMINATION

- Examine the hand closely for any sign of skin puncture, particularly over the third and fourth metacarpophalangeal joints in instances of clenched fist injuries.
- Assess the motor, sensory, and vascular status of the hand and digits.
- If the injury is of a clenched fist type, have the patient make a fist, if possible. This may reveal the underlying soft tissue damage and may facilitate deep wound inspection.
- In clenched fist injuries, the damage to underlying structures is proximal to the skin wound when the fingers are in the extended, anatomic position.

LABORATORY TESTS

Cultures in the acute period before surgical débridement are unlikely to be helpful.

Imaging Procedures

Obtain radiographs of the hand to assess for fracture and tooth fragments.

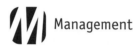 Management

GENERAL MEASURES

The most important therapeutic interventions are aggressive irrigation and débridement, to remove all devitalized tissue and to irrigate the wound copiously with normal saline solution, povidone-iodine (Betadine), or both. The wound may need to be surgically extended to facilitate exposure of the injured tissue. In clenched fist injuries, the skin wound is distal to the zone of deeper injury. After irrigation and débridement, the wound should be packed, and the hand should be immobilized and elevated. *Do not suture bite wounds.* Antibiotics should be commenced; amoxicillin (Augmentin) is a reasonable first-line agent. Antibiotics should be continued for 5 to 7 days in the absence of overt infection. At 24 hours, the packing should be removed, the patient should be reexamined, and warm soaks should be started. If infection is present, the wound should undergo repeat irrigation and débridement, and the patient should be admitted for parenteral antibiotic therapy. For patients presenting late to evaluation and treatment, and for those in whom infection is manifest, urgent irrigation and débridement followed by parenteral antibiotics are essential. Tetanus toxoid should be administered if the patient has not been immunized within the past 10 years. Immediate referral to a hand specialist should be consid-

ered for any patient presenting later than 24 hours after the initial injury, for those who have infected wounds, and for those who have sustained injury to the tendon, capsule, joint, or bone.

SURGICAL TREATMENT

Irrigation and débridement consist of cleaning infected tissues and removing devitalized tissues.

PHYSICAL THERAPY

Physical therapy is not necessary in the acute period. At 1 week after treatment, range of motion should be started to prevent stiffness (especially of the metacarpophalangeal joints).

MEDICAL TREATMENT

See earlier. More than 40 bacterial species have been isolated from infected bite wounds. The most common organisms are *Eikenella corrodens* and group A *Streptococcus* species in human bite wounds, and *Pasteurella multocida* in animal bite wounds. Augmentin provides satisfactory coverage for all of the organisms.

PATIENT EDUCATION

Patients are instructed in the case of open wounds and the signs of infection

—open packing
—soaking
—range of motion
—redness
—pain
—fever
—drainage
—inability to move finger

PREVENTION

Little can be done in terms of prevention, except to counsel patients about fighting. Animal bites are difficult to prevent.

MONITORING

At 24 hours, the packing should be changed. The patient should be followed closely until the wound demonstrates satisfactory healing with no evidence of infection. When doubt exists about the stability of the wound, patients should be followed at 24- to 48-hour intervals.

COMPLICATIONS

- Infection: both soft tissue and bone
- Stiffness

PROGNOSIS

It is usually good if infection is avoided.

RECOMMENDED READING

Abrams RA, Botte MJ. Hand infections: treatment for specific injury types. *J Am Acad Orthop Surg* 1996:4:219–230.

Siverhus DJ, Stern PJ. Avoiding complications of human bite injuries. *J Musculoskel Med* 1996;13:32–44.

Basics

DESCRIPTION

An abnormality of the proximal tibial growth plate causes excessive varus alignment of the knees (bowed legs) in children (Fig. 1).

SYNONYMS

- Infantile tibia vara
- Juvenile or adolescent tibia vara
- Pathologic bowlegs
- Osteochondrosis deformans tibiae

GENETICS

No genetic pattern has been proved. More likely, patients inherit a body habitus that predisposes them to the disorder. The disorder is more common in African-American children.

INCIDENCE

- Infantile tibia vara is the most common cause of pathologic bowing in the young patients, but it accounts for less than 1% of all bowed legs.
- The juvenile form is much less common, with only 60 reports in the literature in the United States.
- The adolescent form is becoming more commonly recognized.
- Infantile tibia vara presents between 2 and 4 years of age.
- Juvenile tibia vara presents between the ages of 6 and 18 years.
- The infantile form is more common in girls.
- The juvenile or adolescent form is more common in boys.

CAUSES

Decreased growth from the proximal tibial physis causes medial angulation and internal rotation of the proximal tibia, possibly from weight-related overload or repetitive trauma to the posteromedial proximal tibial physis.

RISK FACTORS

- African-American ethnicity
- Obesity
- Ligamentous laxity
- Early age of walking

CLASSIFICATION

- The infantile form presents between the ages of 1 and 4 years and has a better prognosis.
- The juvenile form presents after the age 4 to 6 years in obese boys and has a poorer prognosis.

Associated Conditions

- Obesity
- Ligamentous laxity

ICD-9-CM

732.4 Blount's disease

Diagnosis

SIGNS AND SYMPTOMS

- Patients with infantile tibia vara usually present between 14 and 40 months of age with increasingly bowed legs (usually bilateral involvement).
- Juvenile presentation also involves progressive varus deformity (bowing), but many of these patients also have lateral knee pain, and often only one leg is affected.
- The infantile form may progress to become severe if untreated.
- The juvenile form rarely becomes as severe.
- There is usually some internal tibial torsion along with the bowing.

DIFFERENTIAL DIAGNOSIS

- Physiologic bowed legs
- Hypophosphatemic rickets
- Trauma
- Osteochondroma
- Metaphyseal chondrodysplasia
- Focal fibrocartilaginous dysplasia

PHYSICAL EXAMINATION

The patient's height and weight as well as percentiles should be recorded. The finding of short stature suggests a skeletal dysplasia. The distance between the medial sides of the knees should be recorded. Knee range of motion and ligamentous laxity should be checked. Tibial torsion should be assessed by the thigh-foot angle. The routine knee examination should be performed. Gait should be observed, and the foot progression angle should be measured.

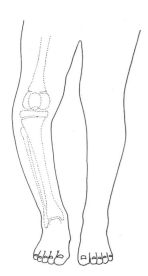

Fig. 1. In Blount's disease, the varus is focal at the upper tibia.

Blount's Disease

LABORATORY TESTS

Testing is indicated if rickets is suspected. In Blount's disease, calcium, phosphorus, alkaline phosphatase, and renal function determinations are all normal.

PATHOLOGIC FINDINGS

The growth plate shows islands of densely packed cartilage cells demonstrating more hypertrophy than normal, islands of almost acellular fibrous cartilage, and abnormal groups of capillaries. Pathologic examination is not usually indicated in patient care, however.

IMAGING PROCEDURES

Appropriate radiographs include a long leg anteroposterior view of the tibia and femur to evaluate the tibiofemoral angle, as well as the mechanical axis. The radiograph should show the whole limb from the hip to the ankle, and it should be a true standing anteroposterior view of the knee. The metaphyseal-diaphyseal angle (MDA) differentiates between Blount's and physiologic varus: an angle of less than 11 degrees is physiologic, and an angle of 16 degrees or greater indicates Blount's disease. More advanced disease reveals a medial physeal bar (fusion of metaphysis and epiphysis). This is not used clinically; however, tomography or magnetic resonance imaging can be useful in delineating the physeal bars that can form later. If a bar is present, the whole growth plate should be fused to prevent recurrent varus. Patients with advanced cases may have a secondary deformity of the distal femur and/or the distal tibia.

Management

GENERAL MEASURES

Children younger than 3 years of age who present with minimal deformity may be braced. This should be a long brace from the hip to the ankle and locked at the knee. Bracing full time (22 of 24 hours a day) puts valgus stress on the knee (more knock-kneed) and decreases the stress on the medial physis. This technique allows the growth plate to "catch up" the growth medially if bracing is begun when the deformity is mild. If the patient is being braced, full weight bearing is encouraged. If osteotomy was performed, the patient is kept non–weight bearing until healing (8 to 12 weeks) of the osteotomy; then full weight bearing can be resumed. If bracing fails to correct the deformity, or if a patient older than 3 years of age presents with moderate to severe deformity, an osteotomy is needed.

SURGICAL TREATMENT

Osteotomy—cutting and realigning the proximal tibia—can also decrease the stress on the medial physis and can allow healing. If a physeal bar has formed, an osteotomy is often combined with completion of the closure of the proximal tibial physis. If significant leg length inequality develops, this may be treated by lengthening the short limb or growth plate closure of the longer limb. Adolescent Blount's disease may be treated with stapling of the lateral sides of the growth plate to allow the bone to correct itself.

PHYSICAL THERAPY

- Crutch training after osteotomy
- Regaining of knee range of motion

PATIENT EDUCATION

The patient's family must understand the benefit of weight reduction. Bracing in patients with infantile Blount's disease must be kept on 22 of 24 hours a day.

PREVENTION

- Weight control
- Extremely early walking should not be encouraged

MONITORING

Patients must be followed until skeletal maturity. The interval between visits is determined by the severity of the disease and the type of intervention.

COMPLICATIONS

- Recurrence of deformity leads to abnormal limb alignment and degenerative joint disease.
- Surgical complications of osteotomy include neurovascular complications and compartment syndrome.

PROGNOSIS

Patients treated after the age of 5 years have high recurrence rate of 70% to 75%, compared with patients treated before age 5, with recurrence rates of 20% to 30%. Therefore, early osteotomy (before age 4) should be performed if bracing is not successful.

RECOMMENDED READING

Greene WB. Infantile tibia vara (instructional course lecture). *J Bone Joint Surg Am* 1993:75:130–143.

Henderson RC, Kemp GJ, Greene WB. Adolescent tibia vara: alternatives for operative treatment. *J Bone Joint Surg Am* 1992:74:342–350.

Tolo VT. The lower limb. In: Morrissy RT, ed. *Lovell and Winter's pediatric orthopaedics,* 3rd ed. Philadelphia: JB Lippincott, 1966:1055–1057.

Basics

DESCRIPTION

Brachial plexus palsy results from injury to the brachial plexus during birth that is caused by downward or upward traction on the arm. Primarily, the brachial plexus is affected. Secondarily, the muscles and bones of the upper extremity become contracted or deformed over time owing to the resultant muscle imbalance. Although the injury occurs at birth, in mild cases it may not be detected until the baby tries to use the extremity.

SYNONYMS

- Birth palsy
- Obstetric palsy
- Erb's palsy
- Klumpke's palsy

INCIDENCE

Currently, the incidence is 0.8 per 1,000 live births. This represents a decline from the rate seen in 1900, when it was reported twice this often. The change most likely results from improved obstetric care. Erb's palsy is about four times as common as Klumpke's palsy. There is no recognized difference in incidence between boys and girls.

CAUSES

- Erb's palsy is due to downward traction on the shoulder or arm or lateral traction against the neck.
- Klumpke's palsy is due to upward traction on the arm.
- Both occur because of the force needed in a difficult extraction.

RISK FACTORS

- Fetal malposition
- Shoulder dystocia
- Cephalopelvic disproportion
- High birth weight: maternal diabetes
- Use of forceps in delivery

CLASSIFICATION

- Type I: Erb's palsy: injury to roots 4 to 6 of the cervical spine
- Type II: whole-plexus palsy: C-4–T-1 involved; also known as Erb-Duchenne-Klumpke palsy
- Type III: Klumpke's palsy: C-8–T-1 involved

ASSOCIATED CONDITIONS

Large birth weight

ICD-9-CM

767.6 Brachial plexus birth palsy

Diagnosis

SIGNS AND SYMPTOMS

Signs

- Decreased active use of the extremity
- Extremity held in internal rotation
- Loss of full active or passive external rotation
- Inability to abduct (raise) the shoulder
- Atrophy of the involved muscles (late) (Fig. 1)
- Possible elbow flexion contracture
- Possible Horner's syndrome in Klumpke's palsy

Symptoms

- The condition is not painful.
- A loss of sensation may be noted with complete plexus injuries.

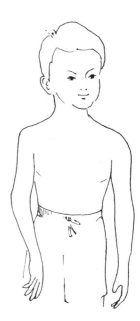

Fig. 1. The most typical deformity after infantile brachial plexus palsy is an internally rotated arm that does not abduct fully or flex at the elbow. This results from damage to the C5-6 roots.

Brachial Plexus Birth Palsy

DIFFERENTIAL DIAGNOSIS

• Clavicle fracture: usually more painful to palpation. Some shoulder motion may be elicited.
• Proximal humeral physeal fracture: same findings as clavicle fracture, with tenderness over the proximal humerus. The abnormality may not show up on radiographs because the proximal humerus is unossified at this age. Ultrasound studies may be diagnostic, as are plain films 7 to 10 days later.
• Septic arthritis of the shoulder: may cause pseudoparalysis. Fever in the newborn may not be pronounced.

PHYSICAL EXAMINATION

Physical examination is the primary means of diagnosis. Palpate for tenderness over the clavicle, proximal humerus, and ribs. Test sensation by responses to light touch or pinch. Test the function of all muscles in the shoulder, elbow, and hand by stimulation and observation. In patient's with Erb's palsy, the shoulder is internally rotated and lacks external rotation and abduction. In Klumpke's palsy, there is loss of finger and interosseous function.

PATHOLOGIC FINDINGS

Pathologic findings vary from stretch to disruption of the nerves at the brachial plexus. This disorder may occur at the cervical foramen, as the nerves exit the spinal canal (poorer prognosis), or farther down in the neck and shoulder. Secondary muscle atrophy ensues.
An electromyogram should be obtained if there is no clinical return of deltoid or biceps function by 3 to 6 months, because this finding may be a relative indication for surgery. Cervical myelography may be helpful to diagnose the level of injury. If meningoceles are seen at the root levels in the cervical spinal cord, this indicates that the roots were avulsed from the cord, and the prognosis is poorer.

IMAGING PROCEDURES

Plain films are often indicated at birth to rule out other injuries. At the time of late reconstruction in an older child who has residual shoulder imbalance, plain radiographs and computed tomography scans are indicated to assess the shape of the glenohumeral joint.

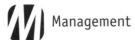 Management

GENERAL MEASURES

• Stretching should be done several times per day by the parents. The patient should be referred to a pediatric orthopaedic surgeon for monitoring and decision making.
• Observation and passive range of motion are indicated for the newborn; approximately 80% of patients recover spontaneously by 1 year of age. Splinting is not necessary, but continued follow-up is needed. Surgery is indicated for the remainder, either with grafting of the injured nerves if there are no meningoceles and the elapsed time is not more than 1 to 2 years or with tendon transfers to improve muscle balance.

SURGICAL TREATMENT

• Reanastomosis is performed using microscopy with direct repair, or grafting of the injured nerves is performed if the patient does not return in about 6 months. The exact timing is controversial.
• Tendon transfers are performed to restore external rotation to the shoulder.
• Release of the tight internal rotators may be indicated as well.
• Humeral osteotomy is another way to restore and externally rotate position.
• Several transfers are available to restore elbow flexion, most notably the latissimus transfer. Transfers for finger and wrist function are least commonly needed.

PHYSICAL THERAPY

An occupational therapist is helpful in teaching the parents how to stretch and what contractures to watch for. Splinting is not needed, but stretching and active range of motion are encouraged.

PATIENT EDUCATION

The prognosis described earlier should be outlined to the parents, so they can plan ahead. The possibility of contractures should be explained to them, so they will be more motivated to continue range-of-motion exercises.

PREVENTION

• Management of gestational diabetes
• Cesarean section if cephalopelvic disproportion is significant

MONITORING

The patient should be seen about every 3 months to look for return of function and to plan for appropriate diagnostic testing.

COMPLICATIONS

• Contracture of shoulder, elbow, or wrist
• Affected extremity smaller in length and girth
• Sensory loss
• Shoulder dislocation

PROGNOSIS

Eighty percent of these patients recover spontaneously. Surgery may help many of the remainder.

RECOMMENDED READING

Boome RS, Kaaye JC. Obstetric traction injuries of the brachial plexus: natural history, indication for surgical repair, and results. *J Bone Joint Surg Br* 1988;70:571–576.

Hoffer MM, Wickenden R, Roper B. Results of tendon transfer to the rotator cuff. *J Bone Joint Surg Am* 1978;60:691–701.

Basics

DESCRIPTION

A bunion is an osseous-cartilaginous enlargement of the medial eminence often combined with swelling of the soft tissues and bursa. Hallux valgus is a lateral deviation of the great toe. The deformity occurs primarily at the metatarsophalangeal joint and is associated with a widening of the angle between the first and second metatarsal (metatarsus primus varus).

GENETICS

There may be an unidentified genetic component. Two-thirds of patients have a positive family history. Hallux valgus also is seen commonly as a component of a hyperlaxity syndrome that is thought to have a genetic component.

INCIDENCE

• It is seen in predominantly middle-aged to elderly patients, although it can be seen in young adults, and a juvenile form exists.
• Women are affected more than men.

CAUSES

• The type of shoe worn, specifically a shoe with a narrow toe box and high heels, is believed to be causative. This is supported by studies that demonstrate higher incidence in shod versus unshod societies and increasing incidence in populations that adopt more westernized shoe styles (Fig. 1).

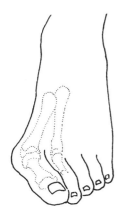

Fig. 1. A bunion is produced by an underlying imbalance of the soft tissues and extrinsic pressure.

• Pes planus is causative, both as part of a laxity syndrome as well as associated with mechanically abnormal pressure on the first metatarsophalangeal joint secondary to a pronated gait.
• Metatarsus primus varus is associated. There is a strong relationship between an increase in the angle between the first and second metatarsal joint and hallux valgus.
• Acquired joint laxity (e.g., from rheumatoid arthritis, gout, or trauma) is causative.
• Other miscellaneous conditions (e.g., amputation of another toe, severe hammering of the toes, Achilles tendon contracture) may also be associated.

RISK FACTORS

• Heredity
• Shoe wear

ICD-9-CM

735.0 Hallux valgus

 Diagnosis

SIGNS AND SYMPTOMS

The patient presents with lateral deviation of great toe with an enlarged medial eminence. When the condition is advanced, "crossover" of the great toe can displace the second toe, which can lead to second toe pain and deformity. This can be associated with pain under the second metatarsal head (transfer metatarsalgia), as well as first metatarsal joint pain and arthritis. Patients' complaints are often cosmetically based and concern difficulty with shoe wear.

PHYSICAL EXAMINATION

A complete neurovascular and musculoskeletal examination of the entire lower extremity should be performed. Subtle neurologic or vascular findings may greatly alter treatment plans or may uncover underlying disorders. Attention must be paid to foot morphology and the status of the arches. Motion should be checked at the ankle, subtalar, midfoot, and metatarsal joints.

PATHOLOGIC FINDINGS

There are two broad categories of hallux valgus: a noncongruent joint and a congruent joint. These are different entities and have different pathoanatomic features.

Incongruent Joint

There are multiple static and dynamic anatomic components. The following is a list of some of the more important findings.

• The first metatarsal head drifts medially (varus). Thus, there is an increase in the angle between the first and second metatarsal.
• The sesamoid complex is held in place by the transverse metatarsal ligament and thus becomes relatively laterally displaced. As the deformity progresses, the fibular sesamoid is pulled into the first web space.
• With progressive deformity, the axis of pull of the adductor hallucis, the flexor hallucis brevis, extensor hallucis longus, and the abductor hallucis all become lateralized. This dynamically contributes to the lateral displacement of the great toe.
• The medial joint capsule and ligaments become attenuated and lax. The lateral joint capsule and ligaments become contracted.

Congruent Joint

There is a lateral sloped articular surface, with no pathologic articulation, so progression of deformity is less likely.

IMAGING PROCEDURES

• Obtain standing anteroposterior and lateral radiographs.
• Assess for the intermetatarsal angle, hallux valgus angle, hallux interphalangeal angle, distal metatarsal articular angle, and the sesamoid incongruence.
• Evaluate for joint incongruence and arthrosis; this greatly influences the treatment plan.
• Evaluate all lesser toes.

Bunion/Hallux Valgus

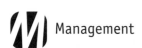 Management

GENERAL MEASURES

- Hallux valgus can be well treated by conservative measures.
- Appropriate shoe wear is necessary. Pointed shoes and high heels must be avoided.
- Lace-up styles have wider forefeet. Soft leather shoes can be stretched to accommodate the bunion. There should be no stitching (which does not stretch) over the medial eminence.
- Prescription shoes, wide with increased depth, should be ordered if necessary.

SURGICAL TREATMENT

The goals of surgery include pain relief with correction of the deformity and biomechanics and maintenance of adequate joint motion.

Indications for Surgery

Indications include failed conservative therapy, with pain and deformity. Decreased function and inability to tolerate footwear are good indicators.

Contraindications to Surgery

- Cosmetic complaints without pain
- Vascular insufficiency
- Degenerative arthritis: contraindication for bunion repair

Relative Contraindications to Surgery

- Spastic muscular conditions
- Severely pronated foot
- Open physis
- Neuropathic joint

Options

Multiple surgical procedures exist. A decision tree for appropriate care is based on multiple factors.

- Age
- The angle between the first and second metatarsal joint (normal, 90 degrees)
- The metatarsophalangeal angle (normal, 90 degrees)
- Joint congruity versus incongruity
- Presence or absence of degenerative joint disease (In the presence of degenerative joint disease, the options are to fuse or to place a prosthesis. Currently, prosthesis technology is associated with high complication and failure rates; it is not recommended.)

Overview of Surgical Procedures

Silver Procedure

This resection of the medial eminence should be used only for elderly patients. The complication rate is low; recurrence rate is high.

Modified McBride Procedure

Soft tissue repair with resection of the medial eminence is often called modified McBride's procedure. It can be used for small deformities. The recurrence rate is high. The procedure is more effective and the indications are expanded when it is performed with a proximal metatarsal osteotomy. Complications include hallux varus.

Distal Chevron Osteotomy

This is usually combined with a medial eminence resection and a capsule plication. The procedure is appropriate for mild deformity in the young patient. It cannot correct for pronation, however, and can be complicated by malunion or nonunion and hallux varus.

Mitchell Procedure

This procedure is a more proximal osteotomy at a right angle to the first metatarsal, lateral displacement of the first metatarsal, and resection of the medial eminence. It is appropriate for moderate deformity. The procedure is associated with shortening of the first metatarsal and can lead to metatarsalgia. It can also be complicated by malunion or nonunion and hallux varus.

Keller Bunionectomy

This procedure involves removal of medial eminence by resection of the proximal portion of the proximal phalanx. It is appropriate only for older patients with limited walking ability. The procedure can be associated with multiple complications, including transfer metatarsalgia and cock-up first toe.

Aiken Procedure

This is an osteotomy of the proximal phalanx. It is performed for deformity in this area.

PHYSICAL THERAPY

No major physical therapy is necessary. Patients must wear a splint for 6 to 12 weeks after surgery.

MONITORING

Patients are followed-up every 2 weeks after surgery to ensure good toe alignment. Shoe wear must be appropriate to prevent recurrence.

RECOMMENDED READING

Myerson MS. Hallux valgus. In: Myerson, MS ed. *Foot and ankle disorders*. Philadelphia: WB Saunders, 2000:225–246.

Basics

DESCRIPTION

• Burners and stingers are injuries to the brachial plexus that cause transient numbness or tingling in the arm (Fig. 1). They affect the neck and shoulder in the area corresponding to the level of the brachial plexus.
• These injuries are common in tackling sports and are usually suffered by teenagers and young adults.
• Males are affected more often than females.

CAUSES

• A traction injury may result from a fall onto the shoulder and neck.
• A direct blow to the supraclavicular area may occur in football and other contact sports, as well as in motorcycle accidents (Fig. 2).

RISK FACTORS

• High-contact sports
• Motorcycle accidents
• Associated conditions
• Horner's syndrome
• Suprascapular nerve compression

ICD-9-CM

767.6 Injury to brachial plexus

 Diagnosis

SIGNS AND SYMPTOMS

• The distribution of symptoms depends on the level of the brachial plexus injury.
• There may be transient numbness or tingling.
• Weakness may occur in the upper extremity.

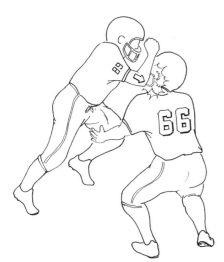

Fig. 1. Burners and stingers are produced by a downward blow to the shoulder or a lateral force to the hand and neck.

DIFFERENTIAL DIAGNOSIS

• Cervical spine injury or stenosis
• Thoracic outlet syndrome
• Long thoracic nerve palsy
• Suprascapular nerve compression

PHYSICAL EXAMINATION

• A complete but brief neurologic examination of all four extremities is indicated. Sensation and movement may be checked by having the patient flex and extend each joint and testing sensation on anterior and posterior surfaces of each limb segment.
• Examination of the cervical spine should be performed.
• Manual muscle testing in the affected upper extremity is done.
• Testing is performed for tenderness in the brachial plexus. Tinel's sign in supraclavicular fossa indicates damage to at least one nerve root.

LABORATORY TESTS

Electromyographic and nerve conduction velocity studies should be obtained if there is no recovery of neurologic function in 2 to 3 weeks. This situation is rare.

IMAGING PROCEDURES

• Plain radiographs of the cervical spine including active flexion and extension views to look for cervical instability and oblique views to visualize the cervical nerve root foramen
• Magnetic resonance imaging of the cervical spine for patients with recurrent stingers
• Scapular anteroposterior and lateral views plus axillary views of the shoulder

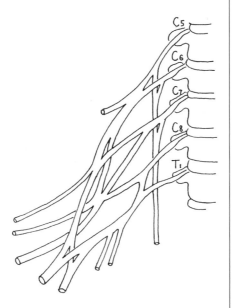

Fig. 2. Burners and stingers are produced by traction in the brachial plexus. The upper roots (C5-6) are the most susceptible.

 Management

GENERAL MEASURES

Patients presenting with persistent neurologic deficits need further imaging. Those with recurrent stingers should be restricted from playing contact sports until further imaging or diagnostic tests can be performed.

• The affected extremity may be placed in a sling for comfort, as needed.
• If symptoms resolve quickly, within a few minutes, the patient may return to competition.
• The patient should be restricted from sports until the symptoms have resolved and any needed workup is complete.
• If stingers are recurrent, a change in sport should be considered.

MEDICAL TREATMENT

Analgesics may be taken, if needed.

SURGICAL TREATMENT

Surgery is not generally indicated.

PATIENT EDUCATION

• Proper tackling technique should be taught.
• The motion and position that produce brachial plexus stretch should be explained.
• Patients should avoid impact on the top of the shoulder or the side of the neck.

COMPLICATIONS

• Incomplete recovery
• Muscle weakness or wasting
• Pain

PROGNOSIS

• True stingers and burners are transient injuries. If symptoms or nerve deficits persist, further workup is needed.
• The prognosis is generally poor for patients with supraclavicular injuries and patients with complete neurologic deficits.
• The prognosis is more favorable for patients with infraclavicular injuries or incomplete neurologic deficits.

RECOMMENDED READING

Rowe CR. *The shoulder.* New York: Churchill Livingstone, 1988:419.

Calcaneus Fracture

 Basics

DESCRIPTION

Calcaneus fractures, which affect the calcaneus (heel) and subtalar joint (between the talus and calcaneus), are extremely difficult injuries to address because of the significant weight-bearing role of this bone and the comminuted (excessive fragmentation) nature of this fracture. These fractures almost always result from a fall from a height and can commonly be associated with a fracture of the lower spine. The difficulty in treating these fractures has been appreciated historically, with poor results commonly cited. Foot and ankle orthopaedists and experienced general orthopaedists are currently operating on these fractures with better results than when these injuries were treated conservatively.

INCIDENCE

Uncommon

CAUSE

Fall from a height

RISK FACTORS

- Osteoporosis
- Jumping activities

CLASSIFICATION

- Two part: two fragments with an oblique fracture line that is anterior to the posterior facet (the key structure that forms most of the surface that articulates with the talus, forming the subtalar joint)
- Three part: the previous fracture line with an additional fracture line through the posterior facet
- Complex fracture: four or more pieces
- Tongue-type: the fragment with the posterior tuberosity (the structure the Achilles tendon inserts into) including the posterior facet

ASSOCIATED CONDITIONS

- Spinal fractures
- Ankle fractures

ICD-9-CM

825.20 Calcaneus fracture

 Diagnosis

SIGNS AND SYMPTOMS

- Extreme hind foot pain and tenderness
- Gross heel widening
- Soft tissue ecchymosis

DIFFERENTIAL DIAGNOSIS

- Subtalar dislocation
- Talar fracture
- Ankle fracture
- Severe ankle sprain

PHYSICAL EXAMINATION

Check for the following:

- Heel ecchymosis
- Extreme heel tenderness
- Ankle tenderness
- Heel widening
- Soft tissue swelling about the heel
- Possible spinous process tenderness in lower spine (if an associated lower spinal fracture is present)

PATHOLOGIC FINDINGS

Fracture patterns depend on the following:

- Force of impact
- Orientation of the heel
- Geometry of the calcaneus

IMAGING PROCEDURES

The x-ray examination includes anteroposterior, lateral, and mortise views of the ankle, as well as a calcaneal axial view (Harris' view). Specialists require a computed tomography scan to decide whether surgery is required. If surgery is needed (displaced fracture), the scan will help to guide the operative reconstruction. When obtaining the computed tomography scan, it is best to specify the need for true axial and true coronal thin slices, to avoid the poor images that reconstructed pictures can create.

Management

GENERAL MEASURES

- Open calcaneal fractures are operative emergencies, as all open fractures are.
- Displaced fractures with heel widening require surgical reconstruction.

SURGICAL TREATMENT

Reconstruction of the calcaneus is performed through a lateral "L" incision. The bone is exposed subcutaneously, and a pin is usually screwed into the posterior fragment to improve the surgeon's ability to reduce the fracture. A plate with multiple holes is placed laterally after the fracture has been reduced, and fixation is provided by placing screws into a stable fragment, commonly the sustentaculum tali. The incision is closed primarily, and the foot is placed into a bulky cotton dressing with a posterior splint postoperatively.

Physical Therapy

Gait training is indicated for non-weight bearing on the affected side until it is healed.

MEDICAL TREATMENT

Closed calcaneal fractures require a bulky Jones dressing (consisting of three layers of Webril (soft cast dressing) around the foot, ankle, and lower leg, bulky cotton, a posterior plaster slab to keep the ankle in 90 degrees, and an overlying elastic [Ace] wrap), ice, and strict, constant elevation of the affected extremity. Nondisplaced fractures can be treated with cast immobilization and non-weight bearing. Analgesics are the drugs of choice. Activity is non-weight bearing until the fracture has healed (a minimum of 6 weeks).

PATIENT EDUCATION

Intraarticular fractures can lead to subtalar arthritis and the late onset of pain.

MONITORING

Serial radiographs are obtained to monitor healing every 6 weeks.

COMPLICATIONS

- Subtalar arthritis
- Heel widening preventing normal shoe wear
- Loss of soft tissue viability
- Inadvertent sural nerve resection (complication of surgery)

PROGNOSIS

Nondisplaced, extraarticular fractures have an excellent prognosis. Patients with displaced intra articular may develop post-traumatic arthritis.

RECOMMENDED READING

Steinberg GG, Akins CM, Baran DT. *Orthopaedics in primary care,* 3rd ed. Philadelphia: Lippincott Williams & Wilkins, 1999:287–288.

Basics

DESCRIPTION

Calcaneovalgus foot is a congenital condition of the foot thought to be due to intrauterine positioning. The hind foot is held in valgus and the foot is markedly dorsiflexed, with the dorsum of the foot approximating the anterior tibia. The condition occurs in neonates; there is no sex predominance.

INCIDENCE

- Most common congenital foot disorder
- Present to varying degrees in 10% of all births

CAUSES

This condition is thought to be due to intrauterine positioning, with the foot placed in extreme dorsiflexion, therefore stretching the Achilles tendon.

ASSOCIATED CONDITIONS

In some cases, this may predispose the patient to the development of pes planus (flatfeet).

ICD-9-CM

754.69 Calcaneovalgus foot

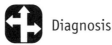 Diagnosis

SIGNS AND SYMPTOMS

- This condition has no symptoms.
- The disorder is present at birth.
- The foot is markedly dorsiflexed, with the dorsum of the foot approximating the anterior tibia.
- The hind foot is held in valgus; occasionally, a contracture of the anterior muscles (dorsiflexors) is present.
- The deformity is usually supple, with the foot easily passively plantar flexed.

DIFFERENTIAL DIAGNOSIS

The appearance of the foot can simulate convex pes valgus (congenital vertical talus). The more serious condition (vertical talus) actually has the more benign appearance, because the forefoot is in a nearly neutral position in a foot with a vertical talus. To differentiate the two conditions, note the position of the calcaneus. In congenital convex pes valgus, the calcaneus is fixed in plantar flexion with contracture of the Achilles tendon and dislocation of the navicular on the dorsal neck of the talus (i.e., the heel points upward). In calcaneovalgus, the calcaneus is dorsiflexed and is somewhat in valgus (i.e., the heel points downward). Another condition to differentiate is the posteromedial bow of the tibia. In this condition, the foot is in the same position (dorsiflexed and everted), but the cause is a bow in the tibia rather than in the joint. Finally, an L-5 paresis as in spina bifida can produce a fixed dorsiflexed foot because of muscle imbalance.

PHYSICAL EXAMINATION

- The appearance of the foot is generally diagnostic.
- The foot is easily plantar flexed and supinated; however, it may not be passively correctable right away.
- Note the orientation of the calcaneus to rule out convex pes planus.

PATHOLOGIC FINDINGS

- The deformity is thought to be due to intrauterine positioning.
- The Achilles tendon is temporarily stretched, but it recovers spontaneously after birth.
- No tarsal abnormalities are present.

IMAGING PROCEDURES

Perform routine anteroposterior and lateral radiographs of the foot and ankle to rule out bony abnormalities if the physical examination alone is not diagnostic.

Management

GENERAL MEASURES

- Reassure the patient's parents that the condition self-corrects with time.
- The parents should perform gentle stretching maneuvers several times per day, to sustain the patient's foot in a corrected position.

SURGICAL TREATMENT

Surgery is never needed for this condition.

MEDICAL TREATMENT

- Treatment often requires repeated counseling to convince the parents that this is not a fixed deformity.
- Parents are encouraged to plantar flex and supinate the patient's feet passively; however, the deformity corrects on its own.
- In the occasional patient, serial casting can be used to speed correction.
- No activity restrictions are indicated.

PATIENT EDUCATION

Inform the family about the benign natural history of the condition and the tendency for the foot to correct on its own.

MONITORING

Newborns with severe deformity or possible congenital covex pes valgus should be referred to an orthopaedist for monitoring.

COMPLICATIONS

On rare occasions, subluxation of the peroneal tendons may occur with this condition. This resolves with serial cast treatment.

PROGNOSIS

- Prognosis is excellent for normal shape, strength, and function.
- This is a benign condition that corrects over time.
- There is no definite evidence that the foot is prone to be flat in later life.

RECOMMENDED READING

Sullivan JA. The child's foot. In: Morrissy RT, Weinstein SL, eds. *Lovell and Winter's pediatric orthopaedics*. Philadelphia: Lippincott–Raven, 1996:1083–1085.

Callus on the Toes and Feet

 Basics

DESCRIPTION

Calluses on the toes and feet are signs of increased pressure on the soft tissues over a bony prominence and can help the clinician to identify an underlying biomechanical abnormality. The skin of the foot responds to an area subjected to elevated pressure with a hyperkeratotic lesion. Calluses on the toes are called "corns." Calluses are not harmful in themselves. They affect the dermis of the foot, the peripheral nervous system, the bones, and the ligaments of the foot.

SYNONYMS

Hyperkeratotic lesions

GENETICS

Several systemic diseases may be underlying causes of calluses (e.g., rheumatoid arthritis).

INCIDENCE

Corns and calluses are the most common foot complaints seen by physicians and podiatrists.

AGE

• Calluses may develop at any age.
• They are more likely to develop with minimal degrees of foot or toe deformity at older ages.
• Skin is more tolerant to pressure at younger ages, without developing corns.
• A young person with a callus is more likely to have a significant underlying muscle imbalance or deformity.

CAUSES

Corns and calluses usually arise on a mallet toe, hammer toe, or clawtoe deformity, which may be a result of neurologic dysfunction such as Charcot-Marie-Tooth disease, a previous compartment syndrome, or a systemic disease such as rheumatoid arthritis. Phalangeal bony prominences are a frequent cause of corns.

RISK FACTORS

• Neuromuscular disorders
• Impaired sensation
• Foot or toe deformities

CLASSIFICATION

• Callus: A large lesion with vague boundaries and no central core
• Corn: A smaller, focal lesion with a well demarcated boundary and central core; usually on toes

ICD-9-CM

700.0 Callus on the toes and feet

 Diagnosis

SIGNS AND SYMPTOMS

Calluses are hyperkeratotic lesions that commonly occur between toes and on the plantar surface of the foot. They have no visible blood vessels and no cores. Calluses are usually not painful until they become large and extensive. Corns are often painful.

DIFFERENTIAL DIAGNOSIS

• Rule out plantar wart. Warts have fine capillaries that diagnostically rise perpendicularly to the surface and exhibit punctate bleeding when they are trimmed.
• Keratosis is thickening of the skin that is not caused by friction and may be inherited.

PHYSICAL EXAMINATION

Hyperkeratotic lesions may or may not be tender. A thorough examination of the foot should be performed to reveal an underlying cause. The involved toe or region should be examined for active and passive range of motion.

PATHOLOGIC FINDINGS

The pattern of the dermis in hyperkeratotic lesions may be analyzed in the dermatopathology laboratory to distinguish corns from warts or other lesions, but this is rarely necessary.

IMAGING PROCEDURES

If foot deformity is seen, standing anteroposterior anterior and lateral radiographs should be taken.

Management

GENERAL MEASURES

Conservative care includes trimming of the lesion with a scalpel or a pumice stone and relief of the affected skin with a pressure-relieving orthotic device such as a toe cap, a metatarsal bar, or a splint. Pressure may also be relieved from toe deformities with a special, custom-made shoe with a large toe box.

SURGICAL TREATMENT

If conservative care fails, treatment of an underlying disorder may be required, such as tendon transfer for a flexible toe deformity, surgical correction of a hallux valgus deformity, or bony prominence resection, such as a metatarsal plantar condyle resection.

PHYSICAL THERAPY

This is usually not required.

PATIENT EDUCATION

Patients should be educated about the causes of corns and calluses and counseled to wear shoes that are neither too tight nor too hard.

MONITORING

Patients who have deficient sensation should return periodically for observation, because they are less able to detect problems.

COMPLICATIONS

Increased pressure on a corn or callus may cause it to break down. This can result in an ulcer, and it is especially common in patients with neuromuscular disorders.

PROGNOSIS

Corns and calluses have a tendency to recur unless underlying causes are removed.

RECOMMENDED READING

Mizel M, ed. *Orthopaedic knowledge update 2*. Rosemont, IL: American Academy of Orthopaedic Surgeons, 1998:170–171.

Mann RA, Couglin MJ, eds. *Surgery of the foot and ankle*, 6th ed. St Louis: CV Mosby, 1993:850–851.

Basics

DESCRIPTION

Camptodactyly is a nontraumatic flexion deformity of the proximal interphalangeal (PIP) joint. It usually involves the little finger alone, but sometimes it affects adjoining fingers as well. It may or may not be associated with a syndrome. Most patients develop the deformity in the first year of life. Some have a "delayed" or "late" form, with onset after age 10 years. The early-onset form affects males and females equally. The delayed form affects mostly females. The best results of treatment occur in children and adolescents. Results in adults are poor.

GENETICS

Many cases are sporadic; others have simple autosomal dominance.

INCIDENCE

Less than 1% of the population is affected.

CAUSES

Camptodactyly is caused by an imbalance between the flexor and extensor mechanisms of the PIP joint. Anatomic anomalies are frequent and include abnormal insertions of the lumbricalis, flexor digitorum superficialis, and retinacular ligaments.

RISK FACTOR

Family history

CLASSIFICATION

Two types of camptodactyly are recognized: one that appears in infancy and affects males and females equally and one, less common, that appears during adolescence and affects mostly females. These have been termed congenital and adolescent, but some clinicians believe the terms early and delayed (or late) should be used, because these manifestations likely represent variations of the same condition.

ASSOCIATED CONDITIONS

- Trisomy 13
- Oculodentodigital syndrome
- Orofaciodigital syndrome
- Aarskog's syndrome
- Cerebrohepatorenal syndrome

ICD-9-CM

755.59 Camptodactyly

 Diagnosis

SIGNS AND SYMPTOMS

- This is a flexion deformity of the PIP joint of the little finger.
- Digital angulation in the anteroposterior plane is not to be confused with clinodactyly, which describes angulation in the radioulnar plane.
- Occasionally, flexion deformity of the PIP joint of adjoining fingers also occurs.
- About two-thirds of patients show bilateral involvement, with the degree of contracture not necessarily symmetric.
- Usually the right hand is involved, when only one hand is affected.
- In children, the deformity usually disappears when the wrist is flexed.
- The metacarpophalangeal joint is usually held in slight hyperextension.
- In severe contractures, with rotatory deformity in the digit, the patient may complain that the finger interferes with tapping or with gripping activities.
- Pain and swelling are usually absent, even with severe flexion contracture.

DIFFERENTIAL DIAGNOSIS

- Clinodactyly, which describes digital angulation in the radioulnar plane
- Trauma residual
- Dupuytren's contracture
- Arthrogryposis
- Absence of an extensor tendon
- Marfan syndrome
- Beal syndrome (contractural arachnodactyly)

Differentiation is based on a thorough history and physical examination.

Camptodactyly

PHYSICAL EXAMINATION

The range of active and passive flexion and extension of the PIP and metacarpophalangeal joints should be quantified, with the wrist in both flexion and extension.

PATHOLOGIC FINDINGS

All structures that could possibly cause flexion deformity at the PIP joint have been considered possible deforming factors. Findings may include the following:

• Absence, atrophy, or abnormal insertion of the lumbricalis muscle into the lumbrical canal
• A band of fibrous tissue arising from the A1 pulley and inserting into the flexor superficialis tendon
• Origination of the flexor superficialis from the palmar fascia in the midaspect of the palm
• Anomalous tendons
• Short flexor digitorum profundus
• Contracture of the collateral ligaments or the volar plate

IMAGING PROCEDURES

Plain films of the digit should be obtained. Radiographic changes that occur with time and growth include broadening of the base of the middle phalanx, indentation of the neck of the proximal phalanx, a narrowed joint space, and dorsal flattening of the condyle of the proximal phalanx with flattening of the palmar surface. These findings bode poorly for chances of correcting the clinodactyly.

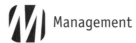 Management

GENERAL MEASURES

No single successful treatment exists, because there is no single cause for the condition. Treatment is designed to restore normal flexor-extensor balance. In the infantile form, normal balance may be best achieved by progressive extension splinting. In the adolescent form, surgery is often indicated if splinting fails and the deformity is severe or progressive. Best results are obtained with surgical treatment in young patients, but the outcome is not completely predictable. Owing to poor results, corrective operations in adults are no longer recommended. For most activities, dysfunction remains so slight that many surgeons discourage surgery, because the results of operative treatment are unpredictable. Splinting or serial plaster casting should be tried before surgery. However, patients with marked contracture may need corrective treatment. The decision should be left up to the patient.
Generally, no limitations are placed on activity. In severe cases, the deformity may pose a problem in sports or occupations requiring fine work with the hands.

SURGICAL TREATMENT

Surgery is designed to correct the aberrant anatomy through release or transfer of abnormal origins or insertions. Unfortunately, the results of these procedures are often disappointing. If radiographs reveal bone and joint changes, corrective extension osteotomy is indicated, rather than procedures designed to increase motion through the joint itself.

PHYSICAL THERAPY

Occupational therapy may help those with infantile or adolescent camptodactyly. The occupational therapist may supervise stretching and splinting.

MEDICAL TREATMENT

• Splinting
• Serial casting

PATIENT EDUCATION

• Skin monitoring around splints is important.
• Stretching should be continued after the splinting or casting program to maintain the gain achieved.

PREVENTION

No effective means of prevention exists.

MONITORING

The deformity may progress with growth spurts. Successful treatment is greatest at younger ages; therefore, it is best to treat early and to monitor the patient's progress.

COMPLICATIONS

Surgery in adults may produce increased joint stiffness and pain.

PROGNOSIS

• Left untreated, the condition will worsen progressively in 80% of cases.
• The deformity often worsens during growth spurts.
• The condition usually does not progress after the age of 18 to 20 years.

RECOMMENDED READING

Kasser JR, ed. *Orthopaedic knowledge update 5.* Rosemont, IL: American Academy of Orthopaedic Surgeons, 1996:298–299.

Milford L. The hand. In: Crenshaw AH, ed. *Campbell's operative orthopaedics,* 7th ed. St. Louis: CV Mosby, 1988:432.

Wood VE. Camptodactyly. In: David P. Green, M.D., ed. New York, Churchill Livingstone, Inc., ed. *Operative hand surgery*. 4th ed: 1998:411–417.

Basics

DESCRIPTION

Carpal tunnel syndrome (CTS) is a neuropathy caused by compression of the median nerve within the carpal tunnel. The floor of the tunnel is formed by the volar radiocarpal and intercarpal ligaments. The transverse carpal ligament forms the roof of the tunnel. Nine long flexors of the wrist and fingers and one nerve (median) run within this spatially limited and relatively rigid tunnel. Thus, any increase in pressure within the tunnel compresses the injury-prone median nerve.

There is a decrease in thenar muscle strength, as well as a numbness or a decrease in sensibility of the palmar surface of the radial three and one-half digits, especially the middle and index fingers.

GENETICS

No genetic predisposing factor to CTS has been described.

INCIDENCE

The prevalence of CTS has been reported to vary between 0.6% and 61% in different occupational groups.

Fifty percent of cases are reported to occur in patients between the ages of 40 and 60 years. CTS occurs predominantly in women (2:1), although the number of men with CTS may be underestimated.

CAUSES

Any factor that increases the pressure within the tunnel compresses the median nerve and leads to CTS. The most common causes include flexor tenosynovitis, trauma to the carpal bones, ganglion, fibroma, or lipoma within the tunnel, rheumatoid cyst, gout, and diabetic neuropathy (Fig. 1).

RISK FACTORS

- Repetitive hand work
- Endocrine imbalance
- History of neuropathy
- Associated conditions
- Rheumatoid arthritis
- Pregnancy
- Thyroid myxedema
- Acromegaly
- Amyloidosis
- Multiple myeloma
- Diabetes
- Trauma
- Alcoholism
- Gout
- Space-occupying lesions within carpal tunnel

ICD-9-CM

354.0 Carpal tunnel syndrome

 Diagnosis

GENERAL MEASURES

CTS can be accurately diagnosed by careful history and physical examination, inspection for thenar atrophy, and detection of sensory disturbance using light touch or a pinwheel. Provocative tests, such as Phalen's, which consists of placing the affected wrist in hyperflexion in an attempt to reproduce the numbness in the hand, or tapping over the course of the nerve in the tunnel to elicit Tinel's sign, also serve to confirm the diagnosis.

SIGNS AND SYMPTOMS

These symptoms can be aggravated with use of the affected hand:

- Paresthesia in the median nerve distribution in the hand
- Weakness or clumsiness in the hand
- Pain in the hand, wrist, or distal forearm
- Awakening from sleep with pain or numbness in the hand

- Tinel's sign: tapping the median nerve over the carpal tunnel with resultant paresthesias in the radial three and one-half fingers
- Phalen's sign: paresthesias in the median nerve distribution with full flexion for at least 1 minute

DIFFERENTIAL DIAGNOSIS

- Thoracic outlet syndrome
- Compression of the lower cervical roots by cervical degenerative disc disease or tumors

PHYSICAL EXAMINATION

The hand should be examined to detect thenar muscle atrophy. Two-point discrimination should be checked at the tips of the fingers on both the radial and ulnar borders (should be less than 5 to 6 mm). Provocative tests such as Phalen's and Tinel's tests should be performed (Figs. 2 and 3).

LABORATORY TESTS

The following basic tests should be ordered to rule out systemic causes of CTS:

- Sedimentation rate
- Serum glucose concentration
- Serum uric acid level
- Thyroid function test

PATHOLOGIC FINDINGS

- Internal fibrosis of the median nerve
- Epineural scarring and constriction
- Reduced nerve conduction velocity

IMAGING PROCEDURES

Plain radiographs of the wrist in patients with previous trauma or in patients with a long history of inflammatory disease should be performed. Cervical spine radiographs can also reveal a cervical rib, if thoracic outlet syndrome is suspected.

Electromyographic studies can help one to rule out proximal injury to the median nerve or to identify peripheral neuropathy.

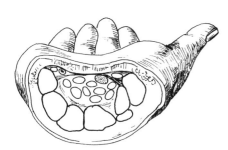

Fig. 1. The median nerve is shown in the carpal tunnel with the finger flexor tendons, under the transverse carpal ligament.

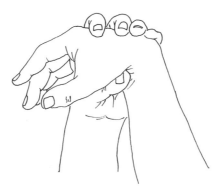

Fig. 2. Phalen's test for median nerve compression in the carpal tunnel is performed by holding the wrist flexed 90 degrees for 30 seconds and checking for paresthesias in the fingers.

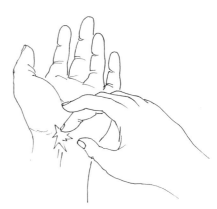

Fig. 3. Tinel's sign indicates an irritated median nerve. It refers to radiating pain down the fingers after percussion of the carpal tunnel.

Carpal Tunnel Syndrome

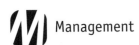 Management

GENERAL MEASURES

Use of hand and flexion and extension exercises of fingers are encouraged after surgery. If conservative therapy is employed, the wrist splint should be worn while the patient works and sleeps.

SURGICAL TREATMENT

Open carpal tunnel release is made through a longitudinal incision that begins on the distal border of the transverse carpal tunnel ligament and extends proximally to the proximal wrist crease, in line with the ulnar border of the axis of the ring finger. The incision is then carried through the palmar fascia to the transverse carpal ligament. The ligament is then carefully divided, using a combination of the scalpel and scissors. Care should be taken to avoid the palmar cutaneous branch or the motor branch of the median nerve. After division of the ligament, the carpal tunnel and the median nerve should be inspected for any space-occupying lesion or any signs of chronic inflammation requiring neurolysis. The skin is then reapproximated using nylon sutures.
The role of endoscopic carpal tunnel release is controversial, but it is expanding and speeds the patient's return to work.

PHYSICAL THERAPY

Occupational or physical therapy should be consulted for activity modification teaching or for various modes of therapy aimed at minimizing the development of painful postoperative scars.

MEDICAL TREATMENT

Conservative therapies consist of cock-up wrist splinting, nonsteroidal antiinflammatory drugs (not proven effective), diuretics, and cortisone injections, which must be performed by an experienced physician to avoid direct injury to the median nerve. Activity modification in work-related CTS is recommended. Surgical release of the transverse carpal ligament is done in patients with failed conservative therapy or in those with constant numbness, motor weakness, or increased distal median nerve latency noted on electromyography.

MEDICATIONS

No effective medication has been described to treat CTS specifically. Corticosteroid injection into the carpal tunnel is indicated when the median nerve compression is predicted to be temporary, as in pregnancy or when the patient's activity can be modified. Injections must be done with great care to avoid injury to the median nerve.

PATIENT EDUCATION

Activity modification teaching is important to prevent recurrence.

PREVENTION

The patient should avoid prolonged and repetitive motions of the wrist.

MONITORING

To obtain maximal beneficial results, the splint should be worn full time for at least 3 to 4 months. After this, the patient can gradually discontinue the use of the splint. If symptoms return with removal of the splint, the patient will become a surgical candidate. The patient usually experiences immediate pain relief after carpal tunnel release, whereas numbness gradually improves over the next several weeks.

COMPLICATIONS

Iatrogenic injuries to the median nerve or its branches may occur with open or endoscopic release. Painful surgical scars may ruin the results of a successful decompression procedure. Flexion tendon bowstringing may occur in a few patients.

PROGNOSIS

Most patients with CTS associated with repetitive trauma commonly seen in the workplace respond to a combination of splinting, cortisone injection into the carpal tunnel, and activity modification. If job modification is not in the patient's conservative treatment program, splinting and cortisone injections may provide only temporary relief. The maximum return of strength after carpal tunnel release can take 6 months or longer.

RECOMMENDED READING

Hanel DP. Wrist and hand: reconstruction. In: Kasser JR, ed. *Orthopaedic knowledge update 5.* Rosemont, IL: American Academy of Orthopaedic Surgeons, 1996:329–347.

Lister G. Compression. In: Saunders *The hand, diagnosis and indications,* 3rd ed. Singapore: Churchill Livingstone, 1993:285–291.

Basics

DESCRIPTION

Cavus feet have an elevation of the longitudinal arch, often with associated deformity of the hind foot or forefoot (Fig. 1).

SYNONYM

High-arched foot

GENETICS

• Many of the disorders causing cavus feet are genetic.
• Isolated cavus feet are only occasionally familial.

INCIDENCE

The condition is common.

CAUSES

• Muscle imbalance, such as peroneus longus and posterior tibialis overpull, can cause the condition.
• Weakness of the intrinsic muscle of the foot, with overpull of the long flexors, is a contributing factor.
• Connective tissue disorders, such as Marfan's syndrome and Beal's syndrome, may also cause cavus foot.

RISK FACTORS

• Neuromuscular disorders
• Trauma
• Connective tissue disorders

CLASSIFICATION

The distinction is between flexible and rigid conditions.

• Cavus: high but unbalanced arch
• Calcaneocavus: heel as main weight-bearing surface
• Cavovarus: high arch, turned inward
• Equinocavovarus: above, with equinus contracture

ASSOCIATED CONDITIONS

• Compartment syndrome of leg or foot

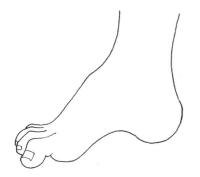

Fig. 1. A relatively high arch characterizes a cavus foot. This may be flexible or rigid.

• Charcot-Marie-Tooth disease
• Friedreich's ataxia
• Spina bifida
• Spinal cord tumor
• Diabetic neuropathy
• Poliomyelitis
• Partially treated clubfoot
• Marfan's syndrome
• Beal's syndrome
• Idiopathic clubfoot

ICD-9-CM

736.70 Cavus
736.75 Cavovarus foot

Diagnosis

SIGNS AND SYMPTOMS

Signs

• High arch
• Calluses on forefoot or hind foot
• May have weak push-off

Symptoms

• May be asymptomatic
• May have pain under forefoot
• Difficulty in fitting or tolerating shoes

DIFFERENTIAL DIAGNOSIS

Muscle atrophy may cause the arch to appear higher.

PHYSICAL EXAMINATION

• Check for flexibility of the foot in weight-bearing versus non–weight-bearing states.
• Check inversion and eversion.
• Measure the strength of all muscles crossing the ankle on both legs.
• Check reflexes and sensation.
• Observe the spine for dimples, markings, and scoliosis.
• Check the upper extremities.
• Perform Coleman's block test for cavovarus to determine whether the hind foot varus is flexible or rigid. In a flexible cavovarus, a lift placed under the lateral forefoot causes the hind foot varus to correct.

LABORATORY TESTS

Electromyography and nerve conduction tests are helpful in diagnosing Charcot-Marie-Tooth disease and hereditary motor and sensory neuropathies.

PATHOLOGIC FINDINGS

In almost all causes of cavus, dissection of the foot reveals some degree of atrophy or fibrosis of the foot, as well as decreased range of motion.

IMAGING PROCEDURES

As part of the workup of an undiagnosed cavus, x-ray studies and magnetic resonance imaging of the spine may be indicated. To assess the foot, standing anteroposterior and lateral radiographs may be obtained. *Calcaneal pitch* is the angle between the calcaneus and the floor. *Meary's angle* is the angle between the talus and the first metatarsal.

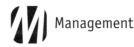

Management

GENERAL MEASURES

• No treatment is indicated if the patient is asymptomatic and the skin is in good condition.
• A padded sole, soft "upper," arch support, or metatarsal bar may help with calluses.
• A brace may help gait in the weakened cavus foot.
• Stretching may help prevent worsening and maintain flexibility.

SURGICAL TREATMENT

• Plantar fasciotomy may improve the flexible cavus foot.
• Osteotomies of the midfoot are needed for the rigid cavus foot.
• If there is rigid hind foot valgus, an osteotomy may be needed for the calcaneus.
• Tendon lengthening procedures or transfers are needed to treat muscle imbalance. A transfer of the long toe extensors to the metatarsal necks is most often performed, along with interphalangeal joint fusion.
• Triple arthrodesis is used mainly as a last resort, especially in patients with painful degenerative joint disease.

PHYSICAL THERAPY

Stretching of the tight plantar fascia, and of other tight muscles, may slow progression of the condition.

PATIENT EDUCATION

• Check skin for calluses or pressure sores.
• Wear shoes that are not too tight.

MONITORING

Patients should be followed once or twice per year to rule out worsening of the cavus. This may be done by an orthopaedist, neurologist, or generalist, depending on the underlying condition.

COMPLICATIONS

• Pain
• Pressure sores
• Toe deformities

PROGNOSIS

Most, but not all, patients with cavus have some degree of foot pain. Treatment should therefore be individualized.

RECOMMENDED READING

Mann RA. Pes cavus. In: Mann RA, Coughlin MJ, eds. *Surgery of the foot and ankle*, 6th ed. St Louis: CV Mosby, 1993:785–801.

Cerebral Palsy

Basics

DESCRIPTION

Cerebral palsy is a static neuropathy developing in the first 3 years of life. The cause may vary, and only the result is typically seen, through its effect on the trunk and extremities. Although the neurologic injury does not change, the function may change as the person grows older. This disorder affects 1% to 2% of all children.

CAUSES

- Prenatal brain dysplasia
- Maternal infection
- Fetal hypoxia
- Vascular event
- Encephalitis
- Trauma
- Kernicterus

RISK FACTORS

- Birth injury
- Difficult delivery
- Prematurity

CLASSIFICATION

Classification is by both anatomic and physiologic types. Anatomically, the types are hemiplegic (ipsilateral arm and leg), diplegic (both legs), and totally involved. Physiologically, the types are spastic, athetoid, mixed, and dystonic.

ASSOCIATED CONDITIONS

Associated defects in some patients may include visual or hearing impairment, seizures, and learning disability.

ICD-9-CM

343.9 Infantile cerebral palsy, unspecified

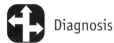

Diagnosis

SIGNS AND SYMPTOMS

Hypotonia followed by spasticity is the most common pattern. Milestones may be delayed and gait is abnormal when and if this condition develops. Deep tendon reflexes are increased after the first year of life, and clonus may develop in certain muscles. Contractures develop, especially in the Achilles tendon, hamstrings, and adductors. Typical findings in the diplegic type are normal intelligence with equinus or equinovalgus feet. Typical findings in the hemiplegic type are normal intelligence with equinovarus feet and upper extremity flexion. Typical findings in the totally involved form are scoliosis, hip dysplasia, and contractures, usually with some cognitive deficit. In the athetoid form, contracture does not develop, and irregular movements occur in the extremities. Intellect may be preserved or mildly impaired.

DIFFERENTIAL DIAGNOSIS

- Brain or upper spinal cord tumor
- Instability of the upper cervical spine
- Neurodegenerative disorder
- Familial spastic paraparesis
- Early stage of myopathy or neuropathy
- Rett's syndrome

PHYSICAL EXAMINATION

The upper extremity should be checked for deformity, sensation, and use. The spine should be checked for scoliosis or dysraphism. Limb lengths should be measured. Contractures at all joints should be documented. Muscle excursion should be documented at all levels, including ankle dorsiflexion, popliteal angle, and hip abduction. Gait should be observed several times, if possible, and with as well as without any braces.

PATHOLOGIC FINDINGS

Peripheral neuropathy is normal. Brain disorders depend on the specific cause. Muscles of the affected limb demonstrate some degree of fibrosis. No biopsy is usually indicated in the typical case.

IMAGING PROCEDURES

The cervical spine may be imaged in some patients with severe diplegia. Magnetic resonance imaging is indicated if there is a diagnostic dilemma or in the hands of an experienced developmental pediatrician. A typical finding in a patient with spastic diplegia is periventricular leukomalacia, the end result of ventricular hemorrhages. However, the magnetic resonance imaging scan may be normal in such patients. Typical findings in spastic hemiplegia are focal infarct or cyst.

Routine films of the hip should be obtained for the child with severe diplegia or total involvement. Scoliosis films should be done for patients with the totally involved variant.

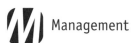

Management

GENERAL MEASURES

Infant stimulation and encouragement of mobility are the most important features. Stretching the at-risk muscles should be done. Intrathecal balcofen may help to decrease peripheral spasticity. Diazepam (Valium) has little benefit except in the perioperative year. Physical therapy is best suited to address specific, short-term goals.

SURGICAL TREATMENT

Foot deformities should almost always be fixed if the patient has even a little ambulatory potential. Lengthening of contracted muscles decreases their spasticity or triggering during gait. This applies especially to the Achilles tendon, hamstrings, and adductors. However, the rectus femoris may also be tight. Hand muscle tightness or dysfunction benefits from surgery much more rarely because of the lack of sensory integration. Hip subluxation should be treated if detected before degenerative changes occur. This includes adductor muscle lengthening, femoral osteotomy, and possibly an iliac osteotomy. Rarely, femoral head removal is indicated.

Scoliosis treatment is indicated if the child has trunk imbalance with difficulty in sitting or back pain. A brace may help the patient to sit more comfortably, but it does not keep the curve from worsening. Surgical correction and fusion are the best choices for those who are having trouble sitting comfortably.

Other surgical treatments for patients with cerebral palsy include rhizotomy and an intrathecal baclofen pump. Dorsal rhizotomy is a procedure to decrease spasticity at a more central level, that of the spinal cord. The dorsal afferent rootlets are checked for their ability to generate a spastic reflex arc, and the most abnormal ones are sectioned. This treatment works for patients with ambulatory diplegia who are less than 10 years old. Intrathecal baclofen also interrupts spasticity at the spinal level by pharmacologic means.

PHYSICAL THERAPY

Physical therapy is useful for gait training, the use of braces, to prevent untracturs, and to aid in activities of daily living.

PATIENT EDUCATION

Patients are encouraged to remain as active as possible and to keep their weight down. They should understand that the condition cannot be totally cured, and they should be aware of any claims that seem impossibly good. They should learn that oral medications offer no significant help for the disease.

MONITORING

Children are seen at least twice a year to check on ambulatory ability and status of activities of daily living.

COMPLICATIONS

Weight gain is a common problem in adulthood and contributes to debility. Fractures are common in this group, especially patients with the totally involved variant. Patients with totally involved cerebral palsy are more likely to have respiratory problems.

PROGNOSIS

The prognosis depends on the extent of cerebral palsy. Patients with totally involved cerebral palsy have a foreshortened life expectancy, but those with other types show no decrease in life expectancy.

RECOMMENDED READING

Renshaw TS. Cerebral palsy. In: Morrisy RT, Weinstein SL, eds. *Pediatric orthopaedics*. Philadelphia: Lippincott–Raven, 1996:469–503.

Basics

DESCRIPTION

Injury to the cervical spine is a diagnostic as well as a therapeutic challenge. Delay in diagnosis and management can lead to significant complications. Early initiation of established treatment protocols can optimize recovery. Neurologic injury is a frequent complication of cervical spine dislocation, but some patients may present to the primary care physician with little more than neck pain. There may be neurologic and vascular sequelae. Although these injuries are most commonly seen in young adults, and more commonly in males, no age is exempt.

Cervical spine instability most frequently has a traumatic cause, but it can be caused by other conditions, as seen in rheumatoid arthritis, Down's syndrome, and bone dysplasias.

In children, a flat board for immobilization of the neck requires a recess for the occipital cranium. Spinal cord injury without radiographic abnormality may be seen in children, and their bony injuries are more likely to heal with immobilization alone.

SYNONYMS

- Neck dislocation
- Jumped facet
- Locked facet
- Rotatory instability

GENETICS

Many skeletal dysplasias have a genetic basis. The atraumatic instabilities can be associated with a genetic predisposition. Down's syndrome is associated with a chromosomal disorder (trisomy 21). Rheumatoid arthritis has a genetic predisposition, which seems to be associated with certain HLA markers. The traumatic cervical dislocations have no genetic predisposition.

INCIDENCE

- Two percent to 5% of patients presenting with blunt trauma have cervical spine injuries.
- Serious diving accidents have a 50% incidence of cervical spine injury.

CAUSES

Traumatic

- Motor vehicle accident
- Diving
- Blunt trauma

Atraumatic

- Rheumatoid arthritis
- Down's syndrome
- Skeletal dysplasias

RISK FACTOR

Young man between 18 and 25 years old

CLASSIFICATION

- Upper cervical injuries
- Occipitocervical dissociation
- Atlantoaxial instability (with hangman's fracture) (Fig. 1)
- Lower cervical injuries
- Facet subluxations
- Facet dislocation (Fig. 2)
- Traumatic spondylolisthesis

ASSOCIATED CONDITIONS

- Neurogenic shock
- Head injury
- Cervical spine fractures
- Chest and abdominal trauma
- Extremity trauma

ICD-9-CM

839.01 C-1 dislocation
839.03 C-3 dislocation
839.05 C-5 dislocation
839.07 C-2 dislocation
839.02 C-2 dislocation
839.04 C-4 dislocation
839.06 C-6 dislocation

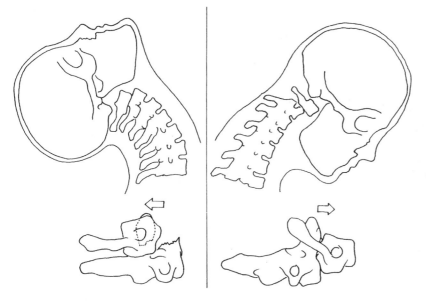

Fig. 1. Atlantoaxial (C-2) dislocations may result from odontoid fracture or transverse ligament disruption.

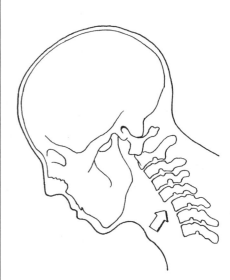

Fig. 2. Facet dislocations are most common in the lower cervical spine.

Cervical Spine Dislocation

 Diagnosis

SIGNS AND SYMPTOMS

• Neck pain after trauma
• Neck deformity is occasionally seen, especially in rotatory subluxations or unilateral facet dislocations.
• Persistent asymmetric posturing or head tilt may be a sign of cervical subluxation or dislocation.
• Neurologic injury may take the form of weakness, numbness, bowel or bladder incontinence, complete quadriplegia, or one of the incomplete spinal cord injury syndromes (Brown-Séquard, central cord, anterior cord, posterior cord).

DIFFERENTIAL DIAGNOSIS

• Pseudosubluxation (a normal, physiologic translation of C-2 only in children, which may be up to 3 mm)
• Cervical spine fractures associated with instability
• Injuries at multiple levels
• Muscular torticollis: contracture or spasm of the sternomastoid muscle

PHYSICAL EXAMINATION

Pain on motion of the head or neck is noted. The head and neck should be examined for tenderness and pain on motion. In the presence of this finding, the head and neck should be carefully immobilized until adequate physical and radiologic examination can be done. Children have a much larger head-to-body ratio; hence neck immobilization in children requires the rest of the body be elevated on blankets to place the neck in an anatomic position. Lacerations, abrasions, or contusions on the scalp, face, neck or shoulders are clues. All voluntary motion of the upper and lower extremities should be observed.

Without moving the patient, one should look for areas of tenderness on the head and back of neck. Any step-off of the spinous processes, or hematoma, may indicate ligament disruption or facet dislocation.

Rapid complete neurologic examination should be performed, including motor, sensory, reflexes, and rectal examination. The following motor and sensory checkpoints are suggested:

Motor

• C-4: diaphragm
• C-5: deltoid and elbow flexors
• C-6: wrist extensors
• C-7: elbow extensors
• C-8: finger flexors (profundus)
• T-1: intrinsics (finger abductors)
• L-2: hip flexors
• L-3: knee extensors
• L-4: ankle dorsiflexors
• L-5: long toe extensors
• S-1: ankle plantar flexors
• S4-5: voluntary anal contraction

Sensory

• C-2: occiput
• C-4: tip of shoulder
• C-5: regimental patch (lateral shoulder)
• C-6: thumb
• C-7: long finger
• C-8: little finger
• T-1: medial epicondyle
• T-4: nipples
• T-10: umbilicus
• L-1: groin
• L-3: patella
• L-4: medial malleolus
• L-5: great toe
• S-1: lateral heel
• S-2: popliteal fossa
• S-3: ischial tuberosity
• S4-5: perianal

LABORATORY TESTS

Estimated vital capacity of at least 20% of predicted is necessary. If it is less than 20% or 1,000 mL, a tracheostomy may be required.

PATHOLOGIC FINDINGS

Cervical spine subluxation involves disruption of facet joint capsule. Dislocation also involves disruption of disc and anteroposterior longitudinal ligaments.

Pathologic examination of spinal cord injury shows edema, hemorrhage, and spinal cord distortion.

IMAGING PROCEDURES

Standard Radiography

These must visualize the occiput to the upper end plate of T-1. One should look for alignment, fractures, prevertebral soft tissue, widening of posterior interspinous distance, vertebral end plate, or facet joint incongruity.

Dynamic Radiography

Flexion-extension views should be ordered only if neurologic examination and plain radiographs are normal and patient has persistent pain and must be supervised by a physician. If the atlas-dens interval is greater than 7 mm, this is a sign of instability and endangers the spinal cord.

Computed Tomography

Indications are evidence or suspicion of cervical injury on plain radiographs if such an injury cannot be diagnosed with certainty from these films. Computed tomography with reconstruction may be used for imaging complex injuries if needed by the orthopaedist or neurosurgeon. The sagittal reconstruction is typically the most useful.

Magnetic Resonance Imaging

Traumatic effects such as hemorrhage, swelling, or edema can also be identified. Indications are incomplete neurologic deficits, worsening neurologic deficits, deficit above the level of skeletal injury, facet dislocations (before attempted reduction) to rule out disc herniation, and epidural hematoma.

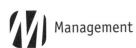 Management

GENERAL MEASURES

Resuscitation and Emergency Measures

• Airway, breathing, and circulation are first priorities.
• Strict immobilization is necessary during extraction and transportation (and intubation if necessary).

Emergency Room Assessment

• A complete examination is performed, including a full neurologic examination as described earlier.
• A full radiographic evaluation is performed.

EMERGENCY TREATMENT

• Traction is indicated for reduction of dislocations (magnetic resonance imaging is necessary for facet dislocations).
• Methylprednisolone started within 8 hours of spinal cord injury helps to preserve neuronal structures; the dose is a 30 mg/kg bolus intravenously followed by 5.4 mg/kg per hour for 23 hours.
• Surgery is performed in patients with irreducible dislocations with neurologic deficit and neurologic deterioration.

DEFINITIVE TREATMENT

• For stable injuries, immobilization may be necessary for a short period.
• The treatment of unstable injuries may vary from immobilization to surgical stabilization.
• Patients with neurologic injuries require long-term rehabilitation, including education, bladder and bowel program, family education, physical and occupational therapy, and psychologic counseling. Once the dislocation is stabilized, activity can be begun and is gradually advanced.

SURGICAL TREATMENT

Occipitocervical Dissociation

This involves an occiput to C-2 posterior fusion with instrumentation.

Atlantoaxial Instability

Procedures include bracing in children and in those with less than 7 mm translation in flexion and fusion in patients with greater than 7 mm translation persisting.

Hangman's Fracture-Dislocation or Traumatic Spondylolisthesis

This injury can be treated with reduction and a Minerva cast in children. Halo immobilization or posterior open reduction and stabilization may be necessary, depending on the type of fracture.

Facet Dislocations

These injuries may require open reduction and stabilization if they are irreducible by closed means.

PHYSICAL THERAPY

• Realistic goals are established.
• Therapy may be helpful after healing to treat residual pain and stiffness.
• Wheelchairs are individualized to the patient.
• Lower extremity bracing may be extremely helpful.
• Orthotics for upper extremity function may be beneficial.

PATIENT EDUCATION

• Skin care and positioning to prevent flexion contractures.
• Education to prevent pressure ulceration, respiratory, and urinary infections.

PREVENTION

• Seatbelts and head rests on car seats.
• Possibly air bags.
• Strict immobilization of the cervical spine mandatory in all patients with unstable cervical spine injury to prevent new-onset or worsening neurologic deficit.

MONITORING

Neurologic monitoring during reduction maneuvers and surgery may increase the safety of the procedure. This includes somatosensory-evoked potentials and motor monitoring.

COMPLICATIONS

Neurologic injury varies from root injuries through incomplete spinal cord lesions to complete spinal cord injuries.

PROGNOSIS

Delay in diagnosis can lead to worsening of the injury.

RECOMMENDED READING

Clark CR, ed. *The cervical spine,* 3rd ed. Philadelphia: Lippincott–Raven, 1998:449–486.

Charcot-Marie-Tooth Disease

 Basics

DESCRIPTION

Charcot-Marie-Tooth disease is the most common of the hereditary motor and sensory neuropathies. Involvement progresses from distal to proximal. Lower extremity wasting, weakness, and cavovarus feet develop, followed in some cases by upper extremity weakness.

GENETICS

Charcot-Marie-Tooth disease is usually autosomal dominant.

CLASSIFICATION

Two basic types of Charcot-Marie-Tooth disease are recognized. Type I, the more common or hypertrophic form, represents 75% of patients. Reflexes are absent, and nerve conduction velocities are slow. Type II, the axonal form, is characterized by a generally severe disease, with presence of reflexes and a mild decrease in nerve conduction velocities. Both types are part of the larger group of similar disorders called hereditary motor and sensory neuropathies, of which there are five additional types.

ASSOCIATED CONDITIONS

- Scoliosis develops in 10% of patients.
- Hip dysplasia develops in 5% of patients.

ICD-9-CM

356.1 Charcot-Marie-Tooth disease

 Diagnosis

SIGNS AND SYMPTOMS

Patients usually present at age 10 to 20 years with a high arch, loss of endurance or coordination, or a steppage gait. Their shoes are worn out rapidly and unevenly. On examination, weakness occurs in the ankle evertors and dorsiflexors before anything else. Sensation and proprioception are diminished. There may be increased circumduction of the extremity.

DIFFERENTIAL DIAGNOSIS

- Tethered cord
- Myelomeningocele, lipomeningocele
- Peroneal nerve palsy
- Early stages of Duchenne's muscular dystrophy
- Other hereditary motor and sensory neuropathies

PHYSICAL EXAMINATION

The calf is usually thin. The strength of the muscles of the foot and ankle should be recorded and monitored for progression. Sensation should be tested. The position of the foot at rest should be examined for the presence of varus of the hind foot. This aspect is most strongly related to functional problems. If present, it should be assessed for rigidity by placing a lift under the lateral side of the forefoot and seeing whether it corrects. This is called Coleman's block test. Alternatively, one can grasp the calcaneus and try to correct it from its varus position. The flexibility of the cavus component should be checked. The relative plantar flexion of the first metatarsals as compared with the others should be noted. The presence or absence of toe clawing should be recorded.

Sensation should be tested. Gait should be observed, including the presence or absence of Trendelenburg's gait. The hips should be examined for abduction. A forward bend test should be done for scoliosis. The upper extremities should be checked for wasting of the ulnar-innervated muscles, including the abductors and the interossei.

LABORATORY TESTS

Electromyography and nerve conduction velocities are typically performed for diagnosis. The electromyogram shows increased duration and decreased amplitude of the motor action potentials. Nerve conduction velocity testing shows decrease in both motor and sensory conduction velocity.

Muscle biopsy shows atrophy, and nerve biopsy shows loss of myelinated fibers. These biopsies are not routinely indicated if the history and electrodiagnostic tests are characteristic.

DNA testing is now available through blood testing for early diagnosis or family analysis. The defect is a duplication or point mutation of the gene for the peripheral myelin protein 22, located on the short arm of chromosome 22. Otherwise, blood testing is not contributory.

PATHOLOGIC FINDINGS

If performed, the muscle biopsy displays diffuse atrophy and replacement of muscle fibers with fibrous and adipose tissue. Nerve biopsy is significant for loss of myelinated fibers and increased fibrous tissue in the endoneurium and perineurium. The pathogenesis of the cavovarus foot is progressive weakness of the lumbricalis or interossei that leaves the long toe flexors and extensors unopposed. Clawtoes develop, and the plantar fascia and intrinsic muscles contract.

IMAGING PROCEDURES

Spinal films are indicated in the index patient without a family history, to rule out spinal disorders. Depending on the index of suspicion, magnetic resonance imaging of the spine may be indicated as well. Once a diagnosis is made, the physician should have a low threshold for ordering pelvic films to rule out dysplasia if there is limitation of abduction.

⚂ Management

GENERAL MEASURES

Patients should be seen on a routine basis to monitor for worsening deformity and to manage it with the least morbidity. Stretching of the Achilles tendon and the plantar fascia is indicated, and use of night splints of the ankle in a neutral position may prevent or slow worsening of the condition.

SURGICAL TREATMENT

Treatment consists of steps in increasing levels of extent, and usually age, as follows:

• Clawtoe correction: flexor-to-extensor transfer or flexor release and proximal interphalangeal fusion
• Plantar release (plantar fascia, abductor hallucis, toe flexors) or plantar-medial release (includes posterior tibialis and long toe flexor lengthening and talonavicular capsulotomy)
• Tendon transfer: split or whole transfer of anterior tibialis or posterior tibialis
• Calcaneal osteotomy for rigid hind foot varus
• Midtarsal osteotomy (dorsolateral closing wedge) for rigid cavus
• Triple arthrodesis

PHYSICAL THERAPY

Therapy involves stretching of the Achilles tendon and plantar fascia.

PATIENT EDUCATION

Stress the importance of stretching and routine follow-up. Counsel on the mode of genetic inheritance so relatives can be screened. DNA testing may be helpful here. Discuss the risks of scoliosis and hip dysplasia.

MONITORING

Patients are checked yearly for ambulatory function.

COMPLICATIONS

Missed hip dysplasia means more difficult or less successful treatment. Recurrence after surgery may occur if soft tissue procedures are performed in patients with a fixed bony deformity. Transfer of stress with degeneration of the ankle or midfoot may occur, especially after triple arthrodesis.

PROGNOSIS

Usually, the foot cannot be made fully normal even after surgery, and the muscle weakness persists. Life expectancy is not shortened.

RECOMMENDED READING

McCluskey WP, Lovell WW, Cummings RJ. The cavovarus foot deformity: etiology and management. *Clin Orthop* 1989;247:27–37.

Miller MJ, Williams LL, Slack SL, et al. The hand in Charcot-Marie-Tooth disease. *J Hand Surg [BR]* 1991;16:191–196.

Palithorpe CA, Benson MK. Hip dysplasia in hereditary motor and sensory neuropathies. *J Bone Joint Surg Br* 1992;74:538–540.

Roper BA, Tibrewal SB. Soft-tissue surgery in Charcot-Marie-Tooth disease. *J Bone Joint Surg Br* 1989;71:17–20.

Sabir M, Lyttle D. Pathogenesis of Charcot-Marie-Tooth disease. *Clin Orthop* 1984;184:223–235.

Westmore RS, Drennan JC. Long-term results of triple arthrodesis in Charcot-Marie-Tooth disease. *J Bone Joint Surg Am* 1989;71:417–422.

Chondroblastoma

 Basics

DESCRIPTION

A chondroblastoma is a benign tumor of cartilaginous origin with a predilection for the epiphysis in skeletally immature patients. It is generally found in the epiphyses of long bones. The humerus is most commonly affected, followed by the tibia and the femur (Fig. 1). Chondroblastoma occurs in all age groups, but the overwhelming predominance is in patients in the second decade of life. There is a slight male predominance (2:1).

SYNONYMS

- Codman's tumor
- Epiphyseal chondromatous giant cell tumor

GENETICS

No known genetic component exists.

INCIDENCE

This tumor is rare. In the largest series, chondroblastoma accounted for 1% of all skeletal neoplasms.

CAUSES

The pathogenesis is unknown. Most authors agree that the neoplastic cells arise from "cartilage-forming matrix cells" or chondroblasts. The tumor may be related to chondromyxoid fibroma.

RISK FACTORS

None known

ASSOCIATED CONDITIONS

Aneurysmal bone cyst

ICD-9-CM

213.4 Chondroblastoma

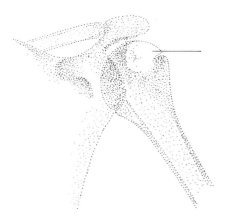

Fig. 1. Chondroblastoma is a lucent lesion in the immature epiphysis, most often the proximal humerus.

 Diagnosis

SIGNS AND SYMPTOMS

Patients usually complain of mild to moderate chronic pain, often months to years in duration. Stiffness and effusion of the adjacent joint are also common. Local swelling is not common.

DIFFERENTIAL DIAGNOSIS

- Enchondroma
- Giant cell tumor
- Osteomyelitis
- Fibrous dysplasia if found in flat bones

PHYSICAL EXAMINATION

The adjacent joint may have an effusion and a decreased range of motion. A soft tissue mass is uncommon. Point tenderness is unusual.

LABORATORY TESTS

Tests are not helpful. All blood tests are within normal limits, including the sedimentation rate.

PATHOLOGIC FINDINGS

The diagnosis requires the presence of chondroblasts on microscopic section. These are small, round or polygonal cells with round or oval nuclei. Cells are described as looking "plump" or like fried eggs. A lattice of calcification extends between the cells. Interspersed giant cells are a common feature and may lead to confusion with giant cell tumor. Areas of aneurysmal bone cyst degeneration may also be present.

IMAGING PROCEDURES

The radiographic appearance is that of a lytic lesion of the epiphysis with a thin sclerotic rim. The sclerotic rim indicates the benign nature of the lesion. It may expand or deform the bone. Occasionally, punctate calcifications may be seen.

The patient's history and plain radiographs are usually sufficient to make the diagnosis. Magnetic resonance imaging may be used if these are not definitive. The boundary of the lesion on magnetic resonance imaging scans should be distinct.

Management

GENERAL MEASURES

Surgical excision is recommended to prevent progressive growth of the lesion with destruction of the epiphysis. Bone grafting is needed. Surgery is sometimes technically demanding, owing to the need to preserve or reconstruct the nearby joint surface.

No restrictions on activity are necessary, because pathologic fracture is not a problem.

SURGICAL TREATMENT

The tumor is considered benign; therefore, local measures suffice. Surgery generally involves curettage and bone grafting.

PHYSICAL THERAPY

Therapy may be used to regain range of motion and strength after surgery.

PATIENT EDUCATION

Patients should be counseled that the lesion is benign and rarely metastasize (less than 2%). However, if the tumor is not removed, local morbidity may occur because of progressive enlargement of the involved epiphysis and destruction of the joint.

MONITORING

Follow-up care is necessary because recurrence is common. Radiographs should be repeated every 6 to 12 months initially after excision for approximately 2 years.

COMPLICATIONS

- Recurrence
- Joint stiffness

PROGNOSIS

The recurrence rate with chondroblastoma alone is 20% at 3 years. If the tumor has an aneurysmal component, the risk of recurrence is higher.

RECOMMENDED READING

Huvos HG. *Bone tumors: diagnosis and treatment.* Philadelphia: WB Saunders, 1971:171–190.

McCarthy EF, Frassica FJ. *Pathology of bone and joint disorders with clinical and radiographic correlation.* Philadelphia: WB Saunders, 1998:221.

Spjut HJ, Dorfman HD, Fechner RE, et al. *Tumors of bone and cartilage.* Washington, DC: Armed Forces Institute of Pathology, 1971:33–50.

Basics

DESCRIPTION

This primary malignant tumor of bone is made of malignant chondrocytes (cartilage cells) and occurs inside a cartilage matrix. It affects the proximal femur, the pelvic girdle, the knee, and the spine.

GENETICS

- In some patients, abnormalities have bone found in the p53 oncogene, located on chromosome 17, in cells isolated from these tumors.
- p53 abnormalities are also found in osteosarcoma, breast, lung, and colon cancers.

INCIDENCE

- Chondrosarcomas comprise 20% of all primary malignant bone tumors, occurring half as often as osteosarcoma.
- The tumor usually occurs in the sixth to eighth decades of life, between 50 and 70 years of age.

CAUSES

Most chondrosarcomas arise *de novo* (primary chondrosarcomas), whereas some arise in preexisting lesions (secondary chondrosarcomas). Secondary chondrosarcomas may arise in preexisting lesions such as in osteochondromas or the enchondromas in patients with Ollier's disease and Maffucci's syndrome. Dedifferentiated chondrosarcomas occur in 10% of patients and are high-grade lesions.

RISK FACTORS

- Multiple exostoses
- Ollier's disease
- Maffucci's syndrome

CLASSIFICATION

This follows the Enneking classification of tumors, also known as Musculoskeletal Tumor Society system:

- Low grade (grade 1): less than a 5% risk of metastasis
- Intermediate grade (grade 2): 20% to 30% risk of metastasis
- Dedifferentiated (grades 3 and 4): 60% to 80% risk of metastasis
- Mesenchymal: greater than a 50% risk of metastasis

ASSOCIATED CONDITIONS

Multiple exostoses or enchondromatosis

ICD-9-CM

170.9 Primary bone neoplasm (malignant)

 Diagnosis

SIGNS AND SYMPTOMS

- The insidious presentation of deep pain often occurs over years to decades.
- Pain is somewhat relieved by nonsteroidal antiinflammatory drugs or narcotic pain medication.
- A red flag is pain occurring at night.
- Pain is not relieved by rest or unloading, as it would with spine disc disorders, hip osteonecrosis, or early osteoarthritis of spine, hips, or knees.
- A soft tissue mass may be palpable in longstanding disease, with soft tissue extension.

DIFFERENTIAL DIAGNOSIS

- Enchondroma
- Bone infarct

PHYSICAL EXAMINATION

Usually, the patient has a large mass causing symptoms of local pressure but not severe pain. Physical examination is not specific.

LABORATORY TESTS

Serum tests are generally not helpful in establishing the diagnosis.

PATHOLOGIC FINDINGS

Histologically, it is difficult to differentiate between well-differentiated chondrosarcomas and chondromas (benign). The radiographic features are correlated with the histologic features to establish the degree of malignancy. Features of chondrosarcoma are as follows:

- Chondroblasts in a chondroid matrix
- Lobular pattern of growth
- Binucleate chondroblasts
- Graded 1 to 3, based on the level of anaplasia

IMAGING PROCEDURES

Plain anteroposterior and lateral radiographs are usually diagnostic of the lesion. Chondrosarcoma is usually described as an intramedullary lesion with stippled and ringlike calcification. In 85%, cortical bone changes are significant: erosions, thickening, and bone destruction. Chest radiographs and computed tomography scans are usually obtained in this age group because of the possibility of metastatic disease. Magnetic resonance imaging of the affected region is helpful to delineate soft tissue extension and to plan the biopsy site and the margins of resection.

Management

GENERAL MEASURES

- Surgery is the mainstay of treatment. Chemotherapy and radiation are not generally used.

- The goal of treatment is resection of entire lesion, to minimize the chance of recurrence.
- For grade I tumors, resection and serial 6-month observation with plain radiographs are all that is necessary. Patients with grade II and III chondrosarcomas are followed with computed tomography scans of the chest at 6-month intervals.
- At the 5-year disease-free interval, the frequency of clinic visits and repeat radiographs may be safely decreased.

SURGICAL TREATMENT

Wide resection involves removal of all the diseased bone with a cuff of normal tissue. The limb can be reconstructed with either an allograft or a custom prosthesis. Muscle flaps are used as necessary to fill in soft tissue defects.

PHYSICAL THERAPY

Physical therapy is used for gait training and to regain range of motion and strength.

PATIENT EDUCATION

The patient should be told that this neoplasm requires correlation of histologic features with radiography for proper diagnosis and that surgery is the mainstay of treatment.

MEDICAL TREATMENT

Patients who develop metastases are treated with chemotherapy, but unfortunately, the results are variable.

MONITORING

Patients are followed at 1- to 3-month intervals until their rehabilitation is complete.

COMPLICATIONS

- Recurrence
- Delayed union or nonunion of resection site
- Fracture through resection site
- Metastases (rare)
- Avascular necrosis of dependent sites (lesions or procedures near the femoral head)

PROGNOSIS

The prognosis in chondrosarcoma depends on the grade of the lesion:

- Low grade (grade I): excellent, less than 5% incidence of metastases
- Medium grade (grade III): very good, less than 30% incidence of metastases
- High grade (dedifferentiated, grade III): poor, more than 70% incidence of metastases

RECOMMENDED READING

Mark DM. *Review of orthopaedics*, 2nd ed. Saunders, Philadelphia, 1996:292–313.

Robbins pathologic basis of disease, 4th ed. Saunders, Philadelpia, 1989:1340–1342.

Simon SR. *Orthopaedic basic science.* American Academy of Orthopaedic Surgeons, Rosemount, Illinois, 1994:237, 265–267.

Clavicle Fracture

 Basics

DESCRIPTION

A fracture of the clavicle involves the shoulder and is also known as a broken collarbone.

INCIDENCE

• This is one of the most common fractures: 85% of cases involve the middle third of the clavicle, 10% the lateral third, and 5% the medial third.
• There is a bimodal distribution with high-energy injuries in young adults and, less commonly, injuries in osteoporotic elderly patients. Injuries also occur in the newborn from birth trauma.
• It appears more commonly in males than in females.

CAUSES

• In the adult, clavicle fractures typically result from sports or motor vehicle accidents and are caused by a direct blow to the shoulder.
• Clavicle fractures can also result from severe chest injuries such as lung trauma or a dissociation of the shoulder complex from the rib cage.
• In the infant, these injuries are frequently related to difficult deliveries.

RISK FACTORS

• Contact sports often lead to trauma to the shoulder girdle.
• A difficult delivery or high birth weight in the newborn may also predispose the newborn to the fracture.
• Age-related factors include

—Newborn: birth injury
—Young adult: high-energy injury
—Elderly adult: osteoporotic fracture with a fall

CLASSIFICATION

The fracture is classified by its location in the clavicle: proximal, middle, or distal third. Lateral clavicle fractures are subclassified as types I, II, and III.

• Type I clavicle fractures are minimally displaced because the coracoclavicular ligaments are not disrupted.
• Type II fractures are associated with ligament injury and can have a large displacement of the proximal fragment.
• Type III injuries are intraarticular and can lead to late arthritis of the acromioclavicular joint.

ASSOCIATED CONDITIONS

• Subclavian vascular injury
• Brachial plexus injury
• Scapular fractures
• Shoulder fracture or dislocation
• Lung or rib injury

ICD-9-CM

767.2 Fracture of clavicle

 Diagnosis

The combination of history, physical examination, and radiographs is nearly always diagnostic.

SIGNS AND SYMPTOMS

• Pain and deformity are present over the clavicular region.
• The patient may splint the shoulder by cradling the affected arm with the contralateral hand.
• There may be a history of direct trauma to the shoulder.
• Infants with birth trauma may show pseudoparalysis of the extremity (i.e., they resist moving it because of pain).

DIFFERENTIAL DIAGNOSIS

A radiograph typically confirms the diagnosis of fracture. However, 3% of these fractures are concurrent with other injuries, including rib fracture, pneumothorax, and humerus fracture.

• Posterior fracture displacement of medial fractures
• Shoulder-proximal humerus fracture or dislocation
• Acromioclavicular separation (tearing of the ligaments without fracture)
• Acromioclavicular arthrosis
• Rotator cuff disorders
• Pneumothorax or hemothorax
• Injury to the brachial plexus
• Injury to the great vessels
• Head injury
• Scapulothoracic dissociation
• "Floating shoulder" (fracture of the clavicle and scapula)

PHYSICAL EXAMINATION

• Assess breathing and neurologic function.
• Check the pulse to assess vascular status.
• Palpate the fracture site for crepitation.
• Determine whether there are any open wounds by examining the skin for tenting or compromise over the area of injury.
• Ensure that no dislocation has occurred by checking the shoulder's range of motion.

LABORATORY TESTS

No laboratory test is needed unless other injuries are suspected.

PATHOLOGIC FINDINGS

This fracture typically occurs in the middle third of the clavicle because of the bone's biomechanics and structure. The middle third of the clavicle experiences the largest bending moment with applied load to the shoulder and has the smallest cross-sectional area.

IMAGING PROCEDURES

• If vascular injury is considered, then an arteriogram can be helpful.
• A standard anteroposterior view of the clavicle and a view with the beam tilted 45 degrees cephalad should be ordered.
• If a shoulder disorder is suspected, then specific shoulder views, including an axillary view, are needed.
• If one suspects posterior displacement of medial fractures, then a computed tomography scan is helpful.

⚡ Management

GENERAL MEASURES

• Analgesics and sling immobilization should be used.
• Therapy for early range of motion of the shoulder (Codman's exercise) should be instituted.
• Most of these injuries can be managed non-operatively.
• Most clavicle fractures do not require reduction maneuvers.
• Immobilization for 1 week in a sling and then gentle range of motion of the shoulder are the treatments of choice for most of these fractures.
• The patient should be referred to an orthopaedic surgeon if there is any question about treatment.
• Midclavicular fractures without large displacements or shortening can be treated with a sling.
• If there is a large displacement of the fracture, attempted reduction and splinting with a figure-of-eight brace can be attempted.
• It is important to ensure that the brace is not causing skin compromise.
• Lateral third fractures can typically be managed nonoperatively, although operative treatment may be preferred for a type II fracture with large displacement.
• Posterior medial clavicle fractures need to be evaluated for the possibility of airway compromise or concurrent injury.

—These may need immediate reduction by an orthopaedic surgeon.
—The medial growth physis does not close for the clavicle until the patient is approximately 21 years old; therefore, medial fractures in the young adult are typically Salter-Harris type II fractures and eventually remodel.

ACTIVITY LEVEL

• The shoulder should be immobilized until comfortable, and then an increasing range of motion exercises should be begun.
• Until tenderness resolves, there should be limited lifting or overhead work.

SURGICAL TREATMENT

Surgery for clavicle fractures may be needed for the following:

• Comminuted or large displacements of fractures
• Open fractures over the clavicle
• Floating shoulders (fractures of the clavicle and scapula)

The treatment of choice is, typically, open reduction and internal fixation with plates and screws. Pin fixation has had the complication of pin migration into the intrathoracic region.

PHYSICAL THERAPY

• Codman's exercises should be instituted early in the course, using a pendulum-type movement of the shoulder with the trunk bent and supported.
• Passive range of motion to the overhead position increases as the pain diminishes in several weeks.
• Strengthening exercises are used when pain resolves.

MEDICAL TREATMENT

Analgesics should be prescribed as appropriate to the level of pain experienced.

PATIENT EDUCATION

The patient should be educated about persistent deformity and occasional functional limitation if significant displacement occurs.

PREVENTION

The patient should avoid activities that can cause a direct blow to the shoulder.

MONITORING

• Order serial radiographs at intervals of 3 to 4 weeks to ensure healing.
• Assess the skin carefully to ensure that it has not been compromised.
• As always, evaluate nerve and vascular function acutely and at follow-up intervals.

COMPLICATIONS

• Skin breakdown over the fracture site
• Nonunion or malunion (which may require future procedures to realign the bone and permit healing)
• Vascular injury
• Nerve injury
• Residual pain
• Decreased shoulder function

PROGNOSIS

• The prognosis is good for patients with minimally displaced fractures.
• Deformity from the fracture typically remains but decreases with time.
• Functional deficit is unusual but can occur with markedly displaced fractures.
• Return to full function should occur by 6 to 12 weeks.
• If the fracture has caused shortening or if there is a type II or III distal clavicle fracture, problems with acromioclavicular arthrosis or function may occur in the future.

RECOMMENDED READING

Cuomo, John F and Goss, Thomas P. Shoulder trauma (bone) In: Kasser JR, ed. *Orthopaedic knowledge update 5*. Rosemont, IL: American Academy of Orthopaedic Surgeons, 217–232.

Ring D, Jupiter J. Clavicle fracture: a guide to basic management. *J Musculoskel Med* 1997;14:65–73.

Clawtoes

 Basics

DESCRIPTION

The term clawtoes describes a flexion deformity of the proximal interphalangeal joint of lesser toes with hyperextension of the metatarsophalangeal joint (Fig. 1). The distal interphalangeal joint may be either flexed or extended. The incidence increases with advancing age. It occurs more frequently in women than in men (5:1).

GENETICS

Clawtoes may have hereditary disposition in patients with hereditary neuropathies such as Charcot-Marie-Tooth disease and Friedreich's ataxia, especially in persons whose muscle imbalance occurs with weakness or loss of intrinsic muscle function.

INCIDENCE

- Ranges from 2% to 20% in industrialized, shoe-wearing countries
- Increases with advancing age

CAUSES

Clawtoes are most commonly due to an imbalance between the intrinsic and extrinsic muscles of the foot. There is simultaneous contracture of the long flexors and extensors of the toes without any balancing force from the intrinsic muscles. Frequent causes are as follows:

- Neuromuscular diseases, including Charcot-Marie-Tooth disease, Friedreich's ataxia, cerebral palsy myelodysplasia, and multiple sclerosis
- Degenerative disc disease
- Diabetes
- Hansen's disease
- Rheumatoid arthritis
- Psoriatic arthritis
- Foot compartment syndrome

RISK FACTORS/ASSOCIATED CONDITIONS

- Cavus foot
- Cock-up deformity of the great toe
- Hallux valgus
- Clawtoe deformity of the other lesser toe
- Neuromuscular disease
- Inflammatory arthritis
- Diabetes mellitus

ICD-9-CM

735.5 Clawtoes

 Diagnosis

SIGNS AND SYMPTOMS

Patients may complain of cosmetic appearance, difficulty with wearing shoes, or a painful bursa over the dorsum of the proximal interphalangeal joint. With hyperextension of the metatarsophalangeal joint, the plantar fat pad subluxates dorsally and causes painful plantar callosities as well as possible ulcerations in insensate feet. Clawtoes often occur in multiple adjacent toes, as well as in bilateral feet. There are also often associated with a cavus foot deformity. A thorough neurovascular examination, as well as an examination for flexibility of the deformity, should be done.

DIFFERENTIAL DIAGNOSIS

- Hammer toes
- Mallet toes

These are disorders of the interphalangeal joint that do not involve the metatarsophalangeal joint.

PHYSICAL EXAMINATION

- Check the strength of the flexors and extensors.
- Test the ankle muscles.
- Stretch the joints to see whether the deformity is fixed.
- Check sensation.

LABORATORY TESTS

Tests may be helpful in diagnosing neuropathies, inflammatory arthropathies, and diabetes. Nerve conduction velocity testing may be helpful if Charcot-Marie-Tooth disease is suspected.

PATHOLOGIC FINDINGS

Weakness of the intrinsic foot muscles, along with the unopposed action of the long flexors and extensors of the toes, causes the hyperextension deformity at the metatarsophalangeal joint, as well as the flexion deformity at the proximal interphalangeal joint.

IMAGING PROCEDURES

Standing anteroposterior and lateral radiographs of the foot can be helpful in assessing the magnitude of the contracture of the interphalangeal joints, as well as subluxation or dislocation of the metatarsophalangeal joints.

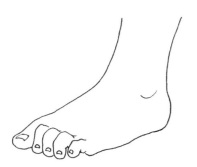

Fig. 1. Clawtoes include hyperextension of the metatarsophalangeal joints and flexion of the distal joints.

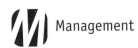 Management

GENERAL MEASURES

Patients in whom conservative management fails may require surgical correction. For fixed clawtoe deformity, Du Vries' arthroplasty of the proximal interphalangeal joint with release of the contracted structures of the metatarsophalangeal joint should be performed. For flexible clawtoes, Girdlestone-Taylor flexor-to-extensor tendon transfers with possible release of the metatarsophalangeal joint should be done.

SURGICAL TREATMENT

Du Vries' arthroplasty-partial phalangectomy of the proximal phalanx through an elliptic dorsal incision followed by Kirschner wire (K-wire) stabilization should be performed. Extensor tenotomy and metatarsophalangeal joint capsulotomy should be performed to realign the metatarsophalangeal joint adequately. With the Girdlestone-Taylor procedure, flexor digitorum longus tendon is passed dorsally and is sutured to the extensor hood. The toe is stabilized, with a K-wire holding it in a reduced position. Release of the metatarsophalangeal joint should be performed as well.

PHYSICAL THERAPY

Daily manipulation of the toes in patients with a flexible deformity may help to keep the toes flexible.

MEDICAL TREATMENT

Patients with clawtoes should receive conservative treatment initially, with better shoes that have wide, high toe boxes. Local treatments with doughnut-shaped cushions or foam toe caps placed over the proximal interphalangeal joint may help with irritation in this area. Patients with pain under the metatarsal heads may need a soft metatarsal support or a metatarsal bar to relieve pressure on the metatarsal head. Patients should ambulate with a postoperative shoe until the K-wire has been removed and the soft tissues have healed.

PATIENT EDUCATION

Wear appropriate shoes that do not crowd the toes and cause them to overlap.

MONITORING

Patients are followed at 2-week intervals after surgery to monitor for early recurrence of the deformity, loss of fixation, swelling, and loss of motion in the ankle and subtalar joints.

COMPLICATIONS

- Failure to correct the deformity
- Recurrence of the deformity
- Persistent pain
- Neurovascular damage

PROGNOSIS

Even with appropriate conservative treatment, most flexible clawtoes become rigid, and, if they are sufficiently symptomatic, they may require surgical correction.

RECOMMENDED READING

Coughlin MJ, Mann RA. Lesser toe deformities. In: Mann RA, Coughlin MJ, eds. *Surgery of the foot and ankle,* 6th ed. St. Louis: CV Mosby 1993:342—350.

Clinodactyly

Basics

DESCRIPTION

Clinodactyly presents as a bent finger in a radial or ulnar direction (Fig. 1), usually the little finger bent in a radial direction. Most often, the finger has a short, delta-shaped middle phalanx. This condition may be associated with mental retardation, especially when clinodactyly is severe.

SYNONYMS

Bent finger

GENETICS

The condition is autosomal dominant with variable expressivity. Some cases are sporadic.

INCIDENCE

- One percent to 10% in otherwise normal children; least common in whites
- Detected at birth
- More common in males, in whom it is usually bilateral

CAUSES

Unknown

RISK FACTORS

In children with Down's syndrome, the incidence of clinodactyly is 35% to 70%. It is also seen in many other syndromes, especially Klinefelter's and trisomy 18.

ASSOCIATED CONDITIONS

- Symphalangism
- Brachydactyly (short fingers)
- Trisomies
- Treacher Collins syndrome
- Silver's syndrome
- Holt-Oram syndrome
- Prader-Willi syndrome

ICD-9-CM

759.59 Clinodactyly

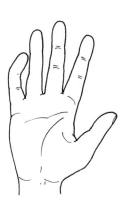

Fig. 1. Clinodactyly refers to bony angulation of a finger, usually the fifth.

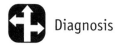 Diagnosis

SIGNS AND SYMPTOMS

- The finger is curved in a radial or ulnar direction, usually the little finger.
- Deviation can occur at proximal phalangeal joint, middle phalanx, and distal interphalangeal joint (Fig. 1).
- It is most common in the distal interphalangeal joint.
- This is a painless condition.

DIFFERENTIAL DIAGNOSIS

- Delta phalanx (a wedge-shaped phalanx with a sloped joint surface)
- Malunion after fractures

PHYSICAL EXAMINATION

- The angle of deviation of a finger at the proximal interphalangeal joint, the middle phalanx, or the distal interphalangeal joint should be measured.
- Active and passive motion at each joint should be recorded.
- The remainder of the skeleton should also be inspected.

LABORATORY TESTS

Chromosome analysis should be undertaken if an underlying syndrome is suspected.

PATHOLOGIC FINDINGS

Maldevelopment of one of the phalanges causes an angulation of the joint surface.

IMAGING PROCEDURES

Conventional plain radiography of the affected finger is recommended, especially when considering surgical correction in a child. Less than 10 degrees of angulation is within normal limits.

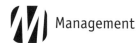 Management

GENERAL MEASURES

Most cases are cosmetic problems. Slight deformity does not need surgical correction. Conservative treatment including manipulation and casting is usually futile, and patients find it difficult to tolerate. Significant deformity persisting after the age of 6 years may call for surgical correction. Surgical procedures are elective, because the problem is mainly cosmetic. There are no restrictions on activity.

SURGICAL TREATMENT

Surgical procedures include osteotomy and growth plate reconstruction with a free fat graft. For a child less than 6 years old, one should perform a fat graft placement after resection of the midportion of the continuous epiphysis and underlying physis (growth plate). After age 6, a simple closing osteotomy can be done easily and with few complications.

PHYSICAL THERAPY

Therapy may be helpful to regain motion after surgery.

PATIENT EDUCATION

Educating patients in the benign nature of the condition is helpful.

PREVENTION

There is no evidence that the deformity may be prevented or its natural history changed by intervention.

MONITORING

Patients may be left to monitor the angulation of the finger clinically and return for surgical treatment if it becomes unacceptable.

PROGNOSIS

The prognosis is good, with no evidence of degenerative joint disease.

RECOMMENDED READING

Green DP, ed. *Operative hand surgery*, 3rd ed. New York: Churchill Livingstone, 1993:455–456.

Basics

DESCRIPTION

Clubfoot, or talipes equinovarus, is a complex deformity of infancy and childhood that can be broken down into three elements: equinus of the heel, varus and internal rotation of the hind foot, and adductus of the forefoot. This is derived from the Latin name: talipes is from *talus* ("ankle bone") and *pes* ("foot") and thus describes the location of the anomaly; *equinus* ("horse") is used to describe a plantar flexed position because horses walk on their toenails with their heels in complete plantar flexion; and *varus* ("turned in") refers to the adducted component to the deformity. The afflicted child thus bears weight along the lateral foot, rather than on the sole.

Clubfoot can be divided into two categories: an isolated, idiopathic type and a type associated with other congenital deformities such as amniotic band syndrome, arthrogryposis, myelodysplasia, and diastrophic dwarfism. Clubfeet of the latter type have a tendency to be more severe and refractory to conservative therapy and nearly always require surgical correction. The talar neck is shortened and deviated medially and in a plantar direction. The foot is smaller than normal, and shortening, usually less than 1 cm from the contralateral, normal side, may occur.

SYNONYMS

Talipes equinovarus

GENETICS

The disorder is widely believed to be polygenic with variable penetrance. When one child has a clubfoot, there is a 2% to 6% chance that the next sibling will have the disorder. Furthermore, if a parent has clubfoot, there is a 10% chance that each child will inherit the disorder.

INCIDENCE

• The incidence of clubfoot is approximately 1.5 of every 1,000 births.
• Clubfoot is approximately twice as common in boys as in girls. When it does occur in girls, it may be more resistant to conservative treatment.

CAUSES

The more common isolated, idiopathic form is thought to be of a genetic origin, although the genetic basis has not been identified. Clubfeet can also be associated with other congenital deformities such as amniotic band syndrome, myelodysplasia, diastrophic dwarfism, and arthrogryposis.

RISK FACTORS

• A parent with the disorder
• To a lesser extent, a sibling with the disorder
• Presence of other disorders associated with clubfoot, including amniotic band syndrome, arthrogryposis, myelodysplasia, Möbius' syndrome, Freeman-Sheldon syndrome, Larsen's syndrome, and diastrophic dwarfism
• Drugs taken during pregnancy, such as aminopterin

CLASSIFICATION

• Idiopathic clubfeet
• Congenital clubfeet associated with other congenital deformities such as amnionic band syndrome, arthrogryposis, myelodysplasia, and diastrophic dwarfism (clubfeet of this type may be more severe)

ASSOCIATED CONDITIONS

• Other congenital deformities, such as amniotic band syndrome, arthrogryposis, certain myelodysplasia, diastrophic dwarfism Larsen's syndrome, Freeman-Sheldon syndrome
• Clubfeet associated with other conditions, rather than the more common idiopathic type, tend to be more severe and refractory to conservative treatment.

ICD-9-CM

754.51 Clubfoot

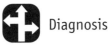

Diagnosis

SIGNS AND SYMPTOMS

Signs and symptoms of clubfoot are related to the findings on physical examination. In general, the newborn's foot looks excessively turned inward. In older children, uncorrected clubfeet may cause gait disturbances, problems with shoe fit, and painful callosities along the lateral border of the foot. The patient may actually be forced to walk on the dorsum (top) of the foot. Pain within the foot may develop in the older child or adult.

DIFFERENTIAL DIAGNOSIS

The differential diagnosis of clubfoot is limited because of the dramatic and characteristic appearance of this deformity. Some cases of metatarsus adductus varus are so severe that they are confused with clubfoot, but the equinus component of clubfoot is absent in metatarsus adductus and should easily enable one to make the distinction.

PHYSICAL EXAMINATION

The physical examination reveals equinus of the heel, supination or varus of the hind foot, and adductus of the midfoot and forefoot. This creates a foot described as "kidney shaped," with a prominent medial crease along the plantar aspect of the foot. The foot projects medially from the leg and resembles a club. The afflicted child is thus forced to walk on the lateral instep rather than on the sole of the foot.

• Check the flexibility of the foot, as well as the ability to correct its position.
• Verify the function of the ankle and toe muscles.
• Note the smallness of the foot, with some shortening, usually less than 1 cm from the nonaffected side.
• Check for significant calf hypoplasia, which is a usual feature.

Clubfoot

PATHOLOGIC FINDINGS

The essential bony change is medial deviation of the talar neck with subluxation of the talonavicular joint. Histologic examination also reveals smaller muscle fibers on cross section. There is also increased thickness of fascia and joint capsules on the medial side of the foot.

IMAGING PROCEDURES

In routine care of clubfoot, radiographs may not be needed unless there is a suspicion of underlying bony fusion or if surgery is contemplated. The most important radiographs to obtain are the simulated standing anteroposterior and lateral views. Because of the deformity caused by clubfoot, these views may be difficult to take and may require multiple attempts. The foot should be corrected as close to neutral as possible and held in this position with a Plexiglas plate. In a normal foot, the anteroposterior view shows the talus to be aligned roughly with the first metatarsal and the calcaneus with roughly the fifth metatarsal; thus, an angle is formed between the axes of these two bones forming the anterior talocalcaneal angle, or Kite's angle. This is normally in the range of 20 to 40 degrees. In clubfoot, the *axes* of the calcaneus and talus are nearly parallel, and thus the angle is much less. Likewise, the talocalcaneal angle on lateral view is normally between 35 and 50 degrees, but in the clubfoot it is significantly less, because the two bones are nearly parallel in all planes. Also noted on the lateral view is the position of the foot in equinus and on the anteroposterior view the forefoot in adduction. The assessment of these radiographic abnormalities in a clubfoot is used to determine whether a correction is acceptable.

Management

GENERAL MEASURES

Clubfoot can be treated so the deformity is reduced and normal function is recovered for the most part. Most clubfeet can be corrected or substantially improved by cast treatment. This should be started as soon after birth as possible. The foot is stretched out as much as possible and is held in place by a cast from above the knee to the toes. This allows the tight tendons to stretch, so further correction may be obtained the next time. Sometimes, an Achilles tenotomy is needed. After the foot is corrected (2 to 4 months), it should be held with reverse shoes and a Denis Browne bar between the legs.

SURGICAL TREATMENT

If cast treatment fails, surgery is needed. Surgery should be reserved until the child is between 4 and 8 months of age. The general principle involves (a) releasing the medial structures by lengthening the flexor tendons and the tibialis posterior tendon and (b) releasing the posterior structures by transecting the posterior joint capsule and lengthening the Achilles tendon. A more extensive release may sometimes be required. The calcaneus can also be repositioned laterally, and a more complete correction can be achieved. Pins are left in place for 6 weeks to help stabilize the correction. Casting should be continued for 2 to 3 months after therapy. About 10% to 20% of children require repeat surgery in later years.

PHYSICAL THERAPY

Some authors believe that certain stretching exercises, particularly of the heel cord and medial ankle structures, may be of some benefit, but exercises alone are usually not sufficient. These exercises are most beneficial in maintaining the correction obtained by cast treatment.

MEDICAL TREATMENT

The first step in management of clubfoot is taping or casting. About one-third of clubfeet, usually the milder cases, will respond to this conservative therapy. Taping or casting should be started as early in life as possible. The heel is firmly stabilized, and the forefoot is brought laterally out of adductus; then the foot is dorsiflexed, and the heel is externally rotated into valgus. By holding the foot in such a position, all three components of clubfoot are essentially corrected. At this point, adhesive tape or a cast is applied to hold the foot in this position. During the immediate postnatal term, the cast or taping is changed every few days; after the first week, the tapings are changed once to twice weekly in the office. By about 8 weeks of age, the foot and leg are large enough that a long leg cast may be applied with the foot in the corrected position. The casts are changed weekly or biweekly until the position of the foot is acceptable or improvement has ceased. Conservative treatment is generally more successful when the deformity is mild.

Drugs are not helpful, except as needed for 2 to 4 days after surgery.

PATIENT EDUCATION

Clubfeet tend to be slightly shorter than normal feet and are less supple. However, parents should be reassured that adequately corrected clubfeet have good long-term function. Parents also need to monitor for signs of recurrence.

MONITORING

Children need regular follow-up care for several years to monitor for recurrence. Idiopathic clubfoot may recur up to age 6 or 7 years. Most recurrences occur in the first few years and may be treated with repeat casting.

COMPLICATIONS

- Residual deformity
- Rocker-bottom foot
- Overcorrection into valgus
- Stiffness
- Pain in later childhood or adulthood

PROGNOSIS

With adequate treatment, whether conservative or surgical, it is likely that the positional deformity can be eliminated, and the ability to ambulate adequately on the affected foot can be achieved. Certain elements of the deformity, such as the smallness of the foot, the calf hypoplasia, and the minimal shortening, cannot be corrected, but these rarely have a large effect on the patient's functional ability.

RECOMMENDED READING

Huurman WW. Congenital foot deformities. In: Mann RA, Coughlin MJ, eds. *Surgery of the foot and ankle,* vol 2, 6th ed. St. Louis, CV Mosby, 1993:1313–1327.

Kasser JR, ed. *Orthopaedic knowledge update 5.* Rosemont, IL: American Academy of Orthopaedic Surgeons, 1996:503–504.

Staheli LT. *Fundamentals of pediatric orthopedics.* New York: Raven, 1992:5.10–5.13.

Basics

DESCRIPTION

Compartment syndrome occurs when an acute or chronic increase in pressure occurs within an enclosed space and results in severely compromised capillary flow to the intracompartmental soft tissues, nerves, and blood vessels.

SYSTEMS AFFECTED

• Undiagnosed or untreated, this condition can lead to necrosis of tissues and nerves within the enclosed space, with resulting ischemic contracture or loss of the involved limb.
• Depending on the amount of muscle injured, massive cell death from hypoperfusion injury can cause acute tubular necrosis, hyperkalemia, and kidney failure.

INCIDENCE

• This condition occurs in 1% to 5% of all tibia fractures.
• It is less common in other injuries such as femoral shaft and forearm fractures.
• It may occur in children or adults.

CAUSES

It can result from any cause of increased intra-compartment volume, including the following:

• Bleeding from fractures
• Crush injury leading to muscle bleeding, massive cell death, and subsequent extravasation of cytoplasmic fluid (hence severe swelling)
• Vascular injury (arterial or venous occlusion) with subsequent hypoxemia and increased vascular permeability
• Iatrogenic causes

—Placement of external fixators
—Open reduction and internal fixation of fractures
—Osteotomy
—Inadvertent extravasation of intravenous fluids
—Tight dressing and casting: exacerbates an increase in intracompartment pressure

RISK FACTORS

• History of trauma, especially high-energy trauma
• Crush injury
• Multiple arterial injections
• Prolonged venous transfusion
• Prolonged unconsciousness
• Associated conditions
• Multiple or high-velocity trauma
• Crush injury

ICD-9-CM

958.8 Compartment syndrome

 Diagnosis

SIGNS AND SYMPTOMS

Five Ps (Pain, Pallor, Paresthesia, Paralysis, and Pulselessness)

• The five Ps signify an established severe compartment syndrome.
• The clinician should have a high index of suspicion for compartment syndrome, because chances for limb salvage are limited if paralysis or pulselessness has evolved.

Involved Limb

The involved limb is tense, firm, and tender to the touch.

Pain

• Pain in passive stretch (i.e., gently stretching the toes or the fingers of the involved limb) is the most reliable clinical sign.
• Pain is severe, even at rest (out of proportion to the injury).
• Paresthesia in the area supplied by the nerves in the compartment is also a common finding.

DIFFERENTIAL DIAGNOSIS

Arterial occlusion (also characterized by pain, pallor, pulselessness)

PHYSICAL EXAMINATION

Careful examination should be performed to assess whether a compartment syndrome is present. The involved compartment should be palpated to assess for swelling to see whether it is hard or soft. The fingers or toes should be passively flexed and extended to see whether this causes severe pain, one of the most sensitive signs. If there is pain with passive stretch, the clinician should suspect a compartment syndrome. One should also carefully check the sensation and motor function supplied by the nerves that traverse the compartment.

Compartment Syndrome

LABORATORY TESTS

- Serial creatine phosphokinase if the clinician suspects significant muscle death
- Routine preoperative laboratory tests

PATHOLOGIC FINDINGS

Intracompartmental edema, causing venous congestion and tissue necrosis if diagnosis is delayed

IMAGING PROCEDURES

Routine radiographs to evaluate skeletal trauma.

SPECIAL TESTS

Two methods of measuring compartment pressure:

1. Hand-held automated measuring device.
2. Insertion of an 18-gauge needle into the compartment.

The needle is connected to a manometer or an arterial pressure monitoring line, and a small amount of fluid (2 to 3 mL) is injected into the compartment. The pressure reading after the fluid injection is the compartment pressure. Compartment pressure of 40 mm Hg or within 30 mm Hg of the diastolic pressure requires fasciotomies (compartment decompression).

Management

GENERAL MEASURES

- Patients suspected of developing a compartment syndrome should have the compartment pressure monitored.
- Immediate splitting or removal of a cast or tight dressing is a must.
- Compartment syndrome is a surgical emergency requiring surgical decompression or fasciotomy to avoid further complications.

SURGICAL TREATMENT

- In general, fascial tissues enveloping the affected compartment are opened in a longitudinal fashion, thereby decompressing the enclosed space and allowing tissue expansion and better perfusion.
- The wound is then left open, and delayed primary closure or skin grafting is done at a later date.
- During the immediate postoperative period, the involved limb should be elevated to minimize swelling.

PATIENT EDUCATION

The patient must be informed about the need for subsequent delayed primary closure or skin grafting.

MONITORING

Intraoperatively, compartment pressure should be measured after fasciotomy to confirm that the compartment is appropriately decompressed.

PREVENTION

A high index of suspicion is needed, especially in dealing with patients with obtunded sensorium because of trauma or pharmacologic agents, or in children in whom the history and physical examinations are often inadequate. Although most cases involve the legs and forearms, compartment syndromes in the thigh, hand, foot, arm (especially in supracondylar fracture of the elbow), and buttock are also well recognized.

COMPLICATIONS

- Motor or sensory deficits
- Kidney failure from rhabdomyolysis
- Volkmann's contracture
- Loss of limb

PROGNOSIS

- Some investigators believe that the prognosis is better in children than in adults; others disagree.
- In general, complications can be minimized with rapid diagnosis and treatments.

RECOMMENDED READING

Ouellette EA, Kelly R. Compartment syndromes of the hand. *J Bone Joint Surg Am* 1996;78:1515–1522.

Pellegrini VD Jr, Evarts CM. Complications. In: Rockwood CA, Green DP, eds. *Rockwood and Green's fractures in adults,* vol 1, 3rd ed. Philadelphia: JB Lippincott, 1991:390–399.

Perry CR. Knee and leg: bone trauma. In: Kasser JR, ed. *Orthopaedic knowledge update 5.* Rosemont, IL: American Academy of Orthopaedic Surgeons, 1996:453–462.

Basics

DESCRIPTION

The foot has nine distinct compartments: medial, lateral, central, calcaneal, four interossei compartments, and the adductor muscle compartment. Because of their unyielding fascial coverings (Fig. 1), the muscles may swell after injury, and a compartment syndrome may develop.

INCIDENCE

The incidence is unknown. However, many cases are missed (not recognized) until clawing of the toes follows the scarring process. The index of suspicion should remain high with any crush injury involving the foot. It may occur at all ages and in both sexes, in children as well as adults.

CAUSES

This condition usually results from high-energy injuries to the foot, most commonly crush injuries. The swelling elevates tissue pressures above capillary perfusion pressure and initiates a vicious cycle of ischemia.

ASSOCIATED CONDITIONS

- Lisfranc's fracture-dislocations
- Multiple metatarsal fractures
- Calcaneus fracture

ICD-9-CM

958.8 Compartment syndrome of the foot

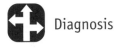

Diagnosis

SIGNS AND SYMPTOMS

No classic signs are diagnostic of foot compartment syndrome, so it is important to have a high index of suspicion. Findings include tense swelling of the foot after trauma, intense pain, pain on passive stretch of the toes, dysesthesia, and diminished pulses. The pain does not abate with elevation of the foot. These findings, however, are inconsistent. The patient with a head injury must be checked more carefully, and pressures measured if there is increased turgor of the foot.

DIFFERENTIAL DIAGNOSIS

- Compartment syndrome of leg
- Posttraumatic or postsurgical swelling and pain without critically elevated compartment pressures
- Isolated nerve laceration or compression

PHYSICAL EXAMINATION

Sensation to light touch should be tested on each of the toes. Active and passive motion of each of the toes should be checked (a measure of interosseous function). The pressure in the muscle compartments can be estimated only roughly by palpation.

LABORATORY TESTS

- Creatine phosphokinase: This may be elevated (later) as a result of myonecrosis.
- Renal function: This can also be affected, 1 to 3 days after the crush.
- Pressure monitoring techniques: This is employed to measure compartment pressures in the compartments described earlier. A measurement of greater than 30 mm Hg, or 30 mm Hg below diastolic blood pressure, is indicative of an ongoing compartment syndrome.

PATHOLOGIC FINDINGS

Myonecrosis is seen on histologic examination if the pressure is allowed to remain elevated for more than 6 hours.

IMAGING PROCEDURES

Plain films may show multiple metatarsal fractures, calcaneal fracture, Lisfranc's fracture-dislocation, and significant soft tissue swelling. Compartment syndrome may also occur without fracture.

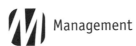

Management

GENERAL MEASURES

- Patients with foot compartment syndrome require emergency surgical decompression with fasciotomies of the compartments to prevent further necrosis.
- Keep the patient's foot at the heart level and remove any occlusive dressings until the patient can be taken to the operating room.

SURGICAL TREATMENT

Two main approaches are used for fasciotomy of the foot compartments. The first uses a double dorsal incision technique, and the second goes through a single longitudinal plantar medial incision. Both are acceptable and adequately relieve the pressure in the respective compartments. If there are coincident metatarsal fractures that require fixation, the dorsal approach is preferred. Fasciotomy wounds are generally left open for 5 to 7 days. The patient is then returned to the operating room for either delayed primary closure or split-thickness skin grafting, once the compartmental swelling has gone down.

The patient should be kept off the affected extremity to avoid further swelling and injury to the foot. The foot should be maintained at heart level.

PHYSICAL THERAPY

Patients may require stretching and other therapeutic modalities after resolution of the acute syndrome to treat any resultant joint contractures.

MEDICAL TREATMENT

Care must be taken to avoid masking the signs and symptoms of compartment syndrome through the use of strong analgesics. Blood pressure should be maintained at normal levels to optimize muscle perfusion.

PATIENT EDUCATION

- Complications of compartment syndrome should be explained.
- Future reconstructive operations of the forefoot, including release of clawtoes and proximal interphalangeal joint arthroplasty, should be outlined.
- Major foot trauma should be avoided.

MONITORING

The foot may be continuously monitored with an indwelling catheter attached to an arterial line monitor by the bedside.

COMPLICATIONS

- Clawtoes, if fasciotomy is insufficient or delayed
- Need for split-thickness skin graft to cover the fasciotomy incisions in 5 to 7 days
- Loss of dorsal skin bridge between fasciotomy incisions

PROGNOSIS

The prognosis is good for feet that undergo timely release by fasciotomies. However, if compartment syndrome is not diagnosed early, patients go on to develop forefoot contractures.

RECOMMENDED READING

Silas IP, Herzenberg JE, Myerson M, et al. Compartment syndrome of the foot in children. *J Bone Joint Surg Am* 1995;77:356–361.

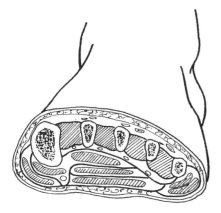

Fig. 1. Compartment syndrome of the foot may damage the many intrinsic and plantar muscles *(shaded)* if prolonged elevation of pressure persists within their thick fascial sheaths.

Congenital Pseudarthrosis

 Basics

DESCRIPTION

Congenital pseudarthrosis is a rare defect of the distal tibia in which the bone is cystic and bowed and eventually fractures. The bone is dysplastic from birth. This condition often increases with age. The abnormality may not be noticed unless anterior bowing becomes prominent or fracture occurs. It has no spontaneous healing potential and requires surgery to attempt union. Multiple surgical procedures are sometimes required. After maturity, the bone behaves more normally. About one-half of cases are associated with neurofibromatosis. Other bones display congenital pseudarthrosis even more rarely, but not in the same patient.

- It affects the tibia, at the junction of the middle and distal third.
- It is almost always unilateral.
- If it is associated with neurofibromatosis, other skeletal findings may be present.
- Congenital pseudarthrosis may also occur in the forearm and the clavicle.
- Congenital pseudarthrosis only affects the right clavicle unless the patient has dextrocardia.

SYNONYMS

- Congenital kyphoscoliotic tibia
- Dysplastic tibia

GENETICS

Neurofibromatosis is an autosomal dominant disorder. Its gene is located on the long arm of chromosome 17 and normally codes for a tumor suppressor. Otherwise, congenital pseudarthrosis in the absence of neurofibromatosis is not an inherited disorder.

INCIDENCE

- Approximately 1 per 100,000 to 1 per 200,000 in the population are affected.
- Males and females are equally affected with all types of congenital pseudarthroses.

CAUSES

- The cause is unknown.
- Fracture usually occurs with minor or unrecognized trauma.
- The location in the tibia (distal segment) is in the most poorly vascularized region of the bone.
- Neurofibromatous tissue is not found in pseudarthrosis.

RISK FACTORS

Neurofibromatosis
Bowing and irregularity of the tibia

CLASSIFICATION

Congenital pseudarthrosis associated in some cases with neurofibromatosis
Isolated congenital pseudarthrosis: further classified by Boyd into dysplastic, cystic, and sclerotic types

ASSOCIATED CONDITION

Neurofibromatosis

ICD-9-CM

733.82 Congenital pseudarthrosis

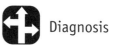 Diagnosis

SIGNS AND SYMPTOMS

Signs

- Increasing anterior and lateral bow of distal tibia
- Mild limp possible
- Possible signs of neurofibromatosis may be present, such as more than five café-au-lait spots, subcutaneous neurofibromas, scoliosis
- In the clavicle, bump in the right midclavicle with clicking
- Mild leg length difference possible

Symptoms

Minimal to absent pain

DIFFERENTIAL DIAGNOSIS

- Ossifying fibroma: a multiply cystic lesion affecting the anterior cortex of the tibia in older children
- Fibrous dysplasia: may produce bowing, but rarely fracture
- Posteromedial bow of the tibia: benign, self-correcting, bow in the same region of the tibia but in the other direction
- Focal fibrocartilaginous dysplasia: rare, usually self-correcting, bow of the proximal tibial metaphysis, which rarely fractures
- Nonunion after fracture or osteotomy of the distal tibia

PHYSICAL EXAMINATION

- Inspect for signs of neurofibromatosis.
- Assess for limb length discrepancy and stability.
- Perform a strength examination.
- Assess the foot for size, stability, and plantigrade status.

LABORATORY TESTS

No characteristic laboratory findings are noted, and no special tests are indicated routinely.

PATHOLOGIC FINDINGS

The pseudarthrosis resembles that of any other cause. A thick cuff of hamartomatous tissue encircles the tibia. This contains inactive fibroblasts, and there are no Schwann cells, axons, or perineural cells.

IMAGING PROCEDURES

- Plain anteroposterior and lateral films display the lesion in the distal tibia and fibula.
- Magnetic resonance imaging is not routinely indicated.
- Even before fracture, one or both of the following signs may be evident:

—Cyst formation and sclerosis in the lesion
—Local tapering

- Once the fracture appears, it may be characterized as atrophic or hypertrophic.
- A search for neurofibromatosis should be conducted. However, the full-blown signs of neurofibromatosis may not appear until later in the first decade of life.
- If vascularized bone grafting is indicated, a preoperative angiogram is useful to demonstrate vascular anatomy.

Management

GENERAL MEASURES

- The leg should be monitored in a splint to rule out increasing deformity.
- Electrical stimulation may help to increase the chances of success.
- If the lesion has not fractured, a brace should be provided for protection.
- If the lesion is fractured, surgery is always required.

SURGICAL TREATMENT

- Intramedullary rod with bone graft: This is left in place until maturity.
- Ilizarov treatment: Distraction and compression of the fracture site stimulate a healing response.
- Free vascularized fibula graft: This involves transporting a living, normal fibula with its blood supply to increase chances of success.
- As a last resort, if many different treatments do not succeed, Syme's amputation through the ankle may be elected by the family to allow the child to proceed with physical activities.

PHYSICAL THERAPY

Physical therapy is not necessary.

MEDICAL TREATMENT

Medications do not affect the success of treatment.

PATIENT EDUCATION

- The family should be educated about the natural history of the lesion, that is, the propensity for fracture, the need for bracing, the tendency to nonunion, treatment options, improvement in biology (increased chance of healing and less likelihood of refracture) after puberty. With this knowledge, they will be more understanding of the multiple procedures sometimes needed for healing.
- Rough play should be avoided as much as possible.
- Prevention of fracture or refracture by use of a brace is commonly practiced.

MONITORING

The patient should be seen every 3 to 6 months to rule out progressive bowing and leg length inequality and to check brace fit.

COMPLICATIONS

- Nonunion of defect after surgical procedure
- Angular deformity, owing to small size and bowing of distal fragment
- Recurrence of fracture, even months to years after apparent healing
- Foot and ankle stiffness
- Limb length inequality

PROGNOSIS

- Good: 80% to 90% may be made to heal.
- Refracture may occur even after union.
- Refracture rate and nonunion rate decline after puberty.

RECOMMENDED READING

Anderson DJ, Schoenecker PL, Sheridan JJ. Use of an intramedullary rod for treatment of congenital pseudarthrosis of the tibia. *J Bone Joint Surg Am* 1992;74:161–168.

Morrissy RT, Riseborough EJ, Hall JE. Congenital pseudarthrosis of the tibia. *J Bone Joint Surg Br* 1981;63:367–375.

Weiland AJ, Weiss APC, Moore JR, et al. Vascularized fibular grafts in treatment of congenital pseudarthrosis of the tibia. *J Bone Joint Surg Am* 1990;72:654–662.

Cubital Tunnel Syndrome

 Basics

DESCRIPTION

Cubital tunnel syndrome consists of pain and paresthesias over the medial border of the forearm and hand, as well as weakness in an ulnar nerve distribution from compression of the ulnar nerve as it passes through the cubital tunnel at the elbow.

It affects the elbow, forearm, and hand in the ulnar nerve distribution and is most commonly seen in adults. Males and females are affected equally.

SYNONYMS

Ulnar tunnel syndrome

INCIDENCE

This is the second most common entrapment neuropathy in the upper extremity (carpal tunnel syndrome is first).

CAUSES

The ulnar nerve is compressed as it passes through the cubital tunnel at the medial side of the elbow. This may compress the blood vessels that feed the nerve and may create symptoms.

Possible causes of the compression include the following:

- Enlarged medial head of the triceps muscle
- Trauma
- Recurrent dislocation of the nerve from the tunnel
- Arthritis (bony spurs)
- Ganglia
- Abnormal muscles (anconeus epitrochlearis)

RISK FACTORS

Diabetes

ASSOCIATED CONDITION

Thoracic outlet syndrome

ICD-9-CM

354.2 Cubital tunnel syndrome

 Diagnosis

The diagnosis is made clinically, with aid from nerve conduction studies.

SIGNS AND SYMPTOMS

- Vague, aching pain
- Paresthesias
- Numbness over the medial forearm, hand, and occasionally, upper arm

DIFFERENTIAL DIAGNOSIS

- Thoracic outlet syndrome
- C-8–T-⊥ cervical root compression
- Compression of the ulnar nerve at the wrist (Guyon's canal)
- Carpal tunnel syndrome

PHYSICAL EXAMINATION

- Note decreased sensation in the ulnar nerve distribution.
- Check for intrinsic weakness by placing a sheet of paper between the patient's thumb and first finger and attempting to pull the paper away as the patient resists.
- Look for intrinsic muscle wasting, especially of the first dorsal interosseous muscle.
- Percussion test (Tinel's sign): Tapping over the ulnar nerve at the elbow causes a reproduction of symptoms.
- Elbow flexion test: Keeping the elbow fully flexed (and the wrist in neutral or extension to avoid carpal tunnel symptoms) for 1 minute causes a reproduction of the symptoms.
- Order nerve conduction studies (slowed across the elbow).

PATHOLOGIC FINDINGS

At decompression, one can usually find specific sites of nerve compression.

IMAGING PROCEDURES

Anteroposterior radiography of the elbow is indicated.

Management

GENERAL MEASURES

Nonoperative treatment involves splinting the elbow in extension to relieve acute symptoms.

SURGICAL TREATMENT

- Consider surgery, if symptoms continue after 3 months of conservative therapy.
- Many procedures have been described.
- Procedures usually consist of some form of decompression of the nerve in the canal.
- Operations often involve transposition of the nerve out of the canal in an anterior direction.

MEDICAL TREATMENT

- Nighttime elbow extension splints with the forearm held in neutral or supination
- Avoid prolonged elbow flexion.

PATIENT EDUCATION

Patients are counseled to avoid activities that exacerbate their symptoms.

MONITORING

Motor and sensory examinations are performed at follow-up visits.

PREVENTION

Repetitive work activities should be avoided if they cause symptoms.

COMPLICATIONS

Reflex sympathetic dystrophy and nerve irritation may occur after surgery.

PROGNOSIS

- Conservative therapy: 50% excellent results
- Surgical therapy: good to excellent results in nearly all patients

RECOMMENDED READING

Eversmann WW. Entrapment in compression neuropathies. In: Green DP, ed. *Operative hand surgery*, 3rd ed. New York: Churchill Livingstone, 1993:1356–1385.

Wright II, Phillip E, Jobe MT. Tardy ulnar nerve palsy and cubital tunnel syndrome. In: Crenshaw AH, ed. *Campbell's operative orthopaedics*. St. Louis: Mosby–Year Book, 1992:2261–2263.

Basics

DESCRIPTION

Deep venous thrombosis (DVT) is thrombosis of deep venous plexus of the legs (Fig. 1). Thrombus may embolize and can result in fatal pulmonary embolism (PE).

INCIDENCE

• Without prophylaxis, orthopaedic patients who have a hip fracture are at highest risk. Risks within this group are as follows:

—40% to 80% risk of calf DVT
—10% to 20% risk of proximal DVT
—1% to 5% risk of fatal PE

• These conditions can affect any age group; however, patients older than 40 years of age are at increased risk.
• DVT and PE affect males and females equally.

CAUSE

The triad of endothelial injury, blood injury, and clotting abnormalities causes these conditions.

RISK FACTORS

• Age greater than 40 years
• Prolonged immobility or paralysis
• History of DVT or PE
• Cancer
• Obesity
• Varicose veins
• Congestive heart failure
• Myocardial infarction
• Stroke
• Fractures of the pelvis, hip, or leg
• High-dose estrogen use
• Hypercoagulable states

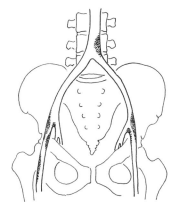

Fig. 1. Deep venous thrombosis is most serious in the iliac veins.

CLASSIFICATION

The clinician should distinguish whether the DVT is above or below the popliteal fossa:

• Thrombi below the popliteal fossa do not embolize.
• Fifty percent of thrombi at or above the popliteal fossa will embolize.

ASSOCIATED CONDITIONS

• Hypercoagulable states
• Cancer
• Prior history of deep venous thrombosis

ICD-9-CM

453.9 Venous embolism and thrombosis, of unspecified site

 Diagnosis

SIGNS AND SYMPTOMS

DVT and PE manifest few specific symptoms, and the clinical diagnosis is neither sensitive nor unreliable.

Deep Venous Thrombosis

• Pain and swelling in the leg and thigh
• Phlebitis also possible

Pulmonary Embolus

• Dyspnea
• Pleuritic chest pain
• Hemoptysis
• Tachypnea
• Acute right ventricular strain
• Rubs or cackles in the lung fields

DIFFERENTIAL DIAGNOSIS

Lower Leg Thrombosis

• Phlebitis
• Cellulitis
• Deep or superficial wound infection
• Ruptured Baker's cyst

Pulmonary Embolus

• Acute myocardial infarction
• Congestive heart failure
• Pneumonia
• Fat emboli syndrome

PHYSICAL EXAMINATION

• Calf pain with increased pain with dorsiflexion of the foot
• Swelling of the calf (may be measured and compared from left to right)
• Swelling of the dorsum of the foot

LABORATORY TESTS

• DVT: none
• PE: arterial blood gas hypoxemia

PATHOLOGIC FINDINGS

• A clot develops in the lower extremity, generally the calf veins, and propagates proximally.
• Clots at or above the popliteal fossa can embolize.
• Most PE are silent; however, there is a 0.2% to 0.4% risk of fatal PE after major orthopaedic procedures.

SPECIAL TESTS

Electrocardiography

• Classic findings after massive PE are those of acute cor pulmonale: S waves in lead I and Q wave with T-wave inversion in lead III.
• In less severe PE, sinus tachycardia and new arrhythmias may be present.

Impedance Plethysmography

• Temporary obstruction to venous outflow by application of a pneumatic cuff around the mid-thigh, followed by rapid deflation, leads to calf volume changes, which also cause changes in electrical resistance (impedance).
• This test is sensitive for proximal DVT.
• It has low sensitivity for detection of distal DVT and cannot be used for detection of pelvic DVT.
• Because of these limitations, it is rarely used.

Deep Venous Thrombosis

IMAGING PROCEDURES

Doppler Ultrasonography

- Sensitivity for detection of DVT is operator dependent.
- It is more sensitive for calf and distal thigh thrombosis.
- Sensitivity decreases in the upper thigh and pelvic veins.

Venography

- This is the current standard for the detection of DVT.
- It is 100% sensitive and specific.
- It provides visualization of the entire deep venous system, but it is expensive and invasive.

Chest Radiography

- It is used to detect PE.
- Results are generally normal; however, a pleural effusion or wedge-shaped pulmonary infarction may be noted.

Ventilation-Perfusion Scan

- A normal ventilation-perfusion scan excludes clinically and hemodynamically significant PE.
- An abnormal scan showing perfusion defects does not necessarily confirm PE.

Pulmonary Angiography

- This is the current gold standard for the detection of PE.
- It is 100% sensitive and specific, but it is expensive and invasive.

Spiral Chest Computed Tomography

- It is sensitive and specific for PE detection.
- It has virtually replaced pulmonary angiography.

Management

GENERAL MEASURES

Prophylaxis

Anticoagulants

- Anticoagulant prophylaxis is indicated with the following agents for all patients undergoing major orthopaedic procedures, to prevent the formation of DVT:

- Aspirin
- Warfarin (Coumadin)
- Low-molecular-weight heparin

All are effective in reducing the incidence of DVT.

Pneumatic Compression

These devices applied intraoperatively and postoperatively have also been shown to be effective.

Vena Cava Filter

A vena cava filter may be placed prophylactically in high-risk patients in whom anticoagulation is contraindicated.

Deep Venous Thrombosis above the Popliteal Fossa

- Patients should be immediately anticoagulated or have a caval filter placed.
- Patients should also be placed on bed rest to decrease the chance of embolization.

Deep Venous Thrombosis below the Popliteal Fossa

- Treatment is controversial.
- Many studies advocate less aggressive anticoagulation (i.e., aspirin and follow-up) and Doppler ultrasonography to rule out propagation of the clot.

Activity

Patients with clots above the knee should be placed on strict bed rest to decrease the chance of embolization.

MEDICAL TREATMENT

Treatment consists of anticoagulants.

PATIENT EDUCATION

Patients at risk are told the warning signs of deep venous thrombosis—calf pain, calf and foot swelling that persists despite elevation and the symptoms of pulmonary embolism—chest pain, cough, and shortness of breath.

PREVENTION

- Chemical prophylaxis
- Mechanical blood flow propagation
- Early mobilization

MONITORING

This varies, depending on the anticoagulant chosen.

COMPLICATIONS

- Increased risk of DVT in the future
- PE
- Death

PROGNOSIS

- Prophylactic anticoagulation and the use of pneumatic compression devices to prevent the formation of DVT have been highly successful.
- Numerous studies have found the incidence of DVT to be less than half in patients treated with these modalities.
- Spinal or epidural anesthesia has been associated with a significantly reduced incidence of DVT when compared with general anesthesia.

RECOMMENDED READING

Clagett GP, Anderson FA, Heit J, et al. Prevention of venous thromboembolism. *Chest* 1995;108:312S–334S.

Kelley MA, Carson JL, Palevsky M, et al. Diagnosing pulmonary embolism: new facts and strategies. *Ann Intern Med* 1991;114:300–306.

Kutty K. Pulmonary embolism. *Postgrad Med* 1990;88:72–88.

Basics

DESCRIPTION

Developmental dysplasia or dislocation of the hip covers a spectrum of varying degrees of superolateral displacement of the femur and deformation of the acetabulum, developing mostly *in utero* or rarely in infancy. It is occasionally first discovered in teens with a limp or pain. This probably represents a mildly subluxed hip that could not be detected on physical examination.

SYNONYMS

- Developmental dysplasia of the hip
- Congenital dislocation of the hip (old term)
- Hip dysplasia
- Unstable hip

GENETICS

Increased risk is noted in persons with a positive family history, but no Mendelian pattern has been established.

INCIDENCE

- The incidence is 1 in 200 births including all degrees of instability and 1 in 1,000 births for full dislocation.
- Females are affected four times as often as males because of increased ligamentous laxity.

CAUSES

- Dysplasia occurs because of unfavorable forces on the hip *in utero*.
- Adduction of the limb, such as with oligohydramnios, directs the femoral head to the edge of the acetabulum.
- Breech position increases hamstring tension and thus the force across the hip.
- Ligamentous laxity, greater in females and in some families, also increases the risk.
- The earlier *in utero* these factors develop, the more severe is the dysplasia.
- Postpartum factors such as a contralateral abduction contracture or swaddling of the limbs have also been reported as causative.

RISK FACTORS

- Breech position
- First-born status
- Female gender
- Oligohydramnios
- Family history

CLASSIFICATION

Dysplasia may present along a spectrum of severity:

- A subluxatable hip is reduced but can be subluxated with pressure and goes back to the reduced position.
- A dislocatable hip can be fully dislocated and reduced.
- A dislocated hip rests in a dislocated position and reduces only with manual effort.

ASSOCIATED CONDITIONS

- Muscular torticollis
- Foot deformities
- Genetic syndromes (especially skeletal dysplasia)

ICD-9-CM

754.31 Congenital dislocation of the hip (unilateral)
754.32 Congenital dislocation of the hip (bilateral)
754.33 Congenital subluxation of the hip (unilateral)
754.34 Congenital subluxation of the hip (bilateral)

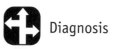 Diagnosis

SIGNS AND SYMPTOMS

No symptoms occur in the first few years of life. Only careful physical examination for a gentle clunk of the hip out of (Barlow's sign), or into (Ortolani's sign), the acetabulum shows the problem. The affected hip may rest in slight adduction and may have a deeper proximal thigh crease, but these signs are not constant. The abduction of the affected limb is usually less than 50 degrees because of the changed center of rotation. This may be noted by the parent while changing the infant's diapers. A click may be felt in the hip, but this is a nonspecific sign, because a click is often felt in normal hips and comes from the meniscus of the knee fascia lata or a synovial fold. The clunk of instability is usually lost after about 6 months, when the dislocation becomes more fixed.

The child with a dysplastic hip may begin to walk on time or just a few months late. After walking age, the thigh crease may become more pronounced and the circumference may be decreased. Trendelenburg's limp may be noted (the pelvis drops when the patient stands on the dysplastic side). If both sides are affected, there may be increased lumbar lordosis. Pain develops only after cartilage degeneration starts at 18 years of age at the earliest, and often much later. Associated conditions should raise the suspicion of hip dysplasia.

DIFFERENTIAL DIAGNOSIS

- Benign soft tissue click from the hip or knee fascia
- Neuromuscular hip dysplasia from muscle imbalance in cerebral palsy or spina bifida, occurring years later and having different treatment options
- Congenital short femur and coxa vara, but with located hip

Developmental Dysplasia of the Hip

PHYSICAL EXAMINATION

- Hip abduction is assessed.
- Ortolani's and Barlow's tests should be documented on all newborns and repeated during well-baby checks:

—Baby warm, quiet, and relaxed on parent's lap
—One hip at a time
—Gentle downward pressure on knee or thigh with adduction
—Feeling whether hip goes partially or fully out (Barlow's test)
—Then abducting to feel it slide back in (Ortolani's test)
—Checking for hip abduction (less than 60 degrees is suspicious)

- With the patient's pelvis flat, note the height of the two knees with the thighs together (Galeazzi's test).
- Check gait in the older child.

PATHOLOGIC FINDINGS

The acetabulum is flattened posterosuperiorly. The femoral head is flattened anteriorly, and femoral anteversion is increased. Cartilage erosion and arthritis develop after the second decade.

IMAGING PROCEDURES

- Ultrasound study is indicated in the first 6 months before cartilage ossifies if abnormal examination or risk factors exist. An ultrasonographer experienced in hips is required.
- Arthrography shows the depth of reduction with a 90% good outcome if there is less than 5 mm space between the femoral head and the acetabulum.
- Plain radiographs are most useful after 5 months. Both the shape of the acetabulum and its relation to the femur should be assessed. Shenton's line should form a smooth arc from the neck of the femur to the superior ramus of the pubis. The femoral epiphysis should be medial to the outer edge of the acetabulum.
- Magnetic resonance imaging and computed tomography have only limited roles in usual cases of developmental hip dysplasia.

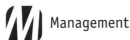 Management

GENERAL MEASURES

The hip should be reduced within the first 6 weeks if the dislocation is recognized. The earlier the diagnosis is made, the easier and safer the treatment will be. Even up until age 6 to 8 years, reduction is worthwhile.

SURGICAL TREATMENT

- A Medial or lateral approach to the hip joint is used to relieve the structures inside the joint that are blocking reduction.
- Osteotomy (cutting the bones) of the pelvis or femur is done to realign the joint surface.

Age 6 to 24 Months

Closed or open reduction is performed with the patient under anesthesia. Many surgeons proceed with a period of skin traction first to stretch the soft tissues. After reduction, a spica cast is applied for 3 to 6 months.

Age More than 24 Months

Open reduction is done, usually including a femoral osteotomy or iliac osteotomy. The results of surgical reduction decline with the increasing age of the child.

PHYSICAL THERAPY

A minimal need exists for physical therapy because children regain strength and motion on their own with time.

MEDICAL TREATMENT

Treatment varies according to age:

Newborn

Click and subluxation are followed with serial examinations. Many patients improve within 1 week.

Newborn to 6 Months

Persistent instability is treated with an abduction brace such as Pavlik's harness, which flexes the hip beyond 90 degrees. Bracing should be done by an orthopaedist familiar with pediatrics. The hip should reduce within 3 weeks, and there should be ultrasound or radiographic confirmation. A full-time brace is used until the hip is clinically stable, then a part-time brace is used until the hip is radiographically normal.

PATIENT EDUCATION

- Skin monitoring around casts and braces is important.
- Infants in Pavlik's harness should wear the device continuously until the hip is stable.
- Older children are treated in a spica (body) cast, so walking is not possible.
- Special car seats and wheelchairs are available.

PREVENTION

- No effective means exists to prevent this problem.
- Early detection is most important.
- Patients with hip dysplasia should have their children carefully examined.

MONITORING

After treatment of a dysplastic hip, follow-up care is needed until the patient reaches maturity. Even after successful reduction of the hip, there is a 10% to 25% chance of incomplete remodeling of the femur and acetabulum that may require osteotomy.

COMPLICATIONS

- Redislocation (5%)
- Residual dysplasia (25%)
- Avascular necrosis (10%) if the blood supply to the upper femur is disturbed by the process of reduction (It may not be possible to fully reverse this process fully.)

PROGNOSIS

Untreated complete dislocation results in a permanent waddling gait and pain by age 30 to 50 years at the latest. Patients with subluxed, but not dislocated, hips may have pain earlier. Hips that are successfully treated early may have normal function.

RECOMMENDED READING

Asher M.A. Screening for congenital dislocation of the hip. *Pediatr Clin North Am* 1986;33:1335–1353.

Churgay CA, Caruthers BS. Diagnosis and treatment of congenital dislocation of the hip. *Am Fam Physician* 1993;45:1217–1228.

Harcke HT, Kumar JS. The role of ultrasound in diagnosis and management of congenital dislocation and dysplasia of the hip. *J Bone Joint Surg Am* 1991;73:622–628.

Ilfeld FW, Westin GW. "Missed" or developmental dislocation of the hip. *Clin Orthop* 1986;203:276–281.

Basics

DESCRIPTION

Discitis is an infection of the disc space and vertebral end plates that is caused by either hematogenous or postoperative inoculation. It affects intervertebral discs of the spine, and the lower lumbar discs are most commonly involved, but the infection may occur in any disc.

INCIDENCE

- Hematogenous infection is uncommon.
- Mean age of occurrence of hematogenous (spontaneous) discitis is 7 years.
- The incidence of infection after discectomy is less than 1%.
- Patients of any age may be affected, however.

CAUSES

Discitis is caused by bacterial infection. The blood supply to the disc comes from the adjacent vertebral body. Vessels cross the cartilaginous end plate in children until about the age of 8 years, and the resultant vascularity renders children of this age more susceptible to infection. The causative organism is most commonly *Staphylococcus,* except in the compromised host or intravenous drug abuser. In these patients, biopsy is indicated.

RISK FACTORS

- Compromised host
- Intravenous drug abuser
- Patient after discectomy

CLASSIFICATION

- Spontaneous (hematogenous)
- Iatrogenic (after discectomy or discogram)

ASSOCIATED CONDITION

Vertebral osteomyelitis

ICD-9-CM

722.90 Discitis

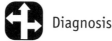 Diagnosis

SIGNS AND SYMPTOMS

Symptoms

- Back pain, usually insidious in onset but increasing with time
- Abdominal pain
- Loss of appetite
- Malaise

Signs

- Back stiffness
- Refusal to walk
- Pain on spinal percussion
- Loss of lordosis
- Fever: usually low-grade, but may be absent

DIFFERENTIAL DIAGNOSIS

- Tuberculosis (usually shows more destruction of adjacent bone)
- Vertebral osteomyelitis (more destruction of bone than disc, but these two entities may merge)

PHYSICAL EXAMINATION

- Note pressure or the absence of normal lumbar lordosis.
- Look for pain or refusal to bend forward.
- Look for pain on paraspinal percussion.
- Look for pain on abdominal palpation in lumbar discitis.
- Neurologic examination remains normal, except in late presentations of fulminant discitis.

LABORATORY TESTS

- White blood count, erythrocyte sedimentation rate, and C-reactive protein are usually mildly elevated but may be normal.
- Blood culture should be done but is positive less than 30% of the time.
- No specific laboratory tests exists for this disorder.

PATHOLOGIC FINDINGS

- Chronic inflammation (Fig. 1)
- Destruction of disc structure and end plates

IMAGING PROCEDURES

- Plain films are positive only after several weeks, and they show irregularity and narrowing of the disc space, with mild bony involvement.
- For suspected cases of discitis, before the radiograph shows abnormalities, a bone scan or magnetic resonance imaging shows the pathologic features. Magnetic resonance imaging gives more detailed anatomic information, but bone scan is an acceptable alternative.

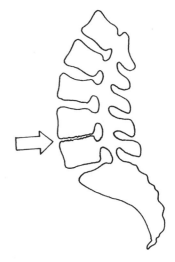

Fig. 1. Discitis produces narrowing or obliteration of the disc and irregularity of the adjacent vertebral surfaces.

Discitis

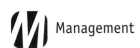 Management

GENERAL MEASURES

- Rest
- Immobilization
- Antibiotics

For childhood spontaneous discitis, no biopsy or débridement is needed, because treatment of staphylococcal infection is virtually always successful. This treatment should be given intravenously if the patient is severely ill or orally if the patient is only mildly symptomatic. Bed rest and bracing may be used if pain is pronounced. For discitis in the compromised host, biopsy and drainage should be done.

SURGICAL TREATMENT

- Biopsy and drainage, if needed. Surgical reconstruction of the spine segment may be indicated in adults with significant disc space or end plate.
- Biopsy may be done from an anterolateral or a posterolateral approach with fluoroscopic guidance.
- Drainage, if indicated, is usually done from an anterior approach to allow adequate visualization, débridement, and safety.

PHYSICAL THERAPY

Therapy is useful in adults with severe back stiffness after treatment has begun.

MEDICAL TREATMENT

- For routine spontaneous discitis, oxacillin, dicloxacillin, and cephalosporin are indicated.
- For complicated cases or in compromised hosts, broad-spectrum antibiotics effective against gram-negative and anaerobic organisms should also be added.
- Nonsteroidal antiinflammatory agents or mild narcotics may help patients with severe pain initially until the infection is controlled.

PATIENT EDUCATION

The patient may resume activity according to symptom level. Activities such as jumping, lifting, and bending forward should be discouraged until symptoms subside.

MONITORING

- Physical examination is the most useful means to monitor healing of the infection.
- The examiner should check for tenderness to percussion, as well as range of forward flexion.
- Radiographs and sedimentation rate lag far behind the clinical course.

COMPLICATIONS

Persistence of infection requires accurate identification of the organism and adequate débridement if symptoms do not improve in the first 1 to 2 weeks.

PROGNOSIS

Prognosis is good once the infection is cleared. After childhood discitis, the vertebrae adjacent to the infected disc usually develop a spontaneous painless fusion. In adults, this does not always occur, and backache may persist.

RECOMMENDED READING

Lifeso RM, Weaver P Harder EH. Tuberculous spondylitis in adults. *J Bone Joint Surg Am* 1985;67:1405–1410.

Morrissy RT. Bone and joint sepsis. In: Morrissy RT, Weinstein SL, eds. *Lovell and Winter's pediatric orthopaedics,* 4th ed. Philadelphia: Lippincott–Raven, 1996:601–604.

Wenger DR, Bobechko WP, Gilday R. The spectrum of intervertebral disc space infections in children. *J Bone Joint Surg Am* 1978;60:100–108.

Basics

DESCRIPTION

Discoid meniscus is a thickened, pancake-shaped lateral meniscus of developmental origin (Fig. 1). It often causes clicking or locking of the knee in childhood or early adulthood. It may be unilateral or bilateral.

SYNONYM

• Wrisberg's meniscus

INCIDENCE

• The approximate prevalence is 4% in United States and higher in Japan.
• Most cases present in late childhood or early adolescence.
• The incidence is equivalent in males and females.

CAUSE

Smillie's Theory

• A lack of resorption of the central cartilaginous disc occurs during normal development.
• This theory is doubtful because no stage of development has an entire disc.

Kaplan's theory

• A normally shaped meniscus with abnormal tibial attachments undergoes a change from the repeated trauma of abnormal mediolateral motion.
• This theory does not explain the stable discoid meniscus.
• The pathogenesis is likely a combination of these two theories.

CLASSIFICATION

• Complete discoid meniscus: covers entire lateral tibial plateau
• Incomplete discoid meniscus: meniscus is larger than normal, but does not cover the entire lateral plateau
• Wrisberg: ligament type; unstable, lacks posterior attachment of meniscus to tibia

ICD-9-CM

717.5 Discoid meniscus

 Diagnosis

SIGNS AND SYMPTOMS

• Many cases are asymptomatic.
• Presentation is highly variable, depending on the type of meniscus and the presence or absence of a tear.
• The classic snapping-knee syndrome (rare) is characterized by a "clunk" at the terminal limits of flexion and extension (Fig. 2)
• It may be associated with pain, clicking, swelling, locking, popping, and blocks to motion.
• The onset is often insidious, without a history of trauma.
• Occasionally, ambulation with flexed stance, quadriceps atrophy, or bulge at anterolateral joint line with full flexion occurs.
• If symptoms are acute or associated with trauma, an acute tear may be the cause.

DIFFERENTIAL DIAGNOSIS

• Acute meniscal tear
• Osteochondritis dissecans or osteochondral fracture
• Physeal fracture
• Fracture of the tibial eminence
• Anterior cruciate ligament tear

PHYSICAL EXAMINATION

• Usually, little to no effusion is present in the knee.
• May be mild tenderness, may occur at the joint line, but it is not as severe as with an acute meniscus tear.
• Often, a pop or click is noted with McMurray's test (rotating the knee in and out in the flexed position).
• The examiner may note a block to full extension or the patient's apprehension when the knee is straightened.
• The classic form may be characterized by a bulge or prominence on the anterior joint line when the knee is straightened, caused by the thickened meniscus bulging out from the knee.
• Some clicking of the knee is normal, as long as there is no locking or pain.

PATHOLOGIC FINDINGS

• Disc-shaped meniscus
• Stable variant: normal tibial ligaments
• Unstable variant: absence of the posterolateral tibial attachments

SPECIAL TESTS

McMurray's test is a knee examination including palpating for clicking or locking at the joint line with flexion and extension.

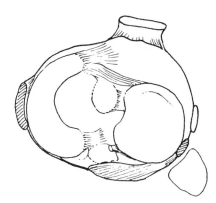

Fig. 1. A diseased lateral meniscus lacks the normal semilunar shape and covers the entire lateral side of the tibia.

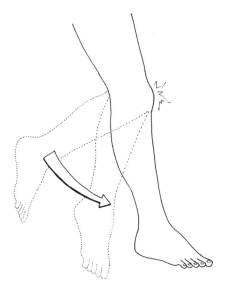

Fig. 2. Clicking in a joint line bulge on extension may be a sign of discoid meniscus.

Discoid Meniscus

IMAGING PROCEDURES

Plain Radiography

- Wide lateral joint space
- Lateral joint lipping
- Cupping of the lateral tibial plateau
- Flattening of the lateral femoral condyle
- Calcification of the meniscus (rarely)
- Obliquity of the joint space or degenerative changes

Magnetic Resonance Imaging

- Three or more contiguous 5-mm sagittal sections demonstrating continuity between the anterior and posterior horns
- Block "bow tie" appearance on the coronal view with increased width of the mid-anteroposterior diameter

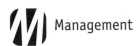 Management

GENERAL MEASURES

- Asymptomatic patients should be observed.
- Symptomatic patients often require surgical treatment, which varies depending on whether a tear is present and whether the meniscus is stable or unstable.
- Conservative methods are rarely helpful in the patient with symptomatic discoid meniscus, although a trial of immobilization may be attempted in patients with acute-onset cases.
- Patients may resume normal activity when symptoms resolve.

SURGICAL TREATMENT

Stable Meniscus

- Formerly, complete meniscectomy was employed.
- Partial meniscectomy or saucerization (trimming) may be done to form a more normal-appearing meniscus; this method has shown improved results.

Unstable Meniscus

- Saucerization and reattachment to the posterolateral capsule are done to attempt to preserve the meniscus.
- Complete meniscectomy is indicated if the patient has degenerative changes or a large meniscal tear.
- Most surgical procedures can be performed arthroscopically.

PATIENT EDUCATION

- Observation, if the discoid meniscus is asymptomatic
- Increased risk of degenerative changes after total meniscectomy

MONITORING

Patients should be followed on an as-needed basis.

COMPLICATIONS

- Degenerative joint disease possible if symptoms continue
- Recurrent meniscal tears

PROGNOSIS

- It depends on the type. Patients with stable discoid meniscus have good results with saucerization.
- Most patients have a good result from surgery, with no long-term sequelae.

RECOMMENDED READING

Dickhaut SC, DeLee JC. The discoid lateral-meniscus syndrome. *J Bone Joint Surg Am* 1982;64:1068–1073.

Fujikawa K, Iseki F, Mikura Y. Partial resection of the discoid meniscus in the child's knee. *J Bone Joint Surg Br* 1981;63:391–395.

Jordan MR. Lateral meniscal variants: evaluation and treatment. *J Am Acad Orthop Surg* 1996;4:191–200.

Nathan PA, Cole SC. Discoid meniscus: a clinical and pathologic study. *Clin Orthop* 1969;64:107–113.

Basics

DESCRIPTION

Dupuytren's contracture is a proliferative disorder of subcutaneous palmar fibrous tissue (fascia) that occurs in the form of nodules and cords and results in contractures of the finger joints (Fig. 1). It occurs typically in men in the fifth to seventh decades. Younger patients are more likely to have rapid progression of disease with poorer long-term results and frequent recurrences. Aggressive, early onset is seen in a subgroup of patients with Dupuytren's diathesis.

SYNONYM

Dupuytren's disease

GENETICS

- The disorder is autosomal dominant with variable penetrance.
- Only 10% of patients with Dupuytren's contractures have a positive family history.

INCIDENCE

- Greatest in Northern Europe and in immigrants of Celtic origin
- Incidence in the United States 2% to 3% of the general population
- Hand dominance not a factor
- More frequent and severe in patients with epilepsy, alcoholism, diabetes, and chronic obstructive pulmonary disease
- More common in men than women: ratios 2:1 to 10:1
- In women, usually later onset and less severe disease

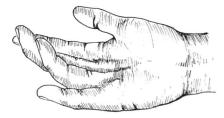

Fig. 1. Dupuytren's contracture most commonly involves the ring and small fingers and produces cordlike tightening over the flexion tendon.

CAUSES

- Unknown
- Strong evidence for hereditary factors, possibly through transmission of defective genes responsible for collagen formation
- Associated with several medical conditions including epilepsy, alcoholism, diabetes, and chronic obstructive pulmonary disease

RISK FACTORS

- White race
- Northern European descent
- Increased age

ASSOCIATED CONDITIONS

- Alcoholism
- Epilepsy
- Diabetes
- Chronic obstructive pulmonary disease

ICD-9-CM

728.6 Dupuytren's contracture

 Diagnosis

SIGNS AND SYMPTOMS

- It usually begins with one or more painful nodules in the palmar fascia of the ring and little finger rays.
- It is often associated with skin dimpling over or around the nodules.
- It is often bilateral (45%).
- It is rarely symmetric.
- As the disease progresses, the digital fascia become involved, usually producing first contractures of the metacarpophalangeal joints and then of the proximal interphalangeal joints (Fig. 2).

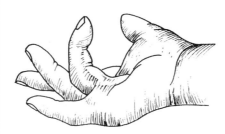

Fig. 2. In advanced Dupuytren's contracture, the finger is drawn up and impairs the use of the hand.

- Web space contractures can occur.
- Knuckle pads over the dorsum of the proximal interphalangeal joints are present in about 20% of patients. They are usually unnoticeable, but if they are large and prominent, they may be painful when hit.
- In the subgroup of patients with Dupuytren's diathesis, the disease involves the hands, feet, and penis. It is often associated with knuckle pads, plantar fibromatosis (Ledderhose's disease), and penile fibromatosis (Peyronie's disease).

DIFFERENTIAL DIAGNOSIS

- Arthritis
- Joint capsule contractures

PHYSICAL EXAMINATION

Hueston's table-top test is positive when the palm is placed on a flat surface and the digits, because of joint contractures, cannot be simultaneously placed fully on the same surface. A positive test is often an indication for the consideration of surgical management.

PATHOLOGIC FINDINGS

Histologically, the important cells are the myofibroblasts, which seem to undergo pathologic proliferation. An increase in the ratio of type III to type I collagen is found in Dupuytren's disease.

Dupuytren's Contracture

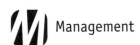 Management

GENERAL MEASURES

In the absence of contracture, or when a contracture is progressing slowly and is not disabling, the patient should be observed every 3 months.

SURGICAL TREATMENT

The five surgical procedures used in treating Dupuytren's contractures are as follows:

- Subcutaneous fasciotomy
- Partial (selective) fasciectomy
- Complete fasciectomy
- Fasciectomy with skin grafting
- Amputation

In choosing the best procedure for a given patient, the degree of contracture, the patient's age, occupation, and general health, the nutritional status of the palmar skin, and the presence or absence of arthritis should all be considered.

PHYSICAL THERAPY

The goals are to maintain the extension gained by the surgical procedure and to restore pre-operative flexion and function of the hand. A comfortable, well-fitted splint is an important adjunct to therapy. Physical therapists play a major role in recovery, and their programs should stress performance of independent exercises.

MEDICAL TREATMENT

Conservative management with vitamin E and splinting has been ineffective. Cortisone injection of nodules that have not yet formed cords has been shown to suppress their development. Currently, surgery is not indicated for static, painless nodules and rarely for knuckle pads. However, any degree of proximal interphalangeal joint involvement is an indication for early surgical intervention.

The frequency and duration of splinting vary with the severity of the disease. However, a minimum of 3 months is usually required, and many patients are instructed to wear a splint at night for an additional period of up to 3 months. Return to normal activity is usually anticipated within 2 months.

PATIENT EDUCATION

Patients should be aware that although metacarpophalangeal deformities can usually be corrected surgically, proximal interphalangeal deformities often may not. The patient must also realize that surgery cannot cure Dupuytren's disease. No effective means of prevention is known.

MONITORING

Patients need to be followed closely, each week during the first postoperative month, to help assess wound healing and to prevent stiffness. Once healed, follow-up may be on an as-needed basis.

COMPLICATIONS

Joint stiffness can usually be prevented with early physical therapy and patient education. Unfortunately, long-term complications often depend on the diathesis of the patient.

PROGNOSIS

The normal postoperative expectation is a full range of flexion and extension in 80% of patients seen primarily. The disease is likely to progress more rapidly and to recur more frequently in young male patients with a strong family history. In addition, patients with epilepsy and alcoholism tend to develop more severe disease. Although long-term recurrence rates vary from 26% to 80%, often only the young patient with a strong diathesis will need multiple repeat procedures.

RECOMMENDED READING

Hueston JT. Dupuytren's contracture. In: Jupiter JB, ed. Flynn's hand surgery. Baltimore: Williams & Wilkins, 1991:864–889.

McFarlane RM. Dupuytren's contracture. In: Green DP, ed. Operative hand surgery, 3rd ed. New York: Churchill Livingstone, 1993:563–591.

Milford L. The hand. In: Crenshaw AH, ed. Campbell's operative orthopaedics, 7th ed. St. Louis: CV Mosby, 1988:111–506.

Basics

DESCRIPTION

Ehlers-Danlos syndrome is a family of disorders involving connective tissue laxity, with many resultant abnormalities in the skeleton, vasculature, and other systems. At least 11 different subtypes of Ehlers-Danlos syndrome have been identified, with varying patterns of inheritance and genetic causes. They affect the skeleton, heart, vessels, coagulation system, eyes, and many other systems. The age at diagnosis varies from infancy to adulthood. Overall, males and females are equally affected.

GENETICS

- Types 1, 4, 8, and 11 are autosomal dominant.
- Types 5 and 9 are X-linked.
- The remainder are autosomal recessive in transmission.
- Many patients present as having a new mutation without a family history.

INCIDENCE

Incidence is impossible to portray accurately, owing to the large number of forms of this disorder and their varying degrees of severity.

CAUSES

- Type IV, the ecchymotic variety, is due to a disorder of type III collagen.
- Type VI (ocular-scoliotic) is the best characterized and is caused by a defect in lysine hydroxylase. This change results in decreased collagen cross-linking.
- Type VII (arthrochalasis multiplex congenita) is due to a defect in type I collagen.
- Type X (with platelet dysfunction) also results from a defect in type I collagen.

RISK FACTORS

A positive family history of the syndrome or of its major manifestations is a risk factor.

CLASSIFICATION

   I. Gravis (classic): aneurysms, rupture of hollow viscus, skin hyperextensibility, bruising, pigmented areas, and hernias
  II. Mitis: similar manifestations but milder
 III. Benign hypermobility syndrome: laxity, joint dislocations, mitral valve prolapse, and positive family history
 IV. Ecchymotic: thin skin, normal joints, aneurysms, and viscus rupture
  V. X-linked: intramuscular hemorrhagea and floppy baby characteristics
 VI. Ocular-scoliotic
VII. Arthrochalasis multiplex congenita: extreme joint laxity, short stature, and hip dislocations
VIII. Periodontosis: progressive periodontal disease
 IX. Occipital horns and skeletal dysplasia
  X. Platelet dysfunction
 XI. Familial joint laxity: patellar and hip dislocation

ICD-9-CM

756.83 Ehlers-Danlos syndrome

 Diagnosis

The diagnosis is made by medical geneticist on a clinical basis, with verification in some types by use of molecular testing.

SIGNS AND SYMPTOMS

Signs

- Lax skin (Fig. 1)
- Joint hypermobility (Fig. 2)
- Joint instability
- Scoliosis
- Ability of some affected persons to perform skeletal contortions impossible for nonaffected persons

Symptoms

- Multiple joint pains
- Vague musculoskeletal pains

DIFFERENTIAL DIAGNOSIS

- Marfan's syndrome is also characterized by laxity of major joints, but this is rarely symptomatic, and it has well-defined diagnostic criteria.
- Larsen's syndrome also presents with multiple joint dislocations, but there are contractures as well, and cervical kyphosis is common.
- Cutis laxa and pseudoxanthoma elasticum should also be ruled out in patients with predominant skin findings.

PHYSICAL EXAMINATION

- Record height.
- Observe the proportions of the skeleton.
- Systematically measure joint range of motion.
- Check the shoulders and knees for stability.
- Feel the quality of the skin.
- Note bruising.
- Pursue an ocular examination if there are any symptoms of deficit.
- Observe the spine for kyphosis.
- Carry out a forward-bend test for scoliosis.

LABORATORY TESTS

Light microscopic examination of the skin shows irregular collagen fibers.

SPECIAL TESTS

Molecular testing is available to confirm many, but not all, of the types of Ehlers-Danlos syndrome. An experienced genetics laboratory should be consulted.

PATHOLOGIC FINDINGS

- Light microscopic examination of the skin shows irregular collagen fibers.
- Gross examination of the aorta may show dis-

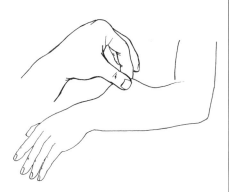

Fig. 1. Ehlers-Danlos syndrome is one of several conditions characterized by cutaneous laxity.

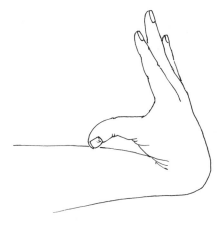

Fig. 2. Hypermobile joints are characteristic of Ehlers-Danlos syndrome.

Ehlers-Danlos Syndrome

secting aneurysms in type I, as well as myxomatous changes in the cardiac valves and redundant chordae tendineae.

IMAGING PROCEDURES

• Imaging of the heart and aorta should be carried out periodically for patients with types I and IV disorders.
• Plain radiographs should be obtained when physical examination suggests scoliosis, kyphosis, or spondyolisthesis.

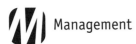 Management

GENERAL MEASURES

• Specialist referral for the systems listed earlier is indicated when problems are manifested by patient.
• One should use caution when recommending surgery for joint instability because the failure rate is higher than normal. Surgical treatment should not be undertaken in Ehlers-Danlos syndrome unless symptoms are severe.
• Fusion of joints may be necessary to provide stability.

SURGICAL TREATMENT

Fusion for scoliosis is indicated if curves exceed approximately 45 degrees and the patient's medical condition is otherwise satisfactory. Physical activity is generally encouraged, but it should be tailored to the patient and focused on low-impact sports.

PHYSICAL THERAPY

• Muscle strengthening may ameliorate some of the symptoms of joint instability, even if these symptoms are not eliminated.
• Physical therapy should also be helpful in educating patients about how to decrease frequency of joint dislocations.

PATIENT EDUCATION

• Genetic counseling should be offered.
• Understanding the nature of any cardiovascular abnormality should be taught, in case of medical emergency.
• Contact or high-impact sports should be discouraged.

PREVENTION

• Prevention of cardiovascular and bleeding emergencies should be goal of treatment.
• Reduction in frequency of joint dislocations may also be possible.

COMPLICATIONS

• Sudden death from cardiovascular complications
• Osteoarthritis of joints
• Visual deficits

PROGNOSIS

The foregoing complications lead to a moderate decline in the mean life expectancy.

RECOMMENDED READING

Badelon O, Bensahel H, Csukonyi Z. Congenital dislocation of the hip in Ehlers-Danlos syndrome. *Clin Orthop* 1990;255:138–142.

Beighton P, Horan F. Orthopaedic implications of the Ehlers-Danlos syndrome. *J Bone Joint Surg* 1969;51:444–448.

McKusick VA. Ehlers-Danlos syndrome. In: *Heritable disorders of connective tissue*. St. Louis: CV Mosby, 1972:292–302.

Basics

DESCRIPTION

The elbow can be affected by both inflammatory and noninflammatory arthropathies. Regardless of the underlying pathologic process, elbow arthritis generally presents with pain on range of motion and weight bearing of the affected extremity.

INCIDENCE

- This disorder is uncommon.
- It can occur in any age group.
- Males and females are affected equally.
- Most authorities recommend reserving total elbow arthroplasty for patients older then 60 years of age; however, a younger age is not a contraindication.

CAUSES

- Inflammatory arthropathies
- Trauma
- Overuse injuries

RISK FACTORS

- Rheumatoid arthritis
- History of septic arthritis
- Previous injury

ICD-9-CM

716.92 Elbow arthritis

 Diagnosis

SIGNS AND SYMPTOMS

Degenerative joint disease of the elbow presents as pain at the extremes of motion that is generally greater in extension than in flexion. A history of overuse or trauma is often present. Carrying of heavy objects, such as a briefcase or groceries, is possible only for short periods. In later stages, pain can be present with any range of motion, and a flexion contracture may develop. The anteroposterior and lateral radiographs show osteophyte formation and bony sclerosis of the elbow.

Inflammatory arthropathy can present with a similar pain profile; additionally, patients have signs of inflammation such as effusion and warmth. Early in the disease, the radiographs may be normal because only intense synovitis and effusion are present.

DIFFERENTIAL DIAGNOSIS

- Septic joint
- Osteomyelitis
- Elbow instability
- Elbow dislocation
- Triceps tendinitis
- Nerve entrapment syndromes

PHYSICAL EXAMINATION

Pain and limited range of motion are the earliest findings. Effusions are most easily palpated on the lateral side of the elbow. Ankylosis of the elbow develops with advanced disease.

LABORATORY TESTS

- Rheumatologic workup is indicated if an inflammatory arthropathy is suspected.
- Joint aspiration with cell count and differential is warranted if a septic joint is a concern.
- Joint fluid may also be sent for crystal analysis if crystalline arthropathy is suspected.

PATHOLOGIC FINDINGS

With rheumatoid arthritis, the synovium proliferates, and there is progressive destruction of the joint. The radial head is often destroyed, and valgus deformity occurs.

IMAGING PROCEDURES

Routine anteroposterior and lateral radiographs of the elbow are obtained.

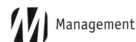 Management

GENERAL MEASURES

Operative treatment should be reserved for those patients in whom conservative measures have failed and who continue to have debilitating pain. Activity should be modified to suit the level of symptoms.

SURGICAL TREATMENT

Patients with osteoarthrosis may benefit from excision of olecranon and coronoid osteophytes, a procedure known as the Outerbridge-Kashiwagi arthroplasty. Patients with inflammatory arthropathies and osteoarthrosis involving more than the ulnohumeral joint may benefit from a total elbow arthroplasty.

PHYSICAL THERAPY

Strengthening and range of motion exercises are helpful in patients who respond to conservative management. A similar physical therapy regimen is critical after operative interventions, to obtain the highest level of functioning possible after arthroplasty or elbow replacement.

MEDICAL TREATMENT

Initial management should be conservative, with nonsteroidal anti-inflammatory medications, rest, and bracing or supportive devices. Caution should be used with bracing and immobilization of the elbow, because elbow stiffness and even ankylosis may occur quickly. Patients who are unresponsive to systemic antiinflammatory drugs may benefit from intraarticular steroid injections. Again, care must be exercised with this treatment option because improper aseptic technique can result in joint infection, and frequent injections can weaken tendinous and ligamentous structures.

PATIENT EDUCATION

Patients are shown how to avoid aggravating activities and are encouraged to maintain a functional range of motion.

MONITORING

Patients with rheumatoid arthritis are followed at 6- to 12-month intervals with anteroposterior and lateral radiographs.

COMPLICATIONS

Nonoperative Treatment

- Ankylosis
- Ulnar nerve palsy

Total Elbow Arthroplasty

- Infection
- Ulnar nerve irritation
- Aseptic loosening

RECOMMENDED READING

Clark CR, Bonfiglio M. *Orthopaedics*. New York: Churchill Livingstone, 1994:176–177.

Crenshaw AH, ed. *Campbell's operative orthopaedics,* 8th ed. St. Louis: CV Mosby, 1992:361–364.

Frymoyer JW, ed. *Orthopaedic knowledge update 4*. Rosemont, IL: American Academy of Orthopaedic Surgeons, 1993:342–347.

Elbow Dislocation

Basics

DESCRIPTION

Dislocation of the elbow mostly results from trauma. Posterior dislocation is most common. It most frequently involves people younger than 20 years of age. Rarely, elbow dislocation can occur in elderly patients after a fall.

INCIDENCE

• The highest incidence is in persons younger than 20 years of age.
• It represents 3% to 6% of all children's fractures and dislocations.

CLASSIFICATION

• Most elbow dislocations occur at the ulnohumeral joint.
• Classifications usually refer to the position of the ulna relative to the humerus after injury.
• Dislocations can be classified as posterior, anterior, medial, lateral, and divergent.

ASSOCIATED CONDITIONS

• Fracture of radius
• Fracture of ulna
• Fracture of humerus

ICD-9-CM

832.0 Elbow dislocation

Diagnosis

SIGNS AND SYMPTOMS

• Elbow dislocation occurs mostly after trauma.
• The patient presents with pain, swelling, elbow deformity, and inability to move the elbow.

DIFFERENTIAL DIAGNOSIS

The main differential diagnosis is whether there is an associated fracture.

PHYSICAL EXAMINATION

• Assess the patient's neurovascular status. The median, ulnar, radial, and anterior interosseous nerves can be injured at the time of dislocation. The radial nerve is least likely to be injured.
• Examine the functions of each nerve. The median nerve can also be injured at time of reduction by becoming entrapped in the joint. It is therefore crucial to check nerve function before and after reduction.
• Evaluate the patient for brachial artery injury. Neurovascular injury is an indication for immediate surgery.
• The upper extremity should be inspected for other injuries, such as Monteggia's fracture-dislocation.

• Check the function of the radial, median, and ulnar nerves.
• Palpate the radial and ulnar pulses.
• Palpate the forearm for increased turgor. Palpation should be done to rule out other injuries of the forearm.

IMAGING PROCEDURES

Anteroposterior and lateral views of the elbow are sufficient for diagnosis. They should be obtained with the elbow out of the splint, to rule out subtle intraarticular fractures and dislocations.

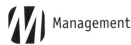

Management

GENERAL MEASURES

• The injured arm should be immobilized and elevated, with ice packs applied to elbow.
• The patient should be sent to the emergency department immediately.
• If any neurovascular injury is detected, a vascular or orthopaedic surgeon should be notified.

SURGICAL TREATMENT

Surgery is indicated for irreducible dislocation, open dislocation, neurovascular entrapment, and certain types of associated fractures. Open reduction and internal fixation are recommended for displaced radial head, olecranon, and supracondylar fractures if they are found with the dislocation. Acute repair of the medial collateral ligament is usually not necessary.

PHYSICAL THERAPY

Therapy involves range of motion and muscle strengthening.

MEDICAL TREATMENT

• The patient's neurovascular status is evaluated before and after reduction.
• The examiner rules out associated fractures.
• Most dislocations can be treated with closed reduction with the patient under sedation.
• Open reduction is indicated in irreducible dislocation, that is, one caused by soft tissue entrapment and free fragment in the joint, or changes in neurovascular status.
• Longitudinal traction, with gradual flexion and downward pressure on the forearm, usually reduces posterior or posterolateral dislocations.
• After reduction, elbow range of motion and stability should be checked with gentle range of motion and valgus and varus stress. Neurovascular function should be examined as well.
• Immobilization of the elbow in 90 degrees of flexion with a posterior splint is recommended.
• Duration of immobilization varies, depending on elbow stability, but in general it is 1 week.
• Prolonged immobilization should be avoided to prevent stiffness.
• Gradual range of motion and strengthening physical therapy should be started as soon as the immobilization device is removed.

• No lifting is allowed for 2 weeks, and the patient can begin gradual passive and active range of motion after immobilization is removed.

PATIENT EDUCATION

• Monitor for signs of compartment syndrome.
• Emphasize range-of-motion exercises at home.

MONITORING

The follow-up frequency varies with the individual surgeon. In general, immobilization should continue for about one week, depending on the stability of elbow. Clinical monitoring of compartment status and of neurovascular function is recommended for the first 12 to 24 hours.

COMPLICATIONS

• Decreased range of motion
• Neurovascular injury
• Persistent pain
• Arthritis

PROGNOSIS

• Most patients do well after closed reduction.
• The most common residual condition after dislocation is decreased range of motion (loss of 10 to 15 degrees of extension).
• Patients treated nonsurgically have a better prognosis.

RECOMMENDED READING

Boerboom AL, de Meyier HE, Verburg AD. Arthrolysis for post-traumatic stiffness of the elbow. *Int Orthop* 1993;17:346–349.

Breen TF, Gelberman RH, Ackerman GN. Elbow flexion contractures: treatment by anterior release and continuous passive motion. *J Hand Surg [Br]* 1988;13:286–287.

Morrey BF. Post-traumatic contracture of the elbow: operative treatment, including distraction arthroplasty. *J Bone Joint Surg Am* 1990;72:601–618.

Basics

DESCRIPTION

An enchondroma is a common benign lesion of mature hyaline cartilage in the medullary canal of the metaphysis or metadiaphysis of bone. Enchondromas most commonly (40%) involve the short tubular bones (usually proximal phalanx) of the hands and feet in adults.

- They may also involve the distal femur, proximmal humerus, and tibia.
- They are rare in the spine and pelvis.
- They do not form in bones that develop by membranous ossification.

INCIDENCE

- They account for 11% of benign bone tumors.
- They are the most common bone tumors of the hand and also are the most cause of destructive bone lesions in the hand.
- Two percent of people have a small cartilaginous island in the medullary canal of the femur.
- The peak age is the second decade, but the tumor is found in all age groups.
- The male-to-female ratio is equal.

CAUSES

- It may be the result of epiphyseal growth cartilage that does not remodel and persists in the metaphysis, or it may be the persistence of the original cartilage anlage.
- Cartilage rests stop growing in adulthood.

ASSOCIATED CONDITIONS

- Enchondroma protuberans: eccentric enchondroma may cause bulging of cortex
- Enchondromatosis (Ollier's disease): multiple enchondromas
- Multiple enchondromas typically occurring in a unilateral distribution
- Male-to-female ratio: equal
- May involve any bone
- Occurrence in multiple siblings documented, but no genetic basis found
- Maffucci's syndrome: multiple enchondromas with soft tissue hemangiomas

ICD-9-CM

756.4 Enchondroma, enchondromatosis, Maffucci's syndrome

Diagnosis

SIGNS AND SYMPTOMS

General Features

- Most lesions are asymptomatic.
- Pain is sometimes present in patients with large enchondromas or enchondromas in the hand from pathologic fractures.
- If lesions occur in the hand, some enlargement of the digit may be noted if the cortex is expanded.
- If there is pain in the absence of a fracture, one should consider low-grade chondrosarcoma.
- The lesion is usually diagnosed incidentally on a routine radiograph or bone scan and is frequently "hot" on a bone scan.
- Rarely, a chondrosarcoma may develop in a preexisting enchondroma (typically in the long bones).

Enchondromatosis

- This condition is similar to that of a solitary lesion.
- It is usually recognized clinically by the age of 10 years because of the development of palpable masses, unilateral shortening of an extremity, or angular deformity.
- Most cases are bilateral, but involvement usually predominates on one side. Within an extremity, the lesions may be asymmetric (i.e., affecting the radial side more than the ulnar side or vice versa).
- Affected bones are shortened or deformed by epiphyseal involvement.
- The disease regresses after puberty.

Maffucci's Syndrome

- This should be considered a premalignant condition.
- Vascular phleboliths are apparent in soft tissue adjacent to enchondromas.

DIFFERENTIAL DIAGNOSIS

Radiographic Features

- Bone infarct
- Chondrosarcoma
- Unicameral bone cyst

Pathologic Features

Benign Lesions

- Fibrocartilaginous dysplasia with prominent chondroid regions
- Cartilage of a prominent costochondral junction

Malignant Lesions

- Low-grade (well differentiated) chondrosarcoma
- Chondroblastic osteosarcoma

Benign Versus Malignant Lesions

Distinguishing a benign latent enchondroma from an active enchondroma or low-grade chondrosarcoma is a common and difficult clinical problem. Because the histologic characteristics of a benign enchondroma overlap those of an active enchondroma or low-grade chondrosarcoma, biopsy is often not helpful. The correct diagnosis relies on observing both the clinical and the radiographic features of the lesion. Is the lesion growing? Is the lesion painful?

Enchondroma

- Painless condition, lack of growth, bone scan variability, uniform matrix calcification, lack of endosteal erosion, uniform small bland cells, low cellularity

Low-Grade Chondrosarcoma

- Painful, slow-growing condition, bone scan variability, presence of lucent regions, endosteal erosion, mild cellular atypia, moderate to high cellularity, Ki-67–positive status

PHYSICAL EXAMINATION

One should palpate the bone for tenderness and a soft tissue mass.

PATHOLOGIC FINDINGS

Microscopic Features

- Nests of cartilage cells without atypia are separated by normal marrow.
- Foci of calcification are usually present.
- Thin layer of lamellar cartilage may be observed.
- Negative Ki-67 stain is noted.
- Evidence of invasive infiltration of bone marrow suggests chondrosarcoma.
- Low magnification: Lesions are hypocellular with a blue-gray aura and inconspicuous nuclei.
- High magnification: Lesions have uniform nuclei (small, regular, darkly stained), and binucleated cells are rare.

Hand Lesions

- These may be hypercellular.
- Slight myxoid change may be seen.
- Cells may be bizarre.
- Double nucleated cells are common.

IMAGING PROCEDURES

Procedures differ according to age.

Children

- Plain radiographs in two planes and bone scan should be obtained, to evaluate for other lesions.

Adults

- Enchondromas are nongrowing lesions.
- Serial radiographs taken every 3 months or review of old radiographs can help to determine whether the lesion is stationary.

Enchondroma

• Small peripheral cartilage tumors tend to be benign, whereas large axial tumors tend to be malignant.
• A computed tomography scan should be obtained to look for the interface between the lesion and endosteal bone (endosteal erosion is often present with malignant degeneration).

Radiography

General Features

• Well-defined, solitary lytic lesions occur in the central portions of the metaphysis or metadiaphysis with occasional endosteal scalloping and intralesional calcifications.
• The calcification pattern is described as ring and stipple, popcornlike, and punctate.
• In small tubular bones (i.e., the hand), the entire shaft is usually involved.
• The cortex is usually intact, but it may be mildly expanded (by lack of remodeling in the metaphysis and not by expansion of the bone by tumor).
• It is radiolucent in the pediatric population (may look like a unicameral bone cyst).
• As patients age, the normally radiolucent cartilage begins to ossify and calcify, and ring and stipple calcifications are observed. Occasionally, the mineralization is so dense that the lesion may suggest a bone infarct.
• No periosteal reaction occurs.

Enchondromatosis

• Radiolucent areas of cartilage are seen in the metaphysis, with irregular calcification in a longitudinal or streaking pattern extending from the physis.
• The cortices are expanded from within, thus inhibiting normal metaphyseal remodeling.
• Affected bones cannot tubulate, so ends have a clubbed appearance.
• It may be located in places other than the centers of the medullary canal.
• It may be intracortical or subcortical or in the epiphysis.
• The tendency is to spare the epiphysis and diaphysis, except in severe cases.

Magnetic Resonance Imaging

• Well-circumscribed lobular lesion that is bright on T_2-weighted images.
• T_1-weighted images show low signal intensity.

Bone Scanning

• Enchondromas take up radionuclide tracer and are "hot" on a bone scan.
• Positive bone scans should be interpreted cautiously.
• Although they do not grow, enchondromas are constantly remodeling.
• Increased uptake and activity are not indications of malignant degeneration unless the lesion had less increased uptake on a prior scan.
• Initial scans are used for baselines if any symptoms change.

⚡ Management

GENERAL MEASURES

The decision to treat is based on clinical features that suggest that the lesion is actively growing, is at risk for fracture, or has become malignant. It is important to differentiate the lesion from a low-grade chondrosarcoma. Lesional growth is marked by increasing lucency in a previously mineralized tumor, cortical erosion, soft tissue mass, and pain. Biopsy is not helpful. The incidence of malignant transformation is extremely low. A benign-appearing, asymptomatic enchondroma that is not structurally weakening the bone, warrants observation (patients should be followed-up with serial radiographs to be certain that the lesion is not growing).
For hand lesions, one should allow the pathologic fracture to heal before surgery.

SURGICAL TREATMENT

General Principles

• If the patient is symptomatic, intralesional curettage and bone grafting should be performed. Local recurrence rates may range from 10% to 15%.
• Local recurrences are managed with repeat curettage, adjuvant treatment, and bone grafting.
• Alternative treatment for local recurrence is wide resection and limb salvage reconstruction.
• If the patient has an associated pathologic fracture, curettage and bone grafting should be delayed until the fracture has healed and the continuity of the bone has been restored.
• Enchondromas of the hand often present with pathologic fracture and should be treated with curettage.

Hand Lesions

• The surgeon should make a small window in the lateral aspect of phalanx, and curettage and bone grafting should be performed. The cortical window is replaced.
• Amputation may be necessary if finger function is compromised by the lesion.

Enchondromatosis

• Surgery may be necessary for angular deformities.
• Osteotomies may be performed through the enchondroma.
• Leg length discrepancy may require epiphysiodesis or limb lengthening procedures.
• Hand lesions may require curettage and bone grafting because of their large size and interference with function.

PATIENT EDUCATION

MONITORING

COMPLICATIONS

General Complications

• Enlarging lesions may fracture.
• Malignant degeneration: look for pain and growth of lesion.
• Incidence of malignant degeneration of enchondroma not known because total number of enchondromas not known (most are asymptomatic).

Enchondramotosis

• Of these patients, 25% to 50% develop low-grade chondrosarcoma.
• It usually occurs with patients in their 30s and 40s.
• One should look for cartilage necrosis or soft tissue invasion.

Maffucci's Syndrome

• Approximately 100% develop low-grade chondrosarcoma.
• Malignant brain tumors and liver and pancreatic carcinomas may also develop.

RECOMMENDED READING

Bullough PG. Atlas of orthopedic pathology with clinical and radiographic correlations, 2nd ed. New York: Gower Medical Publishing, 1992:14.7–14.8.

McCarthy EF, Frassica FJ. Pathology of bone and joint disorders with clinical and radiographic correlation. Philadelphia: WB Saunders, 1998:227–231, 239–240.

Morrissy RT, Weinstein SL, eds. Lovell and Winter's pediatric orthopedics, 4th ed. Philadelphia: JB Lippincott, 1996:133–135, 341–342.

Richards BS, ed. Orthopaedic knowledge update: pediatrics. Rosemont, IL: American Academy of Orthopaedic Surgeons, 1996:58.

Wold LE, McLeod RA, Sim FH, et al. Atlas of orthopaedic pathology. Philadelphia: WB Saunders, 1990:56–61, 74–79.

Basics

DESCRIPTION

Eosinophilic granuloma (EOG) is the bony, and most common, manifestation of a group of non-neoplastic disorders known as reticuloendotheliosis or histiocytosis X. Other forms include Hand-Schüller-Christian disease and Letterer-Siwe syndrome. Hand-Schüller-Christian disease usually presents in patients less than 5 years of age. Letterer-Siwe disease usually presents in patients less than 3 years of age.

These disorders cause an accumulation of abnormal metabolic products of lipids in reticuloendothelial cells (tissue-fixed macrophages). This change produces a granulomatous inflammatory response, which can destroy bone and thereby produce lytic lesions.

EOG commonly affects the skull, ribs, pelvis, spine, diaphysis of long bones, and mandible, but any bone may be involved. It more commonly affects a single bone rather than multiple bones.

SYNONYMS

- Histiocytosis X
- Langerhans' cell hystiocytosis
- Reticuloendotheliosis

INCIDENCE

- Rare
- Usually seen in patients less than 30 years old, with a peak incidence between 5 and 10 years
- Male-to-female ratio of 2:1

CAUSES

The cause of the accumulation of abnormal metabolic products in the reticuloendothelial cells is unknown. An inflammatory response occurs around these cells and produces the lytic destruction of bone.

ASSOCIATED CONDITIONS

Hand-Schüller-Christian Disease

- This is a systemic manifestation of histiocytosis X (multiple bony and visceral lesions).
- The onset usually occurs before age 5 years.
- A single EOG is the usual initial presentation.
- Of patients with EOG, 20% go on to develop this disease.
- Multiple organ systems may be involved.
- Symptoms correspond to the particular organ system (anemia, fatigability, hepatosplenomegaly, lymphadenopathy, weight loss, skin and mouth plaques, and ulcers). Unlike in EOG, bony lesions progress.
- The classic triad (in less than 25% of patients) is exophthalmos (retro-orbital invasion), diabetes insipidus (pituitary involvement), and lytic skull lesions.
- Treatment includes systemic corticosteroids or chemotherapy.

Letterer-Siwe Disease

- Systemic manifestation of histiocytosis X involve almost all organs and tissues of the body. A rare variant is usually seen in infants and young children less than 3 years old.
- It rarely produces significant skeletal lesions.
- Survival largely depends on the age of onset and the use of chemotherapy.

ICD-9-CM

277.8 Eosinophilic granuloma

Diagnosis

SIGNS AND SYMPTOMS

- Local pain
- Swelling, tenderness
- Warmth at the site of involvement
- Occasionally fever

DIFFERENTIAL DIAGNOSIS

- Ewing's sarcoma
- Lymphoma
- Osteomyelitis
- EOG appropriately called the "great imitator," because it may mimic infection or neoplasm

PHYSICAL EXAMINATION

- The skull and skeleton should be palpated for areas of tenderness.
- Note the position of the eyes within the orbit.
- The spine should be percussed for tenderness.
- The patient's gait should be observed for the presence of a limp.

LABORATORY TESTS

- Elevated erythrocyte sedimentation rate
- Peripheral eosinophilia

Eosinophilic Granuloma

PATHOLOGIC FINDINGS

• Sheets of "foamy" (lipid-filled) histiocytes

—Coffee bean–shaped nucleus
—Crisp nuclear membrane
—Abundant pale eosinophilic cytoplasm
—Staining with S-100 stain

• Inflammatory cells found around these histiocytes: predominantly eosinophils, but also a few lymphocytes, neutrophils, and giant cells.

IMAGING PROCEDURES

Plain radiographs show sharply circumscribed, "punched-out" lytic lesions. As the lesion heals, a thick rim of reactive bone forms around the periphery. The cortex may be destroyed with endosteal scalloping, periosteal reaction, and expansion of the bone. If the cortex is destroyed unevenly (EOG attacks cortex from within the canal, but one side of the cortex may be more involved than the other), a "hole within a hole" appearance ensues. In the vertebra, the body may collapse to a slender sclerotic wafer of bone called *vertebra plana*. In the mandible and maxilla, the lytic lesion appears as a "floating tooth."

Bone scanning is not usually recommended, because the lesions may not be "hot" on bone scan.

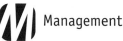 Management

GENERAL MEASURES

Most lesions are self-limiting and resolve spontaneously. Options include the following:

• Observation
• Curettage and bone grafting
• Injection with methylprednisolone

If a pathologic fracture is impending, or the articular surface is in danger, curettage and bone grafting are necessary. Biopsy is often necessary.

SURGICAL TREATMENT

Surgery is unnecessary in most cases. However, curettage and bone grafting with or without internal fixation are indicated if more conservative measures fail and pathologic fracture seems imminent.

MEDICAL TREATMENT

• Methylprednisolone injected into the lesion is effective in more than 90% of patients, with excellent bone healing.
• For patients with systemic disease with constitutional symptoms, chemotherapy is indicated with methylprednisolone, methotrexate, doxorubicin (Adriamycin), and other agents.
• No restrictions are placed on activity unless the patient has an impending pathologic fracture.
• Vertebra plana usually heals itself, and vertebral body height is restored with time.

PATIENT EDUCATION

• Reassure the patient and family about the self-limiting nature of the majority of the lesions.
• Make sure that the child and the parents understand the need for close follow-up care.
• Make sure disease progression is not occurring.
• Ensure that this is not the initial presentation of Hand-Schüller-Christian disease (20%).

MONITORING

Observation with plain radiographs is indicated if the diagnosis is clear-cut and the patient has no impending fracture, until lesions resolve (usually 6 months).

COMPLICATIONS

Pathologic fractures may occur. These usually heal well with closed or operative treatment.

PROGNOSIS

Prognosis is excellent if a second lesion does not appear within 1 year (progression to Hand-Schüller-Christian disease in 20%).

RECOMMENDED READING

Bullough PG. Eosinophilic granuloma. In: *Atlas of orthopaedic pathology,* 2nd ed. New York: Gower Medical Publishing, 1992:8.11–8.13.

Enneking WF. Reticuloendotheliosis. In: *Clinical musculoskeletal pathology,* 3rd rev. ed. Gainesville, FL: University of Florida Press, 1990:288–295.

Greenspan A. Eosinophilic granuloma. In: *Orthopedic radiology,* 2nd ed. Philadelphia: Lippincott–Raven, 1992:17.25–17.26.

Basics

DESCRIPTION

Ewing's sarcoma is a malignant bone tumor of long bones, pelvis, and spine usually seen in childhood. Pain, fever, local tenderness and erythema, and an elevated white blood cell count are associated with this tumor. It most commonly involves the diaphysis or metaphysis of long bones (fibula more commonly than tibia, femur, humerus), although any bone and any location within the bone may be affected. Ewing's sarcoma affects males more than females and is most common in persons less than 25 years old, although it rarely occurs in patients younger than age 3 years. If the patient is less than 5 years old, lymphoma and metastatic neuroblastoma must be excluded.

SYNONYM

Round cell sarcoma

INCIDENCE

This is the second most common malignant bone tumor of childhood, after osteosarcoma.

CAUSES

The causes of this tumor are not known.

RISK FACTORS

• Males more commonly affected than females
• Age more than 3 years and less than 25 years
• White persons more commonly affected than black persons

CLASSIFICATION

Ewing's sarcomas are classified according to the system of the Musculoskeletal Tumor Society. Most are stage II-B (high-grade, extracompartmental tumors); however, up to 20% to 25% of children present with lung or bone metastases.

ICD-9-CM

170.9 Ewing sarcoma

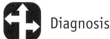 ## Diagnosis

SIGNS AND SYMPTOMS

• A localized mass with pain, tenderness, and erythema for several weeks or months is common.
• The patient often presents with systemic symptoms of fever, malaise, and weight loss.
• Occasionally, the tumor is associated with a pathologic fracture.

DIFFERENTIAL DIAGNOSIS

• This is most commonly confused with osteomyelitis.
• It is histologically similar to metastatic neuroblastoma (especially in patients less than 5 years of age), lymphoma (especially in patients less than 5 years old), and rhabdomyosarcoma.
• One must also consider eosinophilic granuloma and metastatic disease (especially in patients older than 30 years).

PHYSICAL EXAMINATION

In the early course of the disease, the physical examination is often normal. As the soft tissue component of the tumor grows, a soft tissue mass may be palpated.

LABORATORY TESTS

• Complete blood count
• Electrolyte determinations
• Erythrocyte sedimentation rate
• Bone marrow aspiration and biopsy. Surgical biopsy of the soft tissue portion of the lesion (if present) avoids the need to penetrate bone.

PATHOLOGIC FINDINGS

• Numerous small, round cells are blue on hematoxylin and eosin staining.
• The uniform, densely packed cell population has scant cytoplasm.
• The outlines of cells and nuclei are indistinct and may appear "out of focus."
• Special immunochemical stains are used to confirm the diagnosis.

IMAGING PROCEDURES

Plain radiographs are indicated. They often show a large lytic lesion that usually affects the diaphysis or metaphysis of long bones (frequently the fibula). There may be a variable amount of reactive new bone formation. It may show a periosteal reaction, with a characteristic "onion skin" appearance. The tumor often invades the soft tissue. Early in the disease, plain radiographs may appear normal. Patients with lesions suspected of being Ewing's sarcoma should receive staging studies, including magnetic resonance imaging of the primary lesion, chest radiography, chest computed tomography, and bone scanning.

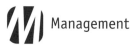 ## Management

GENERAL MEASURES

• Multiagent chemotherapy and external beam irradiation
• Wide surgical resection in certain cases, especially when the bone is "expendable," such as the fibula, iliac, wing, and clavicle

SURGICAL TREATMENT

If surgery is indicated, a wide surgical margin is necessary. Limb salvage is performed in almost all cases.

PHYSICAL THERAPY

Physical therapy is used in patients with surgical and nonoperative cases to maintain range of motion and muscle strength.

MEDICAL TREATMENT

Drugs of choice are various chemotherapeutic agents, according to the most current protocols.

MONITORING

Patients must be monitored closely for both local and metastatic disease recurrence by plain radiographs of the local region and with bone scan.

COMPLICATIONS

• Metastasis
• Pathologic fracture, which may require amputation

PROGNOSIS

• Five-year survival of 60% to 70% with current treatment
• Less favorable with tumor in the pelvis or spine

RECOMMENDED READING

Bullough P. Ewing's sarcoma. In: Atlas of orthopaedic pathology, 2nd ed. New York: Gower Medical Publishing, 1992:17.11–17.14.

Enneking WF. Ewing's sarcoma. In: Clinical musculoskeletal pathology, 3rd rev. ed. Gainesville, FL: University of Florida Press, 1990:375–380.

Pritchard D. Management of Ewings sarcoma. In: Advances in operative orthopaedics, 1993;1:391–400.

Extensor Tendon Laceration

 Basics

DESCRIPTION

Extensor tendon lacerations are common because of the superficial location of the extensor tendons on the back of the hand. The disruption of the tendon is often noted by the change in the posture of the hand or fingers. The most distal injury, at the distal interphalangeal joint, demonstrates a mallet type of deformity. If the injury occurs over the proximal interphalangeal joint, then a boutonnière deformity may result. Extensor injuries are usually repaired surgically, either in the emergency department or in the operating room within 2 weeks of injury.
These injuries affect active finger extension and active wrist extension and are most common in young adults. Males are more commonly affected than females.

INCIDENCE

This laceration is less common than flexor tendon injuries.

CAUSES

• Laceration on dorsum of hand or wrist, coupled with the superficial location of the extensor mechanism
• Possible association with bite injuries

CLASSIFICATION

Partial or complete laceration, as noted during wound exploration

ASSOCIATED CONDITIONS

Open fractures and joints

ICD-9-CM

884.2 Tendon laceration with open wound, upper extremity

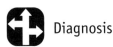 Diagnosis

SIGNS AND SYMPTOMS

Laceration on the Dorsum of the Hand

• Tendon ends frequently visible in wound with minimal exploration
• Change in posture of finger or hand
• Inability actively to extend joints distal to the injury

Mallet Deformity

• Inability to extend the top of the finger: The finger droops downward.
• Boutonnière deformity: The proximal interphalangeal joint goes into flexion while the distal interphalangeal joint extends.
• Decrease in strength or range of motion of either the index or the small finger: Both have small secondary independent extensor muscle and tendon units.

DIFFERENTIAL DIAGNOSIS

Fracture or avulsion injury of extensor mechanism (Fig. 1)

PHYSICAL EXAMINATION

• Examine active extension for all fingers and the wrist for strength and range of motion.
• Carefully explore the wound for evidence of lacerated tendons, either partial or complete.

IMAGING PROCEDURES

Anteroposterior and lateral radiographs are obtained to rule out foreign body or fracture.

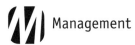 Management

GENERAL MEASURES

• Tetanus booster or toxoid as needed
• Intravenous antibiotics if wound is contaminated
• Skin closure until definitive surgery is performed
• Splint hand in wrist/finger extension (Fig. 1)
• Wound irrigation and débridement as needed
• Orthopaedic surgery or hand surgery consult

SURGICAL TREATMENT

The tendon ends are isolated, approximated, and repaired with either 4-0 nylon or 4-0 Ti-cron (Sherwood-Davis & Geck, St. Louis, MO). Vertical mattress stitches are used. If the injury is at the level of the wrist, then the repair is usually performed in the operating room. The repair is less surgically demanding than a repair of a flexor tendon lacerated at the same level, because there is no tendon pulley around extensor tendons. This anatomy also allows delayed surgical repair for up to 2 weeks without any adverse effects on outcome.

PHYSICAL THERAPY

Physical therapy regimens are based on the type of injury, its location, and the type of repair. The goal is to achieve a repair that allows early range of motion, both active and passive.

MEDICAL TREATMENT

If operative treatment is necessary, standard pre-operative tests are performed depending on the health of the patient.

PATIENT EDUCATION

Patient compliance with splinting, wound care, and physical therapy is critical to good functional outcome. It is important to stress the fact that the tendon will not heal or repair itself for normal function if it is a complete laceration.

COMPLICATIONS

• Infection
• Open joint injuries
• Failure of tendon repair
• Scarring
• Adhesions
• Loss of function

PROGNOSIS

Good with complete surgical repair

References

Ariyan S. The Hand Book. Baltimore, Williams and Wilkin, 1978.

The Hand: Examination and Diagnosis, American Society for Surgery of the Hand, Third Edition, Churchill Livingstone, 1990

The Hand: Primary Care of Common Problems, American Society for Surgery of the Hand, Second Edition, Churchill Livingstone, 1990

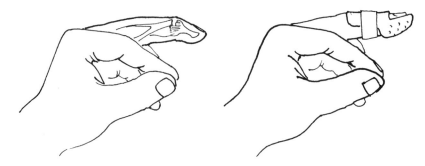

Fig. 1 An extensor tendon laceration or avulsion over the distal interphalangeal joint will heal with a finger splint.

Basics

DESCRIPTION

Femoral anteversion is forward inclination of the femoral neck relative to the distal femur. Stated another way, with the femoral head located in the acetabulum, the extremity is in internal rotation. Abnormal values of anteversion are usually described as more than two standard deviations from the mean for a given age. This condition occurs in young children between 3 and 10 years of age, in boys and girls equally.

SYNONYM

Pigeon toes

INCIDENCE

This condition is common.

CAUSES

The femur *in utero* has a significant amount of anteversion. This usually declines steadily with age, owing to the forces of upright stance. Differences in inheritance and connective tissue account for the variation in anteversion among patients.

RISK FACTORS

Positive family history

ASSOCIATED CONDITION

Tibial torsion

ICD-9-CM

755.63 Femoral anteversion

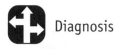 Diagnosis

SIGNS AND SYMPTOMS

In-toeing, tripping, and falling are commonly the original presentations that lead parents to seek medical attention. The primary concern remains the appearance of the child's legs during walking or running. Pain is rare. Physical examination should include an assessment from the hips to the toes. Patients with femoral anteversion usually show a medially directed patella and increased internal rotation compared with external rotation in the prone position. In-toeing and a scissoring gait are also common during walking. Children with a high level of anteversion are most commonly sitting in a "W" or reverse-tailor position, that is, sitting on the legs with the feet placed laterally. Tibial torsion is commonly associated with femoral anteversion.

DIFFERENTIAL DIAGNOSIS

• Tibial torsion
• Associated conditions that may lead to femoral anteversion and should be excluded:

—Developmental dysplasia of the hip
—Cerebral palsy
—Muscular weakness

PHYSICAL EXAMINATION

The amount of in-toeing should be quantitated using the foot progression angle, that is, the inward angle of the foot while walking down a straight-ahead line. The amount of anteversion should be quantitated by measuring the hip's internal and external rotation with the hips extended (out straight). Normally, there should be at least 20 degrees of external rotation in each hip.
In almost all cases, physical examination usually makes the diagnosis. The hip rotation should be checked with the patient prone. If internal rotation is greater than 65 degrees and external rotation is less than 20 degrees, anteversion is likely.

IMAGING PROCEDURES

Physical examination is usually sufficient to establish the diagnosis. A pelvic radiograph is indicated if the patient has markedly asymmetric hip range of motion. Fluoroscopy can be used to quantitate the degree of femoral anteversion. Computed tomography is the most widespread imaging technique used for quantitating femoral rotation and is indicated for planning surgical treatment.

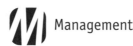 Management

GENERAL MEASURES

Femoral anteversion is the most common cause of in-toeing in children older than 3 years of age. Femoral anteversion at birth is approximately 40 degrees and gradually decreases to the adult value of 10 to 15 degrees by early adolescence. No treatment is necessary. It generally improves with further growth. There is no association between anteversion and early hip osteoarthritis.

SURGICAL TREATMENT

• Femoral derotation osteotomy is the only surgical treatment and is rarely needed.
• Derotation osteotomy should be postponed until the child is at least 8 years of age, to allow natural rotational changes to occur.
• Surgery is indicated if the anteversion is more than 50 degrees and the child is symptomatic.

PHYSICAL THERAPY

Physical exercises do not affect the natural history of anteversion.

PATIENT EDUCATION

• Explanation of the cause of in-toeing and that it normalizes with time
• No limitation of activity
• No evidence that the child's sitting position (i.e., "W" sitting) is causative or harmful

MEDICAL TREATMENT

• No treatment is necessary for physiologic femoral anteversion.
• Underlying pathologic processes may be treated if the patient has other associated conditions, such as cerebral palsy or hip dysplasia.
• Nonsurgical treatment consists primarily of careful explanation to the parents of the cause of in-toeing, including reassurance that it normalizes with time.
• Night splints and special shoes have no significant therapeutic effect.

MONITORING

• Annual or biannual observation and examination are recommended in patients with severe cases, to document expected rotational change with growth.
• Correction occurs slowly, because it depends on growth of the bone.

COMPLICATIONS

The potential complications of derotation osteotomy are as follows:

• Angulation
• Implant prominence
• Overcorrection or undercorrection
• Failure to recognize associated malrotation of the tibia or foot
• Injury to the apophysis

PROGNOSIS

Prognosis is good. Strong evidence shows that these children do not have an increased risk of hip or knee arthritis or athletic difficulty. Femoral anteversion corrects itself by early adolescence, with most improvement occurring before 10 years of age.

RECOMMENDED READING

Eckhoff D, Kramer R, Alongi C. Femoral anteversion and arthritis of the knee. *J Pediatr Orthop* 1994;14:608–610.

Ruwe PA, Gage JR, Ozonoff MB, et al. Clinical determination of femoral anteversion: a comparison with established techniques. *J Bone Joint Surg Am* 1992;74:820–830.

Staheli LT, Corbett M, Wyss C, et al. Lower extremity rotational problems in children: normal v guide management. *J Bone Joint Surg Am* 1985;67:39–47.

Femoral Neck Hip Fracture

 Basics

DESCRIPTION

Femoral neck hip fracture is commonly known as "broken hip." It specifically refers to fracture of the intracapsular portion of the proximal femur. In young patients, femoral neck fractures, although uncommon, can lead to permanent disability.

In patients less than 50 years of age, femoral neck fractures are often the result of high-velocity trauma, and therefore they are associated with major injuries to other organ systems.

The average age of injury is 72 years for men and 77 years for women. In the elderly, immobilization from these injuries can lead to secondary cardiopulmonary complications.

SYNONYMS

- Hip fracture
- Broken hip

INCIDENCE

- The incidence in white women is two to three times higher than that in black or Hispanic women.
- It increases with increasing age, doubling for each decade beyond 50 years. In young patients, more males than females sustain this injury. In elderly patients, women outnumber men 2 to 3:1.

CAUSES

In patients less than 50 years of age, femoral neck fractures are often the result of high-energy trauma with a direct force along the femoral shafts. In the older population, these fractures are caused by seemingly minor trauma, such as a fall from standing height directly on the greater trochanter. Furthermore, cyclic loading on osteoporotic bone can produce microfractures and eventually macrofractures of the femoral necks.

RISK FACTORS

- Osteoporosis, which is the major risk factor for femoral neck fractures in the elderly
- Female sex
- Excessive alcohol or caffeine intake
- Prolonged psychotropic drug use
- Physical inactivity

CLASSIFICATION

Garden classification:

- Type I: Impacted or incomplete fracture
- Type II: Complete fracture but nondisplaced
- Type III: Complete and partially displaced fracture
- Type IV: Complete and 100% displaced fracture

More simple femoral neck fractures can also be classified as either displaced or nondisplaced.

ASSOCIATED CONDITIONS

- Osteoporosis
- Alcoholism
- Generalized poor medical health

ICD-9-CM

820.8 Femoral neck fracture

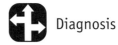 Diagnosis

SIGNS AND SYMPTOMS

- Clinically, these patients have severe pain in the groin area, and the leg is shortened.
- Patients tend to hold their hips slightly flexed and externally rotated.
- Pain is accentuated with attempted range of motion or axial loading.

DIFFERENTIAL DIAGNOSIS

When a fracture is not obviously appreciated on plain films in a patient with hip pain secondary to trauma, an occult (nondisplaced) fracture should be suspected. Other causes of hip pain are as follows:

- Intertrochanteric fracture
- Infection
- Greater trochanter bursitis
- Pathologic fracture, especially in elderly patients

PHYSICAL EXAMINATION

- Perform an examination for pain on range of motion, especially internal rotation.
- The leg is often externally rotated and shortened.
- Examine the pelvis with direct palpation and radiograph to exclude a concomitant pelvic fracture.

LABORATORY TESTS

For patients with an isolated injury and no major medical problems, routine preoperative laboratory tests, blood type and screen, chest radiographs, and an electrocardiogram are needed at time of admission.

PATHOLOGIC FINDINGS

Older patients often have comminution of the femoral neck, especially in the subcapital region.

IMAGING PROCEDURES

- Anteroposterior pelvis radiographs
- Anteroposterior and lateral radiographs of the affected hip and femur
- Magnetic resonance imaging to diagnose occult femoral neck fractures, especially during the first 24 hours, or bone scan 48 to 72 hours after injury

Management

GENERAL MEASURES

• Initially, the patient should be placed in Buck's traction with 3 to 5 lb of weights to minimize pain.
• Avoid decubitus ulcers from prolonged immobilization and decreased sensorium.

—Turn the patient frequently.
—Use heel protectors or specialized beds.

• Because of the high rate of osteonecrosis of the femoral neck associated with this type of injury (up to 33% with appropriate treatments), femoral neck fractures in young patients (less than 50 years of age) are considered orthopaedic emergencies.
• Nondisplaced fractures (Garden I and II) should be internally fixed with cannulated lag screws.
• Treatment of displaced femoral neck fractures is more controversial. In general, displaced fractures in younger, more active patients should be reduced by closed or open means and internally stabilized with pins or screws. In older (physiologic age greater than 70 years) patients, more sedentary patients, or in those with Paget's disease or neurologic diseases such as Parkinson's disease or hemiplegia, primary arthroplasty may be the treatment of choice.
• Hip fractures in elderly patients should be considered a symptom of other medical problems or of decreased overall condition. New or unstable medical problems need to be fully evaluated.
• In the multiply injured patient, attention to other organ systems and simultaneous care with other members of the trauma team are essential. In older patients with isolated femoral neck injuries, rapid medical consultation to optimize surgical outcomes is important. Delayed treatment of femoral neck fractures in elderly patients can lead to major cardiopulmonary complications.

SURGICAL TREATMENT

The patient is placed supine on a fracture table, and the fracture is visualized through a small incision or percutaneously under fluoroscopy. Once the fracture is reduced, three to four pins or screws are placed with the aid of the image intensifier.
Prosthetic replacement can be done through a lateral or posterior approach. In patients with minimal or no osteoarthritis involving the acetabulum, hemiarthroplasty (replacing only the femoral head and neck) is performed. Otherwise, total hip replacement (replacement of both the acetabulum and the femoral head and neck) should be considered.

PHYSICAL THERAPY

Physical therapy should begin on postoperative day 1 if feasible. Weight-bearing status depends on the type of treatment. Minimal or partial weight bearing is indicated for percutaneous pinning or uncemented arthroplasty, and full weight bearing is indicated for cemented femoral replacement.

MEDICAL TREATMENT

Analgesics are given. In the elderly, one should observe for a change in mental status and constipation with the use of narcotic analgesics. Young patients need adequate narcotic doses to facilitate rehabilitation.

PATIENT EDUCATION

Patients should be informed about the high incidence of osteonecrosis (formerly known as avascular necrosis) of the femoral head associated with this type of injury. The risk of osteonecrosis depends on the type of injury, as well as on the timing of diagnosis and treatment. A multiply injured patient has a higher risk of osteonecrosis than a patient with an isolated injury. Fractures treated appropriately still have up to a 33% risk of osteonecrosis. This rate increases to 100% in fractures diagnosed or treated after 72 hours.

PREVENTION

• In elderly persons, calcium or hormonal supplements and physical therapy to preserve bone mass can minimize the risk of femoral neck fracture.
• Ambulatory aids to increase stability are also helpful.

MONITORING

Intensive cardiovascular monitoring in multiply injured patients or in patients with multiple medical problems should be instituted during the perioperative period. In patients with internally fixed fractures, radiographs are taken once a month until union is achieved. In patients who have undergone arthroplasty, radiographs are taken at 3 and 12 months.

COMPLICATIONS

• Osteonecrosis of the femoral head
• Nonunion or malunion of bone
• Prosthetic dislocation or loosening
• Persistent pain
• Infection
• Cardiopulmonary complications

PROGNOSIS

The mortality rate in the elderly population ranges from 14% to 36% at 1 year after hip fracture. It has been estimated that the fracture and its treatment are associated with a death rate at least six times higher than that of an age-matched control population. This rate is highest during the first 6 months and in patients with multiple medical problems or prolonged immobilization.

RECOMMENDED READING

Bentley G. Treatment of nondisplaced fractures of the femoral neck. *Clin Orthop* 1980;152:93–101.

DeLee JC. Fractures and dislocations of the hip. In: Rockwood CA, Green DP, Bucholz RW, et al., eds. *Rockwood and Green's fractures in adults*, vol 2, 3rd ed. Philadelphia: JB Lippincott, 1991.

Gerber C, Strehle J, Ganz R. The treatment of fractures of the femoral neck. *Clin Orthop* 1993;292:77.

Koval KJ. Hip: trauma. In: In: Kasser JR, ed. *Orthopaedic knowledge update 5*. Rosemont, IL: American Academy of Orthopaedic Surgeons, 1996:379–388.

Swiontkowski MF, Winquist RA, Hansen ST. Fractures of the femoral neck in patients between the ages of twelve and forty-nine years. *J Bone Joint Surg Am* 1984;66:837.

Femoral Shaft Fracture

 Basics

DESCRIPTION

Femoral shaft fractures occur below the subtrochanteric region and above the supracondylar region of the femur, namely, the diaphysis.

INCIDENCE

• Approximately 1 fracture occurs per 10,000 persons per year.
• The incidence is higher in urban areas, where vehicular and gunshot wound trauma occurs at a higher rate.
• The age distribution is bimodal, with peaks below 25 years and above 65 years of age.
• Male-to-female ratios approach 2 to 3:1 in some urban areas.

CAUSES

• Vehicular blunt trauma, pedestrian or nonpedestrian
• Gunshot wounds
• Shotgun blasts
• Falls from a height
• Falls from a standing height: occasional causes of shaft fractures in the elderly, but such falls more frequently are the cause of hip fracture

RISK FACTORS

• Being young, male, living in an urban area, highly active
• Previous fractures
• Alcohol or drug abuse

CLASSIFICATION

In general, it is important to distinguish between closed and open fractures. Fractures caused by gunshot trauma are considered closed, so long as the only soft tissue defect is secondary to bullet entry and not exiting bone spikes, and the defect is less than 1 cm. Radiographically, fracture patterns are described as transverse, oblique, spiral, comminuted, segmented (e.g., three-part), or butterfly fragment. More comminuted fractures are indicative of higher forces.
Open fractures are classified with the Gustilo Open Fracture Classification:

Type I: Less than 1 cm external wound at the fracture site, clean
Type II: Greater than 1 cm wound without soft tissue avulsion or flaps
Type IIIA: Extensive laceration, or flaps, with adequate soft tissue coverage; high-energy trauma without regard to the size of the wound defect
Type IIIB: Soft tissue stripping, usually with gross contamination
Type IIIC: Open fracture with arterial injury requiring primary or graft repair. Usually, this classification is made at time of surgery, and extreme precision is not required in the emergency department.

• Neoplasms of bone (pathologic fractures)

—metastatic bone disease
—multiple myeloma
—osteosarcoma
—chondrosarcoma.

ICD-9-CM

821.01 Femoral shaft fracture

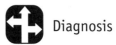 Diagnosis

SIGNS AND SYMPTOMS

• This is an obvious deformity with swelling of the entire affected thigh, sometimes tense.
• Up to 3 liters of blood can be lost in the thigh, so the hemodynamic monitoring of these patients is paramount.
• Thigh circumference compared with that of the contralateral leg can give an indication of the extent of blood loss. The proximal fragment is usually pulled into flexion and abduction, secondary to the pull of proximal musculature.
• Pain is extreme because of muscle spasm and periosteal irritation.
• The affected leg is shortened.

DIFFERENTIAL DIAGNOSIS

Pathologic fractures are due to forces not normally expected to cause injury. This must be ruled out by mechanism of injury, history of neoplasm, and radiographic cues.
One must consider pathologic fractures in several scenarios:

• Spontaneous fracture (no or very low energy trauma)
• History of pain prior to fracture
• Destructive or permeative lesion on radiograph

PHYSICAL EXAMINATION

• Neurovascular status of the lower extremity should be documented.
• The limb should be searched for evidence of open fracture.
• Associated fractures should be sought, especially of the hip and knee.
• Ligament injuries to the knee should be ruled out after the femur is stabilized.

LABORATORY TESTS

All preoperative trauma laboratory tests must be drawn, and blood must be made available by type and crossmatching.

PATHOLOGIC FINDINGS

- Injured tissues: bone, muscle, and fascia
- Rarely, injury to femoral artery or sciatic nerve

IMAGING PROCEDURES

- Anteroposterior and lateral, full-length films of the affected femur are obtained.
- Trauma series is obtained: cervical spine (anterior and lateral views), anteroposterior chest, anteroposterior pelvis, and internal rotation view of ipsilateral femoral neck.
- The neck rigid collar must remain in place until the cervical spine is cleared by radiologist or orthopaedic surgeon and findings of clinical examination do not suggest injury.
- Ipsilateral femoral neck fracture must be excluded.
- Full-length contralateral femur films are useful with comminuted or long oblique fractures of the femur, for length determination at the time of intramedullary fixation.
- Computed tomography with bone windows is helpful if femoral neck fracture is suspected.

Management

GENERAL MEASURES

At present, there are few indications for nonoperative management of femoral shaft fractures. If a patient is too unstable for surgery, balanced traction may be used in short-term management. These fractures almost always require operative fixation. Fractures in medically unstable patients can be stabilized with external fixation. When the patient's condition improves, the external fixator is removed, and the femur is stabilized with an intramedullary nail.

SURGICAL TREATMENT

- Between 6 months and 7 to 8 years of age, spica casting is used.
- Between 7 and 11 years of age (the size of the child is important), external fixation is a useful tool for definitive management.
- For patients aged 12 years to adults, reamed or unreamed intramedullary fixation is the modality of choice. Patients with externally fixed grade III open fractures are often returned to the operating room for delayed intramedullary fixation, once contamination and the possibility of infection have been minimized by several irrigation and débridement procedures. Children should not have intramedullary nails inserted through the piriformis fossa, because this can cause osteonecrosis of the hip.

ACTIVITY

- Generally, patients have 12 to 16 weeks of protected weight bearing (25% to 50%) to the affected extremity with a walker or a crutch before they are allowed full weight bearing with clinical and radiographic evidence of healing.
- The fracture pattern, stable or unstable, determines weight-bearing status and the degree of comminution.

PHYSICAL THERAPY

- Some patients require physical therapy for strengthening and range of motion about the knee, for acquired stiffness.
- With associated contralateral lower or upper extremity injuries, short-term rehabilitation placement and wheelchair use are sometimes indicated, unless in-home therapy and activities of daily living can be accomplished.

MEDICAL TREATMENT

There are few indications for nonoperative management of femoral shaft fractures, as described earlier.

PATIENT EDUCATION

An understanding of the expected course of treatment and therapy is important. Many patients become frustrated at the slow course, particularly when a nonunion or other complication occurs.

PREVENTION

Avoidance of risk factors for extremity injury

MONITORING

Patients are followed at 6-8 week intervals with radiographs to monitor the progress to union.

COMPLICATIONS

- Associated fractures, particularly ipsilateral injury
- Pulmonary fat embolus—incidence decreases with decreased time from injury to fracture stabilization (>24 h).
- Deep-vein thrombosis
- Compartment syndrome—rare (<1%).
- Vascular injury—can occur up to 30% of shaft fractures.

PROGNOSIS

Prognosis is excellent. Approximately 95% of fractures heal uneventfully within 4 months.

REFERENCES

Browner, Jupiter, Levine, Trafton. Skeletal Trauma W.B. Saunders Co., 1992. pp. 1525–1634.

Lovell and Winter, Pediatric Orthopaedics, Lippincott-Raven Pub., 4th Ed., 1996. pp. 1277–1285.

Simon and Koenigsknecht, Emergency Orthopaedics, Appleton and Lange, 3rd Ed., 1995. pp. 263–267.

Fibrous Cortical Defect

 Basics

DESCRIPTION

Fibrous cortical defect is a benign lytic lesion with a sclerotic rim located eccentrically in the metaphysis of long bones in children, most commonly in the distal femur, proximal tibia, or distal tibia. The lesion is seen in children and adolescents and not in adults.

SYNONYMS

- Nonossifying fibroma
- Benign metaphyseal cortical defect
- Metaphyseal fibrous defect
- Benign fibrous histiocytoma

INCIDENCE

- The most common skeletal lesion
- Estimated to occur in 35% of healthy children

CAUSES

The cause is hypothesized to be a focal area of increased periosteal resorption during growth.

CLASSIFICATION

It is classified with other benign lesions as follows:

Stage 1: Latent (approximately 96%)
Stage 2: Active (approximately 2% to 3%)
Stage 3: Aggressive (less than 1%)

Natural History

- Active stage 2 during childhood
- Becoming latent stage 1 at skeletal maturation

ASSOCIATED CONDITIONS

A fibrous cortical defect may "overheal" to form a sclerotic (radiopaque) area of cortical bone in the metaphysis. This healed area is completely benign and does not need to be followed.

ICD-9-CM

213.9 Fibrous cortical defect

 Diagnosis

SIGNS AND SYMPTOMS

Most lesions are asymptomatic and are found incidentally on radiographs.
Occasionally, the condition is painful if a pathologic fracture occurs through the lesion or if such a fracture is impending.

DIFFERENTIAL DIAGNOSIS

- Infection
- Unicameral bone cyst
- Chondroblastoma
- Chondromyxoid fibroma
- Giant cell tumor
- Fibrous dysplasia

PHYSICAL EXAMINATION

- Usually, the lesion is nontender.
- There should not be swelling or tenderness with weight bearing, unless a fracture is impending.

PATHOLOGIC FINDINGS

The lesion is filled with fibrous connective tissue arranged in a whirled, "starry night" pattern. Also seen are multinucleated giant cells, clear histiocytes, and hemosiderin pigmentation. Cystic spaces are not typical.

IMAGING PROCEDURES

On plain radiographs, a lytic (radiolucent) lesion is seen eccentrically in the metaphyses of long bones (usually the distal femur, proximal tibia, or distal tibia). This lesion is surrounded by a scalloped, reactive rim of sclerotic (radiopaque) bone. The lesion often appears multiloculated, producing a "bubbling" appearance. The size ranges from a few millimeters to a few centimeters. The lesion is usually solitary.
If a bone scan is obtained, the lesion will appear "hot" early on from the reactive rim of bone. As the lesion heals, the bone scan will become normal.

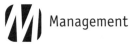 Management

GENERAL MEASURES

In general, full, unrestricted activity is allowed. If weight-bearing pain develops, anteroposterior and lateral radiographs should be obtained to look for stress fractures.

SURGICAL TREATMENT

For impending pathologic fracture, curettage (scraping the lesion) followed by bone grafting (placing bone into the lesion) should be performed. Internal fixation is usually not necessary.

MEDICAL TREATMENT

- Treatment for large lesions is radiographic monitoring according to the physician's judgment because the lesion is self-healing at skeletal maturity.
- Patients with large lesions should be seen every 6 months. This monitoring may continue until growth is complete.
- If more than 50% of the cortex is involved and the patient is symptomatic (pain), a pathologic fracture is possible. In this case, treatment is surgery with curettage and bone grafting. If the lesion is small (less than 25% of the width of the cortex), no monitoring is needed.
- No restrictions are placed on activity unless a pathologic fracture is impending (more than 50% of the cortex is involved in a symptomatic child), in which case the child should be nonweight bearing on the affected extremity.

PATIENT EDUCATION

- This includes reassurance to the child and parents regarding the benign nature of the lesion, the natural course of self-healing, and the prevalence of the lesion in healthy children (35% of healthy children).
- If the lesion is small, no follow-up is needed.
- If it is large, follow-up should be performed every 6 to 12 months.

MONITORING

- Serial radiography
- Anteroposterior and lateral views of the affected part

COMPLICATIONS

- Pathologic fracture is rarely seen.
- Pathologic fractures usually occur only in lesions involving more than 50% of the cortex in symptomatic patients.

PROGNOSIS

All these lesions are self-healing at skeletal maturity.

RECOMMENDED READING

Bullough, PG. Nonossifying fibroma. In: Bullough PG, ed. *Atlas of orthopedic pathology*, 2nd ed. New York: Gower Medical Publishing, 1992:15.15–19.19.

Enneking WF. Nonossifying fibroma. In: *Clinical musculoskeletal pathology*, 3rd rev ed. Gainesville, FL: University of Florida Press, 1990:302–306.

Frassica FJ, McCarthy EF. Metaphyseal fibrous defect. In: Miller MD, ed. *Review of orthopaedics*, 2nd ed. Philadelphia: WB Saunders, 1996:311.

Basics

DESCRIPTION

Fibrous dysplasia affects the skeleton. The condition causes focal defects in bone quality and is characterized by multiple, gradual bone deformities, a risk of endocrinopathy (in the polyostotic variety), and a tendency toward pain in the lesions. Café-au-lait spots are common signs. Physical findings require some time to develop. Precocious puberty may occur as early as the first year of life. Fibrous dysplasia does not display the decrease in severity after maturity that is seen osteogenesis imperfecta. It occurs equally in males and females. McCune-Albright syndrome, the triad of polyostotic fibrous dysplasia, café-au-lait spots, and precocious puberty, is an age-related risk factor.

SYNONYM

Osteitis fibrosa cystica

GENETICS

No reports of familial transmission of this disorder have been published.

INCIDENCE

This condition is rare.

CAUSES

• A defect in the gene occurs for the α subunit of a certain G-protein, a type of protein that couples cell-surface receptors to extracellular signals and activates intracellular synthesis of cyclic adenosine monophosphate.
• The extent and severity of the disease are related to the period in embryonic life when the mutation occurred.

RISK FACTORS

• Endocrine abnormality
• Early femoral bowing
• Café-au-lait spots with irregular borders

CLASSIFICATION

• Monostotic: involving only a single bone
• Polyostotic: multiple bones involved, usually more on one side of the body (McCune-Albright syndrome: triad of polyostotic fibrous dysplasia, café-au-lait spots, and precocious puberty)

ASSOCIATED CONDITIONS

• Endocrinopathy
• Osteosarcoma
• Fibrosarcoma

ICD-9-CM

756.54 Polyostotic fibrous dysplasia
733.29 Monostotic fibrous dysplasia

 ## Diagnosis

SIGNS AND SYMPTOMS

Signs

• Progressive distortion of bone, as in the proximal femur, pelvis, and cranium
• Possible neurologic compromise, caused by cranial or spinal deformity
• Café-au-lait-spots in the polyostotic form (spots have irregular margins likened to the coast of Maine)
• Pain and a waddling gait
• Scoliosis

Symptoms

• Constant aches from bones affected by dysplasia under loading

DIFFERENTIAL DIAGNOSIS

• Unicameral bone cyst
• Fibrous cortical defect
• Osteoporosis
• Osteomalacia

PHYSICAL EXAMINATION

• Measure the patient's height.
• Check for scoliosis, because it may sometimes develop in this condition.
• Measure limb length and angular deformities.
• Check all four extremities for bowing.
• Document the range of motion, especially about the hip.
• Palpate tender areas of bone.
• Observe the patient's gait.

LABORATORY TESTS

Specific tests for any of the described endocrinopathies should be performed if clinically indicated. These may include measurement of growth hormone, thyroid function, and adrenal function.

PATHOLOGIC FINDINGS

• Bone lesions show multiple small, disorganized bony trabeculae, not organized to provide normal mechanical support. They have been likened to "alphabet soup" in their disorganized appearance.
• The marrow is filled with fibrous tissue.
• Osteoblastic rimming of the trabeculae is absent; the bone forms from fibro-osseous metaplasia.

IMAGING PROCEDURES

The internal appearance of bone with fibrous dysplasia on radiographs is so homogeneous that it is called "ground glass." This is not surprising, given the histologic findings of multiple small disorganized trabeculae. Fibrous dysplasia is usually seen occupying a large segment of the diaphysis of a bone, sometimes the entire diaphysis. The classic teaching is that fibrous dysplasia is a "long lesion in a long bone." A characteristic deformity is the "shepherd's crook" appearance of the proximal femur. This is a diffuse, severe bowing of the entire proximal end, owing to weakening of the bone.
Technetium bone scans may be used to locate other lesions of fibrous dysplasia, if needed. The lesions are usually "hot" on bone scans, although not universally so.
Computed tomography is useful for imaging cranial or spinal disorders.

Fibrous Dysplasia

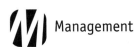 Management

GENERAL MEASURES

- Correct progressive skeletal deformity.
- Treat endocrinopathy appropriately.
- Suggest curettage and bone grafting, which may be useful for symptomatic lesions in the upper extremity, especially in monostotic cases and in skeletally mature individuals. The lesions often recur after curettage and bone grafting, but pain may be relieved and strength may be increased.
- In other settings, recognize the high recurrence rate.
- Perform craniofacial reconstruction in patients with severe deformity.
- Manage pain with analgesics, or consult a pain management specialist. Early trials of diphosphonate agents are promising.

SURGICAL TREATMENT

- Orthopaedic principles are as follows:
- A significant bowing deformity should be straightened to minimize further bending forces. In the proximal femur, this involves a valgus osteotomy or a medial displacement osteotomy.
- Diseased bone should be supported with a stronger material such as cortical bone or a metal implant.
- An intramedullary device is usually better than a plate, because it can protect the length of the bone and is more centrally located and therefore more effective.
- Lesions of fibrous dysplasia often recur after simple bone grafting.
- Lesions often bleed copiously during operation.

PHYSICAL THERAPY

- Therapy is useful for postoperative rehabilitation.
- The involvement of multiple limbs often poses special challenges to the therapist.

MEDICAL TREATMENT

- Pain should be managed with analgesics, or a pain management specialist should be consulted. Early trials of pamidronates are promising.
- There is no evidence that increasing a patient's activity level will strengthen the dysplastic bone.
- Generally, pain should be the patient's guide to what is allowed. High-impact or endurance activities pose an increased risk of fracture.

PATIENT EDUCATION

- Patients should be supported because of the chronic nature of the disease.
- Sports restrictions should be discussed, specific to the patient's individual lesions.
- Career counseling should be given.

PREVENTION

Avoid radiation of the lesions because of the risk of malignant transformation.

MONITORING

Patients should be seen by the same physician or set of specialists periodically to detect progressive deformity. In particular, this regimen should include yearly visits to the orthopaedic surgeon to track femoral bowing and scoliosis. Patients should also be told about the risk and warning signs of malignant transformation to sarcoma. These warning signs include increase in pain, size, or warmth of the lesion.

COMPLICATIONS

- Fracture
- Chronic pain
- Depression
- Malignant transformation, most commonly to osteosarcoma (2.5%)

PROGNOSIS

Progression of dysplasia and new lesions may occur in adulthood. About one-third of patients have chronic pain. Life expectancy is shortened in patients with the polyostotic form, owing to pneumonia, thrombosis, and malignant transformation.

RECOMMENDED READING

Albright F, Butler AM, Hampton AO, et al. Syndrome characterized by osteitis fibrosa disseminata, areas of pigmentation, and endocrine dysfunction. *N Engl J Med* 1937;216:727–746.

Harris WH, Dudley HR, Barry RJ. The natural history of fibrous dysplasia. *J Bone Joint Surg Am* 1962;44:207–227.

Stephenson RB, London MD, Hankin FM, et al. Fibrous dysplasia: an analysis of options for treatment. *J Bone Joint Surg Am* 1987;69:400–409.

Basics

DESCRIPTION

Fractures of the fibula can be divided into three groups:

1. Those that involve the ankle joint
2. Those that involve the fibular shaft without ankle involvement
3. Those that involve the proximal fibula

Distal fibular fractures that involve the ankle joint are by far the most common fibular fractures and are discussed in the chapter on ankle fractures. Fibular shaft fractures and fractures of the head and neck of the proximal fibula are discussed here.

Fractures of the fibular shaft occurring without ankle injury are nearly always associated with tibial shaft fractures. It is essential in these cases to examine the ankle joint fully, particularly medially, to rule out Maisonneuve's fracture (see later). However, isolated fractures involving only the fibula shaft may occur, although rarely, when there is a direct force to the fibula.

Fractures of the proximal head and neck of the fibula are nearly always associated with significant damage to the knee; thus, knee injury must be considered when one is confronted with this fracture. These fractures may be isolated, caused by a direct blow to the area, or an avulsion injury at the insertion of the biceps femoris tendon or lateral collateral ligament. However, in most cases these fractures are associated with injuries to the lateral condyle of the tibial plateau (see the chapter on tibial plateau fractures). Those that are caused by trauma are usually caused by a valgus stress and are thus often associated with damage to the medial collateral ligament of the knee. Like fibular shaft fractures, these, too, may present as Maisonneuve's fractures.

Damage along the medial aspect of the ankle joint by external rotation injuries may be associated with rupture of the deltoid and tibiofibular ligaments, which may, in turn, cause a tear to form in the interosseus membrane between the shafts of the tibia and fibula. As this tear progresses up the interosseus membrane, all the forces are placed more proximally along the fibula at the area where the tear ends. This may cause a proximal fibular fracture. Physical examination of the ankle is essential in determining whether such a fracture is present or whether the proximal fibular fracture is unrelated to an ankle injury. These fractures are more common in adults than in children.

INCIDENCE

Fibular fractures, taken together, are among the most commonly encountered fractures in orthopaedics.

CAUSES

- Trauma
- Falls
- Missteps
- In-line skating

CLASSIFICATION

- Proximal fracture
- Midshaft fracture
- Distal (ankle) fracture

ASSOCIATED CONDITIONS

Fibular shaft fractures are often associated with fractures of the tibial shaft. Thus, they may also be associated with a compartment syndrome of the leg.

Fibular head and neck fractures are often associated with fractures of the lateral tibial condyle. Furthermore, because such fractures imply a lateral, valgus stress, more significant damage to the knee itself, particularly a sprain or tear of the medial collateral ligament, is also commonly encountered. If the fibular head fracture is secondary to an avulsion injury, there may be associated damage to the lateral collateral ligament of the knee or the biceps femoris tendon. Additionally, the common peroneal nerve may be damaged as it wraps around the fibular head laterally.

Oblique proximal fibular neck fractures that suggest structural damage to the medial aspect of the ankle and to the interosseus membrane may also be encountered.

ICD-9-CM

823.8 Fibula Fracture

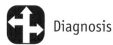

Diagnosis

SIGNS AND SYMPTOMS

- Patients with fibular shaft or head fractures generally present with tenderness and swelling in the area of injury. Numbness or parasthesias may arise if damage to the peroneal nerves has occurred.
- Should a fibular head fracture be noted, there is usually an associated significant knee injury, and patients often have pain and swelling of the knee joint.
- Maisonneuve's fractures present with swelling and pain, not only proximally in the area of the fibular fracture, but also about the medial aspect of the ankle joint.

PHYSICAL EXAMINATION

Physical examination shows point tenderness and swelling in the area of fracture. Stability and medial tenderness of the ankle should always be assessed because a possible deltoid tear with a proximal fibular fracture may be present (Maisonneuve's fracture). Stability and tenderness of the knee, particularly in proximal fibular fractures, should always be assessed as well and should include examination of all ligaments.

LABORATORY TESTS

No serum laboratory tests are indicated.

PATHOLOGIC FINDINGS

The fibular fracture may have several different patterns: spiral, transverse, or comminuted. Fractures secondary to tumors are rare.

IMAGING PROCEDURES

Anteroposterior and lateral views of the shafts of the tibia and fibula should be performed. If a proximal fibular fracture is suspected, anteroposterior and lateral views of the knee are also obtained to look for associated injury to the knee. If on physical examination one suspects an ankle injury and that the fibular fracture may be of Maisonneuve type, three views of the ankle (anteroposterior, lateral, and mortise) are indicated.

Fibula Fracture

⚹ Management

GENERAL MEASURES

Isolated fibular shaft fractures that do not involve the ankle are relatively unimportant because the fibula supports only 16% of body weight and is not essential to stability. The shaft of the fibula tends to heal well on its own, because it is encompassed completely by vascularized muscle. However, the fibula is important distally, where it contributes to the stability of the ankle joint.

If only the fibula is fractured and there is no associated trauma to the ligaments of the ankle, then treatment is symptomatic. A splint or cast may be applied to increase comfort but is not essential; rest, elevation, ice, elastic (Ace) wrap compression, and pain medication may well be sufficient. Weight bearing may be allowed on the involved leg as tolerated by the patient. Pain and swelling are usually diminished in 1 to 2 weeks, and at that time the patient is allowed to return to regular activity as tolerated. Full healing is generally accomplished by 6 to 8 weeks. Nonunion is uncommon.

If a fibular fracture is associated with a tibial shaft fracture or a tibial condylar fracture, then the tibial fracture is repaired, and the fibula will usually heal without fixation. Occasionally, if fixation of the fibular fracture will aid in realignment or length restoration of the tibial fracture, the fibular fracture is repaired as well. Plate fixation is generally performed. Maisonneuve's fractures are much more serious because they imply significant medial injury to the ankle joint. These fractures should be treated operatively.

SURGICAL TREATMENT

Fibular shaft fractures rarely need operative treatment (see earlier). However, when they do, fixation is performed using a 3.5-mm compression plate. Bone grafting is used when the fracture is comminuted with significant fracture gaps.

PHYSICAL THERAPY

Patients are instructed to bear partial weight with isolated fibular shaft fractures, and patients are non–weight bearing with fractures of the distal fibula with ankle instability until the fracture heals.

MEDICAL TREATMENT

- The patient with an isolated fibular shaft fracture or a fracture of the fibular head or neck without an associated injury may wear a splint or cast to increase comfort, but these devices are not essential.
- Weight bearing may be allowed on the involved leg as tolerated by the patient.
- Elevation of the leg, elastic wrap compression, and ice should be used.
- Should the patient have an associated injury such as a tibial fracture or derangement of the knee or ankle joints, the appropriate treatment of the associated injury should be implemented as well.

PATIENT EDUCATION

Patients are counseled that although fibula fractures heal well, tenderness and swelling may persist for several months after injury.

Monitoring

Patients are followed at one-month intervals with plain radiographs until the fractures are healed.

COMPLICATIONS

- Nonunion (rare)
- Chronic pain (rare)
- Malunion (rare)

PROGNOSIS

Generally, these fractures do well, and most patients have normal function on long-term follow-up. Nonunion is uncommon, and when it occurs it is rarely symptomatic. Patients who are symptomatic respond well to operative treatment, as described earlier.

RECOMMENDED READING

Russell TA, Taylor JT, LaVelle DG. Fractures of the tibia and fibula. In: Rockwood CA, Green DP, Bucholz RW, eds. *Rockwood and Green's fractures in adults,* vol 2, 3rd ed. Philadelphia, JB Lippincott, 1991:1915–1982.

Simon RR, Koenigsknecht SJ. *Emergency orthopedics: the extremities,* 2nd ed. Norwalk, CT: Appleton & Lange, 1987:249–251.

Trafton PG. Tibial shaft fractures. In: Browner BD, Jupiter JB, Levine AM, et al., eds. *Skeletal trauma,* vol 2. Philadelphia: WB Saunders, 1992:1771–1869.

Basics

DESCRIPTION

• Flatfoot, or pes planus, is a deformity of the foot in which the normal longitudinal arch of the foot is lost.
• In most cases in which the deformity is symptomatic, an associated anatomic abnormality of the foot is present.
• The foot, ankle, and, in some cases, the heel cord may be affected.
• A flexible flatfoot lacks an arch only when the foot is weight bearing but not when the foot is in a dependent position or when the patient toe-stands.
• A rigid flatfoot lacks an arch at all times, even when the foot is dependent or when the patient toe-stands.

INCIDENCE

• Congenital flexible flatfoot that persists after infancy is a trait that often runs in families, although the pattern of inheritance is not known; it is present in approximately 15% of adults.
• Tarsal coalitions, the most common type of congenital rigid flatfoot, are inherited in an autosomal dominant pattern and demonstrate a 4:1 female-to-male predominance. The overall incidence is unknown but is less than 1%.
• Acquired flatfeet, as the name implies, are not inherited.
• Acquired flexible flatfoot caused by posterior tibial synovitis is the most common cause of acquired flatfoot in adults, although its incidence is not precisely known.
• The exact incidence of other patterns of acquired flatfeet is not known, but they tend to be uncommon and are associated with severe deformity.

CAUSES

• Congenital flexible flatfoot that persists into adulthood is believed to have a genetic origin.
• Congenital rigid flatfoot resulting from tarsal coalitions is caused by genetic mutations that lead to the failure of the formation of synovial joints between the affected tarsal bones.

RISK FACTORS

• Persistent congenital flexible flatfoot: other family members with the same condition, because the condition is inherited
• Congenital rigid flatfoot secondary to tarsal coalition with peroneal spasm: female sex as well as other family members with the same condition
• Acquired flexible flatfoot secondary to posterior tibial tendon synovitis or rupture: hypertension, diabetes, and a history of trauma.
• Other conditions: tight Achilles tendon, neurologic diseases (e.g., poliomyelitis, spina bifida, myelodysplasia, neurofibromatosis, stroke), osteoarthritis, rheumatoid arthritis, calcaneal fracture, Lisfranc's fracture-dislocation, tumors, tuberculosis, genetic diseases (trisomies), and soft tissue dysplasias

CLASSIFICATION

One can separate flatfoot into four categories: congenital flexible flatfoot, congenital rigid flatfoot, acquired flexible flatfoot, and acquired rigid flatfoot.

ICD-9-CM

734 Acquired flat foot
754.61 Congenital flat foot

 ## Diagnosis

SIGNS AND SYMPTOMS

Congenital Flexible Flatfoot

• Congenital flexible flatfoot that is secondary to soft tissue dysplasias such as Marfan's syndrome or Ehlers-Danlos syndrome or that persists after infancy rarely becomes symptomatic. If symptoms appear, they are only minor, most often feet that become tired easily or achy after prolonged standing.

Congenital Rigid Flatfoot

• Congenital rigid flatfoot caused by tarsal conditions with peroneal spastic flatfoot usually presents in adolescence or early adulthood when the bridge between the tarsal bones ossifies.
• Patients with a calcaneonavicular fusion usually present at 8 to 12 years of age, whereas patients with talocalcaneal fusion normally present at 12 to 16 years of age.
• Symptoms may present in both feet.
• The patient complains of a painful, stiff foot and usually reports some history of trauma, often in the form of a twisting of the foot or a forceful fall onto the foot (such as stepping into a hole or missing a stair).
• The associated peroneal spasm is evident as the foot remains fixed in eversion and as attempts at passive or active inversion are met with resistance; this sign is thought to be a response of the patient to restrict hind foot motion and thereby to prevent exacerbation of the symptomatic tarsal bar.

Acquired Flexible Flatfoot

• Acquired flexible flatfoot caused by synovitis or rupture of the posterior tibial tendon presents as a gradual, progressive aching and swelling along the medial aspect of the afflicted person's foot and ankle.
• A history of trauma is noted in about half of the patients; however, the onset of this process is usually gradual.
• The patient may complain of tenderness and swelling along the medial part of the foot, a diminished endurance in the foot, a decreased ability to participate in sports, and eventually a progressive difficulty in ambulating.
• Because the arch is lost, women may mention difficulty in walking in high-heeled shoes.
• Increased wear may be noted along the medial aspect of the shoe.
• Inversion against resistance is absent or diminished, and the patient cannot toe-stand on the affected side or can do so only with pain and difficulty.
• As the condition worsens, a "too many toes" sign is noted on the affected side when the foot is viewed from behind the individual.

Flatfoot

DIFFERENTIAL DIAGNOSIS

• The differential diagnosis should include all the possible causes of the type of flatfoot.
• This diagnosis can usually be sorted out on the basis of history and physical examination.

PHYSICAL EXAMINATION

• Of primary importance is the determination whether the condition is rigid or flexible.

—A rigid flatfoot displays a loss of the normal longitudinal arch of the foot at all times, when the patient is standing or when the foot is in a dependent position.
—A flexible flatfoot displays a loss of arch only on standing on the affected foot, with reappearance when the foot is dependent or when the patient toe-stands.
—The presence of arch should be noted with the patient's foot in these different positions.
—A rigid flatfoot generally displays restricted motion of the ankle, subtalar, or transverse tarsal joints; a flexible flatfoot has normal motion of all these joints.

• The entire foot should be palpated and observed for any deformity, swelling, or areas of tenderness.

—Tenderness and swelling along the medial aspect of the foot and ankle suggest posterior tibial tendon synovitis or rupture.
—A rocker-bottom foot may be present in patients with vertical talus or Charcot's foot.
—Other processes, such as tumors, infection, arthritis, and trauma may also present with swelling, tenderness, and deformity of the foot and ankle.

• The patient's ability to toe-stand indicates the patient's ability to invert the foot actively; patients with posterior tibial tendon synovitis or tarsal coalition with peroneal spasm demonstrate the inability to toe-stand or the ability to do so only with pain and difficulty.
• The patient's ability to ambulate should be noted.

—A "too many toes" sign is present when the invertors or the foot and ankle are not functional and thus throw the hind foot into valgus as the patient bears weight; an observer behind a walking patient notices too many toes projecting laterally.
—An antalgic gait may indicate a painful disease process such as arthritis, infection, or tumor.
—An awkward, foot-slapping gait may suggest a neurologic or neuromuscular disease such as spina bifida, poliomyelitis, or Charcot's foot.
—The Achilles tendon should be examined to test whether the heel cord is tight.

PATHOLOGIC FINDINGS

• Because there are many different causes of flatfoot, the pathologic anatomy of the foot of a patient who presents with the fallen arch may differ according to cause: attenuated or torn posterior tibial tendon, tarsal coalition, lax ligaments.

IMAGING PROCEDURES

• Three plain radiographic views of the patient's ankle (anteroposterior, lateral, and mortise) and three views of the patient's foot (anteroposterior, lateral, and oblique) should be obtained.
• Standing lateral radiographs of the foot and ankle (taken with the patient bearing weight) are useful in quantifying the degree of flatfoot deformity.
• The index generally used is the talus-first metatarsal angle, measured by drawing a line through the longitudinal axis of the talus and through the axis of the first metatarsal and measuring the angle between the two.

—This angle should normally be 0 degrees with the two axes parallel to one another.
—An angle up to 15 degrees represents a minor pes planus deformity, an angle of 15 to 30 degrees represents a moderate deformity, and an angle greater than 30 degrees represents a severe deformity.

• When tarsal coalition is suspected, the following tests are used:

—The oblique radiograph is the study of choice in determining whether a calcaneonavicular bar is present.
—The study of choice to rule out a talocalcaneal fusion is a computed tomography scan; a 45-degree axial view of the subtalar joint (Harris' view) may be obtained; however, this view is not always reliable.

• In patients with a suspected posterior tibial tendon synovitis or rupture, a magnetic resonance imaging scan of the foot and ankle may be useful in visualizing the edematous nature of the tendon or any tears that may be present.

Management

GENERAL MEASURES

Congenital Flexible Flatfoot

• Conservative treatment should be instituted only when the deformity persists in childhood or adulthood and is symptomatic.
• Shoes with good arch supports are used.
• If necessary, the patient should progress to using orthotic devices such as the Thomas heel, or either a custom made or off the shelf soft insert orthosis; however, the efficacy of orthotics has not been proven.
• In the rare instance in which the deformity causes persistent pain and difficulty with weight bearing, operative treatment may be necessary.

Congenital Rigid Flatfoot from Tarsal Coalition With Peroneal Spasm

• This condition is treated when symptomatic.
• Initially, immobilization with a short leg walking cast is attempted for 4 weeks.
• If symptoms do not resolve, operative treatment is usually necessary.

Congenital Flatfoot Secondary to a Tight Achilles Tendon

• This condition may be relieved by physical therapy and stretching exercises.
• Should this approach fail, various tendon lengthening procedures may be used.

Acquired Flatfoot Secondary to Posterior Tibial Tendon Synovitis

• Initial treatment should be conservative.
• The caregiver should institute a regimen of nonsteroidal antiinflammatory drugs and rest to reduce the inflammation and to allow healing.
• If this fails, then a short leg cast or brace should be used for 4 to 6 weeks.
• Injection of corticosteroids is not recommended because it may weaken the already damaged and susceptible tendon and may only expedite rupture.
• Should conservative treatment fail, or should the synovitis recur, operative therapy should be instituted.

SURGICAL TREATMENT

Congenital Flexible Flatfoot

• Surgical treatments usually consist of osteotomies that realign the foot out of valgus so weight bearing is more physiologic.
• One common osteotomy is Evans' anterior calcaneal osteotomy, also known as Evans' opening wedge osteotomy.

Congenital Rigid Flatfoot from Tarsal Coalition With Peroneal Spasm

• The treatment of choice for coalitions in patients who are young and whose symptoms have been present for a short time is to resect the osseus bar with interposition of fat or muscle, usually the extensor digitorum brevis.
• In adults who have had symptoms for years and who have developed extensive degenerative arthritis, subtalar fusion or triple arthrodesis may be necessary.

Congenital Flatfoot Secondary to a Tight Achilles Tendon

• Tendon lengthening involves either a Z-lengthening procedure or partial sectioning of the tendon.

Acquired Flatfoot Secondary to Posterior Tibial Tendon Synovitis

• In early stages of the disease, synovectomy maybe sufficient.

—The surgeon opens the sheath of the tendon, débrides the swollen, degenerative synovial tissue, and repairs the sheath.
—The results are usually satisfactory, and deformity can be prevented if the procedure is carried out early enough.
—If the tendon has significantly degenerated or ruptured, or if synovectomy has failed, a tendon transfer is used, in which the flexor digitorum longus tendon replaces the posterior tibial tendon.

Synovectomy and tendon transfer are ineffective when arthrosis has developed and the hind foot and forefoot have become rigid. Fusion is necessary for alignment and to control pain.

PHYSICAL THERAPY

Physical therapy can be used to increase ankle and foot range of motion and to stretch a tight Achilles tendon. Occupational therapists or podiatrists can help with orthotics.

MEDICAL TREATMENT

Antiinflammatory medications can be used if swelling and pain are significant. These agents are most useful for acute injuries or in patients with posterior tibial tendinitis.

PATIENT EDUCATION

Patient education is important because patients with mild symptoms or those who are asymptomatic should avoid surgery for cosmetic reasons. Stretching exercises can help in patients with tight Achilles tendons, and foot orthoses may be useful for patients who want to be active.

MONITORING

Patients should be followed at 3-month intervals to monitor their discomfort and function and to check whether their deformity is stable or progressive.

COMPLICATIONS

Most patients have little risk of complications with nonoperative treatment. One major exception is patients with posterior tibial dysfunction (acquired flatfoot) because they may develop a rigid flatfoot.

PROGNOSIS

In general, prognosis is excellent. Most patients do not develop progressive deformities and do not need surgery.

RECOMMENDED READING

Bordelon RL. Flatfoot in children and young adults. In: Mann RA, Coughlin MJ, eds. *Surgery of the foot and ankle,* vol 1, 6th ed. St. Louis: Mosby–Year Book, 1993:717–756.

Mann RA. Flatfoot in adults. In: Mann RA, Coughlin MJ, eds. *Surgery of the foot and ankle,* vol 1, 6th ed. St. Louis: Mosby–Year Book, 1993:757–784

Pedowitz WJ, Kovatis P. Flatfoot in the adult. *J Am Acad Orthop Surg* 1995;3:293–302.

Staheli LT. *Fundamentals in pediatric orthopedics.* New York: Raven, 1992:5.14–5.17.

Flexor Tendon Laceration

 Basics

DESCRIPTION

Flexor tendon laceration may require emergency surgical repair, depending on the location of the laceration, hand dominance, and the age and occupation of the patient. Lacerations located between the distal transverse palmar crease and the most distal digit flexor crease represent an area of increased risk from scarring or adhesions and poor functional outcome resulting from the complex and precise anatomy in this area ("no-man's land"). The superficial and deep flexors are at risk at different locations in the hand because each has a superficial course on the palmar surface. Each tendon adds to the strength and independent function of the fingers in flexion.

INCIDENCE

This injury is one of the most common types of tendon lacerations.

CAUSES

The cause of the injury is sharp laceration to the tendon (e.g., knife, glass).

RISK FACTORS

Working with sharp objects

CLASSIFICATION

Classification is by the name of the tendon lacerated (superficial versus deep) and the location of the laceration.
The level of the laceration is most easily described by the zone of the injury:

Zone 1: Fingertip to proximal interphalangeal flexor crease
Zone 2: Proximal interphalangeal flexor crease to distal palmar transverse crease
Zone 3: Distal palmar transverse crease to distal wrist flexor crease

ICD-9-CM

840.9 Upper limb tendon laceration

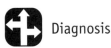 Diagnosis

SIGNS AND SYMPTOMS

• Laceration to the palmar aspect of the hand
• Change in the resting posture of the finger relative to the other fingers, that is, slight extension of the injured finger
• Loss of independent flexion of the distal digital joint flexor function when tested
• Loss of ability to flex the finger
• Decreased strength of finger flexion
• Evidence of tendon injury during wound exploration
• Evidence of tendon sheath or pulley laceration during wound exploration

DIFFERENTIAL DIAGNOSIS

• Fracture-dislocation
• Avulsion injury of tendon
• Rupture of tendon

PHYSICAL EXAMINATION

• Test independent dorsal and proximal interphalangeal flexor flexion (Figs. 1 and 2.)
• Test for lacerations of adjacent nerves.
• Test the strength of each finger.
• Explore the wound for a tendon or pulley injury.

IMAGING PROCEDURES

Obtain radiographs to rule out foreign body, fracture, dislocation, or avulsion injury.

 Management

GENERAL MEASURES

• Tetanus shot
• Wound washout with normal saline
• Antibiotics if the wound is contaminated
• Elevation and splinting of the hand until surgical evaluation is performed
• Orthopaedic consultation and preoperative laboratory tests
• Digital nerve and artery laceration

—Careful and complete neurovascular examination, including two-point discrimination and Doppler study of the neurovascular bundle on each side of the tendon in question

SURGICAL TREATMENT

Flexor tendon repair and results depend on the location, level, and type of injury. Primary acute repair has demonstrated the most functional results. In the presence of a flexor tendon sheath injury, early repair may be done to minimize scarring and adhesions and to give the best functional result.

PHYSICAL THERAPY

Postoperative range of motion depends on the location and type of repair. Usually, the goal is passive range of motion as soon as the skin repair tolerates motion.

MEDICAL TREATMENT

Antibiotic choice is related to the contamination at the time of injury.

PATIENT EDUCATION

• The patient should understand the severity of the injury even though the laceration may appear small.
• Functional outcome strongly depends on the compliance and cooperation of the patient.

PREVENTION

United States Occupational Safety and Health Administration guidelines should be used when working with sharp objects.

COMPLICATIONS

• Infection
• Decreased range of motion secondary to scarring or adhesions
• Loss of strength
• Need for delayed repair or reconstruction

PROGNOSIS

Prognosis greatly depends on the type and location of the injury. Injuries located between the distal transverse palmar crease and the most distal digit flexor crease often result in finger stiffness. In other areas, results are better.

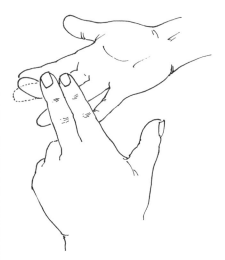

Fig. 1. Testing for an intact profundus tendon is performed by holding the proximal joints straight and asking the patient to flex only the distal joint.

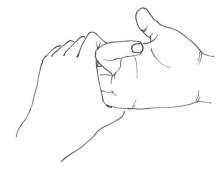

Fig. 2. Testing for an intact sublimis flexor tendon is done by asking patient to flex an individual finger while holding the other fingers in full extension. The finger will then flex only at the proximal joint.

Basics

DESCRIPTION

Forearm fractures involve the bones of the forearm, the radius and ulna, and sometimes the fractures are associated with elbow and wrist injuries. In addition to the bone injury, soft tissue injuries may include compartment syndrome, neuropraxia, and vascular damage. Adult patients are more susceptible to more severe injuries. Adults also require a more exact reduction because they have less potential for bony remodeling. Children younger than 12 years most often do not require anatomic reduction of forearm fractures. There is no particular gender predilection.

SYNONYMS

- Monteggia's fracture (forearm fracture with radial head dislocation)
- Galeazzi's fracture (forearm fractures with distal radioulnar joint dislocation)
- Both-bone forearm fracture

CAUSES

- High-energy trauma (e.g., motor vehicle accidents, fall from a height, crushing injury)
- Low-energy trauma (e.g., falls, gunshot injuries)

RISK FACTORS

- High-energy trauma
- Osteoporosis
- Gunshot wounds

CLASSIFICATION

- Multiple classification schemes
- Important factors: fracture location, fracture configuration, presence of any radioulnar or radiohumeral articular involvement, and status of the surrounding soft tissue

ASSOCIATED CONDITIONS

- Fractures of the ulna may be associated with dislocation of the radial head, an injury called Monteggia's fracture.
- Fractures of the radius may be associated with dislocation of the distal radioulnar joint, an injury also termed Galeazzi's fracture.

ICD-9-CM

813.8 Forearm fractures

 Diagnosis

SIGNS AND SYMPTOMS

- Pain
- Swelling
- Loss of elbow or wrist motion
- Deformity
- Important: assessment of forearm for skin and soft tissue (neurovascular) compromise

DIFFERENTIAL DIAGNOSIS

Look for associated wrist or elbow dislocations and interosseous membrane rupture.

PHYSICAL EXAMINATION

- Careful examination of the entire involved extremity is mandatory, including detailed neurologic and vascular evaluations and assessment of the soft tissues.
- Compartments, anterior (flexor) and posterior (extensor), are checked for evidence of compartment syndrome.
- Compartment pressure is measured if the forearm feels "tight" or if the patient displays pain on passive stretch.

LABORATORY TESTS

No serum tests are indicated.

PATHOLOGIC FINDINGS

Most forearm fractures are either transverse or short oblique in configuration. Comminution is variable from none to moderate.

IMAGING PROCEDURES

Anteroposterior, lateral, and oblique views of the wrist and the entire forearm, as well as anteroposterior and lateral views of the ipsilateral elbow, are mandatory. These may be obtainable on one set of films if the forearm is not too large and the patient allows proper positioning. However, if the foregoing views are not obtained, the physician should not hesitate to repeat them. Fracture of one bone is often accompanied by dislocation of another. Radiographic signs of injury to the distal radioulnar joint include fracture at the base of the ulnar styloid, widening of the joint space on the anteroposterior view, dislocation of the radius relative to the ulna on the lateral view, and radial shortening greater than 5 mm. If the radial head is properly located, a line drawn through the radial head and shaft on any radiographic projection should align with the capitellum of the elbow. If dislocation of the radial head is suspected clinically, a lateral radiograph of the elbow with the arm in supination may be helpful.

 Management

GENERAL MEASURES

Pain medication should be administered only after a careful physical examination, including documentation of neurovascular status. The forearm should be elevated, with application of ice to the fracture site to help to reduce swelling. Again, if ligamentous injury, dislocations, or open fractures are suspected, an orthopaedic surgeon should be consulted immediately.
In general, closed treatment of diaphyseal fractures is best applied to stable (less than 50% of the shaft diameter displaced), isolated fractures of the distal two-thirds of the ulna with 10 degrees or less of angular deformity. Fractures of the proximal one-third of the ulna and fractures of the distal two-thirds of the ulna with more than 10-degree angulation are best treated operatively. In addition, most radial shaft fractures, except those that are nondisplaced, and virtually all bone forearm fractures (prone to shortening and angulation), require surgical management.

SURGICAL TREATMENT

Surgical options include percutaneous Kirschner wire fixation, external fixation, intramedullary nailing, and plate and screw fixation.
For open fractures, irrigation and débridement with the administration of intravenous antibiotics should be performed on an emergency basis. If the open wound is not massively contaminated, the fractures are fixed after débridement (the original wound is left open). With massive contamination, fixation is performed in a delayed fashion. Radial and ulnar fractures are usually rigidly fixed with 3.5-mm dynamic compression plates.

PHYSICAL THERAPY

Early range of motion of the elbow and fingers is important to help to reduce soft tissue scarring and to prevent contractures. With rigid fixation, early forearm rotation is encouraged.

Forearm Fractures

MEDICAL TREATMENT

Closed forearm fractures of one or both bones that are minimally displaced should be splinted in a neutral position to prevent further displacement and possible neurovascular injury. If open fractures or dislocations are suspected, an orthopaedic surgeon should be notified promptly.

In general, forearm fractures with associated ligamentous injuries, either distally (wrist) or proximally (elbow), are unstable injuries. They are not always evident initially, and a high index of suspicion is required. These more severe injuries require early surgical intervention for reduction and stabilization of both the forearm fractures and the associated ligamentous injuries.

The forearm is usually immobilized and held in 90-degree flexion in a sling during the first week after injury to allow the soft tissue to heal. At that time, depending on the type of immobilization and associated elbow injuries, the patient's forearm should be allowed to come out of the sling periodically for early range-of-motion exercises to prevent elbow stiffness.

Acetaminophen plus a mild narcotic is most often used in the immediate postinjury period for pain control. Other nonsteroidal antiinflammatory drugs should be avoided if possible as first-line therapy for pain because of the increased risk of bleeding and hematoma formation immediately after a forearm fracture and the negative effect on fracture healing.

PATIENT EDUCATION

Patients should be told about the potential for posttraumatic arthritis for those fractures extending into the articular surfaces and about partial loss of pronation and supination of the forearm, depending on the severity of the initial injury and the final angulation at the fracture site.

MONITORING

Follow-up care should be arranged within 1 week after injury for repeat physical examination and repeat radiographs before and after the application of a cast, to verify fracture position when cast treatment is chosen. Further follow-up every 2 to 3 weeks is then necessary to assess healing of the fracture site and to guide early range of motion of the fingers and elbow. Healing of closed forearm fractures usually takes 4 to 6 weeks for a child and 6 to 12 weeks for an adult.

COMPLICATIONS

Nonoperative Treatment

- Decreased range of motion (supination and pronation)
- Synostosis (fusion of the radius and ulna)
- Malunion or nonunion (malunion usually defined as any fracture healing with greater than 20-degree angulation or 1 cm shortening)

Operative Treatment

Additional complications include the following:

- Late infections
- Skin breakdown
- Iatrogenic nerve injuries
- Vascular injuries
- Loss of fixation

Compartment Syndrome

Compartment syndrome is a risk in forearm fractures, after either operative or nonoperative treatment. It is manifest by exquisite pain on passive stretch of the digits. Constrictive dressings should be released down to the skin at the first symptom or sign of compartment syndrome.

PROGNOSIS

The prognosis depends on many factors, including the following:

- Fracture location
- Displacement
- Comminution
- Soft tissue condition
- Contamination

In general, most nondisplaced or minimally displaced fractures in children who receive closed treatment heal well, with good return of forearm function. The prognosis in adults with displaced fractures of the radius and ulna and closed treatment is poor. For those fractures treated with open reduction and rigid internal fixation, the prognosis for achieving union is about 95%. Because rigid fixation allows early range of motion, patients who have no associated severe soft tissue injuries should experience only mild loss of forearm rotation.

RECOMMENDED READING

Richards RR, Corley FG Jr. In: Rockwood CA, Green DP, Bucholz RW, et al., eds. *Rockwood and Green's fractures in adults,* vol 1, 4th ed. Philadelphia: Lippincott–Raven, 1996:870–899.

Basics

DESCRIPTION

"Freiberg's infraction" is an eponym for osteonecrosis of the second metatarsal head. The most common presentation is a young or middle-aged adult with a history of well-localized pain to the second metatarsophalangeal (MTP) joint that is aggravated with activities and relieved with rest.

- It primarily affects the second metatarsal head.
- Rarely, the third or other metatarsal heads may be involved.
- It may be unilateral or bilateral.

SYNONYM

Osteonecrosis of second metatarsal head

INCIDENCE

- Relatively rare: incidence less than 1 per 1,000
- Most common in 13 to 18 year olds; symptoms occasionally persisting into adulthood
- Females more commonly affected than males

CAUSES

This disorder is characterized by avascular necrosis of the involved metatarsal head (Fig. 1). Repetitive microtrauma may be a factor. The fact that the second metatarsal is the longest metatarsal places it under increased stress.

RISK FACTORS

- Running
- Dancing
- Long second metatarsal

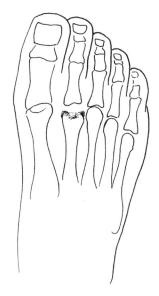

Fig. 1. Freiberg's disease involves avascular necrosis of the second metatarsal head.

CLASSIFICATION

- Early stages of the disease may demonstrate mottling of the metatarsal head or central collapse on radiographs.
- Late stages include loss of joint space and osteolysis.

ICD-9-CM

732.5 Freiberg's disease (flattening metatarsal)

Diagnosis

SIGNS AND SYMPTOMS

- Pain about the second MTP joint is aggravated with activity and alleviated by rest.
- Running appears to be associated with increased symptoms.
- Tenderness and soft tissue thickening about the second MTP joint may occur.
- Reduction in second MTP motion may develop.

DIFFERENTIAL DIAGNOSIS

- Synovitis in juvenile rheumatoid arthritis
- Fracture
- Sprain of joint
- Morton's neuroma

PHYSICAL EXAMINATION

- Joint motion decreased
- Tenderness to palpation
- Swelling after activity
- Pain on toe-raising

PATHOLOGIC FINDINGS

Rarely is a specimen taken. If examined, it shows typical findings of bone osteonecrosis, with fibrosis of the marrow space, bone resorption, and deposition.

IMAGING PROCEDURES

Foot radiographs are obtained: anteroposterior, lateral, and oblique views. The stages seen on plain films progress from osteopenia to a thin line of resorption under the joint surface to flattening of the normal rounded contour of the metatarsal head with sclerosis and cyst formation. Occasionally, in early or occult cases, bone scan or magnetic resonance imaging may be needed to confirm the diagnosis.

Management

GENERAL MEASURES

- Patients should avoid or limit activities that cause pain, especially running, jumping, and dancing.
- Early disease may be treated with a hard-sole shoe or a short leg walking cast.
- Recurrence may be prevented by using a metatarsal pad just proximal to the involved metatarsal head.
- Late stages of the disease may require surgery.

SURGICAL TREATMENT

Surgery is rarely necessary if conservative measures are tried at an appropriate time. Treatment options include the following:

- Joint débridement
- Dorsiflexion osteotomy of the involved metatarsal
- Metatarsal head excision
- Prosthetic joint replacement

MEDICAL TREATMENT

Nonsteroidal antiinflammatory agents may be used in patients who are satisfactory candidates, during periods of acute symptoms.

PATIENT EDUCATION

- Explain the concept of avascular necrosis, including the slow process of revascularization, and warn that joint collapse may occur if weight is borne prematurely.
- Describe activities likely to exacerbate the disorder, such as running and jumping.
- Suggest substitute activities such as swimming.

COMPLICATIONS

- Collapse of joint surface
- Arthritis of the second MTP joint (not common)

PROGNOSIS

In most patients, symptoms abate after the acute period and are replaced by an occasional ache.

RECOMMENDED READING

Coughlin MJ, Mann RA, eds. Surgery of the foot and ankle, 7th ed. St. Louis: Mosby—Yearbook, 1999.

Friedreich's Ataxia

 Basics

DESCRIPTION

Friedreich's ataxia is an uncommon, heritable disorder causing progressive spinocerebellar degeneration. Scoliosis, ataxia, and foot deformities are the most common findings (Fig. 1). Systems affected include the central nervous system, heart, and skeleton.

SYNONYM

Spinocerebellar degeneration

GENETICS

Transmission is autosomal recessive.

INCIDENCE

• Prevalence is approximately 1 in 50,000 population.
• It may become apparent anytime between 5 and 25 years of age.
• Males and females are affected equally.

CAUSES

The cause is a defect in a gene for a protein, frataxin, found on chromosome 9. The pathogenesis of the findings is not well known. Variations in characteristics of the disease, such as age at onset and rate of progression, may be caused by different mutations at one of the loci.

RISK FACTORS

The condition is more common in people of French Canadian descent.

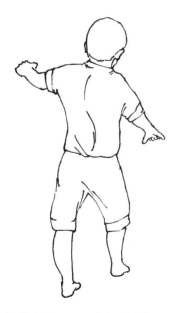

Fig. 1. Scoliosis, cavovarus feet, and ataxia as seen in Friedreich's ataxia.

CLASSIFICATION

There are no subclassifications of Friedreich's ataxia. It is classified under the category spinocerebellar degeneration, and it is the most common example of this class. Another disorder in this class is spinocerebellar ataxia.

ASSOCIATED CONDITIONS

• Diabetes mellitus
• Cardiomyopathy
• Scoliosis
• Foot deformity

ICD-9-CM

334.0 Friedreich ataxia

 Diagnosis

The diagnosis is made on a clinical basis, usually confirmed by a neurologist.

SIGNS AND SYMPTOMS

Common Signs

• Ataxia, wide-based gait, weakness and loss of position sense in the lower extremities, and loss of reflexes in the upper extremities occur frequently.

Less Common Signs

• Pes cavus, optic atrophy, and nystagmus are possible.

Symptoms

• Partial deafness, depression, loss of coordination, painful muscle spasms, and weakness occur.
• Symptoms of diabetes mellitus may also be related, because of the increased coexistence of these disorders.

DIFFERENTIAL DIAGNOSIS

• Cerebellar tumors
• Chiari's malformation
• Muscular dystrophy
• Spinal dysraphism (as a cause of scoliosis and foot deformity)

PHYSICAL EXAMINATION

• Heel-to-toe walking and finger-to-nose testing should be examined (Fig. 2).
• The presence of increased kyphosis on routine standing should be observed.
• The forward-bend test for scoliosis should be performed.
• Reflexes in the upper and lower extremities should be tested.
• The flexibility of the feet and the correctability of any deformity are noted.
• Muscle strength (proximal muscles are affected earlier than distal muscles) should be tested.
• Gluteus maximus is the first muscle to be affected clinically.

LABORATORY TESTS

• Creatine phosphokinase levels are normal.
• Fasting serum glucose for diabetes mellitus should be obtained.

OTHER TESTS

Electrocardiography should be performed before surgery, with echocardiography as indicated, because of the increased incidence of hypertrophic cardiomyopathy. Electromyography shows polyphasic potentials, as well as mild slowing of nerve conduction velocity.

IMAGING PROCEDURES

Standing posteroanterior and lateral radiographs of the spine should be ordered when scoliosis and kyphosis are found. Periodic monitoring is then indicated, even after maturity.

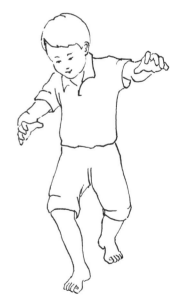

Fig. 2. Ataxia and cavovarus feet in Friedreich's ataxia.

⚂ Management

GENERAL MEASURES

• Foot and spine deformities should be followed by an orthopaedic surgeon, even if surgery is not contemplated.
• Brace treatment of scoliosis is appropriate for curves of 25 to 45 degrees and may slow the rate of progression.
• Stretching and night bracing may be helpful in preventing worsening of the foot deformities.
• Walking should be maintained as long as possible.

SURGICAL TREATMENT

Scoliosis

Posterior fusion with instrumentation using two contoured rods is indicated in curves greater than 50 degrees to prevent progressive decompensation of the spine. If the curve is large, rigid, and unbalanced, an anterior release may also be indicated to increase the correctability. Postoperative immobilization is not usually necessary. A cardiopulmonary evaluation is indicated preoperatively.

Cavovarus Feet

Correction of cavovarus feet may include plantar fasciotomy, Achilles tendon lengthening and transfer or lengthening of the posterior tibialis tendon, and possible osteotomy.

PHYSICAL THERAPY

• Therapy is essential, to keep up strength and skills after surgery.
• Stretching of plantar fascia and ankle muscles will help to prevent deformity.

MEDICAL TREATMENT

• No medical treatment is available at present.
• If painful muscle spasms occur, baclofen or diazepam may be helpful.

PATIENT EDUCATION

• Patients should be counseled about the natural history of the disease, which consists of slow degeneration, so they can plan appropriately.
• Patient support groups are often helpful.
• Genetic counseling should be offered.

MONITORING

This is a progressive disease. Walking distance and status of all physical findings should be monitored every 3 to 6 months. Scoliosis, if present, should be checked every 6 months.

COMPLICATIONS

• Cardiomyopathy
• Calluses or skin breakdown on the foot
• Pneumonia

PROGNOSIS

• If scoliosis develops before 15 years of age, it will most likely become severe and require surgery.
• Most affected individuals stop walking by 20 to 30 years of age and are wheelchair dependent.
• Death usually occurs by fourth or fifth decade; causes most often include pneumonia, aspiration, and cardiomyopathy.

RECOMMENDED READING

Cady RB, Bobechko WP. Incidence, natural history and treatment of scoliosis in Friedreich's ataxia. *J Pediatr Orthop* 1984;4:673–678.

Labelle H, Tohme S, Duhaime M, et al. Natural history of scoliosis in Friedreich's ataxia. *J Bone Joint Surg Am* 1986;68:564–570.

Shapiro F, Bresnan MJ. Current concepts review: orthopaedic management of childhood neuromuscular disease. *J Bone Joint Surg Am* 1982;64:949–960.

Genu Valgum (Knock-Knee)

 Basics

DESCRIPTION

Genu valgum, or knock-knee, is physiologic in children between 2 and 4 years of age. Girls normally have slightly more valgus of the knee than boys. The valgus straightens to achieve the adult position by 6 to 7 years of age. Rickets, trauma, and genetic disorders may also cause genu valgum. Some patients have an idiopathic valgus, not resulting from any of the foregoing disorders, that falls outside the normal limits and persists beyond 10 years of age. Areas affected include the distal femoral and tibial growth plates.

GENETICS

- Many forms of rickets are genetically transmitted.
- Idiopathic valgus may be transmitted in families.

INCIDENCE

- The condition is rare.
- None of the foregoing causes exceed 1 per 1,000.
- It occurs in young children, usually 3 to 11 years of age.
- Physiologic genu valgum is more common in females.

CAUSES

- Physiologic genu valgum
- Metabolic disorder (e.g., rickets)
- Steroid dependence
- Proximal tibia fracture
- Skeletal dysplasias
- Chromosome disorders (e.g., Klinefelter's syndrome)

RISK FACTORS

- Family history of genu valgum
- Proximal tibia metaphysis fracture in children (Cozen's fracture); asymmetric overgrowth occurring and deformity possible (parents should be warned about this)

ASSOCIATED CONDITIONS

- Proximal tibia fracture
- Pseudoachondroplasia
- Renal osteodystrophy
- Metaphyseal dysplasia
- Rickets
- Down's syndrome

ICD-9-CM

736.41 Genu valgum

 Diagnosis

SIGNS AND SYMPTOMS

- Parental concern about the appearance of the child's legs is the most common reason for presentation.
- It is usually asymptomatic.
- The knees are usually not painful; however, the physical appearance is sometimes bothersome. Occasionally, valgus knees are associated with patellar discomfort.
- In adulthood, valgus knees are more likely to produce arthritic symptoms in the outside of the joint.

DIFFERENTIAL DIAGNOSIS

The main differential diagnosis is to determine whether the condition is physiologic or pathologic. Physiologic genu valgum occurs without underlying rickets, dysplasia, or other known cause. The most common skeletal dysplasias causing valgus are metaphyseal dysplasia and pseudoachondroplasia, as well as multiple osteochondromas.

PHYSICAL EXAMINATION

- Measure the range of motion of the knee.
- Determine and plot height and weight percentiles for the patient's age.
- Measure the angle between the tibia and the femur with a goniometer.
- Assess the alignment and range of motion in the adjacent hip and ankle.
- Check the rotation of the limb, as well as the gait.
- Check the collateral ligaments of the knee for laxity.

LABORATORY TESTS

Serum levels of calcium, phosphate, alkaline phosphatase, urea nitrogen, and creatinine should be measured if rickets or a metabolic problem is suspected. The most common type of rickets in developed countries is familial hypophosphatemic rickets. If rickets is to be evaluated, check vitamin D levels (25-hydroxy and 1,25 dihydroxy).

IMAGING PROCEDURES

- Imaging of genu valgum is unnecessary for children younger than 6 years of age, unless the patient has an asymmetric deformity or is suspected to have a pathologic condition.
- An anteroposterior view of the lower extremity from the hip to ankle obtained while the patient is standing should the first imaging study. The knee should be pointing straight ahead. The film cassette should be long enough to accommodate the entire extremity.
- The femorotibial angle should be measured, and the site of the deformity should be identified as femoral, tibial, or both.

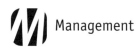 Management

GENERAL MEASURES

Physiologic Condition

No treatment is indicated for physiologic genu valgum in patients less than 7 years of age. If the deformity persists after 7 years of age, later hemiepiphysiodesis (at age 11 to 12 years) may be considered, based on growth-remaining data to achieve straight alignment. Epiphysiodesis consists of slowing or stopping the growth plate on the inside, to allow the outside to catch up to it. This is a relatively simple procedure that does not make the bone unstable and allows early weight bearing.

Pathologic Condition

For metabolic disorders, including renal osteodystrophy, the underlying condition should be treated. Bracing has not been effective in preventing or reversing the deformity. Single- or multiple-level osteotomy may be necessary to correct the deformity; medical control of the disease is needed first. Usually, therapy is directed by a renal or endocrine specialist.

Fracture

Follow-up of proximal tibia fracture should extend for several years after the injury. Early tibial osteotomy should be avoided because of the high incidence of recurrence of valgus deformity. After 1 to 2 years of follow-up, if an unacceptable degree of valgus remains, hemiepiphysiodesis or osteotomy may be indicated.

Dysplasia

Children with pseudoachondroplasia and metaphyseal dysplasias are likely to develop genu valgum. Osteotomy may be necessary to correct the deformity. The child's activity should be as tolerated.

SURGICAL TREATMENT

Two types of surgery are commonly used to correct the valgus deformity: hemiepiphysiodesis and varus osteotomy. Epiphysiodesis is based on growth-remaining data and aims to achieve good mechanical alignment at the end of growth. Proximal tibia osteotomy should be considered if epiphysiodeses is not feasible. It should include fibula osteotomy to prevent recurrence of the valgus deformity. Osteotomy involves a more difficult recovery period than epiphysiodesis, because in the former procedure, the bone is divided completely. The overall success rate of surgery is greater than 90%.

PHYSICAL THERAPY

- This is not indicated.
- Therapy and exercises cannot affect the growth of the limb.

PATIENT EDUCATION

Inform parents that most cases of physiologic genu valgum begin to resolve spontaneously by 7 years of age.

MONITORING

Children with idiopathic genu valgum should be followed every 6 to 12 months to determine whether the deformity is improving before a treatment decision is made.

COMPLICATIONS

Untreated Genu Valgum

If valgus is severe, the patient may develop patellofemoral pain and late degenerative arthritis from stresses on the lateral joint surface.

Surgical Complications

- Infection
- Compartment syndrome
- Recurrence of deformity or overcorrection and neurovascular injury

PROGNOSIS

Physiologic genu valgum resolves by age 7 to 10 years, as long as it is mild (less than 15 degrees) and there are no metabolic problems.

RECOMMENDED READING

Balthazar DA, Pappas AM. Acquired valgus deformity of the tibia in children. *J Pediatr Orthop* 1984;4:538–541.

Bowen JR, Toffes RR, Forlin E. Partial epiphysiodesis to address genu varum or genu valgum. *J Pediatr Orthop* 1992;12:359–364.

Brougham DI, Nicol RO. Valgus deformity after proximal tibial fractures in children. *J Bone Joint Surg Br* 1987;69:482.

Genu Varum (Bowlegs)

 Basics

DESCRIPTION

The knee goes through normal phases of angulation in childhood. Genu varum (bowlegs) is physiologic in infants and young children up to 2 years of age, and its appearance is maximal at 12 to 18 months of age. Bowing is most obvious when children start walking. It may be combined with internal tibial torsion, which makes it appear more pronounced. Bowing may seem greater with weight bearing. This condition usually resolves by 2 years of age and changes to physiologic genu valgum (knock-knees). Tibia vara (Blount's disease), rickets, fibrocartilaginous dysplasia of the proximal tibia, and other genetic disorders can cause pathologic genu varum.

GENETICS

Some causes of bowed legs are familial:

- Blount's disease
- Renal rickets
- Skeletal dysplasia

INCIDENCE

- Physiologic (normal) bowing is approximately 1,000 times more common than pathologic bowing (e.g., Blount's disease).
- It occurs equally in boys and in girls.

CAUSES

Bowing is always a balance between the load and growth plate development. It may be caused by the following:

- Overweight
- Rickets
- Skeletal dysplasia

Physiologic Causes

Normal growth patterns of the femoral and tibial growth plates include a period of normal varus in early infancy.

Pathologic Causes

- Tibia vara (Blount's disease)
- Rickets (nutritional or renal)
- Achondroplasia
- Epiphyseal and metaphyseal dysplasias
- Focal fibrocartilaginous dysplasia

In most of these conditions, the varus results from inability of the growth plate to respond to load normally.

RISK FACTORS

Family history

ASSOCIATED CONDITIONS

- Early walker
- Heavy weight

ICD-9-CM

736.42 Genu varum

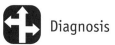 Diagnosis

SIGNS AND SYMPTOMS

- Parental concern about the appearance of the legs is the most common reason for presentation of children.
- The patient should be pain free; if pain exists, another cause should be sought.
- Genu varum may develop spontaneously in the overweight adolescent who previously had straight legs (adolescent Blount's disease), and it usually requires treatment.

DIFFERENTIAL DIAGNOSIS

- Achondroplasia
- Rickets
- Infantile or adolescent Blount's disease
- Metaphyseal or epiphyseal dysplasia

PHYSICAL EXAMINATION

- Obtain a medical, family, and developmental history.
- Determine the patient's height and weight percentiles.
- Estimate the angulation of the knee.
- Check the rotation of the tibia and femur.
- To monitor patient's progress, follow up on the distance between the medial surfaces of the knees.

LABORATORY TESTS

- In routine cases, tests are not indicated if varus appears mild and "physiologic."
- If metabolic causes are suspected, serum calcium, phosphate, alkaline phosphatase, 1,25-vitamin D, and creatinine levels may be measured.

IMAGING PROCEDURES

- Radiographic evaluation of bowlegs in children younger than 18 months of age should be reserved for asymmetric bowing or for patients suspected of having a pathologic condition other than benign physiologic varus.
- A single anteroposterior radiograph of the lower extremity from hip to ankle on a standing film is the most appropriate first imaging study; care should be taken that the knee is pointing straight ahead.
- Widening of physis suggests rickets; delayed ossification of the distal femoral and proximal tibial epiphyses may be a result of excessive pressure on one side of knee.
- The femorotibial angle and the metaphyseal-diaphyseal angle of the tibia should be measured.
- If the metaphyseal-diaphyseal angle is greater than 16 degrees, Blount's disease is likely.

Management

GENERAL MEASURES

Physiologic Conditions

- Physiologic bowing always resolves without treatment; bracing is not needed.
- At 18 months of age, follow-up examination and imaging are needed to differentiate physiologic bowing from tibia vara (may be difficult).

Pathologic Conditions

- Rickets or other metabolic bone disease: The underlying disease is treated, with osteotomy reserved for those patients with persisting varus after treatment.
- Achondroplasia and epiphyseal or metaphyseal dysplasia: The patient may need surgical treatment depending on the degree of deformity.
- Tibia vara (Blount's disease): Brace treatment is appropriate for children younger than 3 years of age. A knee-ankle-foot orthosis brace may be used for walking. If the patient is more than 4 years of age, osteotomy is recommended.

SURGICAL TREATMENT

- The type of osteotomy for correcting varus deformity may include dome, oblique, closing wedge, or opening wedge osteotomy.
- The tibia or the femur may require surgery, depending on the site of the deformity.
- Physeal bar resection or hemiepiphysiodesis may be indicated for some cases.

PHYSICAL THERAPY

- Not necessary for physiologic bowing
- Not an effective treatment for pathologic varus

PATIENT EDUCATION

- Parents should be told that physiologic genu varum will resolve spontaneously and slowly; if it is not at least starting to improve by 2 to 3 years of age, further evaluation is needed.
- No restriction on activity is recommended.
- Exercises do not help genu varum to resolve.

MONITORING

- The frequency of follow-up varies, depending on the individual surgeon or pediatrician.
- Physiologic bowing does not need frequent follow-up unless the condition is not improving; it is a slow process and may take a year.
- Pathologic bowing needs more prolonged follow-up.

COMPLICATIONS

- Untreated genu varum may cause pain on the medial part of the knee and eventual arthritis during adulthood.
- Adolescent genu varum may be painful.
- Complications from surgery include infection, compartment syndrome, recurrence of deformity, and growth disturbance.

PROGNOSIS

- Physiologic genu varum has an excellent prognosis for spontaneous improvement.
- The prognosis of pathologic genu varum varies.
- Knee pain and worsening of the bow are likely in adulthood if the deformity is greater than 10 to 15 degrees.

RECOMMENDED READING

Langenskiold A. Tibia vara: a critical review. *Clin Orthop* 1989;246:195–207.

Morrissy RT, Weinstein SL, eds. *Lovell and Winter's pediatric orthopaedics*, 4th ed. Philadelphia: Lippincott–Raven, 1996:1054–1061.

Salenius P, Vankka E. The development of the tibiofemoral angle in children. *J Bone Joint Surg* 1975;57:259–261.

Giant Cell Tumor

 Basics

DESCRIPTION

This is a benign but often locally aggressive neoplasm, characterized by large numbers of uniformly distributed, osteoclastlike giant cells and a background population of plump, epithelioid-to-spindle mononuclear cells (Fig. 1). More than 75% of these tumors are located near the articular end of a tubular bone; approximately 50% occur in the knee. Additional frequently involved sites include the distal radius, proximal femur, proximal humerus, and distal tibia. Flat bone involvement tends to involve the sacrum and pelvis. Giant cell tumor complicating Paget's disease often involves the flat bones, particularly those of the craniofacial region. Multifocal giant cell tumors are rare.

INCIDENCE

- It accounts for 5% of biopsied primary bone tumors and approximately 20% of benign bone tumors.
- It is the sixth most common primary osseous neoplasm.
- It almost always affects the mature skeleton with closed epiphyseal plates.
- Approximately 10% to 15% of patients are less than 20 years of age, but almost all are skeletally mature.
- The peak incidence is in the third decade of life, with a gradual decline into late adulthood.
- The onset of giant cell tumor after 55 years of age is rare.
- Less than 2% of these tumors occur adjacent to open epiphyses; the diagnosis of giant cell tumor in a skeletally immature patient must therefore be questioned.

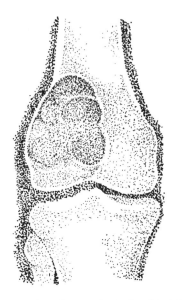

Fig. 1. A giant cell tumor arises in the epiphysis but may expand into the metaphysis. The distal femoral epiphysis is one of the most common sites.

- Females are affected 1.3 to 1.5 times as often as males.

CAUSES

Rare cases may result as a complication of pre-existing Paget's disease of bone.

RISK FACTORS

Paget's disease (rare association)

CLASSIFICATIONS

Muscluloskeletal Tumor Society (MSTS) surgical staging system (also a grading system that may have prognostic importance):

Stage I (less than 5% of patients): It is virtually asymptomatic and often discovered incidentally, occasionally may cause pathologic fracture, has a sclerotic rim on a plain radiograph or computed tomography scan, is relatively inactive on a bone scan, and is histologically benign.

Stage II (70% to 85% of patients): It is symptomatic, may be associated with pathologic fracture, has an expanded cortex but no breakthrough on a plain radiograph, is active on a bone scan, and is histologically benign.

Stage III (10% to 15% of patients): It is a symptomatic, rapidly growing mass, it has cortical perforation with an accompanying soft tissue mass on a plain radiograph or computed tomography scan, its activity on a bone scan extends beyond the lesion seen on a plain radiograph, it shows intense hypervascularity on angiography, and it is histologically benign, although one may see tumor infiltration of peritumoral capsule with violation of the cortex and extension into the surrounding soft tissues.

ASSOCIATED CONDITIONS

- Rarely, giant cell tumors may complicate Paget's disease of bone.
- More frequently, secondary aneurysmal bone cyst formation may be associated with giant cell tumor.

ICD-9-CM

170.9 Giant cell tumor

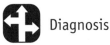 Diagnosis

SIGNS AND SYMPTOMS

- Complaints are generally nonspecific, and patients often have joint symptoms.
- Ninety percent of patients complain of pain, often with accompanying mass or swelling.
- Five to 10% of patients present with pathologic fracture.
- Serum chemistry studies are typically normal.

DIFFERENTIAL DIAGNOSIS

- Giant cell reparative granuloma, or "brown tumor" of hyperparathyroidism (the giant cell reparative granuloma tumor contains a more uniform distribution of larger giant cells with many more nuclei)
- Nonossifying fibroma
- Benign fibrous histiocytoma
- Aneurysmal bone cyst

PHYSICAL EXAMINATION

- Examination is not specific for this condition.
- In general, tenderness over the epiphyseal end of a bone adjacent to a joint is seen.
- There may be an effusion or restriction of joint motion if the tumor has nearly violated the cortex.

LABORATORY TESTS

Serum calcium and phosphate levels should be checked to exclude hyperparathyroidism.

PATHOLOGIC FINDINGS

The tumor has a background of proliferating, homogeneous mononuclear cells. These are round to ovoid, have relatively large nuclei with inconspicuous nucleoli, and display multinucleated giant cells dispersed evenly throughout the tissue. Mitotic figures may be common. It may have an aneurysmal bone cyst component, and it may invade blood vessels. Involutional changes with lipid-filled histiocytes may be observed.

IMAGING PROCEDURES

• Plain radiographs show an eccentric, expanding zone of radiolucency frequently at the end of a long bone.
• Usually, no reactive sclerosis is present.
• The tumor often begins in the metaphysis and extends to the articular surface.
• Almost invariably, it involves the epiphysis, usually with metaphyseal extension.
• If the spine is affected, it usually is anterior vertebral body.
• The tumor is multicentric in only 1% of cases.
• Chest radiography is performed because 2% of patients may have pulmonary metastases.
• A bone scan is often positive, but the lesion may be inactive on a bone scan.

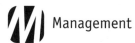 Management

GENERAL MEASURES

Patients with large lesions are placed on crutches until their definitive surgery.

SURGICAL TREATMENT

• Current technique involves a combination of marginal resection and curettage using power burrs on the margins of the cavity, followed by painting with full-strength phenol.
• Polymethyl methacrylate cement augmentation may be applied to fill the cavity and to provide a rigid construct.
• Cancellous bone grafting is used to restore the subchondral surface.
• Internal fixation may be necessary to provide a rigid construct.
• When the tumor is in an expendable bone, such as the fibula, or in recurrent lesions with joint destruction, wide resection is indicated.
• Reconstruction around the knee may involve resection arthrodesis, osteoarticular allograft, or prosthetic implantation.
• Amputation may be indicated for neglected tumors with significant soft tissue extension and, in rare instances, for recurrent tumors.
• Radiotherapy rarely should be used for giant cell tumors because its use increases the risk of malignant behavior of the tumor.

PHYSICAL THERAPY

Patients undergo physical therapy to regain their range of motion and strength.

PATIENT EDUCATION

The patient should understand the frequency of recurrence and the need for continued follow-up. The patient should also understand that the tumor is considered benign, but that in rare instances it may metastasize to the lungs (2% risk).

MONITORING

• Because recurrence is common, patients should be followed closely postoperatively (every 3 months for 2 years).
• A chest radiograph is taken once a year.

COMPLICATIONS

A secondary malignant giant cell tumor results when a sarcoma develops at the site of a previously treated giant cell tumor: 10% to 15% of patients with giant cell tumors treated with irradiation in the past developed postradiation sarcomas; in comparison, approximately 5% of recurrent giant cell tumors not subjected to radiation developed sarcomatous transformation.

PROGNOSIS

Recurrence may occur in 40% to 60% of giant cell tumors treated by simple curettage alone. Most recurrences occur within 2 years, and nearly all occur within 5 years.

RECOMMENDED READING

Bullough PG. *Atlas of orthopedic pathology,* 2nd ed. New York: Gower Medical Publishing, 1992:17.6–17.8.

Campanacci M, Baldini N, Boriani S, et al. Giant cell tumor of bone. *J Bone Joint Surg Am* 1987;69:106–114.

Fechner RE, Mills SE. *Atlas of tumor pathology: tumors of the bones and joints.* Washington, DC: Armed Forces Institute of Pathology, 1992:173–181.

Growing Pains

 Basics

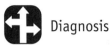 Diagnosis

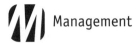 Management

DESCRIPTION

This poorly understood syndrome is characterized by a long history of lower extremity pains, usually occurring at night, and worsened after activity. No objective physical findings are seen. The pain predominantly occurs in the lower extremities.

SYNONYMS

- Leg aches
- Night pains

INCIDENCE

- Very common
- An estimated 15% to 30% of children complaining of these pains at some time
- Occurring in children 3 to 12 years of age
- Slightly more common in girls than in boys

CAUSES

The condition is believed to be due to stretch or fatigue of muscle. Support for this theory includes the beneficial response that many children have to a stretching program.

RISK FACTORS

High activity levels in normal children

ICD-9-CM

729.5 Growing pains

SIGNS AND SYMPTOMS

Signs

- Nonspecific for this condition
- No localized tenderness
- No limp
- Full range of motion

Symptoms

- Pains occur after periods of activity, most often at night.
- Pains come and go spontaneously.
- Pains are most often bilateral, vague, and poorly localized.
- Symptoms are often of long duration, a feature that helps to rule out more serious causes.

DIFFERENTIAL DIAGNOSIS

- Perthes' disease
- Chronic or subacute osteomyelitis
- Leukemia
- Sickle cell anemia
- Juvenile rheumatoid arthritis
- Lyme disease
- Osgood-Schlatter disease (older child)

PHYSICAL EXAMINATION

- Usually with a careful history and physical examination, one can rule out more serious causes and define a typical picture.
- The child should be observed while walking into the office, especially before the child knows that the examiner is watching; there should not be any stiffness or limp.
- The lower extremities should be palpated systematically for tenderness; growing pains do not manifest tenderness.
- The range of motion of the hips, knees, and ankles should be checked.
- The hips, in particular, should show no stiffness or guarding on gentle rolling (the "roll test"). Range of motion should be full and symmetric.

LABORATORY TESTS

- Complete blood count and sedimentation rate may be done if the history is not typical.
- An appropriate workup tailored to the possibilities listed earlier in the differential diagnosis should then be undertaken.

IMAGING PROCEDURES

Bone scans and plain radiographs may help to define the site of pain if the history is not typical.

GENERAL MEASURES

- Reassurance of the parent and child is the first step if the diagnosis of growing pains fits the story.
- A program of stretching for the hamstrings, quadriceps, and calf muscles at night before bed has been shown to decrease the number of complaints; this may work by mechanical means or by virtue of increased parent-child attention.
- Activity levels may need to be modified to bring symptoms into a tolerable range.

PHYSICAL THERAPY

The stretching program described earlier may be guided by parents and does not require a trained therapist.

MEDICAL TREATMENT

Analgesics may be used periodically, but not continuously.

PATIENT EDUCATION

- Describe the nature of the process.
- Instruct in stretching.
- Offer to see the patient any time the symptoms change.

MONITORING

- Several successive office visits may be needed to demonstrate the character of the pain or to determine the direction of the workup.
- The stretching program is maintained and the activity level is adjusted as needed.

PROGNOSIS

Spontaneous resolution is the rule as the patient matures.

RECOMMENDED READING

Baxter MP, Dulberg C. "Growing pains" in childhood: a proposal for treatment. *J Pediatr Orthop* 1988;8:402–406.

Staheli LT. Leg aches. In: Staheli LT, ed. *Fundamentals of pediatric orthopedics*. New York, Raven, 1992:4.1.

Basics

DESCRIPTION

Defined as injury to the growing portion of children's bones, or physeal plate, some growth plate injuries do not produce growth disturbances. Only those causing significant crushing or malalignment of the growth plate cause such sequelae. The most commonly affected bones are the long bones of the growing child. The four most commonly fractured sites are the distal radius, distal tibia, phalanges, and proximal humerus. When injured, the distal femur and the distal tibia are the sites that most commonly show a growth disturbance.

SYNONYMS

- Physeal injuries
- Salter fractures

INCIDENCE

- These injuries account for 15% to 20% of all pediatric fractures.
- These injuries occur most frequently in girls between 11 and 12 years of age and in boys between 12 and 14 years of age, when growth is most rapid and trauma is most serious.
- Growth plate injuries may occur at any age, but adolescents have a higher incidence of physeal fractures.
- Younger patients have a higher risk of serious sequela of a growth plate fracture, because they have more growth remaining.
- Boys are affected twice as frequently as girls.

CAUSES

- Trauma is the most common cause of growth plate injury.
- Other causes that damage the physis include infection, tumors, drugs (e.g., steroids, estrogen, testosterone), and excessive heat or cold.

RISK FACTORS

Adolescent boys

CLASSIFICATION

The Salter-Harris classification describes five patterns of growth plate fractures and is used universally. Types III, IV, and V are at high risk for growth plate damage (Fig. 1).

Type I: Split along the physis without involvement of the metaphysis or epiphysis

Type II: Split along the physis that exits through the metaphysis (most common type)

Type III: An intraarticular fracture of the epiphysis that exits transversely out the physeal plate

Type IV: Fracture of the epiphysis that exits through the metaphysis

Type V: Crush injury to the physis

ASSOCIATED CONDITIONS

- Ligamentous injury
- Chest, abdominal, and head trauma
- Neurovascular injury

ICD-9-CM

813.42 Fracture of distal radial epiphysis
821.22 Fracture of distal femoral epiphysis
824.4 Fracture of distal tibial epiphysis

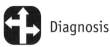 Diagnosis

SIGNS AND SYMPTOMS

- Pain and swelling are the most frequent findings, often accompanied by deformity.
- Sometimes crepitus can be felt.

DIFFERENTIAL DIAGNOSIS

- In the chronic condition, other causes of growth plate injury must be considered.
- Infection may be especially insidious.

PHYSICAL EXAMINATION

The limb should be carefully evaluated for open wounds and distal neurovascular status.

PATHOLOGIC FINDINGS

The growth plate consists of the zone of growth, cartilage transformation, ossification, and the metaphysis. Physeal fractures usually cleave at the zone of cartilage transformation. Fractures through the growth zone may be more prone to growth abnormalities. Permanent injury occurs when a fracture causes malalignment of the edges of the growth plate or when fracture or infection causes the death of cells of the growth plate.

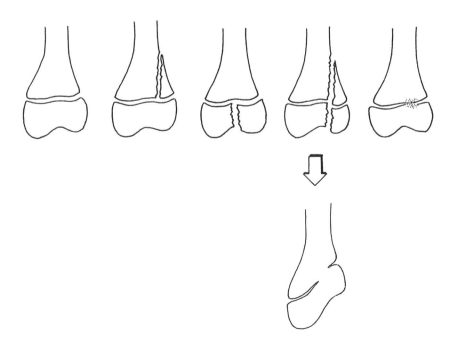

Fig. 1. Salter-Harris classification of growth plate injuries into types I to V (*left to right*). These injuries may result in angular deformity (*lower*).

Growth Plate Injury

IMAGING PROCEDURES

• Anteroposterior and lateral radiographs of the involved area are required.
• Occasionally, tomograms or computed tomography scans may be needed to evaluate more complicated fracture patterns.
• Magnetic resonance imaging is the best method to diagnose an established injury to the growth plate; it shows the cartilage line of the growth plate as distinct from bone. (This should be discussed with the radiologist in advance to select the best settings.)

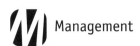 Management

GENERAL MEASURES

• Immediate care for any fracture includes immobilization and ice.
• The neurovascular status of the extremity should be evaluated and treated if necessary.
• Pain medication can be used if compartment syndrome is not a concern.
• Nondisplaced fractures can be splinted immediately.
• Displaced fractures should be reduced using conscious sedation, hematoma block, or general anesthesia; the fracture is then splinted, and reduction is checked with repeat radiographs.
• If a fracture involves the growth plate, patients should be seen within 3 to 5 days. Splints are usually maintained for 1 to 2 weeks and are then replaced by a circumferential cast once edema has mostly resolved.
• The patient is referred to the orthopaedic surgeon for definitive management.
• Non–weight bearing is indicated for lower extremity fractures, and upper extremity fractures are often protected with a sling.

SURGICAL TREATMENT

If closed reduction is not possible, some fractures must be reduced openly in the operating room. These fractures and any other fracture that is not stable after reduction must be pinned percutaneously or internally fixed. All open fractures require operative irrigation and débridement.

MEDICAL TREATMENT

Pain control is indicated.

PATIENT EDUCATION

• The family must understand proper cast care and the possibility of future growth abnormality with physeal injury.
• The family must understand the need to bring the child for 6- to 12-month follow-up of Salter-Harris classification III or IV fracture or any fracture of distal femur or proximal tibia.

PREVENTION

• The adverse effects of growth plate damage may be prevented in some cases, if they are detected early.
• The "bar" of bone that forms in the area of damage may be resected if it is less than 50% to allow normal growth; otherwise, corrective osteotomy for angulation, or lengthening the damaged limb if it is more than 4 cm short, can be done.
• A simple option is to stop the growth in the contralateral growth plate to maintain symmetry.

MONITORING

Patients with growth plate injuries at increased risk of growth disturbance (Salter-Harris classification III to V and all distal femur and distal tibial physeal injuries) should be followed for at least 6 to 12 months to ensure normal growth. At that time, the physician should look for equality of limb length and angulation, for presence of a clean "open" growth plate line on a radiograph, and for a "growth arrest line" of bone that was formed at the time of injury to be separated from the growth plate by an even layer of normal newly formed bone.

COMPLICATIONS

• Growth arrest (physis stops growing)
• Malunion
• Growth disturbance (physis grows abnormally with resultant angulation), a more serious complication than growth acceleration
• Growth acceleration from increased blood flow for healing, which may occur in any child less than 10 years of age with a fracture and usually amounts to only 5 to 10 mm

PROGNOSIS

• Most of physeal fractures heal without difficulty.
• The higher the Salter-Harris classification, the more common is the incidence of growth abnormality.
• The closer patient is to skeletal maturity, the less a growth abnormality will affect growth.

RECOMMENDED READING

Bright RW. Apophyseal injures. In: Rockwood CA, Wilkins KE, King RE, eds. *Fractures in children,* 3rd ed. Philadelphia: JB Lippincott, 1991;170–186.

Rang M. Injuries of the epiphysis. In: Rang M, ed. *Children's fractures,* 2nd ed. Philadelphia: JB Lippincott, 1983;10–25.

Basics

DESCRIPTION

This is a flexion deformity of the proximal interphalangeal joint of the lesser toes with the middle and distal phalanges plantar flexed in relation to the proximal phalanx (Fig. 1).

CAUSES

- The most common cause is prolonged use of shoes with constricting toe boxes.
- Neuromuscular disease, with its associated muscle imbalance, may also be the cause, as in Charcot-Marie-Tooth disease, cerebral palsy, Friedreich's ataxia, myelodysplasia, and multiple sclerosis.

RISK FACTORS

Unusually long second toe

CLASSIFICATION

Flexible versus rigid

ASSOCIATED CONDITIONS

- Painful corn over the dorsal surface of the proximal interphalangeal joint
- Plantar lesion beneath the second metatarsophalangeal joint associated with plantar protrusion of the metatarsal head

ICD-9-CM

735.4 Hammer toe (acquired)

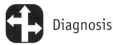 ## Diagnosis

SIGNS AND SYMPTOMS

- Discomfort
- Corn development

DIFFERENTIAL DIAGNOSIS

- Clawtoes
- Mallet toes

PHYSICAL EXAMINATION

- Determine whether the deformities are flexible or rigid. Flexible deformities are passively correctable as the patient stands, whereas a rigid deformity cannot be passively corrected to a neutral position.
- Determine the severity of the deformity. Mild deformities have only a few degrees of flexion; severe deformities involve complete rigid flexion.
- Note any associated forefoot abnormalities such as hallux valgus, multiple toe involvement, and abnormal alignment of adjacent lesser toes that may preclude normal positioning.

PATHOLOGIC FINDINGS

Compartment syndrome can be the underlying disorder, as can neuropathies associated with diabetes mellitus and Hansen's disease.

IMAGING PROCEDURES

Standing radiographs in the anteroposterior, lateral, and oblique views should be obtained.

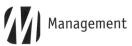 ## Management

GENERAL MEASURES

Shoe modification is indicated to provide ample toe box space to accommodate the deformity. Avoiding high heels helps to prevent toe buckling. Elastic splints, which exert plantar pressure on the proximal phalanx, can be used for flexible deformities. Small felt pads may be worn under the toe to prevent the toe rip from striking the ground.

SURGICAL TREATMENT

Surgical management, reserved for patients in whom conservative treatment fails, for an isolated hammer toe is directed to reestablishing a rectus alignment to the toe, shortening the toe if necessary to place it in appropriate length to its two adjacent toes, and providing sufficient stability and improved leverage for the long and short flexor tendons to assist metatarsophalangeal joint stability.

PHYSICAL THERAPY

Immediate weight bearing is allowed.

PATIENT EDUCATION

Patients are instructed in proper shoe selection.

MONITORING

Monitoring is indicated postoperatively for removal of bolsters, sutures, and splints.

COMPLICATIONS

Some operative treatment may result in inadequate correction. Complications include recurrence and swelling for up to 6 months after surgery.

PROGNOSIS

The prognosis is good.

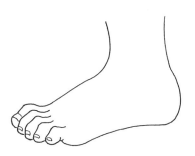

Fig. 1. Hammer toes exhibit a flexion contracture of the proximal interphalangeal joint.

Hamstring Strain

 Basics

DESCRIPTION

The hamstrings are long muscles in the posterior thigh that extend from the ischial tuberosity behind the hip, down to the knee. A hamstring strain is a muscle pull or tear resulting from the sudden change of the hamstring muscle from a stabilizing flexor to an extensor. It is usually caused by quick starts with sudden hamstring contraction.

INCIDENCE

- This injury is common in athletes.
- Athletes of any age may experience a hamstring strain; in young teenagers, however, this usually takes the form of an avulsion of the ischial origin with a rim of bone and cartilage.
- This is more common in males and in younger athletes.

CAUSES

Predisposing Factors

- Poor flexibility
- Inadequate warm-up
- Fatigue
- Deficiency in the reciprocal actions of opposing muscle groups
- Strength imbalance between the quadriceps and hamstring muscles

Movements that Commonly Result in Strain

- Flexing of the leading hip during a hurdle
- Sprinting out of the start-up blocks
- Charging of a football lineman
- Takeoff by a jumper

CLASSIFICATIONS

- Mild strains: These involve muscle spasm only, with no evidence of tear.
- Moderate strains: The athlete often feels a "snap" with immediate pain and loss of function; there may also be a hematoma.
- Severe strains: These generally occur at the origin or insertion of the hamstring into bone.

ICD-9-CM

843.9 Proximal hip strain

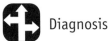 Diagnosis

SIGNS AND SYMPTOMS

- Mild strains: Symptoms may not be noticed until the athlete cools down.
- More severe strains: A "pop" may be felt, with an immediate loss of function; tenderness may be anywhere in the back of the thigh.

DIFFERENTIAL DIAGNOSIS

Femur fracture

PHYSICAL EXAMINATION

- Look for tenderness and swelling in the posterior thigh over one of the hamstring muscles; the most common location is distally in the thigh, over the short head of the biceps femoris.
- Look for pain on resisted knee flexion or hip extension.

PATHOLOGIC FINDINGS

This symptom complex may represent either a partial or a complete tear of one of the hamstring muscles: biceps, semitendinosus, or semimembranosus.

IMAGING PROCEDURES

- Imaging is usually not indicated if the diagnosis is straightforward.
- Radiographs of the pelvis may show an ischial avulsion in a young athlete.
- Radiographs of the knee may show a fibular avulsion if the symptoms are in this area.
- Plain radiographs of the femur may be helpful if a fracture is suspected.
- A bone scan may be needed if the symptoms are compatible with a stress fracture.

Management

GENERAL MEASURES

- Elastic wrap and ice bag initially
- Compressive wrap of injured area; later, taping to provide compression and to restrict stretch
- Rest
- Crutches, if needed
- Analgesics
- Refraining from sports until symptoms allow return
- Finally, physical therapy to regain range of motion and strength
- Similar treatment of bony avulsions

SURGICAL TREATMENT

Surgery is not indicated. This is usually true even for ischial avulsion fractures.

PHYSICAL THERAPY

- Ice massage and ultrasound are advised after swelling is controlled.
- Exercise in water may help range of motion.
- The patient may begin active range of motion followed by knee curls and extensions once soreness is resolved.

MEDICAL TREATMENT

Analgesics of choice are given.

PATIENT EDUCATION

- Explain the importance of hamstring stretch before activity.
- Explain the importance of maintaining strength in these muscles as well as the quadriceps.

PREVENTION

Preventive measures include improved flexibility, adequate warm-up and stretching before rigorous exercise, and muscle strengthening.

PROGNOSIS

- Mild strains heal in a few days to a week.
- Moderate strains heal in 1 to 3 weeks.
- Severe strains involving avulsion fractures at the ischial tuberosity or fibular head may take a month or more to heal.

RECOMMENDED READING

Bull RC. Handbook of sports injuries. New York: McGraw-Hill, 1998.

Kulund D. The torso, hip, and thigh. In: Perrin DH, ed. The injured athlete, 3rd ed. Philadelphia: Lippincott Williams & Wilkins, 1998.

Basics

DESCRIPTION

Although plantar fasciitis can commonly lead to heel pain, it is but one cause to consider when working up a diagnosis in a patient with heel pain. Plantar fasciitis is commonly diagnosed with the history and physical examination alone. Patients commonly complain of heel pain that is worse in the morning with the "first step" and lessens in severity with walking. This heel pain can also occur with the first step after sitting for a prolonged period. Conservative treatment is the cornerstone for this problem, and surgery is hardly ever indicated. Other causes of heel pain include compression of the first branch of the lateral plantar nerve, fat pad atrophy, and pain associated with seronegative spondyloarthropathy. Although these causes should be considered, plantar fasciitis is the more common cause of heel pain. The plantar fascia of the heel is involved, originating from the calcaneus inferiorly.

INCIDENCE

- Extremely common in adults
- Most common in the third to fifth decades

CAUSES

- Foot and ankle experts currently hypothesize that microadhesions form around the plantar fascia, especially during sleep. The pain that is worst with the first step may be associated with tears of these microadhesions.
- Other experts believe that chronic inflammation of the plantar fascia is the cause of plantar fasciitis (Fig. 1).

RISK FACTORS

- Running
- Jumping sports
- Lupus
- Spondyloarthropathy

CLASSIFICATION

- Plantar fasciitis
- Retrocalcaneal bursitis
- Insertional Achilles tendinitis

ICD-9-CM

728.71 Plantar fasciitis
726.79 Heel pain

 Diagnosis

DIFFERENTIAL DIAGNOSIS

- Calcaneal apophysitis or Sever's disease in children
- Tarsal tunnel syndrome
- Reiter's syndrome
- Spinal radiculopathy

PHYSICAL EXAMINATION

- The shape of the patient's foot should be noted on standing; this influences the type of treatment given.
- The patient should then be examined with the foot at rest.
- Palpation just medial to the heel usually elicits tenderness at the base.
- Patients have tenderness along the plantar fascia, which should be considerably worse with the toes dorsiflexed by the examiner, a manuever that stretches the plantar fascia.
- Testing of sensation should be performed as indicated.

LABORATORY TESTS

- HLA-B27 determination may be obtained if spondyloarthropathy is suspected.
- Steroid injection into the plantar fascia insertion may serve both as a diagnostic test and as therapy.

PATHOLOGIC FINDINGS

Chronic inflammation is noted at the base of the plantar fascia insertion.

IMAGING PROCEDURES

- Standing radiographs of the foot should be obtained for patients with persistent pain.
- Bone scans may show increased uptake in the heel. Patients with increased uptake on a bone scan usually have a more severe degree of plantar fasciitis.

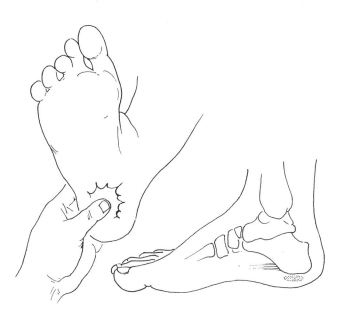

Fig. 1. In a patient with plantar fasciitis, the area of tenderness is in the insertion of the plantar fascia into the calcaneus.

Heel Pain (Plantar Fasciitis)

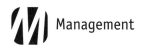 Management

GENERAL MEASURES

- Stretching exercises are recommended. Some patients improve with these; they should be done before sports and on a daily basis.
- Nonsteroidal antiinflammatory agents are given.
- Orthoses are used to cushion the heel and to support the arch if it is flat.
- Injections into the painful area are useful if the condition is localized and if the pain does not respond to other measures.
- Patients may be treated by a night brace (similar to an ankle-foot orthosis) and a stiff-sole shoe (with a custom steel insert in the sole), which reduces strain on the plantar fascia. Patients resistant to this therapy may require casting with a short leg walking cast and an extension beyond the toes to prevent motion at the tarsometatarsal and interphalangeal joints.
- After successful treatment, the patient may be allowed to resume activities gradually; care should be taken not to resume running or jumping sports too early or too strenuously.

SURGICAL TREATMENT

- Depends upon the underlying diagnosis
- For plantar fasciitis, surgery may be indicated for recalcitrant cases. This consists of dividing the plantar fascia, sometimes including osteophytes. It may be done as an outpatient procedure, through a small medial incision.
- For resistant tarsal tunnel syndrome, decompression of the tunnel is indicated.
- For Sever's disease and retrocalcaneal bursitis, surgery is not indicated.

PHYSICAL THERAPY

Physical therapy may be helpful in teaching the patients to stretch and in supervising their return to physical activity.

MEDICAL TREATMENT

Nonsteroidal antiinflammatory agents are useful agents in patients with severe pain.

PATIENT EDUCATION

- Instruct the patient about the anatomy of the plantar fascia and its role in stabilizing the foot.
- Remind the patient about the importance of stretching and of moderation during a return to sports.

PREVENTION

The condition is not always preventable, but it may be limited by avoiding sudden increases in running or jumping stresses.

PROGNOSIS

Most cases of plantar fasciitis resolve by themselves; however, the conservative measures outlined may accelerate healing.

RECOMMENDED READING

Mann RA, Coughlin MJ, eds. *Surgery of the foot and ankle.* St. Louis: CV Mosby, 1993:841–845.

Basics

DESCRIPTION

These sores involve ulceration or breakdown of the skin overlying the heel.

SYNONYMS

- Bedsores
- Heel or foot ulcers

INCIDENCE

- One of the most common complications in the postoperative or rehabilitation setting
- More common in elderly or debilitated patient
- Affecting males and females equally

CAUSES

- These sores generally occur in patients who have limited mobility, neuropathic skin, vascular disease, or diabetes.
- They can also occur in postoperative patients with limited mobility who are bed bound and are subjected to prolonged pressure over the heels.
- They may occur in casts because of excess pressure or decreased padding.

RISK FACTORS

- Diabetes mellitus
- Lower extremity neuropathy
- Lower extremity vascular disease
- Bed-bound status

CLASSIFICATION

Classification by depth is most commonly used:

Grade 0: The at-risk foot with history of ulcer, neuropathy, or a deformity that may cause new ulceration

Grade 1: Superficial skin breakdown or ulceration; not infected

Grade 2: Deep ulceration exposing tendon or other soft tissues; with or without infection

Grade 3: Extensive ulceration with exposed bone or deep infection

ASSOCIATED CONDITIONS

- Paralysis
- Loss of sensation
- Contracture

ICD-9-CM

707 Pressure sore of heel

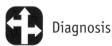 Diagnosis

SIGNS AND SYMPTOMS

- It initially presents as pain and softening over the heel region, often caused by prolonged pressure on the heel.
- It may occur without the warning symptom of pain in the patient with decreased heel sensation.
- If untreated, it can progress to superficial ulceration, deep ulceration, and osteomyelitis.

DIFFERENTIAL DIAGNOSIS

- Osteomyelitis
- Soft tissue abscess
- Cellulitis
- Fracture
- Septic arthritis

PHYSICAL EXAMINATION

- Initially, ulceration may not be present; however, these patients typically complain of pain with palpation of the heel.
- Blistering, softening, and overlying erythema of the heel pad may be noted.
- A dark purple lesion that does not blanch with pressure is a sign that breakdown will eventually occur.
- As the lesion progresses, there is complete skin breakdown with superficial and deep soft tissues visible.
- Grade 3 lesions are characterized by exposed bone; cellulitis or a purulent discharge may be present if the wound is infected.
- The entire foot and ankle should be thoroughly examined to rule out an open joint.
- Pain with range of motion of the joints of the foot or ankle may suggest joint involvement and septic arthritis.

LABORATORY TESTS

- Usually, none are specifically indicated.
- If the wound appears infected, check the complete blood count and sedimentation rate.

PATHOLOGIC FINDINGS

Heel sores are primarily caused by ischemia from prolonged pressure over the heel. As the ischemia and pressure persist, the skin and soft tissues overlying the heel become necrotic, break down, and ulcerate. In chronically debilitated and diabetic patients, these lesions easily become infected and can eventually result in osteomyelitis or septic arthritis.

IMAGING PROCEDURES

- Routine anteroposterior and lateral foot and ankle films are helpful in diagnosing bone destruction.
- Sores confined to soft tissue breakdown may show no radiographic change.

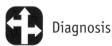 Management

GENERAL MEASURES

- Prevention is key: Patients with neuropathic feet need to be instructed in meticulous foot care and shoe selection.
- Treatment should be initiated at earliest signs of skin breakdown.
- Bed-bound patients need good heel padding and frequent turning.
- Superficial heel sores generally respond to pressure relief and padding over the affected area. Deeper ulcerations may require surgical débridement and meticulous wound care. Prevention of further pressure is key to healing. Most ulcers heal with prolonged pressure relief, usually over the course of several months.
- Broad-spectrum antibiotics are indicated for infected ulcers; one should select antibiotics that cover gram-positive and gram-negative organisms, as well as anaerobes, because these infections tend to be polymicrobial.
- Grade 3 ulcerations generally require surgical débridement and may require removal of infected bone or partial amputation.
- Any complaint of heel pain or burning in a casted patient should lead to cast windowing.

SURGICAL TREATMENT

- Generally soft tissue débridement of the affected tissues is indicated.
- This usually can be done in an outpatient or clinic setting.

PHYSICAL THERAPY

- Whirlpool therapy to débride necrotic tissue may be helpful.
- Physical therapists can be integral in monitoring for pressure relief.

MEDICAL TREATMENT

Antibiotics with broad-spectrum coverage are required to manage the polymicrobial infections associated with these types of foot ulceration.

PATIENT EDUCATION

Patients at risk for heel sores should be educated in foot care and shoe selection.

PREVENTION

- Instruct patients in the early appearance or a pressure sore to prevent it from progressing.
- Have patients avoid prolonged recumbency with the heel on a hard surface.
- Do not allow patients in casts to rest on their heels for a long time.

MONITORING

These lesions need to be closely monitored, because patients are at high risk for disease progression if the ulcer is not aggressively treated.

COMPLICATIONS

- Osteomyelitis
- Septic arthritis

PROGNOSIS

- Grade 1 has a good prognosis.
- Grade 2 has a fair prognosis.
- Grade 3 has a poor prognosis.
- Prognosis also depends on the severity of underlying disease, the age of the patient (younger is better), and the quality of assistance with care.

RECOMMENDED READING

Mann RA, Coughlin MJ, eds. *Surgery of the foot and ankle*. St. Louis: CV Mosby, 1993:896–908.

Hemangioma

 Basics

DESCRIPTION

This benign tumor of vascular origin usually affects the skeletal system, but it may also occur in the soft tissues. Found in all age groups, this tumor is most commonly diagnosed in the middle decades of life.

GENETICS

No known correlation exists.

INCIDENCE

• This tumor is uncommon.
• A Mayo Clinic series described a slight female predominance. Other series have not shown gender predilection.

CAUSES

The cause is unknown. Hemangioma is considered a benign lesion without metastatic potential. Many pathologists consider it a hamartoma, rather than a true neoplasm.

RISK FACTORS

None are known, except the slight female predominance found in one series.

ICD-9-CM

228.0 Hemangioma

 Diagnosis

SIGNS AND SYMPTOMS

• It may present with local pain and swelling of insidious onset and indolent progression.
• Soft tissue hemangioma often presents without pain but with intermittent swelling.
• Occasionally, pathologic fracture may be the initial presentation.
• Hemangioma in the vertebra may lead to vertebral collapse, with local pain and neurologic findings.

DIFFERENTIAL DIAGNOSIS

• Myeloma
• Infection
• Bone cyst
• Malignant primary bone neoplasm
• Metastatic disease

PHYSICAL EXAMINATION

When palpated, hemangiomas have a fluctuant or springy feel to them. They are composed of a large number of blood vessels, which compress when palpated and then refill with blood. Hemangiomas often increase in size when the limb is placed in the dependent position.

LABORATORY TESTS

There are no diagnostic serum tests.

PATHOLOGIC FINDINGS

Tumors are grossly bloody and are traversed by bony trabeculae. Microscopically, conglomerates of thin-walled capillaries filled with red cells are typically seen. Lymphatics may also be prominent.

IMAGING PROCEDURES

• Soft tissue hemangiomas are best imaged with gadolinium contrast-enhanced magnetic resonance imaging.
• Lesions are frequently multiple, expansile, and trabeculated and show little periosteal reaction.
• The typical radiographic appearance is osteopenia with parallel vertical streaks described as a "corduroy cloth" appearance.
• The radiographic appearance is variable; some lesions have a "soap bubble" appearance, and others are purely lytic.
• Lesions in the soft tissue may erode the adjacent bone and may show characteristic "phleboliths" on radiographs. These lesions are easily confused with a variety of other lesions.
• Multiple lesions and lack of periosteal reaction may provide clues to the diagnosis.

Management

GENERAL MEASURES

• Soft tissue hemangiomas can recur after surgical excision.
• Surgery should be avoided when possible.
• Treatment with compressive dressings can aid in nonoperative treatment.
• Angiography and embolization before surgical excision are helpful.
• Sclerosing therapy (with alcohol) is the preferred method of treatment.
• For hemangiomas in bone, surgically accessible lesions may be treated with curettage and bone grafting, with or without radiation.
• Inaccessible lesions are treated with radiation alone.
• Lesions left untreated are occasionally slowly progressive.
• With treatment, prognosis is excellent.

SURGICAL TREATMENT

Surgery should be avoided unless biopsy is needed.

PHYSICAL THERAPY

This is not indicated.

MEDICAL TREATMENT

• Pathologic fractures should be splinted.
• Lesions discovered radiographically occasionally require biopsy for confirmation.
• Lesions should be treated with compressive dressings.
• Surgically inaccessible lesions should be treated with radiation alone.

PATIENT EDUCATION

Patients with soft tissue lesions are instructed to avoid provocative activities such as prolonged standing.

MONITORING

• Patients with bone lesions seldom need treatment unless pathologic fracture occurs.
• Soft tissue lesions are monitored with serial physical examinations and magnetic resonance imaging scans every 3 to 6 months.

COMPLICATIONS

Pathologic fracture

PROGNOSIS

• Good overall
• Recurrence not uncommon

RECOMMENDED READING

Dahlin DC. Vascular tumors. In: *Bone tumors*, 2nd ed. Springfield, IL: Charles C Thomas, 1967:100–109.

Spjut HJ, Dorfman HD, Fechner RE, et al. *Tumors of bone and cartilage*. Washington, DC: Armed Forces Institute of Pathology, 1971:325–328.

Basics

DESCRIPTION

- This disorder of clotting factor results in easy bleeding.
- Secondary effects may occur in any system, most significantly brain, joint, muscle, and nerve, owing to bleeding.
- It is usually diagnosed in early childhood, depending on severity.
- Males are affected much more commonly than females.

SYNONYMS

- Classic hemophilia (factor VIII deficiency)
- Christmas disease (factor IX deficiency)

GENETICS

Hemophilia A (classic hemophilia) and B (Christmas disease) are both inherited as sex-linked recessive disorders. This leads to the typical picture of multiple affected males on the maternal side of a family.

INCIDENCE

- The combined incidence of hemophilia is about 1 per 10,000 population.
- Seventy-five percent of this group have hemophilia A.
- Twelve percent of this group have hemophilia B.
- The rest have rare deficiencies in the other coagulation factors.

CAUSES

- Hemophilia A: defect in gene for factor VIII
- Hemophilia B: defect in gene for factor IX

RISK FACTORS

Positive family history

CLASSIFICATION

- Severe hemophilia: less than 1% clotting factor activity
- Moderate hemophilia: 1% to 5% clotting factor activity
- Mild hemophilia: greater than 5% clotting factor activity

ICD-9-CM

958.2 Hemophilia

 ## Diagnosis

SIGNS AND SYMPTOMS

In patients with severe hemophilia, failure to clot after circumcision, immunizations, or lip lacerations sustained in falls will often bring the diagnosis to light. In persons affected more mildly, major cuts or surgery may be required to show the defect. Later problems include repeated episodes bleeding in a joint or a muscle, possibly with only mild trauma. The joints most affected include the knee, ankle, and elbow. Once a joint has sustained a bleeding episode, it is much more likely to be affected again, and it is called a "target joint." The bleeding episodes are noted first because of pain, before swelling occurs. Muscle bleeding is noted because of swelling and nerve compression, most commonly affecting the psoas muscle and the femoral nerve. Repeated bleeding episodes eventually cause degenerative change with stiffness and pain in a target joint over several years.

DIFFERENTIAL DIAGNOSIS

- von Willebrand's disease
- Pigmented villonodular synovitis
- Transient inhibitor of coagulation
- Thrombocytopenia

PHYSICAL EXAMINATION

- Check all major joints for effusion and range of motion.
- Remember that the knees, ankles, shoulders, and elbows are the joints most commonly involved.
- Note that the presence of an effusion in an ankle is initially heralded by obliteration of the "hollow" around the malleoli.
- In examining the knees, document the symmetry of flexion and the presence or absence of the normal hyperextension of 5 or 10 degrees.
- Look for apparent enlargement of the joints, which is due to either epiphyseal hypertrophy of hyperemia or to atrophy of the surrounding muscles.
- Observe the patient's gait.
- Ask patients to keep a log of joint bleeding to allow detection of a target joint.
- Look for any neurologic sequelae of bleeding, such as hemiparesis from a prior intracranial hemorrhage or neuropathy from a femoral or sciatic hemorrhage.

LABORATORY TESTS

- Factor levels should be quantitated in terms of percentage of normal.
- If factor levels do not rise with replacement as expected, an inhibitor should be suspected. This is an antibody to factor and is a relative contraindication to any elective surgery.
- For all patients with hemophilia, the clinician should be aware of the status of the following: hepatitis, inhibitor, and human immunodeficiency virus.

PATHOLOGIC FINDINGS

- On gross examination of a hemophilic joint, the synovium is brown and appears velvety.
- The joint surface loses its luster and, with advanced disease, becomes eroded in riverlike tracts.
- On light microscopy, the synovial lining of the joint is hypertrophic and hypervascular. This hypervascularity renders it more likely to bleed with further trauma.
- Eventually, the synovium becomes fibrotic, thus accounting for the loss of motion.

IMAGING PROCEDURES

- Plain radiographs show the following sequence of changes in a hemophilic target joint:

—First, soft tissue swelling and osteopenia
—Second, epiphyseal enlargement, followed by joint space narrowing and irregularity
—Finally, degenerative arthritis

Hemophilia

⚡ Management

GENERAL MEASURES

- For acute bleeding episodes
—Factor replacement
—Rest and brief immobilization followed by motion exercises

- Synovectomy for chronic hemarthropathy
- Arthroplasty (or occasionally, arthrodesis) for painful end-stage joint disease
- Factor replacement and observation for psoas bleeding causing femoral neurapraxia
- For compartment syndrome, decompression as in any other situation
- Home maintenance programs, which have shown benefit in terms of decreasing joint bleeding and damage: This type of program should be considered if the patient and family are capable of handling it. When a hemorrhage does occur, factor should be infused immediately. If a large joint effusion develops, aspiration and irrigation should be considered, once adequate factor replacement has been achieved. Rest and compression should also be recommended.

SURGICAL TREATMENT

- Synovectomy is the removal of hypertrophic synovial lining to decrease bleeding in target joints. This may be done through the arthroscope in some joints. It may even be done non-surgically, using injected radioisotopes in high-risk or juvenile patients.
- Knee replacement arthroplasty involves replacement of joint surface with metal and plastic articulation to relieve pain.
- Ankle fusion can be done for end-stage degeneration in this joint.

PHYSICAL THERAPY

- It may assist in monitoring range of motion in target joints
- It is also indicated after a major bleeding episode or surgery

MEDICAL TREATMENT

- Factor replacement
- Rest and brief immobilization
- Factor replacement and observation for a psoas hemorrhage causing femoral neurapraxia
- Decompression for compartment syndrome
- Discouragement of the use of salicylates and other nonsteroidal drugs, except acetaminophen.

PATIENT EDUCATION

- Stress sports restrictions, especially sports involving contact or twisting.
- Advise that the school be notified of the patient's sports restrictions.
- Encourage substitute pastimes.
- Offer genetic counseling early at diagnosis.

PREVENTION

Prevent the development of target joints by a home maintenance program and by observing activity restrictions.

MONITORING

Ideally, patients should be followed in a multi-disciplinary fashion by specialists in hematology, orthopaedics or physical therapy, and dentistry. Social work may be helpful in obtaining needed services and medical coverage.

COMPLICATIONS

- Neurologic: bleeding into the central nervous system or major peripheral nerves
- Joints: stiffness, contracture, and arthritis
- Compartment syndrome
- Blood-borne infections

PROGNOSIS

Life expectancy may be diminished by catastrophic bleeding and infectious diseases.

RECOMMENDED READING

Arnold WD, Hilgartner MW. Hemophilic arthropathy: current concepts of pathogenesis and management. *J Bone Joint Surg Am* 1977;59:287–305.

Greene WB, McMillan CW. *Nonsurgical management of hemophilic arthropathy. American Academy of Orthopaedic Surgeons instructional course lectures.* Chicago: American Academy of Orthopaedic Surgeons, 1989;38:367–381.

Basics

DESCRIPTION

A herniated disc in the neck is a retropulsion of disc material often associated with degeneration in the cervical spine that can cause neck pain, arm pain (radiculopathy), or lower extremity weakness (myelopathy). It affects the spine and neurologic systems. It can occur in any decade of adult life, but it is most commonly seen in the fourth decade.

GENETICS

Increased risk is seen with a positive family history, but no Mendelian pattern is recognized.

INCIDENCE

- Up to 40% of adults will have at least one significant episode of neck pain.
- Ninety-five percent of men and 70% of women aged 60 to 65 years have radiographic evidence of disc degeneration.
- The male-to-female ratio is 1.4:1.

CAUSES

Cervical disc herniations may be either traumatic or nontraumatic.

RISK FACTORS

Cigarette smoking, frequent heavy lifting, and frequent diving from a board have all been strongly correlated with cervical disc herniations.

CLASSIFICATION

The herniation is classified as acute (less than 2 weeks' duration) or chronic. Classification of myelopathy is based on physical function. Nurick's grading system is most commonly used.

ASSOCIATED CONDITIONS

- Congenital cervical stenosis
- Ossified posterior longitudinal ligament

ICD-9-CM

722.0 Displacement, intervertebral disc (with neuritis, pain or radiculitis)
722.71.1 Displacement, intervertebral disc (with myelopathy)

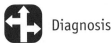 ## Diagnosis

SIGNS AND SYMPTOMS

Symptoms can develop either acutely or insidiously. A spectrum of symptoms including neck pain, occipital pain, shoulder girdle pain, and regional upper extremity symptoms (pain, paresthesias, hypesthesia, or weakness) may be seen. Symptoms are often exacerbated by particular neck motions and positions. Nerve root compression at a specific level may cause "classic" findings of motor, sensory, or reflex symptoms. Spurling's test (axial loading of the neck while the head is rotated and laterally bent toward the affected side) often recreates the radicular symptoms.
Cervical myelopathy usually presents insidiously with a wide variety of symptoms, including gait deterioration (falls), deterioration of manual dexterity (trouble doing buttons), generalized weakness, or bowel and bladder dysfunction. Patients may complain of losing balance or of "jumpy" legs. Babinski's reflex in the lower extremities or Hoffmann's reflex in the upper extremities may be seen.

DIFFERENTIAL DIAGNOSIS

- Intrinsic disease of the shoulder, elbow, or wrist (degenerative joint disease, impingement, rotator cuff disease or instability)
- Peripheral nerve entrapments (carpal tunnel syndrome, cubital tunnel, Guyon's canal, thoracic outlet syndrome)
- Neurologic disorders (brachial plexopathy, multiple sclerosis, amyotrophic lateral sclerosis, spinal cord or neural tumors)
- Infectious discitis
- Vertebral osteomyelitis
- Metastatic cancer

PHYSICAL EXAMINATION

- Quantify neck range of motion.
- Measure muscle strength at each joint in the upper extremities.
- Test sensation at each dermatome.
- Look for spasticity in the lower extremities.

Special Tests

- Spurling's test
- Babinski's reflex
- Hoffmann's reflex

LABORATORY TESTS

Electrodiagnostics including electromyography and nerve conduction velocities can be used as objective diagnostic tools. However, they are recommended only in patients with inconsistencies in history, physical examination, and radiographic studies.

PATHOLOGIC FINDINGS

Disc material (nucleus pulposus) herniates through the disc annulus and compresses either a nerve root, causing radiculopathy, or the spinal cord, causing myelopathy.

IMAGING PROCEDURES

Plain radiographs allow assessment of skeletal alignment and the presence of degenerative changes in disc spaces. Oblique views visualize the neural foramina. Flexion and extension views can be used to assess stability. However, almost 50% of all people in their 40s or older demonstrate degenerative changes, so radiographs should be reserved for patients with acute trauma or failure of conservative therapies.
Computed tomography myelography allows accurate evaluation of the degree of neural compression from both bony and soft tissues. However, myelography is an invasive procedure and should be reserved as a tool for surgical planning.
Magnetic resonance imaging of the cervical spine is noninvasive, involves no radiation exposure, and provides excellent images. Up to 30% of people older than 40 years have either an asymptomatic disc bulge or foraminal stenosis. Thus, magnetic resonance imaging should be reserved for patients who do not respond to nonsurgical treatments.

Herniated Disc in the Neck

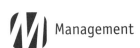 Management

GENERAL MEASURES

Most patients can be treated nonsurgically. However, those patients in whom a minimum of 6 weeks of nonsurgical care fails or who present with a myelopathy or a progressive or severe motor deficit should be referred for possible surgical treatment.

SURGICAL TREATMENT

Either anterior cervical discectomy and fusion or posterior laminotomy and foraminotomy can be used to treat a herniated disc that is refractory to conservative treatment. Both procedures decompress the neural elements, but studies suggest that anterior cervical discectomy with fusion provides better long-term results and is often the preferred procedure.

PHYSICAL THERAPY

Cervical traction, either in therapy or at home, may help to reduce radicular symptoms. Initially, passive modalities may help to decrease acute pain. Then, active stretching and exercises may help patients to return to normal activities.

MEDICAL TREATMENT

Most patients can be treated with a nonoperative program consisting of rest (activity modification), medication (analgesics, nonsteroidal antiinflammatory drugs, and muscle relaxants), intermittent mobilization (soft collar), and physical therapy (exercises or traction). Patients who develop increased symptoms or neurologic deficit during treatment should have treatment discontinued, further diagnostic workup, and referral for surgical care. Cervical epidural steroids have not been clearly shown to benefit patients; however, they may prove beneficial in some individuals. Each practitioner should become familiar with the dosing and side effect of a few nonsteroidal antiinflammatory drugs.

Patients need to limit strenuous physical activity during acute episodes. Modification of the work environment, such as changing the position of computer screens, may be helpful for patients in the long term.

PATIENT EDUCATION

Patients must be educated to look for progressive motor weakness or bowel or bladder dysfunction. Once recovered, patients should be educated on the natural history of degenerative disc disease, as well as on the importance of smoking cessation.

PREVENTION

Cessation of smoking and modification of activity may help to prevent future episodes of neck pain.

MONITORING

No regular monitoring is needed. After resolution of symptoms by nonoperative care, most patients can be expected to have at least one additional episode of neck pain.

COMPLICATIONS

Complications of surgical treatment include infection (1%), persistence of neurologic deficit (5%), and worsening deficit (5%). Moderate and severely myelopathic patients are likely to remain myelopathic. Patients having an anterior cervical discectomy may complain of dysphagia (2%), pain from pseudoarthrosis (2%), or late degeneration at an adjacent disc (4%).

PROGNOSIS

More than 50% of patients will have at least one additional episode of neck pain in their lifetime.

RECOMMENDED READING

Watkins RG. Cervical spine injuries in athletes. In: Clark CC, ed. *The cervical spine.* Philadelphia: Lippincott–Raven Publishers, 1998:373–386.

Basics

DESCRIPTION

Low back pain is one of the most common reasons people seek medical attention. Acute low back pain is sometimes the result of herniation of a lumbar vertebral disc, which can result from trauma or degenerative changes. Treatment is usually nonsurgical, but patients with recalcitrant cases often benefit dramatically from surgery. Herniations affect both the spine and the lower extremities.

Herniated disc in the lower spine is common in all adults, but it is more common in men than in women. Patients older than 50 years are less likely to return to work than are younger patients.

SYNONYMS

- Protruding, extruded in sequestered disc or nucleus pulposus
- "Slipped disc"

GENETICS

No known genetic predisposition is known.

INCIDENCE

- The most common level of herniation is L4-5.
- Incidence increases with age.

CAUSES

- This condition is more commonly secondary to degeneration of the disc and annulus (Fig. 1). High or repetitive loads are factors as well.
- It may be secondary to trauma.

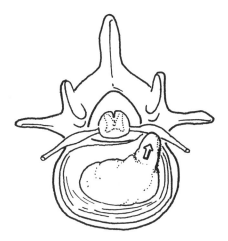

Fig. 1. In a herniated disc in the lumbar spine, material from the nucleus pulposus exerts pressure on the nerve root.

RISK FACTOR

Tobacco smoking is associated with an increased risk of disc herniation.

CLASSIFICATION

Central herniation refers to herniations found in the spinal canal. Lateral herniations are found lateral to the pedicles and may compress the nerve root and exit above the herniated disc. Herniations are described as protruding or sequestered. They may protrude, indicating that the annulus fibrosis is intact, extrude through a hole in the annulus, or become sequestered in the spinal canal.

ICD-9-CM

722 Herniated disc in lower spine

Diagnosis

SIGNS AND SYMPTOMS

- Lower back pain, sometimes severe, may be the only symptom.
- Central herniation of the nucleus pulposus may result in nerve compression, usually of the nerve root, which exits the foramen below the herniated disc.
- L3-4 herniation causes an L-4 root compression characterized by anterior tibialis weakness, decreased knee jerk, and medial knee sensory changes.
- L4-5 herniation results in L-5 symptoms such as altered sensation over the lateral aspect of the calf and the first dorsal web space. Extensor hallicis longus weakness may be evident.

- L-5–S-1 herniation compresses the S-1 nerve root, decreases ankle jerk, and causes decreased plantar flexion strength and diminished sensation over the lateral aspect of the foot.
- Saddle anesthesia and changes in bowel or bladder habits may indicate cauda equina syndrome.
- Cauda equina compression can result from a large herniated disc and should be decompressed on an emergency basis.

DIFFERENTIAL DIAGNOSIS

- Lumbar spinal stenosis
- Sciatic nerve entrapment below the spine
- Spondylolysis
- Muscular back pain
- Degenerative disc disease

PHYSICAL EXAMINATION

A detailed neurologic evaluation is the most important aspect of examination. Sensation in the lower extremity dermatomes and strength of all major muscle groups should be documented. All lower extremity reflexes should be elicited. Rectal examination is important to assess the sacral nerve roots. Rectal tone, perianal sensation, and the anal wink reflex should all be assessed. A straight leg raise that replicates symptoms is a result of stretched nerve roots (Fig. 1). The pain is increased by ankle dorsiflexion. Gait disturbances or foot-drop may be a result of nerve compression and muscular weakness.

Herniated Disc in Lower Spine

PATHOLOGIC FINDINGS

The nucleus pulposus is extruded through defects in the annulus fibrosis. Usually, it remains covered by the thick posterior longitudinal ligament. Symptoms are due to tenting of nerve roots over the herniation. The release of inflammatory mediators may exacerbate the mechanical pressure.

IMAGING PROCEDURES

• Anteroposterior and lateral radiographs are obtained in patients with symptoms lasting longer than 6 weeks.
• Magnetic resonance imaging is used to document the pathologic features if surgery is contemplated or spinal stenosis is suspected. Results may be misleading because false-positive findings are common.
• Magnetic resonance imaging can also be used to confirm the diagnosis of cauda equina syndrome.
• Patients with persistent pain and no obvious disorder may benefit from discograms, which can potentially diagnose discogenic pain.

Management

GENERAL MEASURES

Initial care is directed toward symptomatic relief. A short period of rest followed by activity as tolerated should be prescribed. Nonsteroidal antiinflammatory agents or acetaminophen should be recommended. Diazepam or muscle relaxants have only a limited role in patients suffering from sciatica. Epidural steroids may be helpful for short-term relief but seem to provide no long-term benefit. Manipulation, either manually or in traction, may also be beneficial on a short-term basis. Narcotics should be reserved for only the most severely symptomatic patients.

SURGICAL TREATMENT

Patients having more than 6 weeks of pain or severe pain unresponsive to conservative therapy may benefit from discectomy. This may be performed in an open fashion with formal laminectomy or by a minimally invasive procedure. Chemonucleolysis and endoscopic procedures are under evaluation.

PHYSICAL THERAPY

Physical therapy, including stretching exercises, manipulation, and strengthening of truncal muscles, may be beneficial.

PATIENT EDUCATION

Patients should understand that most herniated discs improve with time and symptomatic treatment. Cessation of smoking also helps to speed the process of healing. Patients should be encouraged to pursue activity as tolerated. Long periods of bed rest may actually delay improvement of symptoms.

PREVENTION

Patients involved in heavy lifting may benefit from instruction in proper lifting technique. This can usually be done by a physical therapist or an occupational medicine specialist.

MONITORING

Monitoring of healing progress is clinical, whether conservative or operative treatment is given. Imaging is needed only for complications during recovery.

COMPLICATIONS

Degenerative disc disease or persistent pain from other causes may follow herniation. Repeat herniation at the same or other levels may occur. Disc infection or arachnoiditis may complicate discectomy.

PROGNOSIS

Prognosis is excellent for complete recovery in most patients. Intermittent back pain may persist in some patients.

RECOMMENDED READING

Kostuik JP, et al. Cauda equina syndrome and lumbar disk herniation. *J Bone Joint Surg Am* 1986:68:386–391.

Weber H. Lumbar disc herniation: a controlled, prospective study with ten years of observation. *Spine* 1993;8:131–140.

Basics

DESCRIPTION

Heterotopic ossification (HO) is pathologic bone formation as a consequence of trauma or central nervous system injuries. It most commonly occurs in proximal joints and limbs such as the hip, elbow, and shoulder. It is less common in children and more common in males.

GENETICS

Currently, no genetic link can successfully predict patients susceptible to HO.

INCIDENCE

It occurs in 10% to 20% of patients with central nervous system or traumatic injuries, with an average onset of 2 months after injury.

CAUSES

- Traumatic brain injury
- Spinal cord injury
- Trauma

RISK FACTORS

- Total hip arthroplasty
- Osteoarthrosis
- Osteophyte formation
- Surgical approach
- Prior surgical procedures
- Trochanteric osteotomy
- Length of surgery
- Ankylosing spondylitis

ASSOCIATED CONDITIONS

- Fibrodysplasia ossificans progressiva
- Primary osteoma cutis

ICD-9-CM

728.89 Heterotopic ossification

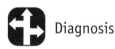

Diagnosis

SIGNS AND SYMPTOMS

- Unexplained increase in pain, spasticity, or muscle guarding
- Decreased motion
- Stiffness
- Radiographic evidence of ectopic bone

DIFFERENTIAL DIAGNOSIS

- Septic joint
- Thrombophlebitis
- Neoplasm in the soft tissues

PHYSICAL EXAMINATION

Limited range of motion is the most common and earliest sign. Erythema, swelling, and signs of inflammation may also be noted.

LABORATORY TESTS

Serum alkaline phosphatase levels are elevated. This value begins to rise 2 to 3 weeks after injury. Although nonspecific and not absolute, elevated serum alkaline phosphatase may be the earliest test for detection.

PATHOLOGIC FINDINGS

Initially, an intense inflammatory response occurs with myofibroblasts and osteoblasts. There is such a high degree of cellular activity that the inflammatory response can be mistaken for a neoplasm.

IMAGING PROCEDURES

- On plain radiographs, new bone formation may be first visible at 3 to 6 weeks; however, radiographs are generally not confirmatory until 3 months.
- Bone scans allow for earlier detection and show intense uptake.
- Computed tomography may be used for preoperative planning and to show the zonal pattern.

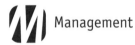

Management

GENERAL MEASURES

Joint motion is maintained to allow normal functioning. Most patients are successfully treated with conservative measures, including physical therapy, analgesics, and antiinflammatory medications. Few patients require surgical excision.

SURGICAL TREATMENT

Surgery is indicated to restore joint motion or to correct contracture. HO should not be resected earlier than 6 months after injury. Excision after 2 years increases the likelihood of permanent contractures. After resection of HO, patients are treated with low doses of radiation (must be delivered within 72 hours). Some patients elect to take antiinflammatory drugs (e.g., indomethacin) for 6 weeks after resection. For effective prophylaxis, the medications must be taken (10% to 20% intolerance rate).

PHYSICAL THERAPY

Use range of motion exercises and treatment modalities that are designed to increase joint mobility.

MEDICAL TREATMENT

- Drugs of choice

—Used to prevent or to lessen the amount of HO formation after the initial insult and to prevent recurrence after surgical excision
—Indomethacin: 25 to 50 P.D.S. mg three times daily for 6 weeks

- Radiation therapy ineffective once HO has been documented

PATIENT EDUCATION

- Joint motion should be encouraged.
- Immobilization is not recommended and can worsen the prognosis.

MONITORING

Serial radiographs are obtained at 1- to 3-month intervals.

COMPLICATIONS

- Loss of mobility
- Ankylosis

PROGNOSIS

Prognosis varies, depending on the location of HO and its cause. Most patients with nonneurogenic HO maintain reasonable function and do not require surgical intervention.

RECOMMENDED READING

Ayers D, Pellegrini V, Evavts CM, et al. Prevention of heterotopic ossification in high-risk patients by radiation therapy. *Clin Orthop* 1991;263:87–93.

Ersgaard-Anderson P, Schmidt SA. The role of antiinflammatory medications in the prevention of heterotopic ossification. *Clin Orthop* 1991;263:78–86.

Garland D. A clinical perspective on common forms of acquired heterotopic ossification. *Clin Orthop* 1991;263:13–29.

Hip Arthritis

 Basics

DESCRIPTION

Hip arthritis is caused by loss of the articular cartilage of the acetabulum and proximal femur. As the cartilage is lost, the subchondral bone of the proximal femur and the acetabulum rub on each other and cause pain and disability.

CAUSES

Primary Osteoarthritis

The cause is unknown.

Inflammatory Arthritis

- Rheumatoid arthritis
- Systemic lupus erythematosus
- Psoriatic arthritis

Secondary Arthritis

- Posttraumatic arthritis
- Avascular necrosis
- Crystalline diseases
- Postinfectious arthritis

RISK FACTORS

- Trauma
- Steroid use (avascular necrosis)
- Infections

CLASSIFICATION

Hip arthritis is classified broadly as follows:

- Primary osteoarthritis
- Inflammatory arthritis
- Secondary osteoarthritis

ASSOCIATED CONDITIONS

- Spine degenerative disc disease
- Knee arthritis

ICD-9-CM

716.95 Arthropathy not otherwise specified (NOS), pelvis

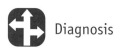 Diagnosis

SIGNS AND SYMPTOMS

Patients present with a diffuse ache over the hip. Classically, pain occurs in the anterior groin. There is often radiation of the pain to the knee, especially the medial side. Knee pain is occasionally the predominant symptom. Patients often describe limping and fatigue with walking. As patients lose their range of motion, they have difficulty tying their shoes and getting in and out of cars.

DIFFERENTIAL DIAGNOSIS

The differential diagnosis is extensive and includes the following:

- Neoplasms

—Young patients: osteosarcoma, Ewing's sarcoma
—Older patients: metastatic bone disease, multiple myeloma

- Stress fractures of the femoral neck: runners and older patients
- Greater trochanteric bursitis: lateral hip pain
- Radiculopathy: pain that travels down past the knee

PHYSICAL EXAMINATION

The major components of physical examination are as follows:

- Assess the patient's range of motion: loss of internal fixation is one of the earliest signs of hip arthritis. Hip flexion is also limited.
- Check for flexion contracture.
- Palpate the greater trochanter to look for trochanteric bursitis.
- Perform a careful neurologic examination and straight leg raising test to look for radicular signs.

LABORATORY TESTS

Rheumatologic screening tests should be ordered if one suspects inflammatory arthritis.

PATHOLOGIC FINDINGS

The major pathologic features include loss of articular cartilage, subchondral cysts and sclerosis, and osteophytes.

IMAGING PROCEDURES

Radiography

Plain radiographs are the first step:

- Anteroposterior view of the pelvis
- Anteroposterior and lateral views of the involved hip
- Anteroposterior and lateral views of the lumbosacral spine if there is any suggestion of radiculopathy

Special Imaging

Technetium bone scans are used if there is severe pain and no apparent areas of disease. The technetium scan screens for occult bone disease over the entire body.
Magnetic resonance imaging of the hip and pelvis is an excellent modality to exclude bone and soft tissue disease of the pelvis and hip. One must ensure that the pathologic area is in the field of the scan.

 Management

GENERAL MEASURES

Weight reduction and activity modification are the major general measures. Initial arthritis care begins with the following:

- Activity modification: avoidance of provocative activities such as running and heavy lifting
- Nonsteroidal antiinflammatory drugs
- Cane support in the opposite hand
- Weight reduction if appropriate

SURGICAL TREATMENT

Total hip replacement is the main surgical procedure. In some young patients with acetabular or proximal femoral dysplasia, acetabular or proximal femoral osteotomy can be used to reduce the joint forces and to improve cartilage physiology.

PHYSICAL THERAPY

Patients are instructed on the use of a cane and on appropriate exercises to prevent contractures.

MEDICAL TREATMENT

- Nonsteroidal antiinflammatory drugs
- Occasional intraarticular steroid injections

PATIENT EDUCATION

Patients are instructed on the importance of compliance with weight reduction, the use of nonsteroidal antiinflammatory drugs, and the avoidance of painful activities. The role of hip replacement is discussed.
Patients can perform activities as tolerated. They should avoid activities that cause pain and may hasten the arthritic changes such as running, racquetball, and heavy lifting.

MONITORING

Patients are followed at 3- to 6-month intervals.

COMPLICATIONS

Contractures of the hip and knee may occur if patients become wheelchair bound.

PROGNOSIS

The prognosis is excellent. Virtually all patients attain pain relief and functional improvement with hip replacement. In patients with early arthritis, nonsteroidal drugs may relieve all pain and may significantly improve function.

RECOMMENDED READING

Hochberg, MC. Osteoarthritis A. Epidemiology, pathology and pathogenesis. B. Clinical features and treatment. In: Klippel JH, Weyand CM, Wortmann RL, eds. *Primer on the rheumatic diseases,* 11th ed. Atlanta: Arthritis Foundation, 1997:216–221.

Basics

DESCRIPTION

Hip avascular necrosis is osteonecrosis or death of the bone in the femoral head. The hip, and all other major joints, can be affected. In the pediatric population, this condition is called Legg-Calvé-Perthes disease and, in general, has a better prognosis than osteonecrosis in the adult.

SYNONYMS

- Avascular necrosis
- Aseptic necrosis

GENETICS

There may be a genetic pattern related to clotting disorder with protein S deficiency.

INCIDENCE

- In the United States, 15,000 new cases appear annually. Patients with hip avascular necrosis also represent approximately 10% of the 500,000 total hip arthroplasties performed each year in the United States.
- This is most common in young adults between the ages of 20 and 40 years and in children aged 6 to 10 years.
- The distribution between men and women is equal.

CAUSES

Idiopathic osteonecrosis is most commonly followed by alcohol-related or corticosteroid-induced osteonecrosis. The threshold of alcohol ingestion reported to be associated with osteonecrosis is the equivalent of 400 mL or more per week of 100% ethyl alcohol. Large incremental and cumulative doses of steroids have also been correlated with a risk of developing osteonecrosis. Some researchers believe that patients who have an idiosyncratic reaction to the steroids, with systemic changes such as acute weight gain or moon faces, have an increased risk of developing osteonecrosis. Other causes include the following:

- Traumatic injuries such as hip fractures
- Subclinical clotting disorders
- Exposure to atmospheric pressure variations

RISK FACTORS

- Femoral neck fractures
- Steroid use
- Alcohol abuse
- Hemoglobinopathies
- Clotting abnormalities
- Dysbarism ("bends")
- Ionizing radiation

CLASSIFICATION

Ficat and Arlet

Ficat and Arlet described four stages:

Stage I: No changes on radiograph, changes noted on magnetic resonance imaging (MRI)
Stage II: Sclerotic or cystic changes on radiographs in the femoral head, no collapse
Stage III: Subchondral fracture, crescent sign on radiographs
Stage IV: Degenerative changes in the hip joint with involvement of the femoral head

Steinberg Modification

Steinberg modified the Ficat and Arlet as follows (all stages except stage 0 represent advanced degenerative changes):

0: Normal radiograph; normal bone scan
Stage I: Normal radiograph; abnormal bone scan
Stage II: Sclerosis or cyst formation in the femoral head
  A. Mild (less than 20%)
  B. Moderate (20% to 40%)
  C. Severe (more than 40%)
Stage III: Subchondral collapse (crescent sign) without flattening
  A. Mild (less than 15%)
  B. Moderate (15% to 30%)
  C. Severe (more than 30%)
Stage IV: Flattening of the head without joint narrowing or acetabular involvement
  A. Mild (less than 15% of surface and less than 2 mm of depression)
  B. Moderate (15% to 30% of surface or 2 to 4 mm of depression)
Stage V: Flattening of head with joint narrowing or acetabular involvement
  A. Mild
  B. Moderate
  C. Severe (acetabular involvement)

One of the most predictive findings on radiography or MRI is the actual size of the lesion.

ASSOCIATED CONDITIONS

- Hip fracture
- Hemoglobinopathy
- Alcohol abuse
- Perthes' disease

ICD-9-CM

733.42 Osteonecrosis (aseptic necrosis), femoral head

 Diagnosis

SIGNS AND SYMPTOMS

Onset of pain in the hip without antecedent trauma is seen. The patient often initially complains of vague pain in the groin for 4 to 6 months before evaluation. Pain increases with internal rotation of the hip. There should be a high index of suspicion in a young patient with hip pain and other risk factors.

DIFFERENTIAL DIAGNOSIS

- Fracture, if history of trauma
- Infection
- Transient osteoporosis of the hip
- Neurogenic pain
- Visceral cause
- Acetabular labral tear
- Psoas bursitis
- Synovitis or adhesions of the capsule

PHYSICAL EXAMINATION

One should look for groin pain with range of motion of the hip (internal rotation), which is not typically tender with direct palpation. The patient has a limp but a normal neurologic examination. The femoral head venous pressure measurement test is not typically done.
The combination of history and physical examination should lead to a suspicion of osteonecrosis of the hip. Plain radiographs should be ordered and reviewed. If these are negative and there is still no diagnosis made, an MRI of the hip is appropriate to evaluate this problem.

LABORATORY TESTS

- Complete blood count
- Erythrocyte sedimentation rate
- Coagulation profile (research tool at present)

PATHOLOGIC FINDINGS

Although osteonecrosis has many possible causes, there is a common final pathway leading to the typical pathologic findings. This includes death of the osteoblast and osteocytes with empty lacunae in the trabecula of the necrotic area. There is also commonly an area of sclerotic margin in the area of necrosis.

Hip Avascular Necrosis

IMAGING PROCEDURES

• Plain radiographs are obtained, including anteroposterior and lateral projections of the hip.
• MRI of the hip is the single best test to diagnose osteonecrosis of the hip with a specificity of 98%. (Patients with atraumatic osteonecrosis of one hip have a greater than 50% chance of developing osteonecrosis of the contralateral side.)

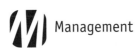 Management

GENERAL MEASURES

The diagnosis of osteonecrosis of the hip should be made as early as possible. Consideration of other joints including the contralateral hip, knees, shoulders, and ankles should be made. Patients with this diagnosis should be evaluated by an orthopaedic surgeon who is experienced in treating osteonecrosis of the hip. Nonoperative treatment is typically not successful, with a failure rate of approximately 80%, depending on the size and classification of the lesion.

SURGICAL TREATMENT

There are multiple surgical procedures for the treatment of osteonecrosis of the hip. Patients with stage I or II disease can be treated with core decompression of the femoral head. This technique decreases pain and may change the natural history of the disease. Vascularized fibular grafts have also been used with some success. Osteotomy and rotation of the affected area of the head away from the weight-bearing portion have had marginal success. Resurfacing arthroplasty and total hip replacement are the definitive treatments. Total hip replacement, however, has a lower success rate for patients with osteonecrosis, compared with patients with osteoarthritis.

PHYSICAL THERAPY

Physical therapy can be useful to maintain range of motion but is generally of little benefit.

MEDICAL TREATMENT

• Nonoperative treatment is typically unsuccessful.
• Anticoagulants: Depending on the origin of the osteonecrosis, anticoagulants may be helpful.

PATIENT EDUCATION

Patients are counseled on the natural history of the disease and are asked to call their physician's attention to bone or joint pain.

PREVENTION

• Limited use of systemic corticosteroid use
• Cessation of steroids with an idiosyncratic reaction
• Avoidance of alcohol-abusive behaviors
• Early fixation of femoral neck fractures or hip dislocations

MONITORING

• Serial radiographs are used to note any progression of joint involvement every 3 to 4 months.
• Clinical symptoms are equally important, especially if nonoperative management is selected with the end point of total hip arthroplasty.

COMPLICATIONS

Progressive collapse of the hip can lead to debilitating arthritis and the need for total hip arthroplasties. Hip arthroplasty in patients with osteonecrosis has a much greater failure rate, owing to loosening, than in patients with osteoarthritis (20% versus 5%, respectively, at 10 years).

PROGNOSIS

The prognosis is good because there are effective arthroplasty procedures for the hip, shoulder, and knee.

RECOMMENDED READING

Frassica FJ, Berry DJ, Morrey BF. Avascular necrosis. In: Morrey BF, ed. *Reconstructive surgery of the joints,* vol 2. New York: Churchill Livingstone, 1996:1085–1110.

Basics

DESCRIPTION

Traumatic hip dislocations are serious, high-energy injuries in which the femoral head becomes completely dislodged from the acetabulum. Associated acetabular or femoral head or neck fractures are common. Because most such dislocations (70% to 90%) are a result of motor vehicle accidents, significant injuries are often present elsewhere in the body (Fig. 1). This injury is most common in young adults after motor vehicle accidents. More males than females are affected. Up to 50% of patients suffer other fractures at the time of injury. Dislocations and fracture dislocations of the hip are orthopaedic emergencies.

INCIDENCE

- Anterior dislocation: 10% to 15%
- Posterior dislocation: 85% to 90%

CAUSES

Most commonly, in 70% to nearly 100% of cases, traumatic hip dislocations are a result of motor vehicle accidents. As the car decelerates, the flexed knee strikes the dashboard, forcing the femoral head out posteriorly. Other mechanisms include automobile versus pedestrian accidents, falls from heights, industrial injuries, and sporting accidents.

RISK FACTORS

- Motor vehicle accidents
- Fall from significant height

CLASSIFICATION

Classification is based on the direction of dislocation (anterior versus posterior) and associated fractures in the femoral head or femoral neck (Fig. 2).

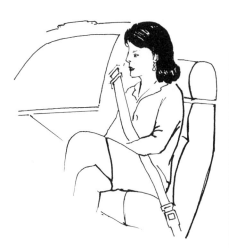

Fig. 1. The most common mechanism for a hip dislocation is a frontal impact with the hip in a flexed, adducted position.

ASSOCIATED CONDITIONS

Because hip dislocations are usually secondary to high-energy trauma, other significant injuries are common and include the following:

- Neurologic injuries: sciatic nerve palsy, herniated discs
- Musculoskeletal injuries: femoral head, neck, and acetabular fractures, midfoot injuries
- Intraabdominal or chest injuries

ICD-9-CM

835.00 Hip dislocation

Diagnosis

SIGNS AND SYMPTOMS

- Severe pain over the hip or numbness along the posterior thigh
- Altered resting lower extremity position: (a) in posterior dislocation (85% to 90%), severe pain, and hip fixed in a position of flexion, internal rotation, and adduction; (b) in anterior dislocation, hip in marked external rotation with mild flexion and abduction
- Shortening of the extremity

Many patients suffering traumatic hip dislocations are obtunded or unconscious when they arrive at the emergency department and, as a result, are unable to assist the physician in the initial evaluation.

DIFFERENTIAL DIAGNOSIS

- Femoral head fracture
- Femoral neck fractures

PHYSICAL EXAMINATION

- Examination must include a full evaluation because concomitant injuries are common, especially other musculoskeletal injuries.
- The affected limb must be carefully examined to detect the presence of partial or complete sciatic nerve injury.
- Classic presentation of anterior versus posterior dislocations (discussed earlier) may be altered by ipsilateral extremity injuries.

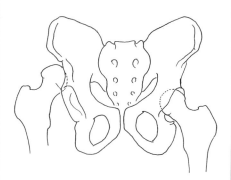

Fig. 2. In an acute hip dislocation, the femoral head is usually displaced posteriorly and superiorly. The acetabulum should be inspected for fractures.

LABORATORY TESTS

There are no diagnostic serum laboratory tests.

IMAGING PROCEDURES

All patients with traumatic hip dislocations should have routine trauma films including cervical spine, chest, and anteroposterior pelvis films. Plain films of painful extremities, or other pelvic views (internal or external oblique-Judet views), should be obtained if associated fractures are suspected.

In a posterior dislocation, the femoral head appears smaller on the anteroposterior radiograph. In an anterior dislocation, the femoral head appears slightly larger than the uninjured hip. Careful evaluation of the femoral neck must rule out the presence of a femoral neck fracture before any manipulative reduction is undertaken. In addition, the acetabulum should be carefully inspected to ascertain the presence or absence of incarcerated osteochondral fragments and the asymmetry of the joint space. Computed tomography scans should be routinely obtained after successful closed reductions, or before surgery, if open reduction is planned. Computed tomography is valuable in demonstrating the presence of small intraarticular fragments and in assessing the congruence of the femoral head and acetabulum.

The role of magnetic resonance imaging in posttraumatic evaluation of the hip has not yet been established, and this technique is not currently used.

Hip Dislocation–Traumatic

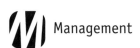 Management

GENERAL MEASURES

It is important to assess patients fully for concomitant injuries because such injuries are often present in these patients with high-energy trauma. The ABCs (airway, breathing, circulation) are still the first steps in management. The management of a patient with a hip dislocation is divided into an initial phase of identifying and reducing the dislocation, followed by a secondary phase of planning and performing definitive care. Once the femoral head has been reduced, the urgency is diminished, and an appropriate diagnostic workup, including computed tomography analysis, can be completed. Surgical intervention, if indicated, can be undertaken after the patient has become hemodynamically stable and safe for operative management.

Regardless of the direction of the dislocation, the reduction can be attempted with in-line traction with the patient lying supine. The preferred approach is to perform a closed reduction with the patient under general anesthesia and with complete muscle paralysis either in the emergency department or the operating room, if one is available. If this is not immediately feasible, an attempt can be made with intravenous sedation in the emergency department.

Emergency orthopaedic consultation should be obtained because urgent reduction of the dislocated hip is necessary to prevent long-term complications.

SURGICAL TREATMENT

If closed reduction cannot be achieved, then open reduction is indicated. The standard posterior approach, or a lateral decubitus position, is used with or without a fracture (traction) table, depending on the surgeon's preference.

PHYSICAL THERAPY

This is often required for gait training with protected weight bearing and range of motion.

MEDICAL TREATMENT

- Assess the patient for concomitant injuries, which are common.
- Determine whether closed reduction can be done.
- Administer medications; the drugs of choice are narcotic analgesics.
- After successful closed reduction and completion of the stability examination, place the patient in traction while awaiting computed tomography evaluation. If the hip has been demonstrated to be stable, simple traction with a Buck's traction boot or skin traction is sufficient. If the hip is unstable, it is preferable to use skeletal traction with a tibial pin.

PATIENT EDUCATION

There is a risk of osteonecrosis of the hip, and even with prompt hip reduction, some degree of posttraumatic arthritis commonly occurs.

PREVENTION

Seat belts should be used in conjunction with air bags.

MONITORING

- Serial hip radiographs in the first year every 3 to 4 months
- Magnetic resonance imaging if concern exists about osteonecrosis

COMPLICATIONS

Posttraumatic Arthritis

Posttraumatic arthritis is the most frequent long-term complication. The incidence of arthritis is significantly increased in patients with associated acetabular or femoral head fractures.

Osteonecrosis

Osteonecrosis (avascular necrosis) occurs in 1% to 17% of these patients. The risk increases when the hip remains dislocated for a period of time. Threshold time is reported to be about 6 to 24 hours. Secondary arthritis may develop as a result of avascular necrosis.

Sciatic Nerve Injury

Sciatic nerve injuries (8% to 19%) are caused by stretching of the nerve from a posteriorly dislocated femoral head or from a displaced fracture fragment. The peroneal component of the nerve is most commonly affected. Electromyography and nerve conduction studies are indicated at 3 to 4 weeks for baseline information, documentation of precise level, and prognostic guidance.

Recurrent Dislocation

Recurrent dislocation is exceedingly rare.

PROGNOSIS

With simple posterior hip dislocations (without associated fractures), most large retrospective studies report a 70% to 80% good or excellent outcome. When posterior dislocations are associated with femoral head fractures or acetabular fractures, the outcome is not favorable. Patients with anterior dislocations have been noted to have a high incidence of femoral head injuries, and long-term outcome is not as good as with posterior dislocations. Only 70% of these patients have good or excellent results.

RECOMMENDED READING

Browner BD, Jupiter JB, Levine AM, et al. *Skeletal trauma*, vol 2. Philadelphia: WB Saunders, 1992:1359–1367.

Rockwood CA, Green DP, Bucholz RW, et al., eds. *Rockwood and Green's fractures in adults*, vol 2, 4th ed. Philadelphia: Lippincott–Raven, 1996:1756–1803.

Basics

DESCRIPTION

Fracture of the femoral neck, intertrochanteric or subtrochanteric region.

INCIDENCE

This injury accounts for less than 1% of all pediatric fractures, far less than the percentage in adults.

CAUSES

Seventy-five percent of pediatric hip fractures are caused by severe trauma and high-velocity injuries (i.e., motor vehicle accidents, falls). The remainder are the result of some underlying pathologic process (i.e., fracture through a unicameral bone cyst, aneurysmal bone cyst, or fibrous dysplasia) or child abuse.

ASSOCIATED CONDITIONS

Infants

Suspect child abuse. If the injury is a result of the child's being run over, look for associated injuries.

Children

Great violence is required. Look for associated injuries.

Adolescents

Acute fracture occurs through the growth plate (slipped capital femoral epiphysis), or it is a pathologic slip (look for hypothyroidism, renal osteodystrophy).

ANATOMY

Epiphysis

Most complications of pediatric hip fractures are influenced by the changing blood supply of the proximal femoral epiphysis. At birth, there is a single physis (growth plate). Between 6 to 12 months, this separates into two centers of ossification, the capital epiphysis and the trochanteric apophysis. By the age of 4 years, the ossific nucleus of the greater trochanter appears.

Blood Supply

At birth, the blood supply to the femoral head travels through the metaphyseal vessels traversing the neck, derived from the medial and lateral femoral circumflex arteries. As the growth plate of the proximal femur develops, it prevents these vessels from significantly penetrating the femoral head. By the age of 4 years, the contribution by the metaphyseal blood supply is negligible, and the retinacular systems derived from the medial femoral circumflex artery provide the major blood supply to the head. As a result, capsulotomy of the hip does not damage the blood supply to the femoral head unless it violates the intertrochanteric notch or damages the posterosuperior or posteroinferior vessels along the femoral neck. The ligamentum teres contributes only a small percentage of the blood supply to the femoral head until the age of 8 years, and in adults it contributes only 20%.

Bone

The periosteal tube in a child is much stronger than in an adult, and about half of pediatric hip fractures are undisplaced. However, if the fracture is displaced, it is likely to be unstable.

CLASSIFICATION

Delbet's classification is as follows:

Type I: Transphyseal separation (i.e., the femoral head separates from the neck through the growth plate); can be undisplaced (widened physis), displaced, or dislocated
Least common type
Occurs in younger children
Many patients with dislocation of the femoral head from the acetabulum
Type II: Transcervical
Type III: Cervicotrochanteric
Type IV: Intertrochanteric

Initial displacement seems to affect the risk of osteonecrosis most directly.

ICD-9-CM

820.08 Pediatric hip fracture

Diagnosis

SIGNS AND SYMPTOMS

- Sudden pain in the hip
- Inability to stand or walk
- Swelling in the inguinal crease, gluteal, proximal thigh
- Limb held in external rotation, flexion, adduction to relieve capsular distention
- Resistance to any movement (active hip motion is impossible if the fracture is displaced and passive motion especially flexion, abduction, and internal rotation are restricted and painful)
- Pain and sometimes crepitation with hip motion
- Pseudoparalysis of the affected limb in infants
- Extremity possibly shortened by 1 to 2 cm

DIFFERENTIAL DIAGNOSIS

- Slipped capital femoral epiphysis
- Developmental coxa vara (This condition has a vertical cleft in the femoral neck.)

IMAGING PROCEDURES

- Radiographs (anteroposterior view of the pelvis and anteroposterior and lateral views of the hip) may show upward and lateral displacement of the femoral shaft.
- Computed tomography scanning can be helpful for determining the direction of the femoral head dislocation.
- In newborns, ultrasound may be helpful in demonstrating a femoral neck fracture.

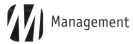

Management

GENERAL PRINCIPLES

- Treatment is aimed at achieving anatomic reduction either open or closed.
- Use smooth pins or cannulated 4.0- to 4.5-mm screws in children and cannulated 6.5- to 7.0-mm screws in older children and teenagers.
- Use a spica cast postoperatively because the smaller diameter of the femoral neck in these younger patients limits the size and number of screws that can be placed.
- If the injury is type I and one must cross the physis, use smooth pins, followed by a spica cast.
- If the hip is dislocated, make one attempt at closed reduction, then try open reduction.
- If open reduction is attempted, the surgical approach should be in the direction of the dislocation: posterior for posterior dislocation, anterior for anterior dislocation.
- Screws should not cross the physis unless the fracture cannot be stabilized without doing so. The physis of the proximal femur only grows 3 mm a year, so fear of limb length discrepancy should not compromise fixation.

SURGICAL TREATMENT

Type I Without Dislocation

Gentle closed reduction and pin fixation are indicated.

Type I With Dislocation

In these patients, 100% develop osteonecrosis, 80% are at risk of developing degenerative joint disease. Attempt gentle closed reduction using longitudinal traction, abduction, and internal rotation; if that is unsuccessful, try immediate open reduction and pin fixation.

Type II

- Most common type
- Most fractures displaced
- Osteonecrosis in about 50% (displaced fractures at higher risk than nondisplaced)
- Closed or open reduction and pin or screw fixation for both displaced and nondisplaced fractures

Type III

- Second most common type
- Osteonecrosis in 25%
- Displaced: gentle closed reduction or open reduction and internal fixation
- Nondisplaced: abduction spica cast possibly adequate in children less than 8 years old, although late displacement or coxa vara possible; close observation necessary

Hip Fractures in Children

Type IV

Skeletal traction is followed by hip abduction spica cast for 12 weeks or open reduction and internal fixation with pediatric hip compression screw fixation for unsuccessful closed reduction in children or older adolescents.

Surgical Pearls

- One should use a fluoroscopy table or a fracture table and an image intensifier.
- A straight lateral approach is used.
- The reduction maneuver includes traction and internal rotation.
- Unacceptable reduction is indicated by a varus position or excessive displacement on anteroposterior and lateral views.
- No displacement exceeding 10% to 20% of the width of the femoral neck should be accepted, because further varus angulation is likely.

Instrumentation

- Types I, II, and III: Use two to three cannulated screws of appropriate size for age.
- Type IV: Use a hip compression screw device with a side plate.
- Nonoperative option: Reduce with 3 to 6 weeks of skeletal traction and then immobilization in hip abduction cast for a total treatment course of 12 weeks.
- If age 7 to 12 years: Use pediatric hip screw fixation, followed by hip spica cast for 8 to 12 weeks after surgery, depending on the stability of fixation.
- Age 13 years and older: Treat like an adult. The hip screw and side plate may cross the physis. No postoperative immobilization is required.

Neonatal Epiphysiolysis

If this is recognized initially, use skin traction to restore alignment. If it is recognized after callus formation is visible radiographically, simple immobilization is used. Open surgical reduction is not advised, because these injuries in newborns tend to remodel if the physis does not close prematurely. Close observation is necessary. There is a low incidence of osteonecrosis.

Timing of Surgery

- Within 24 hours
- Type I fracture with dislocation requiring immediate treatment
- No conclusive data on the effect of timing on osteonecrosis

Hardware Removal

No absolute time limit exists for removal of hardware. Generally, however, it is removed within 12 to 18 months of injury, if the fracture has healed. This is to prevent bony overgrowth or refracture.

COMPLICATIONS

Complications occur in as many as 60% of patients.

Avascular Necrosis (Osteonecrosis)

- Most common, most devastating complication
- May affect epiphysis, epiphysis and metaphysis, or metaphysis alone

Incidence

This develops in 42% of hip fractures in children within 9 to 12 months after injury, as follows:

- Type I: 100%
- Type II: 52%
- Type III: 27%
- Type IV: 14%

Risk Factors

Initial displacement of the fracture, fracture types I and II, and age (greater than 10 years) are associated with increased risk.

Ratliff's Classification of Osteonecrosis in Children

- Type I: Total involvement and collapse of the femoral head; worst prognosis; most common injury to all lateral epiphyseal vessels
- Type 2: Involvement of a portion of the epiphysis and accompanied by minimal collapse of the femoral head; localized injury to the anterolateral femoral head
- Type 3: Increased sclerosis of the femoral neck from the fracture line to the physis, but sparing of the femoral head; injury to the metaphyseal vessels

Treatment

- Motion and containment are maintained.
- Osteotomies to rotate the less deformed or more uninvolved portion into the weight-bearing region may improve congruity and symptoms.

Nonunion

- This occurs in 5% to 8% of fractures (similar to the number in adults).
- Closed treatment of types II and III is associated with an increased incidence of coxa vara and nonunion.
- Internal fixation after acceptable reduction decreases the incidence of nonunion because it does not allow varus angulation or late displacement.

Coxa Vara

- The overall prevalence is less than 20%.
- This is secondary to growth arrest of the proximal femoral physis or to malunion.
- If the neck shaft angle is less than 110 degrees, it will not correct with remodeling.
- Subtrochanteric valgus osteotomy, bone grafting, and internal fixation can give excellent long-term results if no osteonecrosis is present.

Premature Closure of the Physis

- A slight leg length inequality results.
- It occurs even without internal fixation crossing the physis.
- Closure is often related to osteonecrosis.
- The proximal femoral physis contributes to only ⅛ inch per year (about 15% of total length of extremity). However, if osteonecrosis and premature closure occur, a significant limb length discrepancy can develop.
- Follow with yearly scanograms and hand and wrist radiographs for bone age with plotting on Moseley's charts. Consider epiphyseodesis of contralateral limb if significant inequality develops.
- In rare cases, symptomatic trochanteric overgrowth in children older than 8 years can require trochanteric transfer.

PROGNOSIS

- Prognosis is fair to guarded.
- The outcome is determined by the degree of damage to the blood supply.

RECOMMENDED READING

Hensinger RN, ed. *Operative management of lower extremity fractures in children.* American Academy of Orthopaedic Surgeons monograph series. Rosemont, IL: American Academy of Orthopaedic Surgeons, 1992:11–19.

Rang M. *Children's fractures,* 2nd ed. Philadelphia: JB Lippincott, 1983:242–257.

Richards BS, ed. *Orthopaedic knowledge update: pediatrics.* Rosemont, IL: American Academy of Orthopaedic Surgeons, 1996:229–231.

Basics

DESCRIPTION

"Hip pain" is a term used to describe discomfort in the groin, which receives sensory innervation provided by the obturator and femoral nerves. This pain can be produced by a lesion in the region of the hip joint, as follows:

- Capsule and synovial lining
- Bone of the pelvis or proximal femur
- Muscles, nerves, and vascular structures in the region of the hip, buttock, groin, or pelvis

Regardless of cause, the hip pain is usually localized to the region of the anterior groin, the greater trochanter, or the anterolateral thigh down to the knee. Because many of the causes of hip pain need urgent treatment, or carry a poor prognosis if left untreated, it is imperative that hip pain be evaluated thoroughly. In transient synovitis, the average age on onset of symptoms is 6 years, with most cases occurring between 3 and 8 years of age. Approximately two-thirds of all cases of septic arthritis occur before the age of 3 years.
Legg-Perthes disease has a peak incidence at the age of 6 years, whereas slipped capital femoral epiphysis (SCFE) almost always occurs during preadolescence or adolescence.

GENETICS

An association is not clearly shown, except in conditions such as SCFE, in which approximately 4% of patients have a family history.

INCIDENCE

- Transient synovitis is reported to be the most common cause of hip pain in children.
- A 3% risk exists for a child to have at least one episode of transient synovitis of the hip.
- The incidence of Legg-Perthes disease is approximately 1 in 1,500, whereas SCFE occurs 1 in 10,000.
- Septic arthritis is slightly more common in males. There is a male-to-female predominance in transient synovitis (2:1), SCFE (2.5:1), osteomyelitis (4:1), and Legg-Calves-Perthes (6:1).

CAUSES

Transient Synovitis

Transient synovitis is associated with current or recent illness, trauma, or allergic reaction.

Septic Arthritis

Septic arthritis in newborns is most commonly caused by *Haemophilus influenzae* type B, whereas *Staphylococcus aureus* predominates after 6 months. In the adolescent, *Neisseria gonorrhoeae* must be considered. The mechanism of onset is either direct extension of osteomyelitis from the proximal metaphysis of the femur into the hip joint or hematogenous dissemination of organisms through the blood supply of the synovial membrane. During the first 12 to 18 months of life, there is little resistance to the extension of infection across the physis in the proximal femur, owing to vascular channels in the growth plate. As a result, osteomyelitis and septic arthritis are more common.

Legg-Calvé-Perthes Disease

The cause of Legg-Calvé-Perthes disease is unknown, although trauma, hypercoagulability, and thrombosis have all been postulated.

Slipped Capital Femoral Epiphysis

In SCFE, weakness of the physis during the adolescent growth spurt and trauma are probably related. Approximately 80% of patients are obese, and hormonal factors are also most likely involved.

RISK FACTORS

- Rheumatoid arthritis
- Closed trauma
- Impaired host defense
- Obesity, trauma, and age (all shown to be related to the development of SCFE)

CLASSIFICATION

- Infectious
- Traumatic
- Neoplastic
- Idiopathic

ASSOCIATED CONDITIONS

Current or recent illness, trauma, and allergic reactions are associated with transient synovitis.

ICD-9-CM

719.45 Hip pain, not otherwise specified
711.0 Septic arthritis
732.2 Slipped capital femoral epiphysis
732.1 Perthes disease

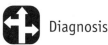 Diagnosis

SIGNS AND SYMPTOMS

- Pain: referable to the groin, trochanter, anterolateral thigh, knee
- Involuntary guarding or spasm of muscles around the hip joint
- Limitation of active and passive hip motion (i.e., loss of internal rotation and abduction in Legg-Perthes disease or hip dysplasia; external rotation of the hip with attempted flexion pathognomonic for SCFE)
- Refusal to walk or bear weight on the affected extremity
- Limp, possibly antalgic or painless, and intermittent
- Atrophy of the thigh or buttock muscles
- Fever in septic arthritis, osteomyelitis

DIFFERENTIAL DIAGNOSIS

- Transient synovitis (although the most common cause of hip pain, should be diagnosis of exclusion only)
- Infections of the hip joint, proximal femur, pelvis, intervertebral discs, sacroiliac joint
- Legg-Calvé-Perthes disease (avascular necrosis of the femoral head)
- SCFE
- Juvenile rheumatoid arthritis, early osteoarthritis
- Tumors of the pelvis, spine, or proximal femur
- Bursitis of psoas or trochanter
- Sickle cell crisis
- Nonarticular processes
- Sacroiliac joint septic arthritis
- Psoas septic bursitis
- Leukemia or lymphoma

PHYSICAL EXAMINATION

- Inspect and palpate the skin around the hip, buttock, lower back, and thigh to detect warmth, erythema, swelling, bruising, or specific areas of point tenderness (e.g., bursae).
- Note the general position of the lower extremity as well as any leg length inequality.
- Measure and document passive and active range of motion of the hip and knee joints, especially internal and external rotation.
- Document a complete neurovascular extremity examination, noting any weakness or numbness.
- If possible, examine the gait, including toe-and-heel walking.
- To rule out septic arthritis, perform hip aspiration, usually under fluoroscopic or sonographic guidance. If no fluid is obtained, an arthrogram should be performed to confirm needle placement.

Hip Pain in a Child

LABORATORY TESTS

In transient synovitis, Legg-Perthes disease, SCFE, and hip dysplasia, results of routine tests are usually nonspecific and are within normal limits. These tests are important to order, however, to rule out infection.

In septic arthritis, the cell count of the aspirated joint fluid is the most sensitive test, with more than 50,000 cells/mm³. The serum leukocyte count is elevated, and a left shift may occur.

Blood cultures are positive in 40% of children with osteomyelitis or septic arthritis. These cultures should always be obtained during the initial stages of the workup.

PATHOLOGIC FINDINGS

In septic arthritis, there is initially synovial hypertrophy and later cartilage destruction. In slipped epiphysis, one sees posterior and inferior displacement of the femoral head on the metaphysis. In Perthes' disease, the femoral head becomes flattened and extruded.

IMAGING PROCEDURES

Transient Synovitis

In transient synovitis, plain films of the hip, anteroposterior and lateral views, are nonspecific, but they may help to rule out other diagnoses. Plain radiographs in septic arthritis may show obliteration of fat planes and soft tissue swelling. With early osteomyelitis, one may see mottling of bone density; later, sclerosis (new bone formation) and lytic lesions (further bony destruction) are more prevalent, with destruction of the femoral head being the end result.

Legg-Perthes Disease

In Legg-Perthes disease, early plain film findings include failure of epiphyseal growth and loss of bone density, whereas later signs include a crescent-shaped subchondral fracture in the femoral head, shortening of the femoral neck, and flattening or ultimately enlargement of the femoral head.

Slipped Capital Femoral Epiphysis

Widening of the growth plate, mild osteopenia of the proximal femur, or displacement of the epiphysis is seen in SCFE.

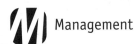 Management

GENERAL MEASURES

Transient Synovitis

• Rapidly resolve underlying inflammation with antiinflammatory agents.
• Prescribe bed rest and full relief of weight bearing on the involved joint until pain resolves and full motion returns.
• Spontaneous resolution is the natural course, because this is usually a self-limiting condition.

Septic Arthritis

• Perform immediate surgical drainage and administer antibiotic therapy.
• Give broad-spectrum antibiotic coverage until culture results are available. Oral antibiotics, if appropriate, are usually given for 3 weeks, until the erythrocyte sedimentation rate has returned to normal.
• Splint hips in abduction if capsular distention has occurred.
• When infection is under control and drainage has ceased, begin range-of-motion exercises.

Legg-Perthes Disease

• Prevent subluxation.
• Preserve the sphericity of the femoral head.
• Order bed rest, if needed, and traction to reduce spasms and synovitis.
• Surgical reconstruction is sometimes necessary to maintain the femoral head within the acetabulum.

Slipped Capital Femoral Epiphysis

• Prevent further slipping while minimizing the risk of avascular necrosis or chondrolysis.
• Provide the necessary immobilization for acute slips with prompt *in situ* pin fixation with threaded screws.

SURGICAL TREATMENT

• Surgical preference for hip drainage is exposure of the hip joint, irrigation of the necrotic debris, fibrin clot, and pus, and insertion of a drain.
• With osteomyelitis, a small window is cut in the bone for curettage of material for culture and open drainage.
• Chronic osteomyelitis, although rare, often requires surgical resection.
• Legg-Perthes disease may require surgical reconstruction of the femur or acetabulum for severe cases.
• *In situ* percutaneous pinning is required for SCFE to prevent further slips and the associated complications.

PHYSICAL THERAPY

This is not usually required.

PATIENT EDUCATION

The parents of a patient who is presumed to have synovitis of the hip should be able to observe the child and ensure that improvement continues. They should maintain regular follow-up and should contact the physician if the child's status worsens.

MEDICAL TREATMENT

Appropriate antibiotics are essential for treatment of septic arthritis and osteomyelitis.

MONITORING

The erythrocyte sedimentation rate or C-reactive protein value has been shown to be a reliable serologic marker to guide the length of antibiotic therapy after surgical management for septic arthritis and osteomyelitis. It should return to within normal limits before antibiotics are discontinued. Observation only is appropriate for all patients with transient synovitis and for patients with Legg-Perthes disease with minimal involvement of the femoral head (less than 50%).

COMPLICATIONS

Untreated septic arthritis and osteomyelitis can be devastating for a growing child and can result in limb shortening, joint surface irregularities, stiffness, and early degenerative changes. (Cartilage destruction begins as early as 8 hours after the onset of infection.)

In SFCE, either the slip itself or reduction attempts may result in avascular necrosis or chondrolysis, a condition in which the cartilage of the femoral head degenerates and produces joint narrowing, stiffness, contracture, pain, and limping. Patients with SCFE have a higher-than-normal risk of developing degenerative arthritis.

PROGNOSIS

If septic arthritis and osteomyelitis are detected early, prognosis may be good. Chronic osteomyelitis often results in residual deformity. In Legg-Perthes disease, the lesser the amount of avascular bone and the younger the child at the onset of disease, the better is the prognosis, although there is always some residual deformity seen on radiographs. Other good prognostic signs include lack of lateralization or extrusion and adequate range of motion. Long-term prognosis of SCFE depends on the amount of displacement. Patients with more severe slips have a greater likelihood of developing degenerative arthritis later in life.

RECOMMENDED READING

Morrissy RT, Weinstein SL, eds. *Lovell and Winter's pediatric orthopaedics*, vol 2, 4th ed. Philadelphia: Lippincott–Raven, 1996:1034–1037.

Renshaw TS. *Pediatric orthopaedics*. Philadelphia: WB Saunders, 1986.

Tachdjian MO. *Pediatric orthopaedics*, vol 2, 2nd ed. Philadelphia: WB Saunders, 1990:1461–1465.

Basics

DESCRIPTION

Many forms of arthritis lead to eventual destruction of the articular cartilage of the hip joint, resulting in pain and loss of function. This end stage, often referred to as degenerative joint disease, can be treated with surgical replacement of the joint with metal and plastic components.

Most hip replacements are performed in patients older than 65 years of age, although the procedure is being performed in younger patients more commonly.

There is a slight predominance of women in patients older than 65 years and in men younger than 45 years.

Elderly patients may have greater risk of cardiac complications and more associated medical problems. Younger patients are likely to need revision surgery, because their life expectancy may far exceed the longevity of the prosthesis. Other treatment options such as medical management, hip fusion, and femoral osteotomy should be strongly considered in the younger, high-demand patient.

SYNONYMS

- Total hip replacement
- Total hip arthroplasty
- Hemiarthroplasty (replacing just the proximal femur)
- Bipolar prosthesis (a type of hemi-arthroplasty)

GENETICS

- Possible familial predisposition to primary osteoarthritis
- No mendelian pattern of inheritance
- More common in whites

INCIDENCE

- More than 200,000 total hip replacements are performed in the United States each year.
- Primary osteoarthritis affects about 5% of the population older than 55 years.

CAUSES

- Primary osteoarthritis is the most common cause of disabling hip arthritis.
- Traumatic arthritis, osteonecrosis, rheumatoid arthritis, sickle cell anemia, recurrent hemarthrosis, Paget's disease, and ankylosing spondylitis may all lead to degenerative destruction of the hip joint.
- Developmental conditions such as slipped capital femoral epiphysis, developmental dysplasia, and Legg-Calvé-Perthes disease may all lead to degenerative joint disease later in life.
- Some acute hip fractures may also be treated with partial or total hip replacement.

RISK FACTORS

- Primary osteoarthritis may be more common in high-demand athletes and in obese patients.
- Osteonecrosis has been linked to prolong steroid use, alcoholism, radiation, and trauma.
- Osteoporosis often leads to femoral neck fractures in elderly patients.

CLASSIFICATION

- Cemented versus uncemented (femoral side only)
- Partial versus total (femoral and acetabular sides)

ASSOCIATED CONDITIONS

Degenerative joint disease of the contralateral hip, either knee, the lumbar spine, and the upper extremity is often seen in patients requiring hip replacement.

ICD-9-CM

715.95 Osteoarthritis

Diagnosis

SIGNS AND SYMPTOMS

- Primary osteoarthritis of the hip may result in pain in the groin, the lateral thigh, or radiating to the knee.
- Pain is more common with activity but may eventually become present at rest and at night.
- In advanced stages, pain may limit the patient to needing rest after walking less than 1 block.
- Limitation of range of motion, especially of flexion, extension, and internal rotation, may be present. With ambulation, abductor lurch may be evident.

DIFFERENTIAL DIAGNOSIS

- Hip pain may be caused by spinal stenosis or a herniated lumbar disc.
- Low back pain of any cause may radiate to the lateral thigh and hip.
- Trochanteric bursitis may result in lateral hip pain.
- Stress fracture must also be considered.
- Occult neoplasms such as metastatic bone disease, multiple myeloma, and primary mesenchymal tumors can also cause hip pain.

PHYSICAL EXAMINATION

- Perform a neurovascular examination of the affected extremity.
- Record the range of motion of the hip.
- Pay special attention to contractures, leg length discrepancy, and gluteal muscle strength.
- Assess the patient's gait.

LABORATORY TESTS

For total hip replacement, order the following before surgery:

- Complete blood count
- Blood chemistry studies
- Coagulation times
- Electrocardiogram, chest radiographs, and urinalysis should be done when appropriate.

Many patients are able to donate autologous units of blood 4 to 6 weeks before surgery.

Hip Replacement

PATHOLOGIC FINDINGS

The common denominators in all forms of arthritis are breakdown of the articular cartilage, loss of the proteoglycan, and gradual dissolution of the cartilage.

IMAGING PROCEDURES

Anteroposterior pelvis and frog-leg lateral hip radiographs are usually adequate to assess the hip joint. Long, standing films of the lower extremities and pelvis may be helpful.
Computed tomography may be performed for patients with severe deformity of the hip.

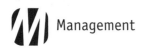 Management

GENERAL MEASURES

Postoperative patients may require prolonged treatment for prophylaxis of deep venous thrombosis such as with warfarin (Coumadin) or low-molecular-weight heparin. Many patients receive home physical therapy or nursing care, and some patients need acute inpatient rehabilitation.

SURGICAL TREATMENT

Total hip replacement consists of a femoral component and a head that replaces the proximal femur and is usually made of chrome-cobalt alloy. The acetabulum is most commonly replaced with a metal shell with a high-density polyethylene plastic insert. The components may be fixed to the bone using cement or by allowing ingrowth of bone into a porous coating on the components. Surgery is performed through a posterior or a lateral approach. Both involve a lateral thigh incision. Some lateral approaches may require a trochanteric osteotomy and repair with wires.
Most patients progress to full weight-bearing activity over 6 weeks to 3 months and are encouraged to ambulate. Most eventually ambulate without external support, but some patients may require a cane or walker on a long-term basis.

PHYSICAL THERAPY

Postoperative patients are instructed in strengthening exercises, especially hip flexion, extension, and abduction. Transfer and gait training with a standup walker are emphasized. Patients are advised not to flex the hip past 90 degrees or to adduct past the midline and to keep internal and external rotation to a minimum during the first 3 months after surgery.

MEDICAL TREATMENT

- Analgesics in the acute postoperative period
- Nonsteroidal antiinflammatory medications for patients who do not desire surgery
- Occasional intraarticular cortisone injections

PATIENT EDUCATION

Patients must understand that hip arthroplasty is a major surgical procedure that requires months of significant limitation of activity and may require a full year to achieve full benefit. They must be prepared to adhere to the hip precautions taught in physical therapy and to contribute to the rehabilitation process.

PREVENTION

Weight loss and limitation of activity may postpone the need for hip replacement.

MONITORING

- Radiographs should be taken at 6 weeks and then at 1-year intervals postoperatively.
- Patients should have long-term follow-up with their surgeons every 1 to 2 years.

COMPLICATIONS

Postoperative patients must be monitored for cardiac complications and pulmonary embolus. Over the long term, patients are at risk for infection of their prosthesis, which may necessitate its removal. The component may also dislocate, a complication that can be treated with bracing or revision surgery. Patients are also at risk of femoral fracture around the prosthesis.

PROGNOSIS

Hip arthroplasty has excellent long-term results, with may patients ambulating without external support and resuming previously impossible activities. The components may eventually become loose, owing to mechanical stress or osteolysis secondary to debris in the joint. The best long-term studies have shown that 85% of cemented prostheses survive for 20 years.

RECOMMENDED READING

Cabanela M. The hip. In: Morry BF, ed. *Reconstructive surgery of the joints*. New York: Churchill Livingstone, 1996:875–1333.

Basics

DESCRIPTION

Transient synovitis of the hip represents the most common cause of hip pain in childhood. The condition's true cause is unknown. It appears to be an immune-mediated inflammation, not an infection. Transient synovitis is characterized by the acute onset of monarticular hip pain, limp, and restricted hip motion. It must be distinguished from septic arthritis. Gradual but complete resolution over several days to weeks is the norm.
Transient synovitis of the hip can occur from 9 months of age to adolescence. Most cases occur in children between 3 and 8 years of age.

SYNONYMS

- Transitory coxitis
- Acute transient epiphysitis
- Toxic synovitis
- Irritable hip

GENETICS

This condition is not recognized to be genetic.

INCIDENCE

Transient synovitis is the most common cause of hip pain in children. Historically, it accounted for 0.4% to 0.9% of annual pediatric hospital admissions. The risk for a child to have at least one episode of transient synovitis of the hip is 1% to 3%. This risk is three times greater in patients with a stocky or obese physique. Right and left involvement is essentially equal, and simultaneous bilateral involvement has not been reported. The incidence is much lower among African-Americans.
The male-to-female ratio is 2:1.

CAUSES

The cause is unknown. It has been proposed that transient synovitis of the hip is associated with active infection elsewhere, trauma, or allergic hypersensitivity. Nonspecific upper respiratory infection, pharyngitis, and otitis media have been associated with the occurrence of transient synovitis in as many as 70% cases. There is an association with minor trauma in up to 30% and with allergic predisposition in up to 25%.

RISK FACTORS

- Male gender
- Upper respiratory infection or other active infection

ASSOCIATED CONDITION

Perthes disease (about 1.5%)

ICD-9-CM

727.0 Synovitis

 Diagnosis

SIGNS AND SYMPTOMS

- An acute onset of unilateral hip pain occurs in an otherwise healthy patient.
- Pain is usually confined to the ipsilateral groin and hip area, but it may present as anterior thigh and knee pain.
- Limp and antalgic gait are common, with some patients refusing to bear weight on the involved extremity.
- The extremity is held in a flexed and externally rotated position and has restricted range of motion.
- The patient may have a low-grade fever.
- Laboratory values are nonspecific and are usually within normal limits.

DIFFERENTIAL DIAGNOSIS

Transient synovitis of the hip is a diagnosis of exclusion.

- Pyogenic arthritis
- Osteomyelitis in the adjacent femoral neck or pelvis
- Tuberculous arthritis
- Psoas abscess
- Juvenile rheumatoid arthritis
- Acute rheumatic fever
- Legg-Calvé-Perthes disease
- Tumor
- Slipped capital femoral epiphysis
- Subluxation
- Dislocation
- Sacroiliac joint infection

PHYSICAL EXAMINATION

- Lower extremity examination usually reveals unilateral hip pain confined to the ipsilateral groin, anterior thigh, or knee.
- The leg is usually held in a flexed and externally rotated position.
- Range of motion is often decreased and painful.
- The patient does not have as much pain as the patient with a septic hip. If the range of motion is tested slowly, it is usually at least 50% of normal.
- While walking, patients often display a limp or an antalgic gait.
- Ipsilateral muscle atrophy is rarely seen, but when present, it usually implies a long-standing duration of symptoms, and a diagnosis other than transient synovitis should be considered.

Hip Transient Synovitis

LABORATORY TESTS

Results are usually nonspecific and within normal limits, but they may help to rule out other diagnoses. The peripheral blood smear usually includes a white blood cell count averaging 10,000 to 14,000 cells/mm³, and the erythrocyte sedimentation rate averages 20 mm/hour, but it may be slightly higher. Urinalysis, blood culture, rheumatoid factor, and tuberculin skin test results are usually within normal limits. Analysis of joint fluid for complement levels or other tests has been nonspecific.

PATHOLOGIC FINDINGS

- This is seen in association with active or current illness, such as upper respiratory infection, pharyngitis, and otitis media, in approximately 70% of cases.
- Biopsy specimens have demonstrated synovial hypertrophy secondary to nonspecific, nonpyogenic inflammatory reaction.
- Hip joint aspirates have shown a culture-negative synovial effusion, usually 1 to 3 mL.

IMAGING PROCEDURES

- Plain films of the hip, anteroposterior and lateral, are nonspecific, but they may help to rule out other diagnoses, such as Legg-Calvé-Perthes disease and slipped capital femoral epiphysis.
- Ultrasound may be useful to determine whether there is an effusion and to guide aspiration.
- Magnetic resonance imaging is useful only in cases of persistent pain, when infection has been excluded. Bone scan is not often helpful because this is not a bony process.

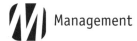 Management

GENERAL MEASURES

- Transient synovitis usually demonstrates a limited duration of symptoms. The average duration is less than 10 days. Most short-term studies report complete resolution of all signs and symptoms with no immediate residual clinical or radiographic abnormalities. Long-term studies have demonstrated mild radiographic changes in the involved hip.
- Bed rest and relief of weight bearing until pain resolves and full motion returns are the treatments of choice, followed by a period of cessation of strenuous activities.
- Antiinflammatory medications can be given to the patient.
- Traction and routine joint aspiration are not recommended. If traction is used, the hip should be in about 30 degrees of flexion to avoid maximum intraarticular pressure.
- The important point in management of this condition is to establish the diagnosis. Pyogenic arthritis must be excluded. Treatment is directed at rapidly resolving the underlying inflammatory synovitis with its symptoms.

PHYSICAL THERAPY

- Usually not necessary
- Parents can moderate child's activity adequately

MEDICAL TREATMENT

- Bed rest, initial acute pain resolves
- Antiinflammatory medications
- No weight bearing until pain resolves and full range of motion returns

PATIENT EDUCATION

Transient hip synovitis is a temporary process without significant consequences. Some authorities have suggested an increased incidence of later Perthes disease in these patients, but this has not been conclusively proven.

MONITORING

- The physician should be available for reevaluation at all times until the possibility of infection is excluded.
- The child should be reexamined in 2 weeks to determine whether there is return of motion before resuming full weight bearing and normal activity.
- Parents should bring the child back if symptoms recur.

COMPLICATIONS

Legg-Perthes disease or avascular necrosis of the femoral head may develop several months after an episode of transient synovitis of the hip.

PROGNOSIS

The prognosis is good, because this condition is usually self-limiting, without any significant sequelae.

RECOMMENDED READING

Haueisen DC, Weiner DS, Weiner SD. The characterization of transient synovitis of the hip in children. *J Pediatr Orthop* 1986; 6:11–17.

Landin LA, Danielsson LG, Wattsgard C. Transient synovitis of the hip: its incidence, epidemic relation to Perthes disease. *J Bone Joint Surg Br* 1987;69:238–242.

Morrissy RT, Weinstein SL, eds. *Lovell and Winter's pediatric orthopaedics,* vol 2, 4th ed. Philadelphia: Lippincott–Raven, 1996:1034–1037.

Tachdjian MO. *Pediatric orthopaedics,* vol 2, 2nd ed. Philadelphia: WB Saunders, 1990:1461–1465.

Wingstrand H. Transient synovitis of the hip in the child. *Acta Orthop Scand* 1986;57:1–61.

Basics

DESCRIPTION

Humeral shaft fractures are fractures of the diaphysis (shaft) of the humerus. They occur in all ages. One should suspect abuse in very young and very old patients. Humeral shaft fractures occur often with high-energy trauma in patients 20 to 50 years old.

SYNONYM

Arm fracture

INCIDENCE

This injury accounts for approximately 1% to 3% of all fractures.

CAUSES

- It usually results from direct violence to the upper extremity.
- It can occur from violent muscle contractions and twisting arm injuries.
- It may happen after relatively insignificant trauma in patients with underlying bone disease.
- It may occur in young adults when throwing balls while playing softball or baseball.

RISK FACTORS

- Osteoporosis in the elderly
- High-energy trauma in younger patients: motor vehicle accident, motorcycle accident, automobile pedestrian accident, falls from heights

CLASSIFICATION

Anatomic Location

- Humeral head or neck
- Proximal third of the shaft
- Medial third of the shaft
- Distal third of the shaft

Fracture Characteristics

- Fracture pattern (transverse versus oblique versus comminuted)
- Fracture open or closed
- Pathologic (secondary to underlying bone disease)

ASSOCIATED CONDITIONS

- Look for other associated upper extremity fractures or injuries.
- Carefully examine the neurovascular status.

ICD-9-CM

812.21 Humeral shaft fracture

 Diagnosis

SIGNS AND SYMPTOMS

- Pain
- Deformity
- Bruising
- Crepitus
- Swelling

DIFFERENTIAL DIAGNOSIS

- Pathologic fracture or through normal bone
- Muscular contusions
- Muscle tear or strain

PHYSICAL EXAMINATION

- Assess for skin integrity (ensure that no open fracture exists).
- Examine the shoulder and elbow joints and the forearm, hand, and clavicle for associated trauma.
- Check the function of the median, ulnar, and, particularly, the radial nerves.
- Assess for the presence of the radial pulse.

LABORATORY TESTS

No serum and laboratory tests are diagnostic.

PATHOLOGIC FINDINGS

High energy absorbed by the humeral shaft causes increased comminution of the fracture and more severe soft tissue injury.

IMAGING PROCEDURES

Anteroposterior and lateral views of the humerus, including the joints below and above the injury, are obtained.

Humeral Shaft Fracture

⚕ Management

GENERAL MEASURES

- In the acute period, apply ice to the region for 20 minutes every 3 to 4 hours to help to decrease swelling.
- Prescribe a moderately strong narcotic for pain control.
- Support the arm in a sling.
- Sensation of movement of the fracture ends is common.

SURGICAL TREATMENT

Surgery involves either intramedullary fixation with a metal rod or fixation of the bone fragments with a plate and screws. If severe soft tissue injury exists, external fixation may be necessary. A 10% complication rate has been reported, including nerve palsy, pseudarthrosis, and implant failure.

PHYSICAL THERAPY

None is required in the initial period. If stiffness results in the elbow or shoulder, physical therapy may assist in range-of-motion exercises.

MEDICAL TREATMENT

Most closed fractures of the humeral shaft may be managed nonoperatively. Treatment in the initial period involves fracture reduction (if indicated) and then splinting the extremity with a "U" splint, which travels from the axilla, under the elbow, and to the top of the shoulder (Fig. 1). This splint is supplemented by a posterior splint, which originates at the proximal humerus and extends behind the elbow to the forearm (Fig. 2). The injured extremity is supported by a sling. Reduction should be attempted if greater than 20 to 30 degrees of angulation, greater than 3 cm of shortening, or greater than 15 degrees of rotational deformity is present. Lesser degrees of shortening or angulation are tolerated satisfactorily. The extremity is then placed in a fracture brace several days to a week after the initial injury, once the acute swelling has subsided. Immobilization by fracture bracing is continued for at least 2 months or until clinical and radiographic evidence of fracture healing is present. With this treatment regimen, union rates of greater than 90% can be attained.

Occasionally, humeral shaft fractures require operative fixation. Indications include the following:

- Open fractures
- Articular injury
- Neurovascular injury
- Ipsilateral forearm fractures
- Impending pathologic fractures
- Segmental fractures
- Patients with multiple extremity fractures
- Fractures in which reduction is unable to be achieved or maintained

Narcotic analgesics should be given acutely, if the patient can tolerate them.

PATIENT EDUCATION

Once in a fracture brace, the patient may commence gentle active range of motion of the shoulder and the elbow. Activities of daily living are encouraged. During the initial healing period, many patients find that sleeping in a chair is more comfortable than sleeping in a bed.

PREVENTION

General safety precautions in the young and elderly are recommended.

MONITORING

Serial radiographs are obtained at 4- to 6-week intervals to ensure progressive healing and angulation less than 30 degrees.

COMPLICATIONS

Complications include injury to the radial nerve at the time of initial injury, during closed reduction, or during operative repair. If radial nerve palsy is identified after fracture reduction, immediate operative exploration is generally recommended. If, however, a patient presents with a radial nerve injury that does not improve after manipulation, observation only is recommended for at least 2 months, at which time formal neurometric studies may be conducted if there is no improvement in nerve function. Most of these injuries are neurapraxias (contusions to the nerve fibers), which improve over time.

PROGNOSIS

The prognosis is good.

RECOMMENDED READING

Rosen H. The treatment of nonunions and pseudarthroses of the humeral shaft. *Orthop Clin North Am* 1990;21:725–742.

Ward EF, Savoie FH, Hughes JL. Fractures of the diaphyseal humerus. In: Browner BD, Jupiter JB, Levine AM, et al., eds. *Skeletal trauma.* Philadelphia: WB Saunders, 1992:1177–1200.

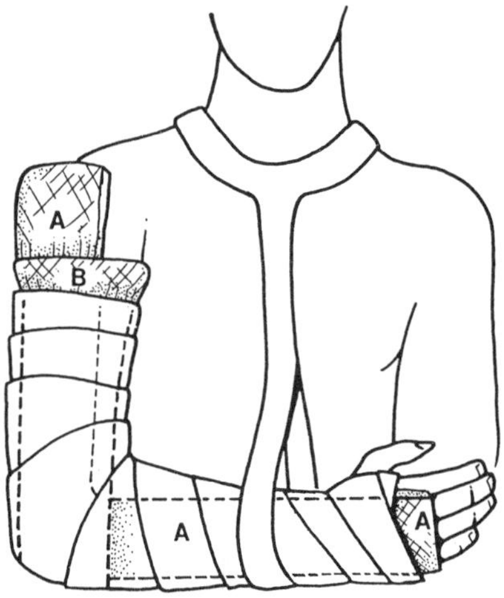

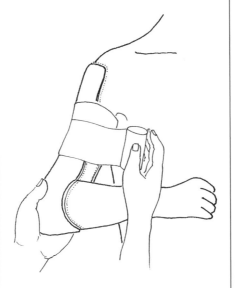

Fig. 1. Immobilization of humeral shaft fractures using a long arm posterior splint **(A)** and a mediolateral splint **(B).** The arm is further supported by a sling or a collar and cuff dressing and is allowed to hang dependently. (From Steinberg GG, Akins CM, Baran DT. *Orthopaedics in primary care,* 3rd ed. Lippincott Williams & Wilkins, 1999, with permission).

Fig. 2. Applying a sugar tong splint for humeral shaft fractures.

Basics

DESCRIPTION

Impingement syndrome and subacromial bursitis are inflammations of the shoulder subacromial bursa and rotator cuff tendons (supraspinatus, infraspinatus, teres minor, and subscapularis muscles). The inflammation is often due to their impingement between the humeral greater tuberosity and the lateral structures of the shoulder (acromion, coracoacromial ligament, coracoid process, and acromioclavicular ligament). The impingement causes a continuum from chronic bursitis to complete rotator cuff tears.
Patients of any age can be affected. However, there is a significant increasing incidence with age, as shown later in the section on classification. An accumulation of wear and impingement over the years leads to an increased incidence with increasing age.

SYNONYMS

- Subacromial bursitis
- Subacromial impingement
- Rotator cuff tendinitis

INCIDENCE

These conditions are common, especially in older age groups and in athletes performing overhead activities (e.g., swimming, tennis).

CAUSES

Impingement of the rotator cuff tendons and subacromial bursa between the humeral head, greater tuberosity and the lateral structures of the shoulder (acromion, coracoacromial ligament, coracoid process, and acromioclavicular ligament) occurs when the arm is elevated.
This causes inflammation and edema and therefore increased impingement, in a self-perpetuating cycle.

- Acromial shape: A hooked lateral surface (as opposed to flat) may increase impingement.
- Posterior shoulder capsule stiffness may force the humeral head upward, thereby increasing impingement.
- Rotator cuff weakness or tear causes a decrease in the humeral head depressor mechanism, thus increasing impingement.

RISK FACTORS

- Middle and older age (40 to 85 years)
- Increased overhead activities (e.g., lifting, swimming, tennis)
- Acromial shape: hooked lateral surface (as opposed to flat) possibly increasing impingement

CLASSIFICATION

Stage I: Patients Less than 25 Years Old
Reversible edema and hemorrhage
Stage II: Patients 25 to 40 Years Old
Fibrosis and tendinitis
Pain recurring with activity
Stage III: Patients More than 45 Years Old
Bone spurs and rotator cuff tendon rupture

ASSOCIATED CONDITIONS

- Rotator cuff tears (95% of cuff tears associated with impingement)
- Calcific tendinitis
- Biceps tendinitis
- Acromioclavicular arthritis
- Frozen shoulder

ICD-9-CM

726.2 Impingement syndrome, shoulder

 Diagnosis

SIGNS AND SYMPTOMS

- Inability to use the arm in the overhead position (flexed and internally rotated) because of pain, stiffness, weakness, and catching
- Pain with sleeping on the affected side
- Pain in the acromial area

DIFFERENTIAL DIAGNOSIS

Many of these conditions are associated with impingement:

Cuff Tears

- Symptoms
—Shoulder pain
—Inability to lift the arm
—Pain with motion
- Identified with magnetic resonance imaging
- Ninety-five percent of cuff tears associated with impingement

Calcific Tendinitis

- Localized tenderness
- Possibly associated with impingement from increased size of the tendon
- Diagnosed with radiographs

Biceps Tendinitis

- Pain to palpation in the biceps groove

Cervical Radiculopathy

- Pain on turning the head

Radiculopathy

- Diagnosed with electromyography

Acromioclavicular Arthritis

- Acromioclavicular joint tenderness to palpation
- Radiographs showing degenerative changes in the joint
- Diagnosed with injection of lidocaine into the acromioclavicular joint

Glenohumeral Instability

- Diagnosed with physical examination

Degeneration of the Glenohumeral Joint

- Diagnosed with radiographs

Stiff or Frozen Shoulder

- Diagnosed with physical examination
- Restricted range of motion with passive range of motion equal to active range of motion

PHYSICAL EXAMINATION

- Atrophy of rotator cuff muscles
- Decreased range of motion, especially internal rotation and cross body adduction, from posterior capsular tightness
- Weakness in flexion and external rotation
- Pain on resisted abduction and external rotation
- Pain on "impingement signs"

—Neer's impingement sign: passive elevation of the arm in the sagittal plane (shoulder flexion)
—Hawkins' impingement sign: with the elbow flexed to 90 degrees, the shoulder passively flexed to 90 degrees and internally rotated

Impingement Syndrome and Subacromial Bursitis

LABORATORY TESTS

• Subacromial injection–impingement test:

—Inject 10 mL of 1% lidocaine into the subacromial bursa. If there is a significant reduction in the patient's pain, this is a positive impingement test.

PATHOLOGIC FINDINGS

Degeneration of the supraspinatus tendon

IMAGING PROCEDURES

Plain Radiography

Anteroposterior

• Subacromial sclerosis ("eyebrow sign")
• Greater tuberosity cyst
• Superior migration of the humeral head

Thirty-Degree Caudad Angled Anteroposterior View

• Subacromial proliferation

Lateral Scapular Supraspinatus Outlet View

• Showing type of acromion (flat, rounded, or hooked)

Magnetic Resonance Imaging

• Used to diagnose a rotator cuff tear

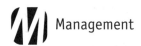 Management

SURGICAL TREATMENT

Acromioplasty

Indications

• No improvement after 6 months of conservative therapy
• Relief of pain with injection

Postoperative Care

• Early range of motion critical to avoid adhesions
• Success rate typically 70% to 90%

Reasons for Failure

• Inadequate or excessive resection of acromion
• Failure of deltoid reattachment
• Incorrect or incomplete diagnosis, such as acromioclavicular arthritis and impingement syndrome
• Postoperative adhesions

Procedure

An incision is made through the skin. The deltoid is then partially incised and is partially elevated off the acromion. The subacromial bursa is then removed. A 2.0 by 0.9 cm wedge is then taken from the anterior undersurface of the acromion including the coracoacromial ligament. The bone is smoothed. The deltoid is repaired to the acromion. The skin is closed. In some cases, this can be done with the arthroscope.

Resect the acromioclavicular joint in the following situations:

• Severe arthritis
• Exposure to the supraspinatus needed
• Impingement felt during the operation
• Repair of torn rotator cuff

PHYSICAL THERAPY

Stretching and Range-of-Motion Exercises

• Relieve posterior capsule tightness
• Avoid frozen shoulder

Strengthening Exercises

• Especially use internal and external rotator exercises
• Strengthen humeral head depressors
• Avoid exercises above the level of the shoulder that could cause impingement

MEDICAL TREATMENT

Initial nonoperative treatment includes the following:

Modalities (No Optimal Protocol but Many Available)

• Rest
• Avoidance of painful and overhead activities that cause impingement
• Modification of work or sport that exacerbates symptoms
• Gradual conditioning before a return to activities

Stretching and Range-of-Motion Exercises

• Relieve posterior capsule tightness
• Avoid frozen shoulder

Strengthening Exercises

• Use internal and external rotator exercises, in particular
• Strengthen humeral head depressors
• Avoid exercises above the level of the shoulder that could cause impingement

Other Measures

• Nonsteroidal antiinflammatory drugs and analgesics
• Ice (20 minutes twice daily), heat, massage
• Corticosteroid injections

The success rate for these treatments is almost 90%.

PATIENT EDUCATION

Patients should understand the impingement syndrome and the need for rest, physical therapy, gradual conditioning before resuming regular activities, and other conservative measures to relieve the symptoms. They should also understand the continuum from chronic bursitis to a rotator cuff tear.

PREVENTION

Avoid overhead and painful activities.

COMPLICATIONS

• Rotator cuff tear
• Frozen shoulder
• Biceps tendon tear

PROGNOSIS

• The success rate with conservative therapy is approximately 90%.
• Of those in whom conservative therapy fails, the surgical success rate is approximately 70% to 90%

RECOMMENDED READING

Matsen FA, Arntz, CT. Subacromial impingement. In: Rockwood CA, Matsen FA, eds. *The shoulder.* Philadelphia: WB Saunders, 1990:623–636.

Rockwood C, Lynons FR, et al. Shoulder impingement syndrome: diagnosis, radiographic evaluation, and treatment with a modified Neer acromioplasty. *J Bone Joint Surg Am* 1993;75:409–424.

Basics

DESCRIPTION

With better understanding of the biomechanics of the distal humerus, the trend is to refer to these injuries as column fractures. Biomechanically and anatomically, the distal humerus forms a triangle composed of a medial column and a lateral column that support the base, the articular surface. (The trochlea articulates with the ulna. The capitellum is the part of the humerus that articulates with the radius and is actually part of the lateral column).
When the distal humerus is fractured, neurovascular compromise of the extremity may occur and must be carefully evaluated and documented. This occurs more commonly in the setting of open distal humerus fractures. Moreover, injury is often the result of high-energy trauma, and the patient should be appropriately evaluated.

SYNONYMS

- Unicondylar fractures
- Bicondylar fractures
- Intraarticular distal humerus fractures

INCIDENCE

Single-Column Fractures

This injury is rare (3% to 4% of fractures of the distal humerus). Lateral column fractures are more common than medial. These injuries are more common in children.

Bicolumn Fractures

This injury is rare overall, but it is the most common distal humerus fracture. The reported incidence varies markedly, ranging from 5% to 62% of all distal humerus fractures.

Age

- This fracture occurs in all age groups.
- Extraarticular distal humerus (supracondylar) single-column (medial or lateral condyle) fractures (not discussed in this chapter) are more common in children.
- Single-column fractures (unicolumnar, unicondylar) are more common in children.
- There appears to be a bimodal age distribution: young, often male, involved in high-velocity trauma, or elderly osteoporotic patients (often female) with a lesser mechanism.
- Concomitant medical issues, soft tissue status, and bone quality (osteoporosis) influence care.

CAUSES

- Falls: from a height; on an outstretched arm
- Automobile pedestrian accidents
- Motor vehicle accidents
- Direct blows to the elbow

RISK FACTORS

- Persons at risk for high-energy trauma
- Elderly persons: risks for falls and osteoporosis

CLASSIFICATION

No single classification system is uniformly accepted or used. Many of the newer classification systems simply substitute the word column for condylar, because this is believed to be more appropriate, given current understanding of the anatomy.

Single-Column Fractures

This classification is divided into medial or lateral fractures. Each fracture is then described as being either high or low, depending on how far proximally the fracture extends. High fractures involve the majority of the trochlea and are unstable.

Milch's Classification

This is based on whether the fracture includes the lateral aspect of the trochlea. A Milch I is analogous to a low single-column fracture, and a Milch II is analogous to a high single-column fracture.

Bicolumn Fractures

A more complex descriptive classification (by Jupiter) is based on the fracture pattern as it traverses the columns and the articular surface: the T pattern, the Y pattern, the H pattern, and the lamda pattern. Some of these classes can be further subdivided.

ASSOCIATED CONDITIONS

- Neurapraxia
- Vascular injury
- Polytrauma

ICD-9-CM

812.41 Closed humerus supracondylar fracture
812.51 Open humerus supracondylar fracture

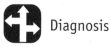 Diagnosis

SIGNS AND SYMPTOMS

- Severe pain, swelling, and a decrease or inability to move the extremity at the elbow
- Ischemia, dysesthesia, or paresthesia also possible (not common but important to assess)

DIFFERENTIAL DIAGNOSIS

- Humerus shaft fracture
- Supracondylar fracture
- Transcondylar fracture
- Elbow dislocation
- Elbow sprain
- Capitellum fracture
- Trochlea fracture
- Olecranon fracture
- Proximal single or both bones of the forearm fracture or dislocation
- Radial head fracture or dislocation
- Monteggia's fracture or dislocation

PHYSICAL EXAMINATION

These injuries are often associated with substantial energy, and the patient requires a thorough examination.

Extremity

Evaluate soft tissues to establish open versus closed fracture status. There is often marked swelling. Assess the limb for vascular status and signs of ischemia (pallor, capillary refill, peripheral pulses).

Neurologic Status

Evaluate and clearly document the neurologic status of the extremity in the ulnar, median (and anterior interossei), and radial (and posterior interossei) nerve distributions, including specific muscle testing and two-point discrimination. Often the patient cannot or will not either move or allow passive movement of the elbow. If the patient does, it is often associated with marked crepitus.

LABORATORY TESTS

- Tests are dictated by the associated injuries.
- If the fracture is displaced, the patient will require age- and institution-appropriate preoperative laboratory tests.

Intercondylar Elbow Fracture

IMAGING PROCEDURES

- Plain radiographs include anteroposterior and lateral views of the elbow and humerus and forearm views if indicated by examination.
- If the clinical suspicion is high and radiographs appear negative, be aware of subtle signs such as posterior or anterior fat pad signs.
- Special views, such as radiocapitellar, can sort out other fractures (e.g., radial head or capitellar fractures).
- In the rare partial articular fracture or in cases with severe comminution, computed tomography can sometimes be useful both with diagnosis and with operative planning. (This is the exception rather than the rule.)

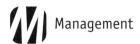 Management

GENERAL MEASURES

- The key to success in all these fractures is stability and early motion. The current trend is to treat most of these injuries surgically.
- Ice, elevation, and immobilization should be initiated even during evaluation.
- If operative care is indicated, surgery is preferably performed early (within 2 to 3 days)

Single-Column Fractures

Nondisplaced fractures are rare and may be treated nonsurgically; however, this requires clinical and radiographic vigilance on the part of the physician. The time of immobilization should be less than 2 weeks. Treatment should include gentle passive motion and placement in a hinged brace with gradually increasing motion. Displaced fractures should be treated surgically.

Bicolumn Fractures

Treat surgically. In rare cases in which the fracture is severely comminuted ("bag of bones" fracture) and the patient is elderly (or for some other reason unable to tolerate surgery), treat with immobilization.

If the limb has a diminished or absent pulse, reduction with immobilization or traction should be performed. If this does not improve the status of the limb, angiography or surgical exploration should be performed. This often requires both an orthopaedist and a vascular surgeon, although some orthopaedists are comfortable with this type of vascular repair. The sequence of angiography versus immediate surgery depends on warm ischemia time, other injuries, availability of angiography, and the surgeon's preference and experience. Associated vascular injuries, although commonly discussed, are rare; when they do occur, they are usually seen in association with open fractures.

Determine whether the fracture is opened or closed. In the case of an open fracture, the patient can be started on appropriate intravenous antibiotics and must be taken to the operating room within 6 hours of the injury.

Activity

Early motion is essential. A period of 10 to 14 days of immobilization is considered by many to be the maximal acceptable duration. Loaded motion (heavy lifting, repetitive loading) must be avoided until adequate fracture healing has occurred.

SURGICAL TREATMENT

Surgical therapy for the different types of intercondylar fractures is similar. Most commonly, a posterior approach is used, and most often this requires olecranon osteotomy (leaves the triceps attached to its insertion). There are different methods of fixation, although plates and screws are currently favored. It has been found clinically and biomechanically superior to use two plates at right angles to each other. The most common configuration is a plate placed posteriorly on the lateral column and medially on the medial column. It is often necessary to reconstruct the articular surface with screws before or concomitantly with plating one or both columns, to use bone graft, and to transpose the ulnar nerve.

Some single-column fractures are far less complex and require simpler constructs, sometimes a single screw or multiple Kirschner wires. Conversely, most of these single-column and bicolumn fractures are complex, and the surgical procedures are often long (4 to 12 hours) and technically demanding. Older patients with severe comminution and osteoporotic bone can be treated with primary total elbow arthroplasty.

PHYSICAL THERAPY

- Therapy is as described earlier.
- Early and carefully monitored range of motion exercises are necessary to regain a functional arc of motion (100 degrees of flexion). A hinged brace is useful to guide motion.

MEDICAL TREATMENT

In the acute setting, the patient requires analgesia and postoperative antibiotics.

PATIENT EDUCATION

The patient must be informed that he or she will lose range of motion at the elbow and that the functional outcome greatly depends on patient compliance with range of motion protocols and strict compliance with lifting and activity restrictions.

PREVENTION

Limit fall and trauma risks.

MONITORING

The patient must be acutely and postoperatively monitored for neurovascular status and compartment syndrome.

COMPLICATIONS

- Loss of range of motion (all patients: usually 10 to 20 degrees of extension 10 to 20 degrees of flexion)
- Nonunion (reported in 1% to 10% of cases)
- Malunion
- Loss of fixation
- Symptomatic hardware (common, especially around the olecranon)
- Osteonecrosis
- Neurovascular injury
- Ulnar neuropathy (one of the most common postoperative problems, reduced with ulnar nerve transposition)
- Infection
- Heterotopic ossification

PROGNOSIS

Despite the technical challenge, studies using the newer techniques report remarkably good results (approximately 75% good to excellent results even with the most complex fractures).

Range of Motion

A good to excellent result is in the range of 15 to 30 degrees to 120 to 130 degrees.

RECOMMENDED READING

Mehne, DK, Jupiter JB et al. Trauma to the adult elbow and fractures of the distal humerus. *Skeletal trauma*, vol 2. Philadelphia: WB Saunders, 1992:1146–1172.

Jupiter JB. Complex fractures of the distal humerus and associated complications. *J Bone Joint Surg Am* 1994;76:1253–1264.

Marsh JL. Elbow and forearm trauma. Levine AM: *Orthopaedic knowledge update: trauma.* Rosemont, IL: American Academy of Orthopaedic Surgeons, 1996: chp. 28 276–277.

Webb LX. Distal humerus fractures in adults. *J Am Acad Orthop Surg* 1996;4:336–344.

Basics

DESCRIPTION

This is a fracture of the proximal femur. Classically, it extends in a line between the greater and lesser trochanters and thus external to the capsule of the hip joint. The greater and lesser trochanters may also be avulsed as separate fragments.

SYNONYM

Trochanteric hip fracture

INCIDENCE

- This is a common injury.
- In 1980, the incidence was estimated to be 98 per 100,000, or four times more common than intracapsular (femoral neck) fractures.
- It is more common in the elderly; patients are an average 10 to 12 years older than patients with femoral neck fractures.
- The increased incidence with advanced age is likely secondary to osteoporosis and the increased risk of falling.
- It is two to eight more times as common in women, presumably because of postmenopausal loss of bone mass

CAUSES

- Nearly all intertrochanteric fractures are the result of falls.
- Motor vehicle accidents comprise the second most common cause of this injury.
- The mechanism is typically direct axial loading of the femur or direct force over the greater trochanter; indirect forces from muscle insertion on the trochanters may also contribute to the injury and deformity.

RISK FACTORS

- Osteoporosis is a significant risk factor.
- Any factor that increases the risk of falling (e.g., unsteady gait) increases the risk.
- Pathologic fractures may occur in the presence of tumor or Paget's disease.

CLASSIFICATION

Several classification systems have been proposed. The modified Evans' system has been shown to be especially useful, because increasing fracture grade correlates with increasing instability and decreasing ability to obtain anatomic reduction.

Evans' Classification

Type I: The main fracture line extends from the greater to the lesser trochanter.
Type II: The fracture extends distally from the lesser trochanter ("reversed obliquity").

Jensen-Michelsen Classification

Jensen and Michelsen subdivided Evans' type I fractures into five classes of progressively increasing instability:

- Type 1 fractures have a single fracture line and are nondisplaced.
- Type 2 is similar, except the two fragments are displaced.
- Types 3 and 4 are three-part fractures involving avulsion of the greater or lesser trochanter, respectively.
- Type 5 is a four-part fracture with avulsion of both trochanters.

ASSOCIATED CONDITIONS

Other fractures and soft tissue injuries of the affected limb, as well as associated neural and vascular injuries, can occur in patients with these fractures.

ICD-9-CM

820.21 Intertrochanteric hip fracture

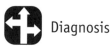

Diagnosis

SIGNS AND SYMPTOMS

- The patient is in significant pain and is unable to ambulate.
- The affected leg is shortened and externally rotated to as much as 90 degrees (more marked than seen with femoral neck fractures) because of the action of the iliopsoas at its insertion distal to the fracture site.
- There may be swelling over the hip and ecchymosis over the greater trochanter (not seen with intracapsular fractures).

DIFFERENTIAL DIAGNOSIS

- Femoral neck fracture
- Subtrochanteric femur fracture
- Femoral shaft fracture
- Isolated avulsion of greater or lesser trochanter

PHYSICAL EXAMINATION

- In addition to assessing the deformity of the proximal femur, the clinician should examine the ipsilateral knee for evidence of ligamentous injury.
- Neurovascular status of the limb should be carefully assessed.

IMAGING PROCEDURES

- Anteroposterior and lateral plain film radiographs should be obtained to determine the degree of comminution and deformity.
- For the anteroposterior view, the hip should be internally rotated.
- The degree of osteoporosis in the proximal femur should be graded using Singh's index, which ranges from grade I (severe loss of trabeculae) to grade VI (normal trabecular architecture).

Intertrochanteric Hip Fracture

 Management

GENERAL MEASURES

• Initially, the limb should be immobilized until definitive treatment can be obtained.
• Treatment typically consists of either closed or open reduction followed by internal fixation, with early mobilization of the patient.
• Patients unable to tolerate operative repair may be treated by traction for 8 to 12 weeks.

Closed Reduction

This is performed by applying direct traction, slight abduction, and slight external rotation to the femur, ideally using fluoroscopy, with the patient anesthetized and on a fracture table. If this approach is unsuccessful, open reduction is performed.

Activity

Early mobilization is the key goal of rehabilitation after operative treatment. Typically, the patient is out of bed on postoperative day 2 and progresses to weight bearing as tolerated, using a walker, crutches, or cane as necessary, by 10 to 14 days after the surgery.

SURGICAL TREATMENT

After open or closed reduction of the fracture, the reduction is maintained by internal fixation using a dynamic hip compression screw or nail plate device. The fixation device, typically with a side plate angle of 135 or 150 degrees, is positioned under fluoroscopy such that the end of the lag screw is well centered within the femoral head. For comminuted fractures, lag screws or cerclage wires may be needed to reattach the trochanteric fragments. Several intramedullary fixation devices (Ender's nails, gamma-locking nail) have also been used but appear to have no clear advantage over the hip screw and may have a higher complication rate. Some surgeons advocate slight valgus overcorrection of the fracture, by either medial cortical overlap or osteotomy, before fixation. Although these techniques improve fracture stability with nail plate devices, they are typically not necessary when a dynamic hip screw is used for fixation.

PHYSICAL THERAPY

Strengthening and ambulation are the main goals.

MEDICAL TREATMENT

Analgesics are given.

PATIENT EDUCATION

• Altering the environment of the elderly person to reduce falls is helpful.
• Measures to reduce osteoporosis (e.g., diet, exercise) may be used.

PREVENTION

• Prevention of osteoporosis (e.g., estrogen replacement, bisphosphonates)
• Prevention of falls in the elderly (e.g., the use of a cane by patients with unsteady gait)

COMPLICATIONS

• The mortality rate in the first year is high, ranging from 10% to 30%. (This high rate is secondary to coexisting morbidities.)
• Mental status change is common during the acute phase of hospitalization.
• Mechanical complications include failure of fixation (usually resulting in impaction or varus angulation), penetration of the fixation device into the hip joint, and stress fractures of the femoral neck resulting from poor positioning of the fixation device within the femoral head.
• Postoperative wound infection rates of 1% to 17% have been reported.
• Nonunion and avascular necrosis are uncommon complications (less than 2%), because these fractures occur through well-vascularized cancellous bone.

PROGNOSIS

• Although most patients can expect satisfactory results of treatment, only about 50% return completely to their prior level of function.
• Morbidity and mortality are significant, mainly because of the age of the patients.

RECOMMENDED READING

Iversen LD, Swiontkowski MF. *Manual of acute orthopaedic therapeutics.* Boston: Little, Brown, 1995:1226–1230.

Jensen JS. Classification of trochanteric fractures. *Acta Orthop Scand* 1980;51:803–810.

Rockwood CA, Green DP, Bucholz RW, eds. *Rockwood and Green's fractures in adults,* 3rd ed. Philadelphia: JB Lippincott, 1991:1538–1560.

Basics

DESCRIPTION

Isolated traumatic dislocation of the radial head is a relatively rare injury seen mainly in children, although several reports have described this injury in adults. Congenital and developmental radial head dislocations are seen more commonly, although they are rarely seen in the absence of other congenital abnormalities of the elbow or forearm. The radial head may be dislocated anteriorly, anterolaterally, posteriorly, or posterolaterally. Isolated radial head subluxation (i.e., nursemaid's elbow and Malgaigne's injury) is much more common, occurring usually between the ages of 1 and 4 years, but true subluxation of the radial head is more frequently associated with fractures of the proximal ulna as part of Monteggia's fracture in adults and children alike.

GENETICS

There does not appear to be a genetic inheritance pattern noted for radial head dislocation. However, because the main restraints to radial head dislocation in the normal elbow are ligamentous, children with ligamentous laxity (e.g., achondroplasia) may have a predisposition to such conditions without associated fractures.

CAUSES

The mechanism of injury is believed to be a fall onto the outstretched hand with the elbow extended and the forearm pronated with a resultant varus stress placed on the elbow.

CLASSIFICATION

• Direction of radial head displacement: anterior, posterior, or lateral
• Pathogenesis: traumatic or congenital

ASSOCIATED CONDITIONS

• In the setting of trauma, this injury may be associated with a proximal ulna fracture, a radial neck fracture, or an elbow dislocation.
• Isolated radial head dislocations, particularly posterior dislocations, may be associated with radial nerve or posterior interosseous nerve stretch injuries.

ICD-9-CM

832.9 Dislocation of radial head

 Diagnosis

SIGNS AND SYMPTOMS

• Pain, swelling, and decreased supination of the forearm are the main symptoms of the traumatic dislocation.
• The congenitally dislocated radial head is normally painless, although it usually is discovered in the young child after elbow trauma. This may also come to attention secondary to painless lateral prominences in the setting of a posterolateral dislocation.

DIFFERENTIAL DIAGNOSIS

• Subluxated elbow
• Congenital dislocation
• Monteggia's fracture with an occult fracture
• Radial neck fracture

PHYSICAL EXAMINATION

• Perform a complete neurovascular examination at presentation and before undertaking any manipulations.
• Direct attention to the radial nerve because it may undergo traction injury.
• Perform an examination of the contralateral elbow to rule out bilateral radial head dislocations, which may suggest a congenital dislocation and preexisting disease in the elbow in question.
• On physical examination, hold the elbow immobile and flexed with the forearm in pronation. The affected child often refuses to use the injured arm. The articular surface of the radial head can usually be palpated, particularly with posterior and posterolateral dislocations, in which there is little overlying soft tissue. Nearly full flexion and extension are usually noted, although there is often some limitation at one extreme, depending on the direction of the dislocation (mildly limited flexion if anteriorly dislocated and extension if posteriorly dislocated).
• Supination and pronation are markedly limited and cause pain.

PATHOLOGIC FINDINGS

• In the normal elbow, the critical restraint to radial head dislocation is the annular ligament. This is usually torn or significantly stretched in the case of a dislocation.
• In the congenitally dislocated radial head, a hypoplastic capitellum and an ovoid radial head are essentially pathognomonic.
• Proximal ulnar bowing is also evident on radiographs, although this is not unique to the congenital dislocation.

IMAGING PROCEDURES

• Anteroposterior and lateral radiographs of the elbow are usually sufficient to make the diagnosis, as well as to assess reduction.
• Abnormalities of the capitellum and radial head may suggest a congenital dislocation.
• Radiographs of the contralateral elbow should be obtained to rule out bilateral involvement, which would also indicate a congenital dislocation.
• Congenital dislocations may be associated with a dysplastic capitellum, a bowed ulna, a relatively long radius, or an ovoid radial head. However, a long-standing traumatic dislocation may have similar radiographic findings unilaterally.
• Heterotopic ossification in the soft tissues about the radial head may suggest an old, unreduced traumatic dislocation.
• Some authors advocate elbow arthrograms if it is difficult to distinguish between congenital and traumatic causes. A congenital dislocation would demonstrate an arthrogram with an ovoid radial head within the joint capsule. A traumatic dislocation would be associated with a normally shaped radial head. In the acute situation, there is extravasation of the arthrogram dye.

Isolated Radial Head Dislocation

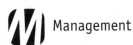 Management

GENERAL MEASURES

• It is important to distinguish a traumatic from a congenital dislocation, because the latter does not require treatment.
• If the condition is judged to be an acute, traumatic dislocation, closed reduction can usually be performed in the acute setting. Reduction is performed with gentle traction and the elbow in full extension with varus stress applied to the elbow joint. The forearm is supinated while direct pressure is applied to the radial head to reduce it. The reduction is then held in 120 degrees of flexion for children or 90 degrees and in supination for adults. A posterior splint usually suffices, although a bivalved cast may be necessary in the young child who may remove the splint.
• If the injury is more than 7 days old, open reduction may be necessary if closed reduction is unsuccessful. After 3 weeks, a successful closed reduction is impossible, and open technique is universally required. For long-standing traumatic dislocations (greater than 2 to 3 years), there may be deformation of the radial head and capitellum, which would preclude a stable reduction.

SURGICAL TREATMENT

• In the unstable reduction, a prolonged period of immobilization may be necessary to allow for fibrous tissue to confer stability. Occasionally, the immobilization may be augmented by a Kirshner wire across the radiocapitellar joint.
• When elbow contractures are of concern (patients greater than 30 years of age, particularly the elderly) or in patients with long-standing dislocations, a radial head resection may be performed to begin early range of motion of the elbow.
• With open reduction of the radiocapitellar joint, most surgeons advocate repair or reconstruction of the annular ligament. This may be successfully done up to 2 years or more after traumatic dislocation. Any ulnar bowing should also be fixed at the same time.

PHYSICAL THERAPY

• Full, pain-free range of motion of the elbow, flexion and extension, and supination and pronation are the goals of treatment of this injury.
• Elbow range of motion is begun as early as possible without compromising the stability of the joint.
• The pediatric elbow is more forgiving than the adults' with respect to regaining full range of motion after prolonged immobilization.

MEDICAL TREATMENT

• Symptomatic treatment for pain is suggested.
• Analgesia is a necessary part of rehabilitation after surgery or cast immobilization.
• In a patient with a history of heterotopic ossification or neurologic injury (which may predispose to heterotopic ossification), prophylaxis with indomethacin may decrease the incidence of heterotopic ossification of the elbow.

PATIENT EDUCATION

Patients are instructed on the need for home range-of-motion exercises. They are also told that they may lose 10 degrees of elbow extension.

MONITORING

Patients are followed at 1 month intervals until they regain their range of motion.

COMPLICATIONS

• Recurrent dislocations
• Decreased range of motion secondary to contracture or heterotopic ossification
• Radial or posterior interosseous nerve palsies and degenerative changes of the radiohumeral joint

PROGNOSIS

• Prognosis is excellent for a functional range of motion of the elbow, forearm, and wrist, particularly in patients less than 30 years of age.
• There may be mild restrictions of range of motion as compared with the contralateral side, but usually none that would be noted by the patient.

RECOMMENDED READING

Burgess RC, Sprague HH. Post-traumatic posterior radial head subluxation: two case reports. *Clin Orthop* 1982;186:192–194.

Heidt RS, Stern PJ. Isolated posterior dislocation of the radial head: a case report. *Clin Orthop* 1982;168:136–137.

Hotchkiss RN. Fractures and dislocations of the elbow. In: Rockwood CA, Bucholz RW, Green DP, et al., eds. *Fractures in adults,* 4th ed. Philadelphia: Lippincott–Raven, 1996;929–1024.

Salama R, Wientroub S, Weissman SL. Recurrent dislocation of the head of the radius. *Clin Orthop* 1977;125:156–158.

Wiley JJ, Pegington J, Horwich JP. Traumatic dislocation of the radius at the elbow. *J Bone and Joint Surg Br* 1974;56:501–507.

Wilkins KE, Beaty JH, Chambers HG, et al. Fractures and dislocations of the elbow region. In: Rockwood CA, Wilkins KE, Beaty JH, eds. *Fractures in children,* 4th ed. Philadelphia: Lippincott–Raven, 1996;653–904.

Basics

DESCRIPTION

This is a fracture of the base of the fifth metatarsal of the foot.

GENETICS

No mendelian pattern is known.

INCIDENCE

• More common in athletes, especially basketball players
• No age predilection, although rare in children
• Occurring equally in males and females

CAUSES

• Avulsion fracture: inversion or internal rotation injury of the foot
• Jones' or diaphyseal fractures: indirect trauma (inversion or internal rotation injuries) or direct trauma, such as dropping a heavy object on the foot

RISK FACTORS

• Athletics
• Falls

CLASSIFICATION

• Tuberosity avulsion fracture: no involvement of the fourth to fifth intermetatarsal joint
• True Jones' fracture: proximal metaphyseal fracture with involvement of fourth to fifth intermetatarsal joint up to the metaphyseal-diaphyseal junction
• Diaphyseal fracture, or pseudo-Jones fracture: at the proximal diaphysis, distal to the tuberosity of the peroneus tertius insertion

ICD-9-CM

825.35 Jones fracture

Diagnosis

SIGNS AND SYMPTOMS

Pain and swelling along the lateral border of the foot occur with point tenderness at the base of the fifth metatarsal.

DIFFERENTIAL DIAGNOSIS

• Lisfranc's injury (dislocation of tarsometatarsal joints)
• Stress fracture of the fifth metatarsal diaphysis (Fig. 1)

PHYSICAL EXAMINATION

• Pain over the lateral forefoot with palpation and weight bearing
• Swelling and redness also common

PATHOLOGIC FINDINGS

The watershed blood supply to metaphyseal-diaphyseal junction makes fractures in this area more susceptible to nonunion and requires more aggressive treatment than other metatarsal fractures.

IMAGING PROCEDURES

Plain, anteroposterior, lateral, and oblique radiographs of the foot are obtained to determine the level and displacement of the fracture.

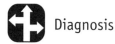

Management

GENERAL MEASURES

Generally, these fractures do well and heal without incident. Treatment varies with fracture classification.

Tuberosity Avulsion

Symptomatic management involves weight bearing as tolerated with a hard-sole shoe, cast, or splint, even with considerable displacement (more than 1 cm). Clinical union often occurs by 3 weeks. Nonunion is rarely symptomatic; if problematic, resect the fragment and reattach the peroneus brevis tendon.

Jones' Fracture

The patient is non-weight bearing in a short leg cast for 4 to 6 weeks.

Diaphyseal Fractures

The patient is non-weight bearing in a short leg cast until radiographic union (usually 8 weeks), followed by 6 weeks of limited activity. Competitive athletes may undergo percutaneous screw fixation with weight bearing after 2 weeks and may return to sports after pain and tenderness have resolved (8 weeks).

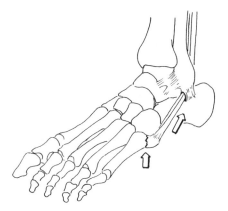

Fig. 1. Avulsion fracture of the fifth metatarsal bone (as shown here) must be differentiated from Jones' fracture, which occurs more distally.

SURGICAL TREATMENT

• Diaphyseal fractures may be treated with percutaneous placement of a malleolar screw for earlier return to activity; this fixation method after takedown of nonunion with bone grafting of the nonunion site is also used.
• Screw fixation of widely displaced avulsion fractures in competitive athletes may also be used.
• Symptomatic nonunions of avulsion fractures may be treated with excision of the fragment and reattachment of the peroneus brevis tendon.

PHYSICAL THERAPY

This is rarely indicated.

PATIENT EDUCATION

Stress the importance of following weight limitations to prevent nonunion and delay in return to normal activities.

PREVENTION

Proceed to radiographs early in athletes complaining of lateral foot pain, so treatment measures can be initiated to decrease prolonged symptoms.

ACTIVITY

Activity is as tolerated with the previously mentioned external supports, except in diaphyseal fractures, in which patients should remain non-weight bearing for 6 to 8 weeks

MONITORING

Patients are followed at 1-month intervals until the fracture heals and they return to full weight bearing. Delayed union occurs when the healing at the fracture site is delayed. The fracture is judged to be a nonunion if there is no evidence of further healing and there is pain at the fracture site.

COMPLICATIONS

Nonunion of fracture or recurrent fractures (more common in highly competitive athletes) may occur.

PROGNOSIS

The prognosis is good overall, although many diaphyseal fractures have been reported to require surgical intervention.

RECOMMENDED READING

Lawrence SJ, Botte MJ. Jones fractures and related fractures of the proximal fifth metatarsal. *Foot Ankle* 1993;13:358–365.

Rockwood CA, Green DP, Bucholz RW, eds. *Rockwood and Green's fractures in adults*, vol 2, 3rd ed. Philadelphia: JB Lippincott, 1991:2155–2156.

Torg JS, Balduini FC, Zelko RR, et al. Fractures of the base of the fifth metatarsal distal to the tuberosity: classification and guidelines for nonsurgical and surgical management. *J Bone Joint Surg Am* 1984;66:209–214.

Jumper's Knee (Patellar Tendinitis)

 Basics

 Diagnosis

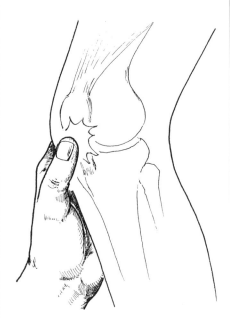

Basics

DESCRIPTION

Jumper's knee, or patellar tendinitis, is inflammation of the patellar tendon, generally caused by overuse. Its prevalence is unknown. It occurs primarily in adults. Children develop a related condition known as Osgood-Schlatter disease.

CAUSES

• Overuse injury
• Often occurring in athletes who engage in frequent jumping on unyielding surfaces, such as gymnasium floors or stiff dance surfaces

RISK FACTORS

• Repetitive jumping on unyielding surfaces
• Resisted knee extension exercises

ICD-9-CM

726.64 Patellar tendinitis

Diagnosis

SIGNS AND SYMPTOMS

Dull, aching pain over the patellar tendon, exacerbated by active and resisted knee extension. Peritendinous synovitis may be palpable

DIFFERENTIAL DIAGNOSIS

• Anterior horn meniscal injuries
• Patellar tracking problems
• Patellofemoral osteoarthrosis
• Stress fracture of the tibia

PHYSICAL EXAMINATION

• Patients complain of anterior knee pain (Fig. 1).
• Rule out patellofemoral stress syndrome. (In this condition, patients have pain underneath the kneecap itself, not over the patellar tendon.)

IMAGING PROCEDURES

Anteroposterior and lateral radiographs of the knee should be performed to rule out fracture, arthritis, or neoplasm.

Fig. 1. Jumper's knee is characterized by pain on the inferior pole of the patella.

Management

GENERAL MEASURES

• The mainstays of treatment are activity modification, antiinflammatory agents, rest, and ice.
• As the symptoms improve, patients often benefit from quadriceps and hamstring stretching exercises, followed by strengthening.
• Acute activity should be decreased, especially jumping and knee extension exercises.
• As symptoms improve, patients can gradually resume activity; however, non–impact-loading sports (e.g., swimming, cycling) are recommended at first.
• Diet is regular.

MEDICAL TREATMENT

Nonsteroidal antiinflammatory agents are given.

PATIENT EDUCATION

Patients should be educated regarding activities that may aggravate their patellar tendinitis (e.g., deep knee squats, open chain quadriceps exercises, jumping activities on hard surfaces).

MONITORING

Patients should have a follow-up examination approximately 6 weeks after diagnosis. This allows time for the inflammation to subside and for quadriceps and hamstring strengthening and stretching to start. Once symptoms have completely resolved, patients may return to their regular activities.

COMPLICATIONS

There is a theoretically increased risk of patellar tendon rupture in patients with chronic patellar tendinitis.

PROGNOSIS

• Patients who are compliant with activity modification and physical therapy generally do well.
• It is important to educate patients about which activities to avoid because these patients are at increased risk for a recurrence of their patellar tendinitis.

RECOMMENDED READING

An HS. *Synopsis of orthopaedics.* New York: Thieme, 1991:246–249.

Clark CR, Bonfiglio M, eds. *Orthopaedics: essentials of diagnosis and treatment.* New York: Churchill Livingstone, 1994:242.

Fu FH, Stone DA, eds. *Sports injuries: mechanisms, prevention, treatment.* Baltimore: Williams & Wilkins, 1994:302.

Basics

DESCRIPTION

Kienböck's disease is avascular necrosis of the lunate of the wrist with collapse of the bone and arthritis in the advanced stage. (Fig. 1).

SYNONYMS

Lunatomalacia

GENETICS

No known correlation exists.

INCIDENCE

- Approximately 1 per 1,000
- Most common in young adults (20 to 40 years of age)
- Sex predominance uncertain
- Disease onset usually in young to middle adulthood

CAUSES

Although this disease was originally described by Kienböck in 1910, the precise cause has yet to be determined. Theories proposing a primary ischemic or traumatic origin are supported in the literature. Current consensus supports repetitive microtrauma in the lunate at risk.

RISK FACTORS

- Ulnar-negative wrist: The carpal bones of the wrist are supported by the distal radius and ulna. They should be the same length. The term "ulnar-negative wrist" refers to a short ulna, which causes more pressure to be borne by the radial side of the wrist. The ulnar-negative variant wrist is thought to overload the lunate and predispose to Kienböck's disease. Simi-larly, the lunate is perfused through a single nutrient artery so it is thought to be at higher risk.
- Disorders leading to ischemia of the lunate, such as sickle cell anemia
- Traumatic ligamentous disruption of the intercarpal ligaments

CLASSIFICATION

The classification of Kienböck's disease by Stahl and later modified by Lichtman and Weis is based on the radiographic appearance of the lunate:

Stage 1: This is either radiographically normal or may show evidence small fracture lines in the lunate.
Stage 2: This shows sclerosis of the lunate.
Stage 3a: This demonstrates collapse of the lunate.
Stage 3b: This shows collapse accompanied by proximal migration of the capitate and fixed rotation of the scaphoid.
Stage 4: This shows generalized wrist arthrosis.

A stage 0 lesion, with magnetic resonance imaging evidence of avascular necrosis of the lunate and no physical findings, has been added to this classification.

ICD-9-CM

732.3 Kienböck's disease

 Diagnosis

SIGNS AND SYMPTOMS

- Most patients complain of pain and stiffness with tenderness over the dorsal lunate (middle of the wrist) on physical examination.
- Alternatively, patients may have little pain, but markedly decreased grip strength.
- Many patients give a history of a recent hyperextension injury of the wrist.
- If untreated, the pain may increase progressively and develop into arthritis of the wrist.

DIFFERENTIAL DIAGNOSIS

- Scapholunate ligament tear
- Scaphoid fracture
- Perilunate dislocation
- Wrist arthritis

PHYSICAL EXAMINATION

Tenderness with palpation over the anatomic snuffbox is noted.

PATHOLOGIC FINDINGS

A transverse internal fracture of the lunate has been described in 75% of cases. This is rarely recognized clinically. Changes characteristic of avascular necrosis are seen in biopsy specimens.

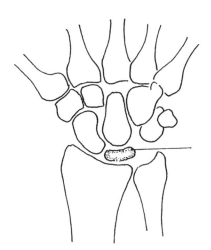

Fig. 1. Kienböck's disease is avascular necrosis of the lunate, usually followed by flattering of this bone (*stippled*).

Kienböck's Disease

IMAGING PROCEDURES

- Plain anteroposterior radiographs of the wrist often establish the diagnosis. The lunate may show a lucent line; in more advanced cases, sclerosis or collapse may be seen.
- In cases with a strong clinical suspicion and normal radiographs, magnetic resonance imaging may demonstrate characteristic changes of avascular necrosis.
- An ulnar variance view with the shoulder in 90 degrees of abduction, the elbow in 90 degrees of flexion, and the wrist in neutral rotation should be obtained.
- Bone scanning is sometimes used to establish the diagnosis, and it shows a cold spot (less technetium uptake) over the lunate.

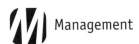 Management

GENERAL MEASURES

The optimal treatment for patients with Kienböck's disease is debated:

- The wrist should be splinted and the patient referred to a hand specialist for further treatment.
- Untreated, the condition may follow a course of relentless radiologic progression; however, the clinical course is variable.
- Most practitioners favor some surgical intervention in the young, active patient with early-stage disease.
- Ulnar lengthening may be considered if the ulna is short.
- Arthroplasty or another reconstructive procedure may be considered for advanced cases.

SURGICAL TREATMENT

Stage 1 and 2 Disease

Surgery is aimed at reduction of the load on the lunate or improvement of lunate perfusion. Load reduction may be achieved by joint leveling procedures (in the case of the ulnar-negative wrist) or limited intercarpal fusion. Perfusion may be improved through vascularized muscle pedicle bone grafts.

Stage 3 Disease

A proximal row corpectomy may provide symptomatic relief while maintaining range of motion.

Stage 4 Disease

Wrist fusion is the treatment of choice.

PHYSICAL THERAPY

This is usually not necessary. Splinting of the wrist helps to relieve discomfort.

PATIENT EDUCATION

The patient should be counseled about the natural history of the disease and the need for rest or activity restriction.

MONITORING

Even if no surgery is performed initially, the patient should be followed periodically to determine whether collapse and arthritis are progressive.

COMPLICATIONS

- Increasing pain, clicking
- Wrist arthritis

PROGNOSIS

Degenerative arthritis usually results over 1 to 2 decades.

RECOMMENDED READING

Altnquist EE. Kienböck's disease. *Hand Clin* 1987;3:141–148.

Amadio PC, Taleisnik J. Fractures of the carpal bones. In: *Operative hand surgery,* 3rd ed. New York: Churchill Livingstone, 1991:832–842.

Weiland AJ. Avascular necrosis of the carpus. In: *Hand surgery update.* Rosemont, IL: American Academy of Orthopaedic Surgery, 1994:85–92.

Klippel-Feil Syndrome

Basics

DESCRIPTION

Klippel-Feil syndrome consists of congenital fusions of the cervical vertebrae, clinically exhibited by the triad of a low occipital hairline, a short neck, and limited neck motion (Fig. 1).

SYSTEMS AFFECTED

• Musculoskeletal: cervical spine, thoracolumbar spine, and sometimes the scapula
• Associated anomalies possibly involving the genitourinary, cardiovascular, pulmonary, and central nervous systems

SYNONYM

Brevicollis

GENETICS

• This condition is phenotypically heterogeneous and may be sporadic, but familial autosomal dominant patterns have been observed.
• A chromosomal inversion—(8) (q22.2q23.3)—has been found to segregate with Klippel-Feil syndrome in some families.

INCIDENCE

• The incidence in the general population is unknown, because there have been no screening studies.
• The incidence of congenital cervical fusions is approximately 0.7%.
• The anomaly itself develops in embryogenesis.

• The age of presentation is variable: massive fusions are usually noted earlier (2 to 4 years), whereas degenerative changes present later (after age 4 years).
• The female-to-male ratio is 1.5:1.
• Most young patients are asymptomatic and present incidentally.
• Symptomatic stenosis occurs only in older persons with weakness, numbness, or tingling of the arms or legs.

CAUSES

• One hypothesis involves incomplete segmentation of a sclerotome during embryologic development.
• Other hypotheses include abnormal facet joint segmentation, multiple or global insults to the fetus (i.e., hypoxia), and vascular disruptions or malformations.

RISK FACTORS

• Spina bifida
• Congenital renal anomalies

CLASSIFICATION

Type I: Fusions involving cervical and upper thoracic vertebrae
Type II: Fusions of cervical vertebrae only; several segments may be fused
Type III: Type I or II with lower thoracic or lumbar vertebrae involvement in addition

ASSOCIATED CONDITIONS

• Musculoskeletal: Sprengel's deformity (failure of normal descent of the scapula), scoliosis

(both congenital and idiopathic in up to 60% of patients), spinal stenosis, spina bifida occulta
• Craniofacial: hearing abnormalities, extraocular palsy
• Genitourinary: renal abnormalities (up to 30% of patients), including unilateral renal agenesis
• Cardiovascular: various congenital heart malformations

ICD-9-CM

756.16 Klippel-Feil syndrome

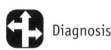

Diagnosis

SIGNS AND SYMPTOMS

• The clinical triad consists of a low occipital hairline, a short neck, and limited neck motion.
• The clinical triad is seen in 40% to 50% of patients, with decreased neck motion in up to 75% of patients and shortening of neck (with resulting lowering of posterior hairline) in fewer than 50%.
• Many patients present incidentally, because a radiograph was taken for other reasons.
• Other findings may include scoliosis, deafness, and renal and cardiac anomalies.

DIFFERENTIAL DIAGNOSIS

• Cervical fusion after a prior operation
• Torticollis from muscular causes
• Cervical spinal stenosis

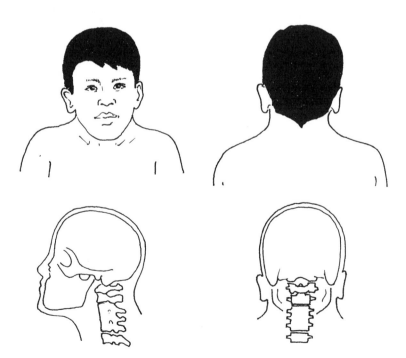

Fig. 1. Klippel-Feil syndrome is congenital cervical fusion. It is evidenced by a short, stiff neck and a low hairline.

Klippel-Feil Syndrome

PHYSICAL EXAMINATION

• Careful and thorough examination of cervical spine, focusing on resting appearance, posture, range of motion, as well as a general neurologic examination
• Complete physical examination to evaluate associated anomalies in other organ systems

PATHOLOGIC FINDINGS

• Congenital cervical fusions, which may be associated with instability
• Discs in the area of fusion narrow or absent, and the remaining mobile discs showing degeneration from overuse
• Degenerative joint disease
• Stenosis of the spinal cord
• Subluxation possible over time

IMAGING PROCEDURES

• Plain radiographs of the neck show various patterns and degrees of vertebral fusion ranging from simple block vertebrae to multiple anomalies. Up to 50% show anterior, posterior, and lateral portions of vertebrae fused. Vertebral bodies alone are fused in about 20% of cases, posterior fusion alone in 9%, and lateral in 3% of cases. Spina bifida occulta is seen in many patients. Spinal stenosis at the level of the segmentation defect is sometimes observed and may develop with aging because of degenerative changes from adjacent segment hypermobility.
• Flexion and extension radiographs are important to assess any potential instability, especially before undergoing intubation and surgery.
• Computed tomography may be helpful, especially with the presence of scoliosis and multiple anomalous vertebrae.
• Magnetic resonance imaging in flexion and extension is indicated if there is neurologic compromise.

Management

GENERAL MEASURES

Evaluation

All children with Klippel-Feil syndrome should be further evaluated for other organ system problems, including congenital cardiac, renal, or neurologic abnormalities. Renal imaging (a simple renal ultrasonogram) should be done in all children. A magnetic resonance imaging scan should be obtained whenever any concern for neurologic involvement exists on a clinical basis and before any orthopaedic spinal procedure. Plain flexion and extension lateral radiographs should be taken before any general anesthetic to rule out occult instability of the cervical spine.

Treatment

The course of treatment depends heavily on the severity of the associated renal or cardiac problems. In general, it is important to determine those patients with an increased risk of neurologic injury. Surgical fusion is indicated when instability results in neurologic symptoms or in patients with documented (e.g., magnetic resonance imaging) stenosis. Nonsurgical treatment includes cervical collars, bracing, and analgesics. Patients should avoid strenuous activities and contact sports, as well as occupations and recreational activities that increase the risk of head trauma.

SURGICAL TREATMENT

Surgery is rarely indicated. Compensatory curves below the level of primary congenital fusions, whether symptomatic or not, should be carefully monitored and treated with bracing or fusion, because these curves are more likely to progress and to cause major deformities. In addition, these patients may require surgery for associated anomalies, such as Sprengel's deformity, scoliosis, or cervical rib resection.

PHYSICAL THERAPY

This is not indicated.

PATIENT EDUCATION

Patients with extensive fusion (at more than one level) should be evaluated by a spinal specialist and most likely counseled to avoid high-impact contact sports because of the increased risk of neurologic damage. Each case should be taken individually, however.

MONITORING

These patients should be followed regularly by an orthopaedic surgeon.

COMPLICATIONS

• Spinal stenosis is often associated and may become symptomatic.
• Paralysis or paraparesis may occur from neck trauma in patients with extensive lesions.

PROGNOSIS

Some patients develop neck pain or extremity weakness with time.

RECOMMENDED READING

Baba H, Maezawa Y, Furasawa N, et al. The cervical spine in the Klippel-Feil syndrome: a report of 57 cases. *Int Orthop* 1995;19:204–208.

Guille JT, Miller A, Bowen JR, et al. The natural history of Klippel-Feil syndrome: clinical, roentgenographic and magnetic resonance imaging findings at adulthood. *J Pediatr Orthop* 1995;15:617–626.

Morrissy R, Weinstein SL, eds. *Lovell and Winter's pediatric orthopaedics,* 4th ed. Philadelphia: Lippincott–Raven, 1996:755.

Basics

DESCRIPTION

Dislocation of the knee is an orthopaedic emergency. It is mostly due to trauma, and anterior dislocation is the most common manifestation. The incidence is rare. Motor vehicle accident is the most common cause of this injury, and sports-related injury is the second most common.

CLASSIFICATION

Classification of knee dislocations is based on the relationship of the tibia with the femur.

- Anterior
- Posterior
- Medial
- Lateral
- Rotary: subclassified as anteromedial, anterolateral, posteromedial, and posterolateral

ASSOCIATED CONDITIONS

- Neurovascular injury
- Fractures of the tibia and femur
- Rupture of the collateral ligaments and the cruciate ligaments

ICD-9-CM

836.5 Closed knee dislocation
836.6 Open knee dislocation

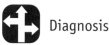 Diagnosis

SIGNS AND SYMPTOMS

- Patients with knee dislocations present with obvious deformity, swelling, pain, and inability to move the knee.
- Many knee dislocations are reduced before examination by a physician, and thus obvious deformity may not be present.
- Arterial injury, namely, popliteal artery, occurs in 20% to 35% of cases, and nerve injuries, most commonly peroneal nerve, occur in 25% to 35% of cases. It is therefore critical to assess the neurovascular status of all patients with possible knee dislocations (Fig. 1).
- Absent pulses, ecchymosis in the popliteal fossa, a cold, cyanotic extremity, and loss of sensorimotor function are danger signals.
- Neurovascular injury is an indication for immediate surgery.

DIFFERENTIAL DIAGNOSIS

The main differential diagnosis is an associated neurovascular injury, fracture, or dislocation of the patella.

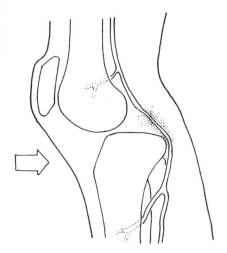

Fig. 1. Knee dislocation may produce vascular damage, resulting from the vascular tether to the tibia.

PHYSICAL EXAMINATION

- The extremity should be inspected for obvious deformity, swelling, and ecchymosis in the popliteal region.
- Careful attention should be paid to the neurovascular status.
- Pulses should be palpated, warmth of skin noted, and sensory and motor function examined. Examination for laxity of the knee should be performed carefully, because further neurovascular injury could occur.

SPECIAL TESTS

Arteriograms are performed in all patients who have diminished pulses or neurologic injuries.

IMAGING PROCEDURES

Anteroposterior and lateral views are sufficient but should not delay reduction of an obvious dislocation.

Knee Dislocation

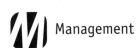 Management

GENERAL MEASURES

Reduction

- Immediate reduction is recommended.
- Anterior dislocations are reduced with longitudinal traction and the lifting of the femur anteriorly until located.
- Posterior dislocations are reduced with longitudinal traction and the lifting upward of the proximal tibia while extending the knee.
- Medial and lateral dislocations are reduced with longitudinal traction and appropriate mediolateral pressure on the tibia and femur.

Splint

- The knee should then be immobilized in a posterior splint with 15 degrees of flexion with careful attention to the neurovascular status.
- In patients who are going to undergo nonoperative treatment, this should be followed by 5 weeks in a long leg cast with 15 degrees of flexion.

Exercises

- Early exercises should be encouraged with a formal rehabilitation program for motion and strength after cast removal.

Neurovascular Status

- This should be examined before and after reduction.
- An orthopaedic or vascular surgeon should be notified.
- Immediate surgical intervention is indicated for open or unreducible dislocations and dislocations with vascular injury.

Activity

- A regimen of 6 weeks of immobilization is prescribed, with early start of quadriceps setting exercises followed by active leg lifting exercises.
- A rehabilitation program for motion and strength should be started after the cast is removed.

SURGICAL TREATMENT

Immediate

- Most patients (less than 50 years of age) are treated with reconstruction of the major knee ligaments. Surgery is indicated for open dislocations, unreducible dislocations, and vascular injuries.
- Open dislocations require copious irrigation and débridement.
- Unreducible dislocations require open reduction with the removal of trapped soft tissue.
- Vascular injury requires repair by a vascular surgeon (usually saphenous vein bypass graft).
- Ligament repair should be performed at time of initial surgery unless other factors preclude it.

PHYSICAL THERAPY

- An early start of quadriceps setting exercises is followed by active leg lifting exercises.
- A rehabilitation program for motion and strength should be started after the cast is removed.
- Patients who have undergone ligament reconstructions require intensive physical therapy to regain strength and motion.

PATIENT EDUCATION

Emphasize range-of-motion and strength exercises.

MONITORING

Patients are followed at 4- to 8-week intervals until they achieve maximum improvement.

COMPLICATIONS

- Loss of limb
- Decreased range of motion
- Neurologic deficit
- Knee instability
- Posttraumatic arthritis

PROGNOSIS

- Prognosis depends on the associated injuries and on the rapidity of intervention of these injuries.
- The most common residual effects are knee stiffness and early arthritis.

Basics

DESCRIPTION

Knee pain has many causes, including pathologic processes in the knee as well as disorders in distant locations with radiation to the knee area. Knee pain can be diffuse or located in a specific region of the knee. A characteristic history and physical examination will frequently narrow the diagnosis, with advanced testing used to confirm the clinical suspicion.

CAUSES

The knee is generally considered a hinge joint between the femur and the tibia. The ends of the two bones as well as the patella are coated with articular cartilage to provide a smooth surface for the joints to move. The joint is held together with the strong collateral and cruciate ligaments. The meniscus is a C-shaped structure between the medial and lateral sides of the joint to act as an additional cushion between the bones. The patella functions to extend the lower leg by transmitting the force from the quadriceps tendon to the patellar tendon. Pathologic processes in any of these areas can lead to knee pain.

RISK FACTORS

- Age
- Activity
- Obesity
- Sedentary lifestyle

CLASSIFICATION

- Traumatic
- Acquired

ASSOCIATED CONDITIONS

- Rheumatoid arthritis
- Active lifestyle

ICD-9-CM

719.46 Pain in joint
719.6 Knee Pain

 Diagnosis

SIGNS AND SYMPTOMS

- Swelling
- Locking
- Popping
- Difficulty on stairs and rising from a chair
- Chronic pain with increased activity

Patellofemoral Conditions

Patellofemoral Syndrome

This typically occurs in young adults and involves softening and degeneration of the articular cartilage. Pain is most frequent in the anterior knee and is worse with stair climbing. Knee range of motion often has a grating sensation, and pain is elicited by pressing firmly on the deep surface of the patella.

Patellar Subluxation-Dislocation

This is most frequent in young girls and is related to a combination of structural variations in the knee and leg. The femur may have more anteversion, and the lateral femoral condyle is flatter. The leg may be more knock-knee than typical, a configuration that increases the Q angle. The patella moves laterally as the knee is extended, causing a "J sign."

Articular Cartilage Injury

This is frequently related to a traumatic event. Pain is worse with activity.

Meniscal Disorders

Meniscal tears can be degenerative, with an obscure initial event, or traumatic, with a clear twisting injury. Swelling occurs slowly over the next day. Symptoms of pain improve somewhat with time. Locking or giving way of the knee along with medial or lateral joint line pain is common.

Arthritis

Symptoms are frequently gradual in onset and progressive. Pain is worse with increased activity and improves with rest. Pain at night after an active day is common. Increasing leg deformity is associated with the side of knee involvement.

Ligament Tears

Anterior Cruciate Ligament

The anterior cruciate ligament (ACL) prevents anterior translation of the tibia on the femur. ACL injuries occur predominantly from noncontact decelerations such as stopping suddenly, pivoting, or landing after jumping. These injuries can range from mild sprains, with no resultant functional abnormalities, to complete ruptures. In the pediatric patient, injury to this ligament most often occurs at the ligament-bone interface, whereas in the adult, rupture of the midsubstance of the ligament is more common.

Posterior Cruciate Ligament

The posterior cruciate ligament is the primary stabilizer to posterior translation of the tibia on the femur. Knee pain and swelling occur after the injury, with improvement in generalized pain symptoms at several weeks. Patients then note instability, especially when climbing steps, and they may develop posterior knee pain. Late findings can be knee recurvatum.

Medial Collateral Ligament

The medial collateral ligament (MCL) is the primary restraint to valgus stress on the knee. Pain is felt along the medial aspect of the knee. Typically, the pain extends proximally and distally along the region of the MCL. There can be a knee effusion. This injury can also be associated with an ACL tear as well as a medial meniscal tear. Patients also complain of increased pain with valgus loading. Patients occasionally recall a pop or snap at the time of the injury.

Knee Pain

Lateral Collateral Ligament

The lateral collateral ligament (LCL) extends from the lateral femoral condyle to the fibular head. Injury to this ligament is frequently associated with extensive soft tissue injury. Assessment of the cruciate ligaments and meniscus is important.

Tendon Ruptures

Rupture of the quadriceps or patellar tendon causes a loss of extension of the leg. Symptoms include the inability to extend the knee actively, pain, knee effusion, and ecchymosis about the knee. Quadriceps tendon ruptures often have a palpable defect proximal to the patella, and the patella appears more distal than normal. The most frequent cause is direct trauma to the knee or forced flexion of the knee that is resisted by maximal quadriceps contraction.

Bursitis and Tendinitis

Inflammatory changes occur in the bursa or tendon insertions around the knee, with typical tenderness to direct palpation over the anatomic location.

Osteochondritis Dissecans

This condition is more frequent in children and young adults who are active and participate in sports. The condition is the result of localized bone necrosis with overlying cartilage injury. Symptoms include knee pain, effusion (often hemarthrosis), thigh atrophy, tenderness over the lesion, and, occasionally, locking or catching of the knee if the fragment has become a loose body in the joint. Pain is often insidious and is related to activity.

Osgood-Schlatter Disease

This disturbance in the apophysis of the tibial tubercle in active children causes pain and enlargement of the patellar tendon insertion. This may be an overuse syndrome with repetitive stress on the tubercle, with a resultant partial avulsion.

Baker's Cyst

Popliteal cyst is caused by a distended bursa in the posterior fossa of the knee often directly connected to the joint space. It is most often associated with intraarticular disease and presents as a mass in the popliteal fossa of the knee, usually on the medial side, and occasionally associated with knee effusion and tenderness. The intraarticular disorder may not be symptomatic, and therefore the patient may only complain of posterior knee stiffness.

Fracture

Fracture about the knee should be ruled out in any patient with a traumatic injury. Fracture can occur in the distal femur, proximal tibia, and patella. Typically, plain radiographs in anteroposterior and lateral views are sufficient. Avulsion fractures are more common in children than are ligamentous injuries.

Tumor

Bone tumors are rare; however, they should always be kept on the list of differential diagnoses in patients with pain. Most patients with bone tumors present with musculoskeletal pain. The pain is typically described as dull, deep, and aching. The pain often becomes constant, and many patients experience pain at night. Patients may also complain of swelling, loss of function at the involved site, weight loss, or the acute symptoms of a pathologic fracture. The pain may not be related to activity.

DIFFERENTIAL DIAGNOSIS

A complete differential diagnosis is beyond the scope of this chapter. However, it is possible to cover the most frequent knee problems and their diagnosis. The onset and type of symptoms are helpful in determining an appropriate differential diagnosis:

- Patellofemoral conditions
- Articular cartilage injury
- Meniscal disorders
- Arthritis
- Ligament tears
- Tendon ruptures
- Osteochondritis dissecans
- Neurologic causes
- Osgood-Schlatter disease
- Baker's cyst
- Gouty attack
- Fracture
- Tumor

By Location of Pain

Anterior Knee

- Patellofemoral syndrome
- Patellar subluxation-dislocation
- Articular cartilage injury
- Patellofemoral arthritis

Posterior Knee

- Baker's cyst
- Posterior cruciate ligament
- ACL

Medial Knee

- Medial meniscus
- Medial compartment arthritis
- Medial plica

Lateral Knee

- LCL
- Lateral meniscus
- Lateral arthritis

The diagnosis can be made by the patient's symptoms and history in conjunction with the location of the pain (Table 1).

PHYSICAL EXAMINATION

Physical examination can provide many clues to the correct diagnosis by palpation, visualization, and testing.

Palpation

- Check joint effusion and synovial thickening by palpating the suprapatellar pouch (almost always indicates joint disease).
- Check joint line tenderness. Tenderness medially and laterally often suggests a meniscal tear.

Visualization

- Range of motion: The normal knee should bend from 0 degrees to 130 to 140 degrees.
- Patellar tracking: Observe for smooth patellar motion as the knee is ranged from extension to flexion.

Test

- Check the medial, lateral, and anterior stability of the joint (MCL, LCL, and ACL).

Table 1

SYMPTOM/HISTORY	LOCATION OF PAIN	DIAGNOSIS
Locking	Medial or lateral knee	Meniscus tear
Pop and sudden turn	Entire knee with swelling	Anterior Cruciate Ligament
Stairs and getting out of chair	Anterior knee	Patellofemoral cause
Striking knee hard against dashboard	Entire knee with swelling	Posterior Cruciate Ligament
Side contact to knee	Medial or lateral knee	Collateral ligament
Chronic pain with increased activity	Medial or lateral knee	Arthritis

LABORATORY TESTS

Order serum laboratory tests based on the level of suspicion for specific clinical entities, as follows:

- Septic arthritis: complete blood count with differential erythrocyte sedimentation rate
- Rheumatoid arthritis or other inflammatory arthritis: rheumatoid screen including rheumatoid factor and antinuclear antibody
- Gout: serum uric acid level

Arthrocentesis is often the best and only method to establish a definitive diagnosis. In the case of septic arthritis, findings include positive culture, most commonly *Staphylococcus aureus*. In the case of gout, findings include urate crystals.

PATHOLOGIC FINDINGS

- Loss of the articular cartilage (thinning, fragmentation, and eventually bone-on-bone articulation)
- Subchondral cysts and sclerosis
- Osteophytes

IMAGING PROCEDURES

Radiography

Plain radiographs are the first step in imaging. Two views detect most forms of arthritis, fractures, and tumors, as follows: the weight-bearing anteroposterior view and the lateral view.

Magnetic Resonance Imaging

Magnetic resonance imaging is used to detect meniscal tears, ligament disease, synovial proliferative disorders, tumors, and avascular necrosis. This imaging technique is so sensitive that a normal appearance of bone cartilage and ligaments virtually excludes a major structural problem.

Bone Scanning

Technetium bone scans are used only to detect occult bone disorders. If a patient has diffuse and severe discomfort and the clinician has not identified the site of disease, then the bone scan is an excellent imaging modality to localize the problem area.

Management

GENERAL MEASURES

- Patellofemoral syndrome: antiinflammatory medication and exercise
- Patellar subluxation-dislocation: often improved by extensive physical therapy and increasing age
- Arthritis: initially, analgesics, activity modification, injections, bracing
- MCL tear: typically bracing
- LCL: treatment depending on the degree of instability
- Bursitis and tendinitis: analgesics, topical treatments, activity modification, occasionally by injection into bursa
- Osgood-Schlatter Disease: rest and activity modification

SURGICAL TREATMENT

There are three main categories of knee surgery:

- Arthritis management: arthroscopic débridement of meniscal and cartilage disease, tibial and femoral osteotomy, knee replacement
- Sports medicine: meniscal repair, ligament reconstruction, patellar mechanism realignment
- Trauma: internal fixation of fractures, external fixation of fractures, arthroscopic repairs

PHYSICAL THERAPY

Physical therapy is an excellent modality for treating patients with knee pain. Therapists concentrate on range of motion, quadriceps strengthening, and stretching of tight structures. Weight bearing is delayed in patients who have fractures until healing has occurred. The emphasis on regaining strength and endurance of the entire lower extremity through isometric, isotonic, and closed- and open-chained isokinetic exercises facilitates rapid rehabilitation.

MEDICAL TREATMENT

- Nonsteroidal antiinflammatory drugs
- Acetaminophen
- Mild narcotic analgesics

PATIENT EDUCATION

Patients are carefully counseled to maintain their range of motion and to prevent contractures of the knee. Quadriceps strengthening and stretching exercises must be done to facilitate rehabilitation.

MONITORING

Patients are followed at 4- to 6-week intervals until they regain their strength and range of motion.

COMPLICATIONS

The main complication of knee pain is ankylosis through arthrofibrosis of the joint. In ankylosis, the articular joint undergoes irreversible degenerative changes. Reflex sympathetic dystrophy may also occur in patients with both acute and chronic pain syndromes.

PROGNOSIS

The prognosis is excellent, with well-defined diagnoses and many methods of effective surgical and nonsurgical treatment.

Knee Replacement

 Basics

DESCRIPTION

Total knee arthroplasty, resurfacing of the articular surfaces of the knee with metal and interposed plastic components, is a highly effective treatment for patients with disabling knee arthritis. The components are shaped to conform to the previous joint geometry. The ligaments, muscles, and tendons generally are not replaced.

CAUSES

- Osteoarthritis: often idiopathic
- Posttraumatic: athletic injuries, falls, motor vehicle accidents
- Inflammatory arthritis: rheumatoid arthritis, pseudogout or gout

RISK FACTORS

- Trauma
- Meniscectomy
- Obesity

CLASSIFICATION

Classification is by involved compartment:

- Medial compartment (tibial femoral)
- Lateral compartment (tibial femoral)
- Patellofemoral

ASSOCIATED CONDITIONS

Many patients have associated hip arthritis. Foot and ankle arthritis with and without significant deformity is common in patients with rheumatoid arthritis.

ICD-9-CM

Not applicable

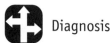 Diagnosis

SIGNS AND SYMPTOMS

Signs

- Effusions
- Medial joint line tenderness
- Varus (osteoarthritis) or valgus (rheumatoid arthritis)
- Deformity
- Limp

Symptoms

- Pain, especially on the medial side of the knee
- Swelling
- Catching
- Giving way

DIFFERENTIAL DIAGNOSIS

- Arthritis
- Infections: septic arthritis or osteomyelitis
- Patellofemoral syndrome or patellofemoral instability
- Meniscal tears
- Tumors

PHYSICAL EXAMINATION

The knee is easily examined and provides many clues to diagnosis.

- Palpation
- Effusions
- Joint line tenderness: suggests meniscal disorder
- Areas of tenderness
- Range of motion

LABORATORY TESTS

When infectious causes are considered, the white blood cell count and erythrocyte sedimentation rate are useful tests. Serum uric acid levels are determined if the clinician suspects gouty arthritis.

SPECIAL TEST

Arthrocentesis is an easy and effective method to screen for septic arthritis and gout or pseudogout.

PATHOLOGIC FINDINGS

The common denominator in all forms of arthritis is breakdown of the articular cartilage with loss of the proteoglycan and gradual loss of thickness. As the cartilage thins, the joint deformity increases, and patients often experience the sensation of bone rubbing on bone.

IMAGING PROCEDURES

Plain radiographs are the first step in imaging:

- Standing anteroposterior view of both knees: One can detect subtle loss of the articular cartilage thickness.
- Lateral view: One can assess for arthritic changes in the patellofemoral joint.

Magnetic resonance imaging can be used to detect meniscal tears, synovial proliferative disorders such as pigmented villonodular synovitis, and cartilage loss.

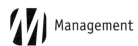 Management

GENERAL MEASURES

Patients are prepared for knee replacement with a careful medical examination, and they generally donate 2 U of blood preoperatively. Antiinflammatory medications are halted 6 to 7 days before the procedure.

SURGICAL TREATMENT

Knee replacement is performed by removing 8 to 12 mm of the cartilage and underlying bone that forms the surface of the joint. The surfaces of the bone are cut after aligning the cutting surface with special jigs. The components are either cemented onto the bone or press fit (the bone will then grow into the pores). The patellofemoral joint is also resurfaced. The actual joint articulation is between metal and high-density polyethylene.

PHYSICAL THERAPY

The focus of this integral component of care after knee replacement is on the following:

• Range of motion (attaining 0 to 110 degrees within 4 to 8 weeks)
• Quadriceps strengthening
• Full weight bearing

MEDICAL TREATMENT

After knee reconstruction, adequate narcotic analgesics are necessary to allow patients to participate fully in physical therapy. Most patients do not require long-term analgesics, although intermittent courses of nonsteroidal antiinflammatory drugs may be used for minor aches and pains about the knee.

PATIENT EDUCATION

Early on, patients must rigorously perform their range-of-motion exercises to attain functional arc and to prevent contractures.
To ensure the longevity of the replacement, patients must modify their activities. Activities can be grouped as follows:

Good Activities

• Walking
• Bicycling
• Golf
• Swimming

Bad Activities

• Running
• Racquetball
• Heavy lifting
• Singles tennis

MONITORING

After surgery, patients are followed at 1-month intervals until they attain a functional range of motion, and then they are followed once a year.
Plain radiographs are used to monitor the metal and cement interfaces with the bone and to check for polyethylene wear.

COMPLICATIONS

The major complications of knee replacement are infection, aseptic loosening, and patellofemoral problems (quadriceps mechanism). Quadriceps mechanism problems include subluxation, dislocation, patellar fracture, and quadriceps and patellar tendon ruptures.

PROGNOSIS

The long-term results of total knee replacement are excellent. Fewer than 5% of patients will require a revision for loosening 10 years after knee arthroplasty.

RECOMMENDED READING

Heck, DA, Blaha, JD, Windsor, RE, Kasser JR, ed. *Orthopaedic knowledge update 5.* Rosemont, IL: American Academy of Orthopaedic Surgeons, 1996:481–492.

Morrey BF, ed. *Reconstructive surgery of the joints,* 2nd ed. New York: Churchill Livingstone, 1996:1389–1400.

Rand JR. Cemented total knee arthroplasty: 1389–1400

Knee Supracondylar Fracture

 Basics

DESCRIPTION

Fractures involve the supracondylar (metaphyseal) or intracondylar (epiphyseal) areas, generally the distal 9 cm of the femur.

SYNONYMS

- Distal femur fractures
- Intercondylar femur fractures

INCIDENCE

- These comprise 4% to 7% of all femur fractures.
- Two peaks occur: young (less than 35 years of age), high-energy fractures and older (more than 50 years of age), low-energy fractures.
- Males are more commonly affected than females in patients with young, high-energy fractures: females are more often affected than males in those with older, low-energy fractures.
- Osteopenia occurs in the older, low-energy group.

CAUSES

- Younger group: high-energy trauma (e.g., motor vehicle accident, falls from heights)
- Older group: low-energy trauma (e.g., falls on flexed knee)

RISK FACTORS

Risk factors in the older group are osteopenia and previous age-related fractures.

CLASSIFICATION

These fractures are classified as displaced and nondisplaced:

Type A. Extraarticular (supracondylar)
Type B. Unicondylar
Type C. Bicondylar

ASSOCIATED CONDITIONS

- Acetabular fractures
- Hip dislocations
- Femoral neck and shaft fractures
- Knee ligamentous injuries
- Tibial plateau and shaft fractures
- Femoral artery disruptions

ICD-9-CM

821.23 Femur supracondylar fracture

 Diagnosis

SIGNS AND SYMPTOMS

- Pain
- Tenderness to palpation
- Edema
- Deformity
- Inability to walk

DIFFERENTIAL DIAGNOSIS

- Bruise
- Knee ligamentous injury
- Fracture of the patella or proximal tibia

PHYSICAL EXAMINATION

Complete musculoskeletal and neurovascular examination is essential.

PATHOLOGIC FINDINGS

- Muscle spasm often leads to shortening of the femur and limb.
- The femoral shaft often overrides anteriorly as the gastrocnemius pulls the distal fragment posteriorly and rotates the separated condylar fragments.
- The adductors often cause a varus deformity.

SPECIAL TESTS

- Angiogram if distal vascular status is questionable
- Knee: anteroposterior and lateral radiographs of the knee and supracondylar region; 45-degree oblique radiographs if there is intercondylar involvement
- Pelvis: anteroposterior radiograph (to rule out other fractures) in major trauma settings
- Hip and femur: anteroposterior and lateral radiographs of the hip and the whole femur (to rule out other fractures) in major trauma settings

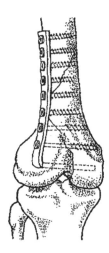 Management

GENERAL MEASURES

- Anatomic articular alignment is paramount.
- For nondisplaced and impacted fractures, a splint, cast, or fracture brace is used.
- For extraarticular fractures and medically unstable patients, skeletal traction is an option.
- For severe (grade III) open fractures, external fixation is performed across the knee with limited internal fixation to restore the articular surface; this is converted to internal fixation when soft tissue injuries are controlled.
- Open reduction internal fixation is used for the majority.

SURGICAL TREATMENT

Typical surgical techniques include:

- open reduction internal fixation technique
- open reduction internal fixation with plate and screws

or

- retrograde intramedullary rod fixation
- A lateral incision is used.
- Fracture reduction is performed.
- Lag screws are placed across the condyles.
- A 95-degree fixed angle device (blade plate, or dynamic condylar screw) is placed if possible (Fig. 1).
- If the fracture is too comminuted or too distal, use a condylar buttress plate.
- Bone grafting (form iliac crest) is often necessary.
- Other internal fixation devices are used less frequently.

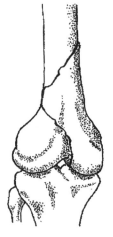
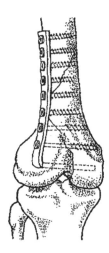

Fig. 1. A supracondryal fracture of the knee with intercondylar extension is treated with a plate.

PHYSICAL THERAPY

- Quadriceps and hamstring strengthening beginning on postoperative day 2
- Gait training on postoperative day 3 (minimal weight bearing)
- Progressive weight bearing and resistance exercises when there is clinical and radiographic evidence of healing (usually 2 to 3 months)
- Progressive weight bearing until solid union (usually 4 to 6 months)

MEDICAL TREATMENT

Analgesics are given.

MONITORING

- Patients are followed once a month until their fracture heals and they regain their range of motion.
- Clinical (pain to palpation) and radiographic (callus) monitoring is done until the fracture is healed.

COMPLICATIONS

- Knee stiffness (most common complication)
- Infection (0% to 7%)
- Nonunion
- Malunion
- Loss of fixation
- Traumatic arthritis

PROGNOSIS

- The prognosis depends on the type and severity of the fracture.
- In general, 70% to 85% of patients have a good to excellent result.

RECOMMENDED READING

Helfet DL. Fractures of the distal femur. In: Browner BD, Jupiter JB, Levine AM, eds. *Skeletal trauma,* vol 2. Philadelphia: WB Saunders, 1992:1643–1683.

Taylor JC. Fractures of the lower extremities: distal femur. In: Crenshaw AH, ed. *Campbell's operative orthopaedics,* vol 2. St. Louis: CV Mosby, 1992:947–858.

Wiss DA. Supracondylar and intercondylar fractures of the femur. In: Rockwood CA, Green DP, Bucholz RW, et al., eds. *Rockwood and Green's fractures in adults,* vol 2, 4th ed. Philadelphia: Lippincott—Raven, 1996:1973–1999.

Köhler's Disease

 Basics

DESCRIPTION

Köhler's disease is an eponym for osteonecrosis of the tarsal navicular (scaphoid) bone (Fig. 1). Pain in the medial midfoot in a young boy (aged 3 to 7 years) is the typical clinical presentation. It is usually worsened with activity and is relieved with rest. Clinical outcome is generally good after healing. There is a male predominance; it is two to three times more common in males than in females.

SYNONYMS

Osteonecrosis, osteochondrosis, and osteochondritis of the tarsal navicular

GENETICS

No known genetic transmission of this disorder exists.

INCIDENCE

This disease is uncommon.

CAUSES

The most likely cause is mechanical compression of the navicular, thus impairing vascularity. The navicular forms the apex of the longitudinal arch of the foot and is subject to constant compression during walking. These forces appear to cause vascular interruption during a critical phase early in the ossification of the navicular.

RISK FACTORS

- Male gender
- High activity level

CLASSIFICATION

This disorder is one of multiple disorders, termed "osteochondroses," which are characterized by transient vascular impairment of developing bones. Others in this category include the following:

- Perthes' disease
- Freiberg's disease
- Panner's disease

ASSOCIATED CONDITIONS

There seems to be a slight association with Perthes' disease (childhood osteonecrosis of the femoral head).

ICD-9-CM

732.5 Juvenile osteochondrosis of foot

 Diagnosis

SIGNS AND SYMPTOMS

- Medial midfoot pain worsening with activity
- Tenderness to palpation
- Walking on the outside of the foot to avoid stress on the navicular

DIFFERENTIAL DIAGNOSIS

- Ankle fracture
- Ankle sprain
- Accessory navicular
- Soft tissue infection

PHYSICAL EXAMINATION

Look for tenderness over the navicular with soft tissue swelling about the navicular and an antalgic gait. Some patients walk on the outer border of the foot to minimize compression of the navicular.

PATHOLOGIC FINDINGS

Pathologic specimens are not routinely obtained, nor are they necessary for diagnosis. Some specimens reported in the literature show areas of necrosis, resorption of dead bone, and formation of new bone; these are general findings of healing osteonecrosis.

IMAGING PROCEDURES

Plain films are sufficient to make the diagnosis. The normal navicular begins to ossify at age 2 to 3 years. It may normally start from several small ossification centers that eventually coalesce. In Köhler's disease, the navicular is flattened in its anteroposterior diameter and may show irregular sclerosis. It may be bilateral. With healing, increased ossification and resumption of normal growth occur.

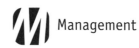 Management

GENERAL MEASURES

- Rest
- Arch support
- Casting
- Return to activity, based more on physical examination than on radiographs

Measures used depend on the level of symptoms. For minimally symptomatic cases, refraining from strenuous activities or the use of an arch support may be all that is needed. For more pronounced cases, a short leg cast with the arch well molded, worn for 4 to 12 weeks, usually provides relief. If the symptoms are severe, the patient may need to avoid weight bearing in the cast. After casting, if tenderness is minimal, use of an arch support and gradual resumption of activities are advised.

SURGICAL TREATMENT

Surgery is hardly ever needed. There are a few reports of persistent symptoms after maturity that required fusion of the talonavicular joint.

PHYSICAL THERAPY

Physical therapy is not needed. Parents may be placed in charge of timing the return to activities, based on the child's symptoms.

ACTIVITY

Activities that produce the pain should be avoided in the acute phase. These usually include sports involving running, jumping, and kicking. After symptoms resolve, these activities may be resumed gradually, with use of an arch support.

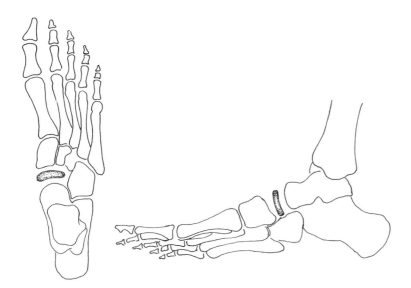

Fig. 1. Köhler's disease is avascular necrosis of the tarsal navicular, which usually produces compression of this bone (*stippled*).

MEDICAL TREATMENT

- Rest
- Arch support
- Acetaminophen or nonsteroidal antiinflammatory agents as needed

PATIENT EDUCATION

- Patients should be counseled about the benign, self-resolving nature of this condition and its relation to activity so they may moderate activities accordingly.
- Prevention is not effective or practical in this rare disease.

MONITORING

The course of the disease should be followed by clinical examination (tenderness, limp), rather than by radiography.

COMPLICATIONS

Rarely, ache or tenderness may persist. These symptoms may be treated in the same fashion, by rest, arch support, or, rarely, surgery.

PROGNOSIS

Prognosis is good. In 2 to 4 years, the radiographic appearance of the navicular usually returns to normal, and the patient's symptoms resolve.

RECOMMENDED READING

Coughlin MJ, Mann RA, eds. *Surgery of the foot and ankle,* 7th ed. Philadelphia: CV Mosby, 1997.

Kyphosis

Basics

DESCRIPTION

Kyphosis is the normal curve of the thoracic spine when viewed from the side. It is normal when it occurs within a certain range (20 to 49 degrees). It may be increased because of postural factors, Scheuermann's kyphosis (apophysitis), fracture, infection, osteoporosis, neurologic disorders, malignancy, or other conditions. It may also occur in other areas of the spine, where it is always abnormal. Scheuermann's kyphosis has its onset in early adolescence and is slightly more common in boys (Fig. 1). Postural kyphosis usually develops in the early teen years.

Osteoporosis is more common in older women. Kyphosis tends to increase with age in most persons due to narrowing of discs, and this process is accelerated by osteoporosis. Life expectancy is not compromised by kyphosis.

SYNONYMS

- Round back
- Hunched back
- Scheuermann's disease
- Scheuermann's apophysitis

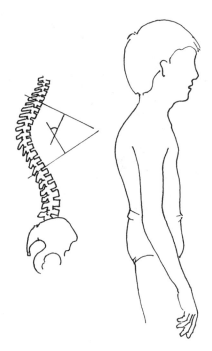

Fig. 1. Kyphosis is measured by the angle between the uppermost and lowermost inclined vertebrae on the lateral view.

GENETICS

- Kyphosis usually occurs sporadically.
- Some causes of kyphosis may be inherited, including the following:

—Ankylosing spondylitis
—Osteoporosis
—Some cases of Scheuermann's disease

INCIDENCE

- Mild increases in kyphosis are common, occurring in at least 2% to 5% of the population.
- Symptomatic, severe kyphosis is much less common.

CAUSES

Postural kyphosis results from stretching of the ligaments, with the vertebrae themselves normally formed. Scheuermann's kyphosis is kyphosis caused by wedging of the vertebrae, which usually develops during early adolescence. It is possibly caused by increased loading on the growing vertebrae, or in other cases, mild osteoporosis or abnormalities of vertebral growth cartilage. Congenital kyphosis is present starting from birth and is characterized by hemivertebrae or by fusion of the vertebrae in front. Other causes of kyphosis include healed vertebral fractures, ankylosing spondylitis, and tuberculosis. An increasingly prevalent cause is osteoporosis, especially in elderly persons or those taking steroids.

RISK FACTORS

- Osteoporosis
- Positive family history of kyphosis
- History of spine fracture
- Heavy loading of the spine during adolescence (e.g., butterfly stroke in swimming or repeated heavy lifting)
- Exposure to tuberculosis
- Malignancy
- Both pregnancy and kyphosis are risk factors for back pain, and they may be additive.

ASSOCIATED CONDITIONS

- Lumbar lordosis
- Spondylolysis
- Mild scoliosis

ICD-9-CM

737.10 Postural kyphosis
732.0 Scheuermann kyphosis
733.0 Congenital kyphosis
737.41 Tuberculosis

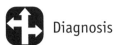

Diagnosis

SIGNS AND SYMPTOMS

The patient, the parents, and others note "poor posture." It may be more noticeable when the patient bends forward, when the spine assumes a sharp angulation at the apex of the kyphosis. Back pain may or may not be present, but if present is rarely disabling. It is located over the apex of the curve. Usually, the remainder of the spine assumes compensatory reverse curvatures, such as cervical and lumbar lordosis. The hamstrings are often tight. Slight scoliosis often coexists but is of no consequence. If the kyphosis is severe and sharp, it may compress the spinal cord. This usually occurs only in congenital kyphosis, fracture, or tuberculosis.

DIFFERENTIAL DIAGNOSIS

- Scoliosis may resemble kyphosis because of the rib deformity on the convex side, but in fact, most patients with thoracic scoliosis have less than normal kyphosis.
- The various causes of kyphosis must be differentiated from one another (see earlier). Neuromuscular disorders may cause kyphosis because of low muscle tone.
- Surgical laminectomy of the spine in a growing child may cause kyphosis to develop afterward.

PHYSICAL EXAMINATION

The patient should be examined when he or she is in the neutral standing position and bending forward. Flexibility of the curve should be assessed by prone hyperextension. Neurologic examination should be completed.

LABORATORY TESTS

- If infection is suspected, it should be worked up by obtaining a complete blood count, sedimentation rate, and possibly blood cultures. Magnetic resonance imaging should be considered. Biopsy may be indicated if the organism is not known.
- Results of routine laboratory studies are normal in most cases of kyphosis, even if there is osteoporosis.
- In ankylosing spondylitis, patients may have antibodies to HLA-B27, although the diagnosis remains largely clinical.
- In cases of suspected tuberculosis, a tubercular skin test should be performed, followed by a biopsy if the result is abnormal.

PATHOLOGIC FINDINGS

Gross anatomy of the spine is abnormal in kyphosis in several respects. In most cases, the posterior elements of the spine are relatively elongated; the laminae and facets appear "stretched out." In Scheuermann's kyphosis, the discs are flattened and irregular, and the anterior longitudinal ligament is thickened and contracted. The vertebral bodies are wedged into a triangular shape at several levels in ankylosing spondylitis, the spine is stiff, and eventually the involved vertebrae become fused. In kyphosis from infection or tumor, there may be a soft tissue mass posterior to the vertebrae that narrows the spinal cord.

IMAGING PROCEDURES

Initial plain radiographs to assess and measure kyphosis should be taken with the patient standing, because the degree of curve decreases when the patient lies supine. The films should include the entire spine on one cassette ideally and should be taken with the arms gently elevated forward. If a bony abnormality is seen on the initial films, a coned (focused) film of the abnormal area should then be taken. A hyperextension film (lying supine with the apex on a soft bolster) may be done to determine the flexibility of the curve, which may assist with treatment decisions. The bony maturity of an adolescent may be determined by measuring the amount of the iliac apophysis that has ossified (Risser's sign). If there is any question of neurologic abnormality, the spinal cord may be assessed with magnetic resonance imaging. If the kyphosis is congenital, other congenital malformations such as renal abnormalities should be ruled out with an ultrasound scan.

Management

GENERAL MEASURES

Bracing is indicated for growing adolescents with Scheuermann's kyphosis with an apex below the eighth thoracic vertebrae. It consists of wearing a plastic brace for the thoracic and lumbar spine under the clothes. It corrects the curve by relieving the deforming forces. If the brace is worn full time until maturity, it may provide permanent correction. It is not effective for large curves, such as those measuring more than 70 degrees. Exercises are described later. Surgery, if indicated, usually includes correction with posterior rods and fusion, sometimes supplemented by anterior disc excision and fusion.

SURGICAL TREATMENT

Surgery is indicated for various types of kyphosis if deformity or pain is unacceptable and unresponsive to conservative measures. If indicated, surgery usually includes correction with posterior rods and fusion, sometimes supplemented by anterior disc excision and fusion. Significant correction is usually possible.

For congenital kyphosis, surgery should be performed if the patient is still growing, because there is a significant chance of neurologic compromise if the curve is allowed to worsen.

PHYSICAL THERAPY

- Exercises provide benefit for pain in many types of kyphosis.
- The three components include strengthening, stretching, and general conditioning.
- Stretch the hamstrings, the tight structures on the anterior part of the kyphosis, and the tight muscles in the lumbar lordosis.
- Strengthening should include abdominal muscles and the back extensors.
- Conditioning should be done for cardiovascular purposes and should include activities that do not make the pain worse.

MEDICAL TREATMENT

- Kyphosis (except the congenital variety) rarely produces deleterious effects on vital structures, so treatment should be based on the patient's chief complaint.
- For those complaining of pain, exercises and analgesics are the mainstay of treatment.
- For those concerned with deformity, bracing during adolescence or postural exercises during adulthood may be offered.
- In either case, surgical correction may be used for severe cases.
- For patients who have no complaints about pain or deformity, no treatment is needed.

- For congenital kyphosis, surgery should be performed if the patient is still growing, because there is a significant chance of neurologic compromise if the curve is allowed to worsen.
- Analgesics may be used if back pain recurs; usually, treatment is with nonsteroidal agents or acetaminophen.
- Estrogens or alendronate may be considered as part of a program to prevent or treat osteoporosis in appropriate patients.

PATIENT EDUCATION

The nature of the potential problems with kyphosis should be explained to the patient, to determine the desired level of treatment. The patient should be shown the exercises and given the option of learning them from a physical therapist or on his or her own. If exercises are instituted, they should become a permanent part of the patient's daily routine. Smoking should be avoided.

The importance of diet should be discussed. Although it may not play a role in the causes of most types of kyphosis, osteoporosis may later affect many patients and may worsen the kyphosis. Therefore, adequate daily calcium intake should be stressed.

MONITORING

In growing patients, the curve should be monitored every 4 to 6 months. Adults may be seen as needed.

COMPLICATIONS

Patients with severe, sharp kyphosis may have neurologic compromise from the apex of the curve. This may be triggered by a fall or fracture.

PROGNOSIS

Kyphosis, particularly if greater than normal, tends to worsen with age. The back and neck pain it causes may range from minor to persistent. Pulmonary function and life expectancy are not affected. Patients are usually able to carry out full-time jobs, although physical work may need to be limited.

RECOMMENDED READING

Fon GT, Pitt MG, Thies AC. Thoracic kyphosis: range in normal subjects. *Am J Roentgenol* 1980;134:979–983.

Murray PM, Weinstein SL, Spratt KF. The natural history and long-term follow-up of Scheuermann kyphosis. *J Bone Joint Surg Am* 1993;75-A:236–248.

Lisfranc Dislocation

Basics

DESCRIPTION

This is a dislocation of the tarsometatarsal joints of the foot (Fig. 1). It can occur in all ages.

CAUSES

The mechanism of injury includes a wide spectrum of causes from low-energy compression and twisting to high-energy crush injuries. Indirect causes are common, especially an axial load on the plantar flexed foot.

CLASSIFICATION

Hardcastle's classification is as follows:

Type A. Total incongruity of tarsometatarsal joint
Type B. Partial incongruity of tarsometatarsal joint complex, either medial or lateral
Type C. Divergent (first metatarsal medial, second to fifth lateral)

ASSOCIATED CONDITIONS

- Comminuted fractures of the metatarsal bases or cuneiforms
- Severe soft tissue injury
- Compartment syndrome
- Open fractures

ICD-9-CM

825.25 Metatarsal fracture

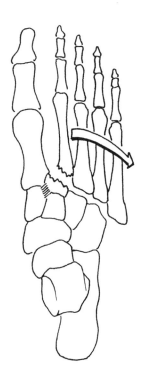

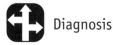

Diagnosis

SIGNS AND SYMPTOMS

- Pain
- Swelling
- Deformity
- Ecchymosis
- Difficulty bearing weight
- Tenderness over midfoot
- Possible spontaneous reduction

DIFFERENTIAL DIAGNOSIS

- Soft tissue contusion
- Ligament sprain
- Isolated metatarsal or midfoot fractures

PHYSICAL EXAMINATION

- Rotational stress on the forefoot will cause pain at Lisfranc joint.
- Palpation over the second metatarsal base can also cause pain.

LABORATORY TESTS

There are no laboratory tests.

IMAGING PROCEDURES

Plain films are usually diagnostic. Anteroposterior, lateral, and oblique projections are mandatory. On the anteroposterior view, the medial margin of the second metatarsal base should be aligned with the middle cuneiform. On the oblique view, the medial base of the fourth metatarsal should be aligned with the medial margin of the cuboid. On the lateral view, there should be an unbroken line from the dorsum of the first and second metatarsals to the corresponding cuneiform. Avulsion fracture of the second metatarsal base ("fleck" fracture) and compression fracture of the cuboid are pathognomonic of this condition.
If the diagnosis is uncertain on plain film, especially if Lisfranc joint has spontaneously reduced, stress radiography with fluoroscopy may be helpful in further defining the instability pattern.
Computed tomography and technetium bone scans may also provide information if the diagnosis is still unclear.

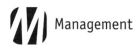

Management

GENERAL MEASURES

Before the patient is taken to the operating room, compartment syndrome and neurovascular injury should be assessed. The foot is splinted and is kept elevated until surgery.

SURGICAL TREATMENT

Open reduction and internal fixation of the joints are done through two to three dorsal longitudinal incisions. Fixation may consist of either Kirschner wires (K-wires) or 3.5-mm cortical screws.
If K-wires are used as fixation, they can be removed in the office at 6 weeks, and the patient may begin protected weight bearing. However, if screws are used in the surgery, unprotected weight bearing is not permitted until the screws have been removed, at 10 to 12 weeks postoperatively.

PHYSICAL THERAPY

Patients should be referred for gait training on a non–weight-bearing basis postoperatively.

MEDICAL TREATMENT

The goal of treatment is to achieve and maintain anatomic reduction of the joints while the ligaments heal. This usually requires surgical intervention.
General measures before and after surgery are ice elevation and a compression dressing.

PATIENT EDUCATION

Patients must be warned about the risks of traumatic arthritis as well as fixed deformity, which may require an arthrodesis later.

MONITORING

Follow-up radiographs should be taken to check for maintained alignment of Lisfranc complex. Radiographs are taken at 1-month intervals.

COMPLICATIONS

- Traumatic arthritis
- Fixed deformity
- Injuries diagnosed late (7 to 8 weeks): poor prognosis; patients may be candidates for primary arthrodesis

PROGNOSIS

- Patients with anatomic reduction generally have good to excellent results.
- Outcomes are worse with nonanatomic reduction and extensive joint injury. Patients with posttraumatic arthritis can undergo salvage procedures with arthrodesis.

RECOMMENDED READING

Heckman, JD. Fractures and dislocations of the foot. In: Rockwood CA, Green DP, Bucholz RW, et al., eds. *Rockwood and Green's fractures in adults*, 4th ed. Philadelphia: Lippincott-Raven, 1996:2362–2372.

Rockwood CA, Green DP, Bucholz RW, et al., eds. *Rockwood and Green's fractures in adults*, 4th ed. Philadelphia: Lippincott-Raven, 1996:491–496.

Fig. 1. Lisfranc dislocation occurs at the midfoot joints, usually with significant trauma.

Basics

DESCRIPTION

"Little League elbow" refers to a group of injuries about the elbow that arise from repetitive throwing or striking with a racquet in children and adolescents (Fig. 1). These injuries affect young children to young adults (ages 7 to 20). Younger patients (7 to 11 years old) often have an injury of the physis, whereas older adolescents (15 to 19 years old) are subject to avulsion fractures or ligament tears. Little League elbow occurs more frequently in younger athletes, who are involved in sporting events associated with throwing or striking.

SYNONYMS

- Tennis elbow
- Osteochondritis (or osteochondrosis) of the radial head or capitellum

GENETICS

No mendelian inheritance pattern is known.

INCIDENCE

The incidence increases with the intensity of competition.

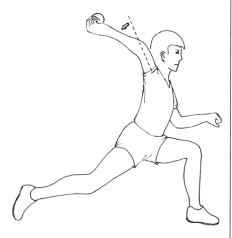

Fig. 1. Little League elbow results from valgus strain, which may cause tendinitis medially or osteochondritis laterally in the growing elbow.

CAUSES

- Medial epicondylar fragmentation or avulsion
- Delayed or accelerated growth of the medial epicondyle
- Delayed closure of the medial epicondylar growth plate
- Osteochondritis of the capitellum
- Deformation and osteochondritis of the radial head
- Olecranon apophysitis with or without delayed closure of the olecranon apophysis

RISK FACTORS

Throwing or serving sports in young children and adolescents (e.g., baseball, football, javelin, and tennis) are risk factors.

CLASSIFICATION

- Medial disease involves the medial collateral ligament, the medial epicondyle, and surrounding soft tissues.
- Lateral disease involves the radial head, the capitellum, the lateral epicondyle, and surrounding soft tissues.

ICD-9-CM

726.32 Little League elbow

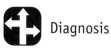

Diagnosis

SIGNS AND SYMPTOMS

Most patients present with medial elbow pain, although some have lateral pain, with diminished throwing distance and decreased throwing effectiveness. Pain is aggravated by throwing. Examination demonstrates point tenderness over the medial epicondyle, swelling, and a flexion contracture often greater than 30 degrees. The injury most often involves the dominant elbow. Nocturnal pain is uncommon, and possible neoplastic lesions must be excluded. Burning around the medial elbow associated with paresthesias or dysesthesias in ulnar digits signifies ulnar nerve involvement. Duration of symptoms can help to delineate injuries such as ulnar collateral ligament ruptures (acute) from medial epicondylitis (chronic).

The patient may present with vague lateral elbow pain and swelling—capitellar necrosis (Panner's disease) (ages 7 to 12 years)—versus osteochondritis dissecans of the capitellum (ages 13 to 16 years). Late-presenting lateral symptoms include locking, catching, and severe pain. Posterior pathology involves the olecranon and surrounding soft tissues.

DIFFERENTIAL DIAGNOSIS

- Elbow fracture (supracondylar humerus, olecranon)
- Neoplasm
- Ulnar nerve entrapment or posterior interosseous nerve entrapment
- Tendinitis of medial or lateral elbow muscle origin
- Loose bodies in the joint

Little League Elbow

PHYSICAL EXAMINATION

- Document the range of elbow motion, including flexion, extension, pronation, and supination.
- Look for an effusion, as signified by loss of the normal lateral soft tissue recen.
- Pinpoint the location of tenderness.
- Perform a neurovascular examination of the extremity.
- Observe the patient performing the causative motion.
- Stability of the elbow to valgus stress with the elbow in 25 degrees of flexion helps to assess the collateral ligaments.

PATHOLOGIC FINDINGS

- Weak physis in growing children makes injuries to this area (fracture or osteochondritis) common, whereas young adults with fused physes tend to develop more soft tissue injuries.
- The pathologic process of Panner's disease and osteochondritis dissecans is unknown but thought to arise from repetitive trauma. Osteochondritis dissecans may progress to loose bodies with painful locking.

IMAGING PROCEDURES

- Plain radiographs (anteroposterior and lateral) are obtained to rule out fractures, loose bodies, or osteochondritis dissecans.
- Stress radiographs may be helpful.
- Bone scan is useful to rule out physeal injury or apophysitis.
- Magnetic resonance imaging may be useful in evaluating injury to cartilage, physis, tendons, muscles, and ligaments.

Management

MEDICAL TREATMENT

- Most injuries resolve with 4 to 6 weeks' rest.
- With severe pain, a regimen of 1 to 2 weeks of splint immobilization is helpful, followed by active motion exercises.
- Loose bodies often require surgical removal.
- Occasionally, large osteochondritis dissecans fragments and avulsion fragments with more than 2 mm displacement require surgical fixation.
- Nonsteroidal antiinflammatory agents are the drugs of choice.
- Steroid injections rarely indicated.
- Stability of the elbow should be assessed before the patient returns to competitive throwing. If symptoms resume with activity after 6 weeks of rest, further investigation into causes should be pursued (computed tomography, magnetic resonance imaging).

SURGICAL TREATMENT

Many of these conditions may be treated arthroscopically, including pinning of osteochondritis dissecans fragments, removal of loose bodies, and removal of osteophytes. Occasional open reduction with internal fixation of avulsion fractures with wires is necessary or open reconstruction or repair of the ulnar collateral ligament.

PHYSICAL THERAPY

After 6 weeks of rest, when the patient is asymptomatic and has pain-free range of motion, begin elbow strengthening exercises with a progressive throwing program beginning over 6 to 8 weeks after injury. The therapist may be effective in supervising the patient's return to sport more closely than the physician is able to do.

PATIENT EDUCATION

- Instruct the patient in proper throwing mechanics.
- Recognize symptoms early.
- Rest from throwing activities (4 to 6 weeks) to avoid further injury.
- Advise a gradual return to competitive sports when the patient is asymptomatic.
- Recurrence of symptoms often requires longer rest followed by strengthening exercises.

MONITORING

Patients with Panner's disease should have follow-up radiographs to assess healing of the capitellum every 3 to 4 months on the average.

COMPLICATIONS

- Rare: Panner's disease may lead to late deformity and collapse of the capitellum articular surface.
- Osteochondritis dissecans may displace and become a loose body in the joint that requires removal.
- Epicondyle fractures may form a nonunion, but this is usually asymptomatic.

PROGNOSIS

Overall, most patients do well with rest. Occasionally, one may develop slight flexion contractures and valgus deformity of throwing arm, which is rarely symptomatic.

RECOMMENDED READING

DeLee JC, Drez D Jr, eds. *Orthopaedic sports medicine: principles and practice,* vol 2. Philadelphia: WB Saunders, 1994:250–260.

Hunter SC. Little League elbow. In: Zarins B, Andrews JR, Carson WG, eds. *Injuries to the throwing arm.* Philadelphia: WB Saunders, 1995.

Pappas AM. Elbow problems associated with baseball during childhood and adolescence. *Clin Orthop* 1982;164:30–41.

Yocum LA. The diagnosis and non-operative treatment of elbow problems in the athlete. *Clin Sports Med* 1989;8:439–451.

Basics

DESCRIPTION

Lyme disease is an immune-mediated disorder in reaction to infection by the spirochete *Borrelia burgdorferi*. It may include rash, arthritis, synovitis, carditis, or neurologic manifestations. Both children and adults are affected equally.

SYNONYMS

Deer tick disease

GENETICS

The HLA-DR4 haplotype predicts increased risk of disease.

INCIDENCE

• The incidence varies with region of the country, but it has been reported in most states.
• There are three major endemic areas in the United States:

—Upper mid-Atlantic area from Massachusetts to Maryland
—Upper Midwest (especially Wisconsin and Minnesota)
—Western states of Oregon, Utah, Nevada, and California

CAUSES

Lyme disease is a reaction to an infection by the spirochete *Borrelia burgdorferi*, which is transmitted by the deer tick, *Ixodes dammini*. The disease was first characterized after an epidemic of involvement in Old Lyme, Connecticut in the mid-1970s. Since then, other endemic areas have been identified.

RISK FACTORS

• Endemic area
• Deer tick exposure
• HLA-DR4 antigen haplotype

CLASSIFICATION

Acute Stage

• Rash
• Early arthritis

Chronic Stage

• Arthritis
• Carditis
• Neuritis

ICD-9-CM

714.0 Inflammatory arthritis
727.0 Synovitis

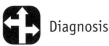

Diagnosis

SIGNS AND SYMPTOMS

Acute

• Spreading rash known as erythema chronicum migrans, beginning 3 to 30 days after a tick bite
• Fever
• Headache
• Malaise
• Migratory arthralgias and myalgias

Chronic

• Swelling of large joints, most commonly the knee
• Involvement of one or more joints
• Pain, which may be minimal, as in juvenile rheumatoid arthritis, or acute, resembling bacterial arthritis
• Cardiac involvement, possibly including atrioventricular block or myocarditis
• Neurologic involvement, possibly including seventh cranial nerve (facial) palsy, meningoencephalitis, or peripheral neuropathy

DIFFERENTIAL DIAGNOSIS

• The diagnosis of juvenile rheumatoid arthritis requires at least 6 weeks of continued arthritis, but the arthritis does not respond to antibiotics, in contrast to Lyme disease.
• Bacterial arthritis usually produces more acute pain and fever and does not have a characteristic prodromal rash.
• Rheumatic fever should be excluded.

Lyme Disease

PHYSICAL EXAMINATION

- Inspect the patient's skin for the spreading, oval rash.
- Question about a rash occurring earlier.
- Examine for cranial nerve or peripheral nerve palsy.
- Examine all joints for effusion, even if painless.
- Listen to the patient's heart.

LABORATORY TESTS

Erythrocyte sedimentation rate is usually elevated. Tests for Lyme disease include two methods of antibody detection. Enzyme-linked immunosorbent assay for spirochete is sensitive but not specific. A titer of more than 1:80 is considered positive. If positive, this should be followed up by Western blot test, a gel electrophoresis technique, which is more specific. Arthrocentesis is not a specific test for Lyme disease, but it is often performed to rule out other disorders. The white blood cell count is 25,000 to 90,000 and may include up to 95% polymorphonuclear leukocytes. The spirochete is not recoverable from joint fluid. Electrocardiography may be indicated to demonstrate atrioventricular block.

PATHOLOGIC FINDINGS

- No pathologic specimens are usually taken or required for diagnosis.
- When the joint lining is examined by biopsy, it shows nonspecific synovitis.

IMAGING PROCEDURES

- Plain radiographs of the affected area are indicated.
- Joint changes may include soft tissue swelling in early stages, osteopenia if the inflammation has been present for several weeks, and joint space narrowing if it has been chronic.

Management

GENERAL MEASURES

Consult other specialists, such as those in infectious disease, neurology, rheumatology, or cardiology, as appropriate.

SURGICAL TREATMENT

Synovectomy is a rare option for chronic disease that does not respond to initial antibiotic therapy.

PHYSICAL THERAPY

Physical therapy may be helpful to teach crutch walking in early stages when joint rest is important. In later stages when effective treatment is under way, therapy may be helpful to deal with weakness or any joint contractures that have occurred.

MEDICAL TREATMENT

- Arrange diagnostic testing.
- Start treatment with oral (early stages of disease) penicillin or amoxicillin empirically.
- Administer these drugs intravenously if disease is treated later.
- Tetracycline is also an option for children who are more than 8 years old. It should not be used in younger children because of potential discoloration of teeth.
- Restrict the patient's activity in the presence of significant joint, cardiac, or neurologic involvement.

PATIENT EDUCATION

Patients should be educated about prevention of reexposure, and the family should be so counseled. They should also be informed about the late signs and symptoms of cardiac and neurologic involvement.

PREVENTION

- Awareness of endemic areas
- Avoidance of deer tick exposure

MONITORING

- Follow patients daily to weekly to monitor response to therapy.
- Possibly admit patients to the hospital if cardiac or neurologic involvement is severe.

COMPLICATIONS

- Carditis (conduction block, myocarditis)
- Neurologic involvement (e.g., cranial or peripheral nerve palsy, meningoencephalitis)

PROGNOSIS

Prognosis is usually good, unless late joint changes or neurologic complications have occurred.

RECOMMENDED READING

Cristofaro RO, Appet MH, Gelb RI, et al.: Musculoskeletal manifestations of Lyme disease in children. *J Pediatr Orthop* 1987;7:527.

Rose CD, Fawcett PT, Eppes SC, et al. Pediatric Lyme arthritis: clinical spectrum and outcome. *J Pediatr Orthop* 1994;14:238–241.

Steere AC. Lyme disease. *N Engl J Med* 1989;329:586.

Basics

DESCRIPTION

Macrodactyly is overgrowth of one or several adjacent digits or rays of a hand or foot that produces the appearance of localized gigantism (Fig. 1). Virtually all cases are present at birth, although in some progressive cases it is not until further enlargement occurs that the condition is clinically recognizable. Growth of the enlarged digits ceases when the patient reaches skeletal maturity. No predilection is known for increased frequency in one sex.

SYNONYM

Localized gigantism

GENETICS

Isolated macrodactyly is not a heritable condition. Only if it is associated with neurofibromatosis is there a familial tendency.

INCIDENCE

- Less than 1 in 10,000
- Upper extremity more commonly affected than lower extremity
- Most cases (95%) unilateral

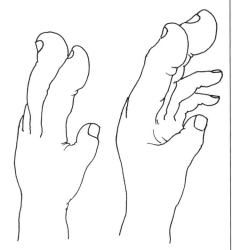

Fig. 1. Macrodactyly is generalized enlargement of one or two digits of the hand or foot.

CAUSES

In idiopathic macrodactyly, the cause is unknown. It may be due to a localized disturbance of growth factors in the ectodermal ridge. Other cases of macrodactyly occur in patients with neurofibromatosis, Proteus syndrome, lymphedema, and hemangiomas.

RISK FACTORS

- Neurofibromatosis
- Proteus syndrome
- Klippel-Trenaunay syndrome

CLASSIFICATION

- Static: Enlargement remains proportionate to other digits.
- Dynamic: Enlargement increases with time, even by proportion.

ASSOCIATED CONDITIONS

- Proteus syndrome (multiple hamartomatous abnormalities)
- Neurofibromatosis
- Klippel-Trenaunay syndrome

ICD-9-CM

755.57 Macrodactyly of fingers or thumb
755.65 Macrodactyly of toes

 ## Diagnosis

SIGNS AND SYMPTOMS

- Generalized overgrowth of all tissues in the affected digits occurs.
- Enlargement is greater distally than proximally.
- The nail is especially enlarged.
- Tissues on the plantar or palmar surface of the digit are more greatly enlarged than those on the dorsal side, thus causing the digit to become hyperextended.
- The second ray is most commonly affected, followed by the third, first, and fourth.
- Syndactyly may coexist.
- If two digits are involved, they grow away from each other.
- In some cases, the enlargement becomes proportionately greater with time (the dynamic type).
- Main clinical symptoms are related to overgrowth, such as clumsiness in the hand or difficulty with shoe wear.
- Pain may occasionally develop in adulthood, because degeneration of the involved joints is premature.

DIFFERENTIAL DIAGNOSIS

- Hemihypertrophy, in which all digits in a hand or foot are uniformly overgrown
- Acrodactyly, in which overgrowth of all digits is greatest distally
- Growth hormone overabundance (hypersecretion)

Macrodactyly

PHYSICAL EXAMINATION

- Diagnosis is made purely by physical examination.
- Inspect the patient's hands and feet for hemangiomas and other signs of Proteus syndrome and neurofibromatosis.
- Compare limb lengths. They are rarely uneven in idiopathic macrodactyly.
- Check the motion of the affected digits.
- Compare the widths and lengths of the two hands or feet.
- Progression of growth of the hand or foot may be tracked clinically by making tracings or prints of both hands or feet over time, so length and width may be measured and compared.

LABORATORY TESTS

Genetic testing is available for Proteus syndrome and neurofibromatosis.

PATHOLOGIC FINDINGS

- All tissue types are overgown in the affected digit.
- Fibrofatty proliferation accounts for the greatest bulk.
- Vessel, bone, subcutaneous tissue and dermis are enlarged, and the changes are greatest distally.
- Pathologic changes are greatest in the digital nerves.

IMAGING PROCEDURES

Plain films should be made to help assess the extent of overgrowth and the segments involved. Soft tissue enlargement may also be quantified from these films. The extent of skeletal maturity may also be judged; it is often advanced in the enlarged rays.

Magnetic resonance imaging is rarely necessary.

Management

GENERAL MEASURES

- Serial follow-up
- Measurements of length and width
- Surgery

The pattern of growth should be determined by serial follow-up. In this way, the static and the progressive types may be distinguished, and the appropriate treatment may be chosen: observation, shoe modification, or surgery.

SURGICAL TREATMENT

- Surgery may involve resection of the most enlarged ray, if the width of the hand or foot is greatly increased. This is the fastest way to make an important difference.
- In other cases, phalangectomy may make the length more even.
- Epiphysiodesis (closure of the growth plates) is another way of evening length; the correction occurs more gradually with time, and it may not completely correct the length inequality.
- Debulking of fat may improve the appearance, especially of the plantar fat hypertrophy.

MEDICAL TREATMENT

- No drugs are known to help this condition.
- No restrictions are placed on activity.

PATIENT EDUCATION

- Show radiographs to help explain the nature of the condition.
- Advise that macrodactyly often requires several surgical procedures to achieve an optimal result.
- Benefits of ray resection, if appropriate, should be emphasized.

PREVENTION

No means of prevention are known.

MONITORING

Serial follow-up appointments every 6 to 12 months are needed to develop and monitor a treatment plan. To keep records, tracings or radiographs should be made at each visit. Follow-up should be continued up to, and past, maturity.

COMPLICATIONS

- Stiffness and aching in the joints of the enlarged digits often develop in adulthood.
- Persistent enlargement, especially in the width of the involved digits, is the norm.
- Circulatory disturbance may occur if both sides of an involved digit are operated on at once.

PROGNOSIS

Most patients are made significantly better by judicious surgery. At the same time, it is important to realize that the parts will not be completely normal.

RECOMMENDED READING

Barsky AJ. Macrodactyly. *J Bone Joint Surg Am* 1967;49:1255–1266.

Dennyson WG, Bear JN, Bhoola KD. Macrodactyly in the foot. *J Bone Joint Surg Am* 1977;59:355–359.

Basics

DESCRIPTION

Malignant fibrous histiocytoma (MFH) is an uncommon, malignant, primary mesenchymal tumor of soft tissue or bone that resembles fibrosarcoma. In primary MFH of bone, the long bones are most commonly affected. Any age can be affected, but the tumor mainly occurs in the fifth to seventh decades. There is no real sex predominance. Both of the largest series show a slight male predominance.

SYNONYM

Malignant (fibrous) histiocytoma

GENETICS

No known correlation exists.

INCIDENCE

This is an uncommon primary bone tumor. In the Mayo Clinic (Rochester, MN) files, there are 83 cases of MFH in 8,591 primary bone tumors. In contrast, MFH is the most common soft tissue sarcoma in adults.

CAUSES

The cause is unknown.

RISK FACTORS

This tumor may arise as a complication of pre-existing bone disease, such as Paget's disease, within a bone infarct, or from radiation. Up to one-fourth of cases are believed to be secondary.

CLASSIFICATION

Several subtypes have been described, but typing has not been shown to have prognostic implications.

ICD-9-CM

171.3 Malignant fibrous histiocytoma

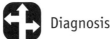 Diagnosis

SIGNS AND SYMPTOMS

- Identical to other primary bone tumors
- Insidious onset with slow progression
- Symptoms including pain and swelling, which is slowly worsening
- Patients often symptomatic for 6 months or longer before diagnosis

DIFFERENTIAL DIAGNOSIS

- Metastatic disease
- Myeloma
- Lymphoma
- Other primary mesenchymal tumors
- Ewing's sarcoma
- Osteosarcoma
- Fibrosarcoma

PHYSICAL EXAMINATION

The physical examination may be normal or may show only subtle findings. When the tumor has penetrated the bone, a soft tissue mass may be felt. Muscle atrophy is common in the involved extremity.

LABORATORY TESTS

The serum alkaline phosphate level may be increased secondary to bone destruction.

PATHOLOGIC FINDINGS

- Grossly, these tumors appear fibrous.
- Light microscopy reveals spindle cell stroma with a characteristic "storiform pattern" (irregularly whirled).
- Histiocytes with slightly foamy cytoplasm and multinucleated giant cells are also prominent features.
- Any chondroid or osteoid matrix production by the tumor cells excludes the diagnosis of MFH.

IMAGING PROCEDURES

- Lytic bone destruction has a moth-eaten pattern. There may be reactive bone formation.
- Large lesions may show soft tissue extension or may be complicated by a pathologic fracture. Occasionally, lesions may show focal areas of calcification.

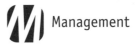 Management

GENERAL MEASURES

- MFH is typically radioresistant; however, preoperative chemotherapy may improve the surgical outcome.
- Any patient in whom the diagnosis of MFH is suspected should be referred to a musculoskeletal oncologist for further evaluation and treatment.

SURGICAL TREATMENT

In the past, amputation was the mainstay of therapy for lesions in the appendicular skeleton. With recent refinements in surgical technique, limb salvage surgery with prosthetic or allograft reconstruction is frequently an option.

PHYSICAL THERAPY

Physical therapy is used extensively after limb salvage surgery or amputation.

MEDICAL TREATMENT

Preoperative and postoperative chemotherapy is used to minimize the risk of systemic metastases.

PATIENT EDUCATION

Patients with lower extremity lesions should be limited to partial weight bearing until referral to an oncologist, to avoid the possibility of pathologic fracture.

PREVENTION

No preventive measures are known.

COMPLICATIONS

Recurrence and metastasis are the most feared complications.

RECOMMENDED READING

Huvo AC, Heilweil M, Brodsky SS. The pathology of malignant fibrous histiocytoma of bone: a study of 130 patients. *Am J Surg Pathol* 1981;9:853–871.

Krishnan Unni K. *Dahlin's bone tumors: general aspects and data on 11,087 cases,* 5th ed. Philadelphia: Lippincott–Raven, 1996:217–224.

Mallet Finger

 Basics

DESCRIPTION

Mallet finger is a loss of continuity of the conjoined lateral bands at the distal joint of the finger that results in a characteristic flexion deformity of the distal joint.

It may occur at any age. Many studies show the highest age incidence in males to be in the adolescent and young adult group (11 to 40 years), whereas in females the incidence is higher in middle age (41 to 60 years). Males are affected more often than females, but the numbers vary with the population studied. Mallet finger deformity resulting from a fracture of a child's distal phalanx is usually a transepiphyseal fracture of the phalanx.

SYNONYMS

- Drop finger
- Baseball finger

GENETICS

A familial predisposition may exist.

INCIDENCE

- Varies with the population studied
- Progressive increase in incidence from the radial to ulnar side of the hand noted.

CAUSES

Mallet finger may be secondary to a variety of sports, occupational, or home activities. Open injuries may be caused by sharp or crush-type lacerations, but closed injuries are more common. The usual mechanism of injury is sudden, acute, forceful flexion of the extended digit, which results in rupture of the extensor tendon or avulsion of the tendon with or without a small fragment of bone from its dorsal insertion. Forced hyperextension of the distal joint may result in a fracture at the dorsal base of the distal phalanx involving one-third or more of the phalanx. Although a mallet deformity is associated with this injury, the lesion should be considered a fracture with a secondary mallet finger deformity.

The microvascular anatomy of the distal digital extensor tendon reveals an area of deficient blood supply in the region of insertion over the distal interphalangeal joint (DIP), and this vascularity may have implications in the cause of mallet finger.

CLASSIFICATION

Classifications are used as an aid in establishing an appropriate treatment plan.

- Type I (most common). Closed or blunt trauma with loss of tendon continuity with or without a small avulsion fracture
- Type II. Laceration at or proximal to the DIP joint with loss of tendon continuity
- Type III. Deep abrasion with long vein subcutaneous tissue tendon
- Type IV.

—a. Transepiphyseal plate fracture in children
—b. Hyperflexion injury with fracture of the articular surface of 20% to 50%
—c. Hyperextension injury with fracture of the articular surface usually greater than 50% and with early or late volar subluxation of the distal phalanx

ICD-9-CM

736.1 Mallet finger

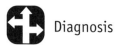 Diagnosis

SIGNS AND SYMPTOMS

- The DIP joint of the involved finger is held in flexion, and active extension is lost. Full passive extension is usually present.
- Hyperextension of the proximal interphalangeal joint may also be observed.

DIFFERENTIAL DIAGNOSIS

- Fracture of the dorsal base of the distal phalanx with secondary mallet finger deformity
- Transepiphyseal plate fracture of the distal phalanx

PHYSICAL EXAMINATION

- Document the integrity of the skin and nail bed.
- Note active and passive extension (and flexion if not acute).
- Observe the status of the proximal joints.
- Diagnosis is based on physical examination with radiographs to assess for fracture.

LABORATORY TESTS

There are no laboratory tests to aid in this diagnosis.

PATHOLOGIC FINDINGS

The lateral bands of the extensor tendon from each side of the digit merge and join to form a single tendon on the proximal portion of the middle phalanx. This tendon continues distally to form a wide unit for insertion into the dorsal base of the distal phalanx.

Loss of continuity of the conjoined lateral bands at the distal joint of the finger results in a characteristic flexion deformity of the distal joint. A study of the microvascular anatomy of the distal digital extension tendon noted an area of deficient blood supply here and suggested that this zone of avascularity could have implications in the cause and treatment of mallet finger.

IMAGING PROCEDURES

Anteroposterior and lateral radiographs of the involved finger are mandatory to assess for fracture, because this influences classification and treatment options.

Management

GENERAL MEASURES

These injuries require a minimum of 6 weeks of continuous DIP joint immobilization. Partial recurrence of the extension lag is common, and a regimen of at least 2 to 3 weeks of night splinting of the DIP joint in extension is mandatory after the continuous splint has been discontinued. Careful follow-up is required, and if recurrent extension lag is severe, a second course of full-time splinting for 8 weeks may be considered. Surgical treatment is frequently recommended for type IV injuries, but splinting is often adequate treatment.

Management of chronic mallet deformities seen late includes arthrodesis or secondary extension tendon reconstruction. Mallet deformities not seen until 2 to 3 months after injury have been improved with prolonged splinting of the distal joint. If the patient has significant symptoms, surgical options should be considered.

SURGICAL TREATMENT

The joint is reduced, the fracture fragment is manipulated into place, and a Kirschner wire is passed longitudinally across the joint, to hold it in full extension. Surgical options for chronic mallet finger include plication or reefing of the scarred tendon, arthrodesis, tenodermodesis, and even DIP disarticulation.

PHYSICAL THERAPY

Occupational therapy may benefit the patient who has a difficult time regaining flexion after the splinting is completed or the surgical Kirschner wire is removed.

MEDICAL TREATMENT

Type I

This is treated with a dorsal or volar prefabricated splint such as the stack splint. Excellent to good results can be anticipated in nearly 80% of these patients if treated early. Fair to poor results are to be anticipated in patients treated on a delayed basis or in those who wear the splints incorrectly. Continuous maintenance of the extended position of the DIP joint must be achieved for a minimum of 6 weeks for the splint to be effective. Some recommend 8 weeks of splinting, followed by 2 weeks of night splinting. Direct repair of type I injuries is to be avoided, because the extensor tendon at this level is extremely thin and has a poor blood supply. Conservative treatment of these injuries yields a more satisfactory result than operative repair. A transarticular Kirschner wire may be placed in patients who cannot

wear a splint for 6 weeks, but physical activities must be limited and a splint worn most of the time to protect the pin from breakage. Dorsal ulceration and maceration have been noted with the use of dorsal aluminum foam splints; if these splints are used, place tubular gauze or moleskin beneath the splint. Full-thickness skin necrosis over the DIP joint has been noted after dorsal splint immobilization in hyperextension. Therefore, the distal joint should be splinted with minimal hyperextension. The amount of hyperextension that produces blanching should not be exceeded.

Types I and III

Repair is done with a simple figure-of-eight or roll-type suture, which reapproximates the skin and tendon simultaneously. Apply a small dressing, incorporating a splint, which maintains the distal joint in full extension. The suture is removed in about 10 to 12 days, and the distal joint is maintained in the extended position by the stack or aluminum foam splint, as used in treatment of type I injuries.

Maintain the splint in position continuously for a minimum of 6 weeks, followed by protective range of motion. Reapply the splint if any extension loss is noted after its removal.

Type III mallet deformities with loss of tendon substance and soft tissue coverage require reconstructive surgery to provide skin coverage, with late reconstruction by free tendon graft to restore tendon continuity or arthrodesis of the joint.

Mallet finger resulting from a distal phalanx fracture in a child is usually a transepiphyseal fracture of the phalanx. Closed reduction of the fracture usually results in correction of the deformity. Continuous external splinting of the distal joint in full extension for 3 to 4 weeks results in union of the fracture and correction of the deformity.

Type IV

In an adult, type IV injuries are associated with significant fracture fragments. This type of fracture with an associated mallet finger deformity is a relatively uncommon injury. Operative treatment has been recommended for fracture fragments greater than one-third of the articular surface. An accurate reduction is advocated to prevent joint deformity with secondary arthritis and stiffness. However, excellent results have been reported with splinting alone, and nonoperative treatment avoids all potential complications of surgery. Indications for surgery are controversial and may depend on the amount of volar subluxation of the distal phalanx.

At the end of 6 to 10 weeks of continuous splinting, the patient is allowed to begin guarded flexion exercises, but the extension splint is still continued at night.

PATIENT EDUCATION

Patients should understand the importance of the continuous maintenance of the extended position of the DIP joint for a minimum of 6 weeks for the splint to be effective.

PREVENTION

- No effective means of prevention is known.
- Early detection is associated with a better prognosis.

MONITORING

A high complication rate (up to 45%) has been reported with splinting, represented mostly by transient skin problems. Most patients require two visits during the first week of treatment, and weekly visits thereafter, to monitor their progress and check their skin. At the end of 6 to 10 weeks, the splint is removed and the finger inspected. Night splinting is begun, and careful follow-up is required to monitor for recurrence and to individualize treatment as needed.

COMPLICATIONS

- Skin problems: dorsal maceration, skin ulceration, tape allergy
- Transverse nail grooves
- Pain from the splint
- More than 50% complication rate noted in patients treated surgically for mallet finger (permanent nail deformities, joint incongruities, infection, pin or pullout wire failure, radial or ulnar prominence, deviation of the DIP joint)
- Loss of surgical reduction, requiring additional surgery

PROGNOSIS

Poor prognostic factors are as follows:

- Age older than 60 years
- Delay in treatment of more than 4 weeks
- Initial active extension lag
- More than 4 weeks of immobilization
- Patients with short, stubby fingers

RECOMMENDED READING

Doyle JR. Extension tendons: acute injuries. In: Green, DP, ed. *Green's operative hand surgery.* 1993:1925–1943.

Green DP, Butler TE. Fractures and dislocations in the hand. In: Rockwood CA, Green DP, Bucholz RW, et al. *Rockwood and Green's fractures in adults,* vol 1, 4th ed. Philadelphia: Lippincott–Raven, 1996:416–419.

Marfan Syndrome

 Basics

DESCRIPTION

Marfan syndrome is a familial disorder of elastic connective tissue that is characterized by aortic root dilatation and dissection, valvular insufficiency, lens dislocation, and arachnodactyly, among other findings. It affects the cardiovascular, ocular, skeletal, and neurologic systems and has caused sudden death in several prominent basketball and volleyball players. Although the disorder is inherited at birth, some of the manifestations, such as aortic dilatation, scoliosis, and sternal deformity, take time to develop. This may cause the diagnosis to be delayed until later in childhood. Males and females are affected equally.

GENETICS

The syndrome is autosomal dominant with variable expressivity. Some patients are affected by a *de novo* mutation, and these are more likely to have severe cases or be diagnosed in the neonatal period. Even among families with high penetrance, manifestations may vary from member to member.

INCIDENCE

Approximately 1 in 10,000 persons is affected.

CAUSES

Marfan syndrome results from a defect in the fibrillin gene, which is found on chromosome 15. Multiple different deletions have been found that result in Marfan syndrome and probably explain the condition's heterogeneity. Fibrillin is found in the zonules that suspend the lens of the eye, as well as in the arterial walls. The explanation for other findings is still being sought.

RISK FACTORS

- Positive family history of Marfan syndrome
- Aortic dissection or unexplained sudden death
- Tall, slender habitus

CLASSIFICATION

- Classic Marfan syndrome
- MASS phenotype (mitral prolapse, aortic dilatation, skin and skeletal findings), which is a forme fruste of the syndrome

ICD-9-CM

759.82 Marfan syndrome

 Diagnosis

The diagnosis is made mainly by clinical criteria. The patient must have at least two systems involved, at least one major criterion (ascending aortic enlargement or dissection, ectopia lentis, dural ectasia), or four skeletal findings.

SIGNS AND SYMPTOMS

Symptoms

- Relatively few; rarely the means for diagnosis
- Delay in walking or coordination, fatiguability, poor vision, chest pain (at aortic dissection)
- Dislocations of knees or shoulders (rare)

Signs

- Tendency to tall stature
- Long limbs in relation to the trunk
- Scoliosis
- Kyphosis
- Multiple foot deformities
- Pectus excavatum or carinatum
- Slender cranium
- Joint hypermobility, which is usually moderate and is considerably less than in Ehlers-Danlos syndrome
- Often, a positive thumb sign, in which the clenched thumb protrudes beyond the ulnar border of the closed fist

DIFFERENTIAL DIAGNOSIS

- Congenital contractural arachnodactyly (caused by a fibrillin defect coded on chromosome 5), which is distinguished by multiple joint contractures in the presence of arachnodactyly
- Stickler's syndrome (hereditary arthroophthalmopathy)
- Homocystinuria (characterized by mental delay and inferior dislocation of the lens)
- Ehlers-Danlos syndrome (generalized ligamentous laxity more extreme than in Marfan syndrome, with more cutaneous laxity)
- MASS phenotype
- Familial aortic dissection

PHYSICAL EXAMINATION

- Measure the patient's height. The upper-to-lower segment ratio (head to symphysis over symphysis to floor) is less than 0.85.
- Check for kyphosis, scoliosis, and pectus deformity.
- Thumb and wrist signs should be sought.
- Leg length inequality should also be assessed.
- Slit-lamp examination by an experienced ophthalmologist is also helpful in making the diagnosis and in following the patient's course.

LABORATORY TESTS

Results of routine laboratory tests are normal, but genetic testing for mutations in fibrillin is now available. False-negative results are still possible with this test.

PATHOLOGIC FINDINGS

The aortic root shows dissection of the medial layer in some patients. The dura of the lower lumbar spine sometimes shows dilatation and saclike protrusions from the sides and front of the spinal canal.

IMAGING PROCEDURES

- Echocardiography is key to assessing main structures at risk in this syndrome, the heart valves and ascending aorta. This test should be performed as a baseline at time of diagnosis and periodically afterward, according to the judgment of the cardiologist.
- Magnetic resonance imaging is useful for imaging entire aorta. It also can be used to evaluate spine for dural ectasia or neural impingement.
- Plain radiographs of the spine are adequate for diagnosis of scoliosis, if it is suspected. Patients with aching or pain in the hip should also have an anteroposterior radiograph of the pelvis to rule out protrusio acetabuli, which is an excessive deepening of the hip sockets.
- Plain films of the hands can be used to calculate a metacarpal index, but this is not specific and is not clinically necessary.

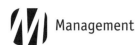 Management

GENERAL MEASURES

- Medication for aortic dilatation
- Support group in the United States: National Marfan Foundation, Port Washington NY (tel. 800-4-MARFAN)
- Genetic counseling

SURGICAL TREATMENT

- Spinal fusion is occasionally indicated for severe scoliosis or kyphosis. This involves correction with rods and bone graft for fusion.
- Spinal fusion is sometimes indicated for severe or symptomatic spondylolisthesis of L-5 on S-1.
- Hip replacement is occasionally indicated for arthritis related to protrusio acetabuli.
- Aortic root and valve replacement with a composite graft are indicated when the dilatation reaches a certain size; this is highly successful and is preferable to waiting for aortic dissection to occur!

ACTIVITY

Persons with Marfan syndrome should keep active, but they should avoid high-impact or high-stress sports. A cardiologist should be consulted if there are specific questions.

PHYSICAL THERAPY

- May help an infant who is significantly delayed in walking or other motor milestones
- Also useful as part of a conservative program for back pain

MEDICAL TREATMENT

- Periodic cardiology follow-up is done with ultrasound, as indicated. If aortic enlargement is suspected, a beta-2 blocking drug may be started to minimize pressure in the aorta; this has been shown to be effective in clinical trials.
- Patients should avoid sports that cause high impact or cardiac stress.
- Bracing or surgery for spinal deformities may occasionally be appropriate.
- Procedures to deal with a partially dislocated lens or a retinal detachment are available.
- Atenolol is the beta-2 blocker most commonly used for this syndrome.
- No current drug or therapy can correct the basic defect in fibrillin.

PATIENT EDUCATION

- Describe the warning signs of aortic dissection and retinal detachment.
- Stress the importance of taking beta blockers, when prescribed.
- Offer genetic counseling.
- There is evidence that the risk of aortic dissection or critical dilatation may be decreased by cardioselective beta blockade.

MONITORING

- Coordinate care by a geneticist and a cardiologist.
- See other specialists seen as needed.
- Routine checkups may prevent catastrophes.

COMPLICATIONS

- Aortic dissection
- Valvular insufficiency
- Retinal detachment
- Spontaneous pneumothorax

PROGNOSIS

Without modern cardiovascular management, the life expectancy for patients with this condition would be less than 50 years. Now, this can be significantly prolonged, and many patients live into or past the seventh decade.

RECOMMENDED READING

De Paepe A, Devereux RB, Dietz HC, et al. Revised diagnostic criteria for the Marfan syndrome. *Am J Med Genet* 1996;62:417–426.

Finkbohner R, Johnston DJ, Crawford S, et al. Marfan syndrome: long-term survival and complications after aortic aneurysm repair. *Circulation* 1995;91:728–733.

Pyeritz RE. The Marfan syndrome. In: Royce PM, Steinmann B, eds. *Connective tissue and its heritable disorders*. New York: Wiley–Liss, 1993:437–460.

Medial Collateral Ligament Injury

 Basics

DESCRIPTION

Medial collateral ligament injury is a disruption of the medial collateral ligament of the knee, which is the primary restraint to valgus stress on the knee. It occurs commonly, in teenagers and young adults, and equally among men and women.

CAUSES

The cause is overload of the ligament with valgus overload.

RISK FACTORS

- Contact sports
- Falls

CLASSIFICATION

This injury is classified as follows (Fig. 1):

   I. Microscopic strain
  II. Partial tear
 III. Complete tear

ICD-9-CM

844.1 Medial collateral ligament

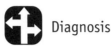 Diagnosis

SIGNS AND SYMPTOMS

- Pain is felt along the medial aspect of the knee, typically extending proximally and distally along the region of the medial collateral ligament.
- Knee effusion is possible.
- This injury is associated with an anterior cruciate ligament tear as well as a medial meniscus tear.
- Patients also complain of increased pain with valgus loading.
- Patients occasionally recall a "pop" or "snap" at the time of the injury.

DIFFERENTIAL DIAGNOSIS

- Anterior cruciate ligament rupture
- Medial meniscal tears
- Posterior cruciate ligament rupture
- Tibial plateau fractures
- Tibial spine avulsions

PHYSICAL EXAMINATION

- Medial collateral ligament ruptures are frequently associated with other injuries; physical examination and diagnostic workup should reflect a high suspicion for adult injuries.
- Test the stability of the medial collateral ligament by flexing the patient's knee 30 degrees and applying a valgus force (Fig. 2). An estimate of the degree of opening and the character of the end point (soft, solid) should be attained.
- Perform a complete neurovascular examination distal to the knee.
- Perform Lachman's test and the posterior drawer test to rule out associated anterior or posterior cruciate ligament injury.
- Examine the contralateral knee for comparison.

IMAGING PROCEDURES

- Anteroposterior and lateral plain radiographs should be obtained initially to rule out fractures.
- Magnetic resonance imaging is an appropriate study because of its sensitivity to other ligamentous or meniscal disease.

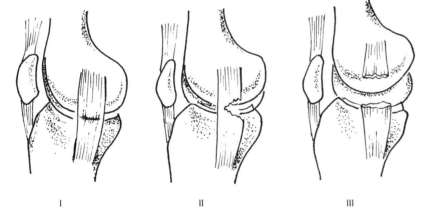

      I   II   III

Fig. 1. Medial collateral ligament injuries may be graded as follows: I (microscopic strain), II partial tear, or III complete tear.

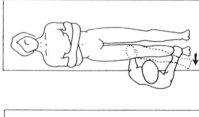
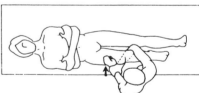

Fig. 2. Examination for collateral ligament injuries. Applying valgus stress.

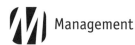 Management

GENERAL MEASURES

Combined medial collateral ligament and anterior cruciate ligament injuries have had high success rates with hinged bracing, hamstring or quadriceps strengthening, and anterior cruciate ligament reconstruction without medial collateral ligament repair.

SURGICAL TREATMENT

Chronic medial collateral ligament tears unresponsive to conservative treatment need surgical augmentation or advancement.

PHYSICAL THERAPY

After ligament healing, begin range of motion and quadriceps strengthening exercises.

MEDICAL TREATMENT

- Hinged bracing
- Non-weight bearing with braced early range of motion
- Analgesics

PATIENT EDUCATION

Most medial collateral ligament injuries heal completely without surgery. Patients are instructed in range-of-motion and quadriceps strengthening exercises.

PREVENTION

Prevention is best accomplished through careful conditioning before sport activities.

MONITORING

- Adequate initial radiographs are obtained.
- Patients are followed at 4 to 6 weeks to check range of motion and quadriceps strength.
- Repeat radiographs if symptoms persist.

PROGNOSIS

Most patients with medial collateral ligament injuries respond to nonoperative treatment (bracing and early range of motion). Prophylactic bracing should be considered for patients returning to contact sports.

RECOMMENDED READING

Indelicato PA, Hermansdorter J, Huegel M, et al. Nonoperative management of complete tears of the medial collateral ligament of the knee in intercollegiate football player. *Clin Orthop* 1990;256:174–177.

Shelbourne KD, Nitz PA. The O'Donoghue triad revisited: combined injuries involving the anterior cruciate and medial collateral ligament tears. *Am J Sports Med* 1991;19:474–477.

Meniscus Tear

 Basics

DESCRIPTION

A meniscus tear is an acute or degenerative injury to the meniscal fibrocartilage of the knee. Acute tears occur mainly in adolescents and young adults, and degenerative tears predominate in the 40- to 60-year-old population. These injuries occur equally in males and females.

GENETICS

No mendelian inheritance is known.

INCIDENCE

- Acute tears in one study reported to be 61 in 100,000
- Degenerative tears in 60% of cadavers at age 65 years
- Sports-related injuries accounting for one-third of acute tears
- Eighty to 90% rate of associated anterior cruciate ligament tear with acute injury
- Medial tears more frequent than lateral meniscal tears

CAUSES

- Acute: often during athletic activities, most commonly football, basketball, and wrestling, usually after twisting injury or rapid change in motion at the knee, often associated with anterior ligament disruption
- Degenerative: chronic breakdown of collagen fibers, often associated with arthritis

RISK FACTORS

Sports participation is a risk factor.

CLASSIFICATION

Acute Tear

- Longitudinal (50% to 90%)
- Radial (6%)
- Flap (4%)

Degenerative Tear

- Mostly horizontal cleavage or complex tears

ASSOCIATED CONDITION

Ligamentous injury (anterior cruciate ligament, collateral ligaments) in acute tears

ICD-9-CM

836.2 Meniscus tear

 Diagnosis

SIGNS AND SYMPTOMS

- Pain localized to the joint line or popliteal region with knee flexion
- Possible popping, locking, or buckling with large, unstable tears
- Examination often noting knee effusion, tenderness at joint line, and pain at terminal flexion or extension
- With a displaced bucket-handle tear, possible locking of the joint that blocks full extension

DIFFERENTIAL DIAGNOSIS

- Discoid lateral meniscus (adolescent population)
- Osteochondral fracture
- Osteonecrosis
- Anterior cruciate ligament tear
- Collateral ligament tear
- Osteoarthritis
- Malignant disease

PHYSICAL EXAMINATION

- Assess knee stability and rule out hip disease during the examination.
- Palpate for joint line tenderness; rotate the leg back and forth to feel for a palpable click.
- McMurray's test: External rotation with valgus stress. Bring the knee from flexion to extension and feel for "pop" in the posterolateral corner of the knee. Flex the knee; check external rotation of the leg (medial meniscus); check internal rotation of the leg (lateral meniscus); slowly extend the knee and palpate for a click.
- Apley's grind test: The patient is prone; internally and externally rotate the leg with traction and compression.

PATHOLOGIC FINDINGS

- The meniscus is only well vascularized in the anteroposterior horns and the peripheral third.
- Tears in inner two-thirds heal poorly, owing to the lack of blood supply.
- Collagen fibers are oriented circumferentially with interposed proteoglycan and are resistant to compressive forces; they may tear under shear stresses.
- Degeneration from repeated microtrauma occurs, with gradual loss of collagen and integrity that leads to tears.

IMAGING PROCEDURES

- Plain radiographs (anteroposterior and lateral) to rule out fractures
- Double-contrast arthrography: 60% to 97% accurate (seldom done with refinement of magnetic resonance imaging [MRI])
- MRI: 90% to 98% accurate; can give a high rate of false-positive results
- Grades I to IV, with III and higher representing significant injury

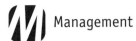 Management

GENERAL MEASURES

Partial-thickness splits, degenerative tears in a knee with osteoarthritis, and stable tears that displace less than 3 to 5 mm when they are probed should be left alone at arthroscopy.

SURGICAL TREATMENT

- Nearly all treatments are now performed arthroscopically.
- Complex tears and those in the avascular zone are resected.
- Vertical longitudinal tears within 5 mm of the meniscocapsular junction are repaired.
- Repairs fare better when they are done simultaneously with needed anterior cruciate ligament reconstructions.
- Total meniscectomy is not recommended, owing to the increased risk of degenerative arthritis.

PHYSICAL THERAPY

After meniscal repair, initiate a gradual strengthening program, limiting deep squats for 3 to 6 months with eventual sports-specific activities and return to sports after 5 to 6 months.

MEDICAL TREATMENT

Begin with a trial of rest and protected weight bearing, often with a knee immobilizer (2 to 4 weeks) for acute injuries. If there is significant locking, obtain urgent arthroscopy or MRI. In patients with degenerative changes or in older patients, consider intraarticular injection and nonoperative treatment for 6 weeks. If the patient remains symptomatic, offer MRI or arthroscopic evaluation and treatment. Drugs of choice are analgesics or nonsteroidal antiinflammatory drugs.

PATIENT EDUCATION

- Braces are rarely needed, except for a knee immobilizer in the acute period.
- Weight bearing is allowed as tolerated after partial meniscectomy or arthroscopy alone.
- Patients often return to full activities in 2 to 3 weeks.
- Partial weight bearing and limited motion are allowed after meniscal repair.

MONITORING

Patients are checked at 4- to 6-week intervals to monitor range of motion and quadriceps rehabilitation.

COMPLICATIONS

Complications are uncommon, but they include the following:

- Injury to neurovascular structures (infrapatellar branch of saphenous nerve, causing pain, dysesthesias at the portal site)
- Infection
- Deep venous thrombosis
- Arthritis

PROGNOSIS

- Degenerative tears often improve with partial meniscectomies, and 93% of repaired menisci were clinically stable when studied on follow-up.
- Partial meniscectomy is effective in relieving pain and mechanical blocking from tears in the avascular regions.

RECOMMENDED READING

Andrish JT. Meniscal injuries in children and adolescents: diagnosis and management. *J Am Acad Orthop Surg* 1996;4:231–237.

DeLee JC, Drez D Jr, eds. *Orthopaedic sports medicine: principles and practice,* vol 2. Philadelphia: WB Saunders, 1994:1146–1162.

Hardin GT, Farr J, Bach BR Jr. Meniscal tears: diagnosis, evaluation and treatment. *Orthop Rev* 1992;21:1311–1317.

Weiss CB, Lundberg M, Hamburg P, et al. Nonoperative treatment of meniscal tears. *J Bone Joint Surg Am* 1989;71:811–822.

Metacarpal Fracture

 Basics

DESCRIPTION

This is a fracture of the metacarpal bone, the small tubular bone in the hand.

SYNONYMS

- Boxer's fracture
- Bennett's fracture
- Rolando's fracture

INCIDENCE

- Metacarpal fractures account for 1.6% of fractures evaluated in emergency departments.
- In males, the greatest incidence is in patients aged 10 to 39 years.
- In females, the greatest incidence is in those 50 to 60 years old.
- The male-to-female ratio is 2:1.

CAUSES

Mechanisms of metacarpal fractures include direct trauma and crush injuries, but most occur from axial loading applied at the metacarpal head. A common injury, the boxer's fracture, is a fracture of the fifth metacarpal neck sustained while striking the fifth metacarpophalangeal (MCP) joint of the clenched fist against an opponent.

RISK FACTORS

In extremely young and old patients, the increased incidence of falls increases the percentage of these fractures.

CLASSIFICATION

These fractures are classified according to their anatomic location. They may be at the head (intraarticular), neck, base, or along the shaft. Metacarpal fractures of the thumb constitute 25% of all metacarpal fractures, second in frequency only to that of the fifth digit. In the thumb, 80% of metacarpal fractures occur at the base. These are classified into four patterns, according to whether they are intraarticular or extraarticular.

Type I. Bennett's fracture, in which the fracture line creates a volar lip fragment at the carpometacarpal joint of variable size, and the remainder of the base is displaced from the joint.

Type II. Rolando's fracture classically involves a dorsal lip fragment in addition to the volar fragment. There may be more comminution, to create more than three fracture fragments.

Type III. Extraarticular fractures of the first metacarpal base are often transverse or oblique.

Type IV. Fractures of the base of the first metacarpal involve the growth plate in children.

ASSOCIATED CONDITIONS

Conditions that cause a propensity for falls and decreased bone mass are associated with these injuries.

ICD-9-CM

815.00 Metacarpal fracture

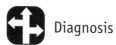 Diagnosis

SIGNS AND SYMPTOMS

- The combination of history, physical examination, and radiographic views is nearly always diagnostic.
- Pain and swelling are mainly demonstrated in the dorsum of the hand.
- Malrotated digits may also be evident on physical examination.

DIFFERENTIAL DIAGNOSIS

- Dislocation of the MCP joint
- Extensor or flexor tendon injury
- Contusion or soft tissue trauma

PHYSICAL EXAMINATION

- Patients present with pain, swelling, and deformity at the location of the fracture.
- Assess the shortening and malrotation of the affected digit.
- Document the neurologic examination with two-point discrimination, as well as capillary refill.
- Examine any break in the skin to ensure that the fracture is not open or that an intraarticular injury did not occur.

LABORATORY TESTS

There are no laboratory tests to aid in the diagnosis.

PATHOLOGIC FINDINGS

The findings are typical for bone fractures:

- Disruption of the bone cortex and periosteum
- Hematoma formation
- Later callus formation with eventual healing

IMAGING PROCEDURES

Obtain anteroposterior, lateral, and oblique plain radiographic views. Coned-down views on the expected metacarpal can give better detail of the fracture pattern.

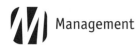 Management

GENERAL MEASURES

As with any fracture, one must determine whether it is open or closed. (Is there a skin wound such that the outside environment communicates with the fracture site?) Additionally, the neurovascular status of the affected extremity must be documented before and after any manipulation is performed. Open fractures are treated with operative irrigation and débridement and pin fixation.

Most often, metacarpal fractures can be treated by splinting and casting, unless the fracture pattern is unstable, intraarticular, or including multiple digits. Other reasons for operative repair include the inability to obtain a satisfactory reduction including malrotation of the digits.

SURGICAL TREATMENT

• Treatment of metacarpal fractures includes the use of pins, plates, and screws or a combination of all.
• Oblique and spiral fractures of the shaft, intraarticular fractures, and open fractures typically require surgery.
• Fractures with significant bone loss, such as a gunshot wound, occasionally require an external fixator to be placed.

PHYSICAL THERAPY

Gentle active and passive range-of-motion exercises typically can be performed.

MEDICAL TREATMENT

The metacarpal fracture should be reduced and splinted or casted. The patient should be instructed about the possibility of surgery if the fracture reduction cannot be maintained with splinting. Ice, elevation, and analgesics are important adjuvants in the initial treatment. The hand should be splinted with the wrist in approximately 20 degrees of dorsal angulation and the MCP joints of both the affected and adjacent finger at 70 to 90 degrees of flexion. The proximal and distal interphalangeal joints are kept in full extension. Reasonable guidelines to permissible apex-dorsal angulation of the fractures are 10 degrees for index, 20 degrees for middle, 30 degrees for ring, and 40 degrees for the small fingers. Rotatory displacements in general are not acceptable and require further treatment. Intra-articular fractures need to be anatomically reduced. Most metacarpal fractures heal by 4 weeks.

PATIENT EDUCATION

• Intra-articular fractures have a higher incidence of stiffness and pain after healing.
• Early range-of-motion activities are begun when the fracture is stable.

MONITORING

• Obtain radiographs 1 week after closed or open reduction, and repeat in another 2 to 3 weeks.
• Begin early motion when appropriate.

COMPLICATIONS

• Soft tissue damage results from the initial injury or secondary to overzealous reduction attempts.
• Flexor or extensor tendons may be damaged or develop decreased excursion.
• Malunion is another complication, with rotation the worst.
• MCP stiffness is the result of immobilizing the joint in extension and allowing the collateral ligaments to shorten.
• Surgical complications include infection, delayed wound healing, and sensory nerve injury.

PROGNOSIS

• The prognosis is good to excellent.
• Comminuted intra-articular fractures have the worst prognosis, with subsequent joint pain and decreased function.
• Otherwise, near-anatomic position offers nearly normal to normal strength, mobility, and function.

RECOMMENDED READING

Green DP, Butler TE. Fractures & dislocations of the hand. In: Rockwood CA, Green D eds: *Rockwood & Green's fractures in adults*. Philadelphia: Lippincott–Raven, 1996:658–674.

Metatarsal Fracture

 Basics

DESCRIPTION

These are fractures of the forefoot. They occur in both sexes at all ages.

SYNONYMS

- Jones' fracture
- Pseudo-Jones' fracture
- March fracture

INCIDENCE

These injuries are common, especially fifth metatarsal fractures in athletes.

CAUSES

The injury is usually a result of a direct blow, inversion injury, or overuse.

RISK FACTORS

Stress fractures of the metatarsals occur with excessive training or repetitive stress in athletes or with a sudden increase in the level of exercise of any person.

CLASSIFICATION

- These are classified as metatarsal head, neck, or shaft fractures.
- Stress (march) fractures most commonly involve the second metatarsal and result from repetitive overuse.
- Fifth metatarsal fractures can be further subdivided into the following: avulsion fractures (pseudo-Jones' fractures), which are proximal to the region of the fourth to fifth intermetatarsal articulation; Jones' fractures, which are located within the region of the fourth to fifth intermetatarsal articulation; and diaphyseal stress fractures, which are distal to this juncture.

ASSOCIATED CONDITION

Compartment syndrome (rarely)

ICD-9-CM

825.25 Fracture of metatarsal bones

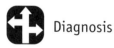 Diagnosis

SIGNS AND SYMPTOMS

- Pain
- Swelling
- Deformity
- Ecchymosis
- Difficulty bearing weight
- Tenderness over the affected metatarsals

DIFFERENTIAL DIAGNOSIS

- Soft tissue contusion
- Sprain
- Lisfranc's dislocation

PHYSICAL EXAMINATION

Physical examination usually reveals point tenderness over the involved metatarsal. Severe swelling of the entire forefoot commonly occurs.

LABORATORY TESTS

There are no laboratory tests to aid in the diagnosis.

PATHOLOGIC FINDINGS

- Different stages of bone healing may be seen with metatarsal fractures.
- Long-standing fractures may show signs of delayed union or nonunion.

IMAGING PROCEDURES

Plain films are usually diagnostic. Anteroposterior, lateral, and oblique projections are mandatory. Alignment in the lateral film is the most important aspect in management of these injuries. If plain radiographs are inconclusive, bone scanning or magnetic resonance imaging may be helpful.

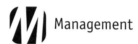 Management

GENERAL MEASURES

Isolated metatarsal neck or shaft fractures can be treated with a well fitted short leg cast and weight-bearing as tolerated for 4 to 6 weeks until healed. Injuries with multiple metatarsal fractures are often unstable and require open reduction and internal fixation with small fragment plates or Kirschner wires. Metatarsal head fractures are rare, and if they are unstable after reduction, they may require open reduction and internal fixation.

SURGICAL TREATMENT

- Open reduction and internal fixation of metatarsal fractures are done through a dorsal incision with one-third tubular plates and 3.5-mm cortical screws on the tension side.
- Other techniques involve intramedullary fixation with Kirschner wires extending out the distal tip of the toe.
- Jones' fractures may be treated with open reduction and internal fixation with a long intramedullary malleolar screw, owing to the increased tendency to nonunion.
- Nonunions should be treated with bone grafting.

PHYSICAL THERAPY

Once healed, patients usually have little difficulty in returning to activities of daily living.

MEDICAL TREATMENT

- Most metatarsal shaft and neck fractures can be treated conservatively with a walking cast or a postoperative shoe. However, if angulation is greater than 10 degrees, closed reduction may be required. The most important alignment is the sagittal alignment, because malunion in this plane may cause metatarsalgia, transfer metatarsalgia, or pain on the dorsum of the foot. Displacement in the transverse plane is usually well tolerated, although this may cause a painful neuroma or difficulty with shoe wear.
- Recommended drugs are pain medications of choice initially. Avoid nonsteroidal antiinflammatory drugs.
- Closed management consists of 4 to 6 weeks of a short leg walking cast.
- Patients with Jones' fractures that are treated closed should remain non–weight bearing for 8 weeks.
- Diaphyseal stress fractures may take longer to heal.
- Patients with Jones' fractures treated by open reduction with internal fixation can be gradually advanced in weight bearing after 2 weeks.
- Avulsion fracture of the fifth metatarsal can be cared for symptomatically with a postoperative (wooden-soled) shoe only.
- Patients with march fractures (stress fractures) need activity modification and protection in a cast or orthosis.

PATIENT EDUCATION

Patients should be warned about the risks of nonunion and possible metatarsalgia.

PREVENTION

- Avoid foot trauma.
- Modify training regimens.

MONITORING

Follow-up radiographs should show callus and healing of the metatarsal fractures. Clinically, the patient should no longer be tender over the fracture site when healed. Follow-up radiographs should be performed 1 week after reduction to ensure satisfactory alignment, and a second set should be obtained 4 to 5 weeks after injury.

COMPLICATIONS

- Transfer metatarsalgia
- Neuroma
- Delayed union
- Nonunion
- Difficulty with shoe wear

PROGNOSIS

The prognosis is good if there is no significant sagittal displacement at the time of healing.

RECOMMENDED READING

Rockwood CA, Green DP. In: *Fractures and dislocations of the foot.* Philadelphia: JB Lippincott, 1984:1807–1814.

Basics

DESCRIPTION

Metatarsus adductus is a deformity in which the forepart of the foot is adducted or medially deviated (Fig. 1). The heel is in neutral or mild valgus position. This is the most common foot condition seen by those caring for children. It appears in the newborn and is equally distributed between males and females.

SYNONYMS

- Metatarsus varus
- Pes varus
- Metatarsus internus
- Pes varus
- Hooked forefoot; Z-foot or C-foot

GENETICS

The risk is increased for those with first-degree relatives who have metatarsus adductus.

INCIDENCE

The incidence is 1 to 10 per 1,000 infants.

CAUSES

- Unknown
- No association with birth order, gestational age, or maternal age
- Most accepted theory: metatarsus adductus a possible result of tight intrauterine packing

RISK FACTORS

- Family history
- Hip dysplasia

CLASSIFICATION

- Types of feet: flexible (correctable with manipulation) or rigid
- Degree of deformity: mild, moderate, or severe, based on heel bisector method (The line bisecting the heel is drawn by visual examination of the sole of the foot. It normally crosses between second and third toes.)

—Mild heel bisector crosses the third toe.
—Moderate: heel bisector crosses between third and fourth toes.
—Severe: heel bisector crosses between fourth and fifth toes.

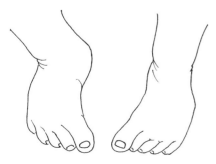

Fig. 1. Metatarsus adductus is characterized by a deviated forefoot but a normal hind foot and ankle.

ASSOCIATED CONDITION

Developmental dysplasia of the hip occurs in 1% to 5% of patients with metatarsus adductus.

ICD-9-CM

754.53 Metatarsus adductus

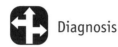

Diagnosis

SIGNS AND SYMPTOMS

- Adduction (medial deviation) of the forefoot, with various degrees of supination. One sees concave medial border and convex lateral border of the foot, with prominence at the base of the fifth metatarsal.
- The heel is in neutral or slightly valgus position, but not in equinus (foot-drop).
- The flexible deformity may persist until 1 to 2 years of age.
- Most feet (86% in one study) become normal, 10% are mildly adducted, and 4% remain stiff and deformed without treatment.
- A deep medial crease suggests moderate deformity.

DIFFERENTIAL DIAGNOSIS

- Clubfoot: heel varus and foot equinus

—More rigid
—Whole foot turned inward

PHYSICAL EXAMINATION

The flexibility of the forefoot adduction should be determined by trying to correct it. The ankle range of motion should be determined. The forefoot is medially deviated but is flexible. The hind foot is normal, and the foot may be dorsiflexed to a flat position. The hips should also be checked.

PATHOLOGIC FINDINGS

All structures of the foot are normal, just medially deviated.

IMAGING PROCEDURES

- Radiographic evaluation of most patients is unnecessary.
- If congenital anomalies are suspected or the foot is stiff, anteroposterior and lateral views of foot should be obtained.

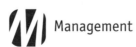

Management

GENERAL MEASURES

This condition resolves spontaneously in most patients. Parents should be educated about this deformity.

SURGICAL TREATMENT

Surgery is an option, but it is rarely indicted and then only for children older than 4 years of age who have residual metatarsus adductus. Fewer than 1% of children require surgery. Procedures include the following:

- Multiple metatarsal osteotomies
- Lateral shortening osteotomy
- Medial cuneiform opening wedge osteotomy

PHYSICAL THERAPY

Stretching of the foot is recommended for patients with a flexible deformity. This may be done by parents during diaper changes.

MEDICAL TREATMENT

Most children with metatarsus adductus at birth do not require treatment. For severe deformity, serial manipulation and casting may be offered. The appropriate age to start casting is between 6 months and 1 year. The duration of cast treatment is several months. Children may be placed in straight- or reverse-last shoes for several months after the foot is straightened by cast treatment. Because most of these cases improve spontaneously, early cast treatment before 6 months is not recommended. Patients may participate in weight-bearing activity as tolerated.

PATIENT EDUCATION

Stress the benign nature of this condition. Even if a mild degree of adduction persists, it has no functionally negative consequences.

PREVENTION

There is no effective means of preventing this deformity.

MONITORING

Frequency of follow-up varies by the individual. It should be more frequent in patients with moderate and severe deformity and in those undergoing treatment.

COMPLICATIONS

- Failure to correct the deformity completely (uncommon)
- Avascular necrosis of the cuneiform

PROGNOSIS

More than 95% patients with mild and moderate deformity have done well in long-term, follow-up studies. Patients with severe and rigid deformities that require surgery do less well; one study reported a 41% failure rate.

RECOMMENDED READING

Cook DA, Breed AL, Cook T. Observer variability in the radiographic measurement and classification of metatarsus adductus. *J Pediatr Orthop* 1992;12:86–89.

Farsetti P, Weinstein SL, Ponseti IV. The long-term functional and radiographic outcomes of untreated and non-operatively treated metatarsus adductus. *J Bone Joint Surg Am* 1994;76:257–265.

Monteggia Fracture

 Basics

DESCRIPTION

Because the radius and ulna are bound by ligaments and an interosseous membrane, a displaced fracture of the ulna is often accompanied by dislocation of the radial head (Fig. 1). The different types reflect different directions of dislocation. The diagnosis is sometimes missed. Reduction of both the fracture and the dislocation must be achieved.

Peak incidence is between the ages of 4 and 10 years. However, this lesion may occur at any age, including adulthood. Males are more commonly affected because they have a generally increased fracture rate.

INCIDENCE

• These injuries are relatively uncommon and comprise approximately 0.05% of all fractures in children.
• In children, the proximal radioulnar joint is more commonly disrupted in association with an ulnar fracture.
• In adults, the distal radioulnar joint is more commonly disrupted.

CAUSES

The ligamentous connections between the radius and ulna cause the radial head dislocation to occur when the ulna fractures, or vice versa. The mechanism of the common type I fracture is either hyperpronation or hyperextension. The mechanism of type II fractures is axial loading of a partially flexed elbow.

RISK FACTORS

Any child or adult with a fracture of the proximal or middle of the ulnar shaft should be considered at risk for this fracture, and the radiograph should be made to show the joint above (elbow) as well as the fracture itself and the joint below (wrist). This also includes greenstick fractures and plastic deformation (bowing).

CLASSIFICATION

Bado's classification, the most commonly used, is based on the direction of the dislocation of the radial head. This is also the same as the direction of the apex of the ulnar fracture.

Type I. Anterior dislocation of the radial head; most common type
Type II. Posterior dislocation of the radial head
Type III. Lateral dislocation of the radial head; second most common pattern in childhood
Type IV. Anterior dislocation of the radial head in combination with a proximal radial fracture

ICD-9-CM

813.03 Closed Monteggia fracture
813.13 Open Monteggia fracture

 Diagnosis

SIGNS AND SYMPTOMS

Signs

• Swelling both in forearm and elbow
• In cases diagnosed late, a bump possibly present over the elbow at the time a cast is removed for treatment of an ulnar fracture, indicating the dislocated radial head

Symptoms

• Acutely, tenderness over the elbow, as well as the more obvious fracture
• If diagnosed late, the unreduced radial head possibly blocking the full range of flexion or extension or causing clicking with pronation and supination

DIFFERENTIAL DIAGNOSIS

• An isolated ulnar fracture may occur without radial head dislocation.
• The status of the radial head may be determined by drawing a line through the radial shaft. This line should fall in the center of the capitellum of the distal humerus.
• An isolated radial head dislocation may occur but is rare.
• Congenital dislocation of the radial head does occur. This may be distinguished by changes in the shape of the radial head: overgrowth and loss of the normal concave reciprocal articular surface.

PHYSICAL EXAMINATION

In acute cases, diagnosis should be made primarily by radiography showing both the ulnar fracture and the radial head dislocation. In chronic cases, one sees a prominence of the radial head when the arm is out of the cast. This represents the dislocated radial head and may be compared with the opposite side.

PATHOLOGIC FINDINGS

At the time of injury, the annular ligament of the radius is torn and has become infolded. If the radial head is left out after several years, it becomes degenerated as the cartilage becomes worn away.

IMAGING PROCEDURES

Plain radiographs are sufficient for diagnosis. All forearm fractures should include visualization of the elbow joint and the wrist joint. These should be true anteroposterior and lateral shots. If they cannot be obtained on the same film, separate films should be ordered of these regions. The physician should be available to help in positioning if needed.

Magnetic resonance imaging is not required for diagnosis of these lesions.

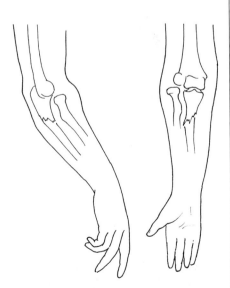

Fig. 1. An angulated, isolated ulna fracture causes the radial head to dislocate. This combination is called Monteggia fracture.

⍟ Management

GENERAL MEASURES

• Closed reduction is usually successful for children to treat both the dislocated radial head and the ulnar fracture.
• Open reduction is needed for adults.
• Patients should be given the usual directions about fracture care.
• Follow-up should be performed in 1 week.
• If Monteggia fracture is detected late (after 1 week), then the radial head may require open reduction even in children.
• If it is detected later than 3 weeks after injury, a reconstruction of the annular ligament of the radial head may be necessary.

SURGICAL TREATMENT

In a child, closed reduction of the ulna fracture and radial head dislocation by a knowledgeable orthopaedic surgeon are usually successful. The mechanism used to reduce the ulnar fracture is also used to maintain reduction of the radial head fracture.

• Type I fractures: The forearm should be in supination to midposition, and the elbow should be in flexion of over 110 degrees.
• In type II fractures, the elbow should be in extension.
• In both cases, the radial head may require a push to place it properly. A long arm cast should be applied, and a bivalved cast should be used if there is significant swelling. A radiograph should be obtained after reduction to confirm that alignment is satisfactory. If the ulnar fracture cannot be held reduced, open reduction and internal fixation should be performed. This usually causes the radial head to become and remain located. If it is not located, then an open reduction of the radial head should be performed. This is done only if all the aforementioned measures fail, because open reduction causes a risk of stiffness.

• In adults, Monteggia fracture should be treated directly with open reduction and internal fixation of the ulna. Radial head reduction should be performed only if needed.
• In a child, internal fixation of the ulna may be done with an intramedullary rod if needed because of a failure of closed reduction.
• In an adult with an extremely proximal fracture, a plate is used more often.
• Late reconstruction of the annular ligament of the ulna is done by the Bell-Tawse technique: A strip of triceps fascia is used to reconstruct the ligament and is anchored to the ulna.
• In children, immobilization is continued for 6 weeks.
• In adults, because of a greater risk of stiffness, carefully supervised range of motion may be started earlier.

PHYSICAL THERAPY

• Therapy is often needed in adults to regain optimal motion.
• There may be a slight residual loss, but it is rarely functionally significant.
• In children, physical therapy is not needed. Parents can do the necessary exercises with them.

MEDICAL TREATMENT

• Closed reduction is usually successful for children.
• Open reduction is needed for adults.
• Patients should be given the usual directions about fracture care.
• Follow-up should be performed in 1 week.
• If Monteggia fracture is detected late (after 1 week), then the radial head will require open reduction. If it is detected later than 3 weeks after injury, reconstruction of the annular ligament of the radial head is necessary.
• Missed cases may be prevented by carefully scrutinizing the elbow joint in all patients with ulnar fracture.

PATIENT EDUCATION

At the time of initial consultation, patients should be counseled about the risk of redislocation. This will help to encourage compliance with follow-up care and exercises.

MONITORING

• The patient should be seen 1 week after injury to rule out redisplacement.
• Further follow-up should be continued until range of motion is satisfactory.

COMPLICATIONS

• Redislocation
• Stiffness
• Nerve injury (usually radial) at time of radial head dislocation, about 5% to 10%

PROGNOSIS

The prognosis is excellent with careful reduction and follow-up.

RECOMMENDED READING

Bado JL. The Monteggia lesion. *Clin Orthop* 1967;50:71–86.

Bell-Tawse AJS. The treatment of malunited anterior Monteggia fractures in children. *J Bone Joint Surg Br* 1965;47:718–723.

Stanley E, de la Garza JF. Monteggia fracture-dislocation in children. In: Rockwood CA, Wilkins KE, Beaty JH, eds: *Fractures in children*, 4th ed. Philadelphia: Lippincott–Raven, 1996:548–580.

Multiple Myeloma

 Basics

DESCRIPTION

Multiple myeloma is the most common of the plasma cell dyscrasias, usually with a monoclonal gammopathy, affecting the hematopoietic, musculoskeletal, and renal systems. The peak age is the sixth decade of life, and it is rare in patients less than 40 years of age. The male-to-female ratio is approximately 2:1.

SYNONYMS

- Myeloma
- Plasmacytoma

INCIDENCE

It affects approximately 10% of elderly patients with evidence of malignant bone disease. There are approximately 13,000 new cases in the United States each year.

CAUSES

The cause is unknown.

RISK FACTORS

Age greater than 40 years is a risk factor.

CLASSIFICATION

Plasma cell dyscrasias are classified as follows:

- Solitary myeloma
- Multiple myeloma
- Osteosclerotic myeloma

ICD-9-CM

302.0 Multiple myeloma
238.6 Solitary myeloma

 Diagnosis

SIGNS AND SYMPTOMS

- Bone pain is the most frequent complaint at the time of diagnosis, and it is usually of less than 6 months' duration.
- Constitutional symptoms of weakness, lethargy, and weight loss often occur.
- Back pain and rib pain are the two most frequent initial symptoms of disease at presentation.
- Pathologic fracture usually results in sudden-onset pain.
- Peripheral neuropathy may be present.
- A tendency toward bleeding and fever may be experienced.
- Hypercalcemia occurs in about one-third of patients.
- Monoclonal gammopathy is revealed by serum electrophoresis and immunoelectrophoresis.

DIFFERENTIAL DIAGNOSIS

- Metastatic bone disease
- Malignant lymphoma
- Fibrosarcoma

PHYSICAL EXAMINATION

- Local pain and tenderness are common.
- A palpable mass may be found, owing to extraosseous extension of the tumor or hemorrhage related to it.
- Anemia with hemoglobin is less than 12 mg/dL in two-thirds of patients.
- Elevated erythrocyte sedimentation rates are greater than 50 mm per hour in two-thirds of patients.
- Peripheral neuropathy may be detected in some patients with osteosclerotic myeloma.

LABORATORY TESTS

- Hypercalcemia is seen in one-third of cases.
- Serum creatinine levels are elevated in about 50% of patients.
- Serum electrophoresis and immunoelectrophoresis generally reveal monoclonal gammopathy.
- Bence Jones proteinuria is noted.
- Hypergammaglobulinemia may manifest itself as rouleaux formation appreciable on a peripheral blood smear.

PATHOLOGIC FINDINGS

Monoclonal plasma cells are found in the bone marrow.

IMAGING PROCEDURES

Plain film radiographs reveal multiple small, discrete, lytic lesions most commonly involving the axial skeleton (skull, spine, ribs). The surrounding bone does not show a sclerotic reaction, nor is there a periosteal reaction. Expansion of the affected bone and associated soft tissue mass are common.
Bone scanning can be helpful in detecting lesions at other sites; however, this is unpredictable because the lesions may not have increased activity. A skeletal survey to evaluate for distant involvement is often a better study.

 Management

GENERAL MEASURES

The mainstay of treatment is chemotherapy. Surgical stabilization with irradiation is used for impending or complete pathologic fractures. External-beam irradiation is used for painful lesions that do not meet the criteria for pathologic fracture.

SURGICAL TREATMENT

- This consists mostly of internal fixation for stabilization of the long bones.
- Decompression with spinal instrumentation may be necessary in patients with pathologic fractures and neurologic deficits.

MEDICAL TREATMENT

- Antiinflammatory drugs or narcotic analgesics for pain control
- Chemotherapeutics (prednisone and alkylating agents)
- Early use of crutches or a walker for painful lesions in the lower extremity to lessen the risk of fracture
- Orthopaedic surgery consultation to consider surgical stabilization
- Limited activity, according to the level of symptoms and the nature of the bony lesions
- Selected patients treated with bone marrow transplantation

MONITORING

Monitor closely for impending pathologic fractures, so appropriate surgical intervention can occur before completion of pathologic fractures. Patients undergoing chemotherapy are monitored for changes in their serum protein levels to access the response to treatment.

COMPLICATIONS

- Pathologic fractures
- Spinal stenosis with compressive myelopathy
- Renal failure
- Amyloidosis (carpal tunnel syndrome)

PROGNOSIS

Prognosis is related to the stage of the disease, with an overall median survival of 18 to 24 months. Virtually all patients eventually die of the disease. Bone marrow transplantation is currently being tried in an attempt to cure selected patients.

RECOMMENDED READING

Frassica FJ, Frassia DA, Sim FH. Advances in orthopedic surgery: myeloma of bone. St. Louis: CV Mosby, 1994:357–378.

Kyle RA. Multiple myeloma: review of 869 cases. Mayo Clin Proc 1975;50:29–40.

McCarthy EF, Frassica FJ. Pathology of bone and joint disorders. Philadelphia: WB Saunders, 1998:185–191.

Basics

DESCRIPTION

Muscular dystrophies are a group of noninflammatory inherited disorders characterized by progressive degeneration and weakness of skeletal muscle without apparent cause in the nervous system. Skeletal and cardiac muscles are affected, and there are secondary effects on lungs, skeleton, and many other systems. These conditions have been divided by clinical distribution, severity of muscle weakness, and pattern of genetic inheritance. Owing to limited space, only Duchenne's muscular dystrophy (DMD) is described in detail (Fig. 1). DMD occurs in young children and affects more boys than girls.

GENETICS

DMD is sex-linked, as is Becker-type tardive dystrophy. Other dystrophies are autosomal recessive and autosomal dominant.

INCIDENCE

- DMD occurs in 1 in 3,500 live male births.
- Becker's dystrophy occurs in about 1 in 30,000 live male births.

CAUSES

A single gene defect in the short arm of the X chromosome has been identified as being responsible for DMD and Becker's muscular dystrophy. The gene encodes the protein dystrophin, which is a component of the cell membrane cytoskeleton.

RISK FACTORS

Male gender is a risk factor.

CLASSIFICATION

- Sex-linked muscular dystrophy: DMD, Becker's, Emery-Dreifuss
- Autosomal recessive muscular dystrophy: limb-girdle, infantile fascioscapulohumeral
- Autosomal dominant muscular dystrophy: fascioscapulohumeral, distal, ocular, oculopharyngeal

ICD-9-CM

359.1 Duchenne muscular dystrophy

 Diagnosis

SIGNS AND SYMPTOMS

Duchenne's Muscular Dystrophy

- The disease occurs only in males, and it is generally evident between 3 and 6 years of age.
- Common presentations include the following:
—Delayed walking
—"Waddling," Trendelenburg's gait, or lordotic gait
—Frequent tripping and falling
—Inability to hop and jump
- Progressive weakness occurs in the proximal muscle groups including the gluteus, quadriceps, abdominal muscle, and shoulder girdle muscles.

- Pseudohypertrophy of calf muscle is common.
- Most patients have cardiac involvement, most commonly tachycardia and right ventricular hypertrophy.
- Many also have static encephalopathy with mental retardation.
- Death from pulmonary and cardiac failure occurs during the second or third decades of life. Owing to weakness of hip muscles, patients compensate by carrying the head and shoulders behind the pelvis during gait, thus producing an anterior pelvic tilt and increased lumbar lordosis.
- A waddling, wide-based gait is also a sign of the condition.
- Weakness in the shoulder girdle occurs 3 to 5 years later; it is difficult to lift the patient under the arms because of the weakness. This has been termed Meryon's sign.
- No sensory deficits are detected.
- Children are usually unable to ambulate effectively beyond 10 years of age.

Becker's Muscular Dystrophy

- This is similar to DMD in clinical appearance and distribution of weakness, but it is less severe.
- The onset is usually after the age of 7 years.
- The rate of progression is slower.

There are many more types of muscular dystrophy, but they are not described here.

DIFFERENTIAL DIAGNOSIS

- Peripheral neuropathy
- Anterior horn cell disease
- Poliomyelitis

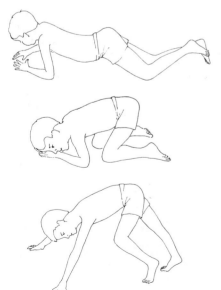
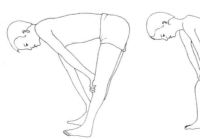
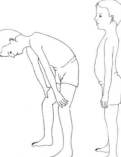
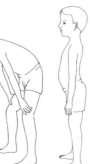

Fig. 1. This series of six drawings illustrates the Gower maneuver of a 7-year-old child with Duchenne muscular dystrophy.

Muscular Dystrophies

PHYSICAL EXAMINATION

History, physical examination, measurement of creatine phosphokinase and dystrophin, and electromyography help in making diagnosis. Electromyography shows a myopathic pattern, with reduced amplitude, short duration, and polyphasic muscle action potentials. Muscle biopsy may also be performed.

- Evaluate muscle bulk, to look for pseudo-hypertrophy of the calves.
- Observe the patient's gait, and look for Trendelenburg's gait.
- Look for muscle weakness, starting proximally.
- Evaluate the patient's ability to stabilize the shoulder; test for Meryon's sign.
- Note contracture, developing later, followed by scoliosis.

LABORATORY TESTS

- Serum creatine phosphokinase is markedly elevated in the early stages of DMD.
- It may be 200 times normal, but it later declines as muscle degeneration becomes complete. Dystrophin is completely absent in DMD and is decreased in Becker's dystrophy.

PATHOLOGIC FINDINGS

- Muscle degeneration, with subsequent loss of fibers
- Variation in fiber size
- Proliferation of connective tissue

Management

GENERAL MEASURES

Most patients with DMD die in their second or third decade of life. The goal of orthopaedic treatment should be designed to improve or maintain the functional capacity of the involved adolescent.

SURGICAL TREATMENT

- Contracture release (Achilles, fascia lata) may be indicated.
- Correction of scoliosis involves fusion of nearly the entire thoracic and lumbar spine (T-2 to L-5 or sacrum). Rods are used to straighten and hold the spine. This should be done when the curve reaches 30 degrees or greater.

PHYSICAL THERAPY

Physical therapy is directed toward prolongation of functional muscle strength, prevention or correction of contractures by passive stretching, gait training with orthoses, and wheelchair and equipment measurements.

MEDICAL TREATMENT

- Test muscle strength to assess the rate of deterioration.
- Use ankle-foot orthoses for correctable deformities.
- The best treatment for fractures is closed reduction and immobilization.
- Fractures of the lower extremities occur frequently in children with DMD, especially in children who are wheelchair bound.
- Contractures of both lower and upper extremities may occur. Surgical release of contractures is sometimes indicated to improve function.
- About 95% of patients with DMD develop progressive scoliosis. Surgical correction of scoliosis improves sitting balance and minimizes pelvic obliquity. Posterior spinal fusion is recommended for curves greater than 20 to 30 degrees. Programs of vigorous respiratory therapy and the use of home negative-pressure and positive-pressure ventilators may allow patients to extend their life. Proper diagnosis and early genetic counseling may help parents to be aware of the risk of additional male infants with DMD.

- There are no restrictions on activity. Activity is to be encouraged as much as possible.
- No drugs have been proven effective. Steroids have some short-term benefit, but they are also associated with long-term problems, including weight gain, osteoporosis, and myopathy.

PATIENT EDUCATION

Genetic counseling is important, to warn of the risk of additional affected infants.

MONITORING

Patients need to be followed frequently every 4 to 6 months by a neurologist to assess their progression.

COMPLICATIONS

- Respiratory failure
- Cardiac failure
- Fracture
- Scoliosis

PROGNOSIS

DMD is fatal in the second or third decade of life. Becker's dystrophy is more slowly progressive, and life expectancy is greater.

RECOMMENDED READING

Darras BT. Molecular genetics of Duchenne and Becker muscular dystrophy. *J Pediatr* 1990;117:1–16.

Duggan DJ, Gorospe JR, Fannen M et al: Mutations in the sarcoglycangenes in patients with myopathy. *N Engl J Med* 1997;336:618–624.

Morrissy PT, Weinstein SL. *Lovell and Winter's pediatric orthopaedics,* 4th ed. Philadelphia: Lippincott–Raven, 1996:540–550.

Shapiro F, Specht L. Current concepts review: the diagnosis and orthopaedic treatment of inherited diseases of childhood. *J Bone Joint Surg AM* 1993;75:439–459.

Basics

DESCRIPTION

Neck pain is common in adults and is usually secondary to degenerative disc disease and arthritis. In contrast, neck pain is less common in children and adolescents, and when it does occur, the pain is often secondary to a neoplasm or infection. Neck pain also occurs after trauma and is extremely common after motor vehicle accidents.

CAUSES

There are many different causes, and they can be broadly divided into traumatic and atraumatic.

Traumatic

- Soft tissue sprains
- Fractures
- Subluxations and dislocations
- Herniated discs

Atraumatic

- Arthritis
- Degenerative disc disease
- Neoplasms
- Infections

RISK FACTORS

Congenital fusions of the spine (Klippel-Feil syndrome) are risk factors.

CLASSIFICATION

- Traumatic
- Atraumatic

ASSOCIATED CONDITIONS

Inflammatory Arthritides

- Rheumatoid arthritis
- Ankylosing spondylitis

Congenital Syndrome

- Klippel-Feil Syndrome

ICD-9-CM

723.1 Cervicalgia

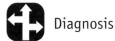 Diagnosis

SIGNS AND SYMPTOMS

- Pain well localized to the neck
- Stiffness
- Arm

DIFFERENTIAL DIAGNOSIS

The differential diagnosis is long in patients with neck pain. One can conveniently separate the differential diagnosis into adults and children and traumatic and atraumatic.

Adults

Atraumatic

- Degenerative disc disease
- Inflammatory arthritis

—Rheumatoid arthritis
—Ankylosing spondylitis

- Infections

—Disc space infections
—Vertebral osteomyelitis

Traumatic

- Ligament sprains
- Fractures
- Subluxations and dislocations
- Herniated discs

Children

Atraumatic

- Rotatory subluxation
- Abscess or osteomyelitis
- Meningitis
- Neoplasm

Traumatic

- Ligament disruption
- Foot dislocation
- Fracture

PHYSICAL EXAMINATION

- Physical examination should focus on range of motion, areas of tenderness, and neurologic examination.
- Loss of flexion, extension, and rotation should be noted.
- One should palpate the posterior ligamentous structures to detect tenderness and the paraspinal muscles for spasm.
- A careful neurologic examination should be performed including motor testing, deep tendon reflexes, and sensation.

LABORATORY TESTS

Laboratory tests are of limited value. If one suspects infection, white blood cell count and erythrocyte sedimentation rate should be obtained.

PATHOLOGIC FINDINGS

No findings are applicable.

IMAGING PROCEDURES

Radiography

- Anteroposterior and lateral radiographs are the first step in imaging. Other useful views include the following:
- Oblique views: to check the neural foramen if one suspects osteophytic nerve root impingement or facet dislocations
- Open mouth view: to check for C-1 fractures (atlas) or odontoid fractures

Magnetic Resonance Imaging and Computed Tomography

Magnetic resonance imaging and computed tomography are sensitive modalities to detect structural problems. They may be used singly or in combination.

- Computed tomography is most useful to detect bone abnormalities such as fractures, facet dislocations, and osteoid osteomas.
- Magnetic resonance imaging is useful to detect abnormalities in the marrow or soft tissue processes such as nerve root impingement or spinal cord compression.

Neck Pain

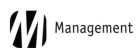 Management

GENERAL MEASURES

Most patients with neck pain suffer from an inflammatory process. Rest and nonsteroidal antiinflammatory measures are the mainstays of treatment. Soft cervical collars are useful for support.

SURGICAL TREATMENT

The most common surgical procedures are to remove nerve root or spinal cord compression from degenerative disease, trauma, and neoplasms. Once the vertebral body has been removed, or a major portion of the posterior elements, fusion is necessary.

PHYSICAL THERAPY

Physical therapy is useful to regain range of motion and strength of the paraspinal muscles. Gentle traction of the spine can be useful to decrease nerve root irritation.

MEDICAL TREATMENT

Nonsteroidal antiinflammatory agents are the drug of choice to decrease inflammation. They are generally prescribed for an initial 4- to 6-week period. If the pain has resolved at that time, the medication is discontinued.

PATIENT EDUCATION

Patients with neck strains (whiplash injuries) are counseled that full recovery can be expected in the motivated patient. Patients with significant cervical degenerative disease generally improve but may have chronic mild to moderate symptoms.

PREVENTION

There are no definite methods of prevention. General measures such as the use of seatbelts and avoidance of motorcycles are recommended.

MONITORING

Patients are followed at 4- to 6-week intervals until their discomfort resolves.

COMPLICATIONS

The major complication that must be recognized is progressive neural deficit from nerve root or spinal cord compression. Symptoms of nerve root or spinal cord compression include the following:

- Weakness in the arms and hands
- Sensory deficits in the upper extremities
- Difficulty in walking
- Bladder and bowel abnormalities

PROGNOSIS

The prognosis is generally good unless the cause is a malignant bone tumor such as metastatic bone disease, myeloma, or primary bone tumor.

RECOMMENDED READING

Hardin JG, Halla JT. Cervical spine syndromes. In: McCarty DJ, Koopman WJ, eds. *Arthritis and allied conditions,* 4th ed. Malvern, PA: Lea & Febiger, 1993:1563–1572.

White AA. *Your aching back: a doctor's guide to relief.* New York: Simon & Schuster, 1990:160–169.

Neurofibromatosis

 ## Basics

DESCRIPTION

Neurofibromatosis (NF) is the most common single gene disorder found in humans. The disease involves multiple organ systems; among them, the skeletal and nervous systems account for the greatest number of clinical features. The most common form is NF1, which is discussed here. NF2 refers to bilateral acoustic neuromas. The manifestations of NF1 may not develop until late childhood. Many signs are present at birth, but neurofibromas may take years to become apparent. Males and females are affected equally.

SYNONYM

von Recklinghausen's disease

GENETICS

- Inherited in an autosomal dominant pattern with about one-half of patients presenting as new mutations
- Thought to occur with complete penetrance

INCIDENCE

This disease occurs in approximately 1 in 3,000 newborns.

RISK FACTORS

No known risk factors exist, except advanced paternal age has been associated with an increased incidence of NF.

ASSOCIATED CONDITIONS

- Nearly 50% of people have mental handicaps ranging from severe retardation to slight learning disabilities.
- A few patients seem to develop metabolic bone disease that results in a type of osteomalacia.
- Hypertension on the basis of renal artery stenosis or pheochromocytoma may be encountered.

ICD-9-CM

237.7 Neurofibromatosis

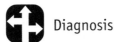 ## Diagnosis

SIGNS AND SYMPTOMS

The following are the characteristics that make up the diagnostic criteria. Two of these criteria must be met to establish the diagnosis (Fig. 1). Symptoms vary, depending on the criteria. Plexiform neurofibromas are often associated with pain and neurologic deficit in the distribution of the particular nerve. Cutaneous neurofibromas typically cause few symptoms.

- Six café-au-lait spots measuring 5 mm or more in children and 15 mm or more in adults
- One optic glioma
- Two or more Lisch's nodules on the iris
- One osseous lesion typically seen in NF, including vertebral scalloping or pseudarthrosis of a long bone
- A first-degree relative with the disease
- Axillary or inguinal freckling
- Cutaneous or plexiform neurofibromas

DIFFERENTIAL DIAGNOSIS

Proteus syndrome most closely resembles NF in its manifestations. Patients with isolated congenital pseudarthrosis must be monitored for NF, because the café-au-lait spots may develop later NF. NF2 consists of only bilateral acoustic neuromas.

PHYSICAL EXAMINATION

- The neck and spine should be examined for deformity.
- The skin should be inspected all over the body, including the axillae.

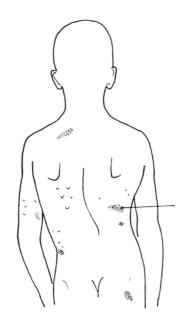

Fig. 1. This patient displays multiple café-au-lait spots, subcutaneous neurofibromas, and scoliosis characteristic of neurofibromatosis.

- The eyes should be examined with a slit lamp for Lisch's nodules and optic glioma.
- Limb lengths should be measured.

LABORATORY TESTS

No laboratory tests reveal abnormalities specific for NF.

PATHOLOGIC FINDINGS

The disorder is one of cells of neural crest origin. The cells of the embryonic neural crest are destined to form tissue in many different organ systems, and this accounts for the diverse manifestations of the disease. Lisch's nodules of the iris are hamartomatous deposits. The bone in pseudarthrosis is typically fibrotic, with few osteoblasts. Cutaneous neurofibromas are composed of Schwann's cells and connective tissue.

IMAGING PROCEDURES

The skeletal manifestations usually can be identified on plain radiographs. Posterior vertebral body scalloping may be noted. The dystrophic type of scoliosis is characterized by penciling of the ribs, severe apical rotation, short, segmented thoracic curves, and congenitally malformed vertebrae. The features of the pseudarthrosis that can occur in long bones can include anything from a cystic appearance to a severely thinned and pointed pseudarthrosis, which fractures at birth. Sclerosis and constriction can also be found at the pseudarthrosis site. Dural ectasia and pseudomeningocele can also affect the spine.

When instrumentation is planned to correct a spinal deformity, magnetic resonance imaging should be obtained to evaluate the spinal canal for these changes. Curious long bone lesions can include anything from benign scalloping of cortices to permeative lesions that resemble malignant disease radiographically.

Neurofibromatosis

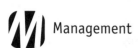 Management

GENERAL MEASURES

Patients should be seen regularly by a geneticist or primary physician to rule out growth disturbance, scoliosis, or neurologic deterioration. Patients usually are functional, except those who are severely mentally handicapped.

SURGICAL TREATMENT

• Dystrophic scoliosis should be treated surgically if any evidence of progression is seen.
• Anterior and posterior fusions are usually recommended if there is focal kyphosis or a curve greater than 50 to 60 degrees.
• Patients with dystrophic tibial changes should be braced when diagnosed, and the bracing should be protected until skeletal maturity.
• If fracture occurs, use either intramedullary rods and bone grafting or vascularized fibula bone grafting or compression and distraction (Ilizarov) treatment with ring fixators. All treatment should be protected after union occurs until the end of growth.
• Plexiform neurofibromas should not be treated surgically, because total removal is nearly impossible and neurologic deficits typically occur.
• Leg length inequality should be charted and followed with serial scanograms to ascertain the timing of either contralateral leg epiphysiodesis or limb lengthening.

MEDICAL TREATMENT

• Although speculative, angiogenesis inhibitors may be used to decrease the vascularity of plexiform neurofibromas and allow easier removal surgically.
• Bracing for pre-pseudarthrosis is recommended by most authors until fracture occurs. Otherwise, activity should not be unnecessarily restricted.
• No specific dietary requirements exist.

PATIENT EDUCATION

The incidence of tumors, especially those of the nervous system, including optic gliomas, astrocytomas, and acoustic neuromas, is increased. Education about the early signs of auditory, visual, or motor disturbances should be discussed with patients. Educate the patient regarding the need to protect pseudarthrosis of the tibia until skeletal maturity. Discuss the potential for limb length discrepancy when either pseudarthrosis of the lower extremity or limb gigantism is present. Typical discrepancy in both disorders rarely exceeds 6 cm.

• If possible, bracing of pseudarthrosis in the tibia should be attempted.
• Bracing for dystrophic scoliosis is not effective.
• Bracing for the more commonly encountered idiopathic type of scoliosis should be instituted when the regular indications for idiopathic scoliosis are met.

MONITORING

• Annual scanograms are indicated for limb length discrepancy.
• Physical examinations for detection of scoliosis should be performed on a yearly basis while the child is growing.
• Hypertension is a common finding in patients with NF and should be monitored regularly.

COMPLICATIONS

• Patients with NF1 have a high incidence of malignancy.
• Usually, these are tumors of the central nervous system.
• Plexiform neurofibromas can degenerate as well into neurofibrosarcomas.

• Amputation of a pseudarthrosis in the extremity may still be necessary despite treatment, because a few of these lesions are not amenable to current methods designed to promote healing.
• The function of the patient may be best served in rare instances with amputation.
• Some patients with dystrophic scoliosis have malformed vertebrae.
• If significant kyphosis exists, correction can cause neurologic compromise.
• Spinal cord monitoring should be performed during all spinal procedures.

PROGNOSIS

Life expectancy is normal in the absence of severe mental retardation and malignant disease.

RECOMMENDED READING

Akbarnia BA, Gabriel KR, Beckman E, Chalk D, et al. Prevalence of scoliosis in neurofibromatosis. *Spine* 1992;17:S244.

Crawford AH, Bagamery N. Osseous manifestations of neurofibromatosis in childhood. *J Pediatr Orthop* 1986;6:72–88.

Goldberg MJ. Syndromes of orthopaedic importance. In: Morrissy RT, Weinstein SL, eds. *Lovell and Winter's pediatric orthopaedics.* Philadelphia: Lippincott–Raven 1996:255–260.

Joseph KN, Bowen JR, MacEwen GD, et al. Unusual orthopaedic manifestations in neurofibromatosis. *Clin Orthop* 1992;278:17–28.

Sponseller PD. Localized disorders of bone and soft tissue. In: Morrissy RT, Weinstein SL, eds. *Lovell and Winter's pediatric orthopaedics,* 4th ed. Philadelphia: Lippincott–Raven, 1996:322–329.

Basics

DESCRIPTION

A fracture nonunion is the presence of a post-fracture defect in a long bone, well past any reasonable estimate of healing time. Children, because of their active healing potential, rarely develop a nonunion unless other predisposing conditions are present.

CAUSES

• Injury-related causes include segmental bone loss, extensive soft tissue damage, and loss of adequate blood supply.
• Treatment-related factors include quality of reduction, amount of distraction, and period of immobilization.

INCIDENCE

The incidence depends on the fracture type. Tibial shaft and scaphoid fractures have a higher risk of nonunion, owing to a more tenuous blood supply than other bones (this blood supply is often damaged with the injury).

RISK FACTORS

• Poor nutritional status
• Poor bone quantity and quality
• Suppressed immune system
• Presence of bone infection may contribute to development of a nonunion.

CLASSIFICATION

• Atrophic
• Hypertrophic
• Atrophic nonunions often have poor blood supply, and when they are visualized on radiographs, they often show poor bone quality with tapered edges.
• Hypertrophic nonunions have good blood supply. Most of these go on to heal if adequate stabilization can be achieved.

ICD-9-CM

733.82 Nonunion fracture

 Diagnosis

SIGNS AND SYMPTOMS

Patients have continued pain and instability at a fracture site.

DIFFERENTIAL DIAGNOSIS

• Delayed union, which is characterized by some tenderness and motion at the fracture site with variable amounts of callus present after a period in which most fractures would be clinically healed
• Synovial pseudarthrosis, in which a fluid-filled gap exists between two bones

PHYSICAL EXAMINATION

• Patients have continued tenderness at the fracture site.
• Motion of the bony fragments may or may not be evident.

PATHOLOGIC FINDINGS

Thick fibrous tissue with areas of uncalcified callus formation is noted.

IMAGING PROCEDURES

• Plain anteroposterior and lateral radiographs, to determine the presence of callus formation
• Serial radiographs, to ensure callus progression
• Bone scans, to help determine whether there is increased blood flow and subsequently increased bone turnover at the fracture site

 Management

GENERAL MEASURES

Patients should avoid medications and environmental conditions that inhibit fracture healing.

SURGICAL TREATMENT

Surgical treatment of nonunions includes the following:

• Placing bone graft (autogenous, allogenic, or synthetic) in the fracture site
• Stabilizing fractures that have excessive motion at the nonunion site

PHYSICAL THERAPY

• Protected weight bearing or range of motion while the fracture heals
• Plate fixation: range of motion only
• Rod fixation: protected weight bearing

MEDICAL TREATMENT

Treatment varies depending on the location of the fracture and the cause of the nonunion. Possible therapy includes the following:

• Prolonged immobilization
• Increased or decreased activity of the involved bone
• Operative intervention
• Bone stimulators
• Combination of these modalities
• Calcium supplementation and vitamin D
• Level of activity depending on location and fracture type

PATIENT EDUCATION

Strict adherence to the recommendations of the orthopaedic surgeon regarding activity and care of the fracture may reduce the likelihood of developing a nonunion, particularly in problematic fractures.

MONITORING

Serial radiographs are obtained once a month, to assess the development of callus.

COMPLICATIONS

Orthopaedic hardware, such as plates, screws, and rods, will eventually fail if the bone does not heal.

PROGNOSIS

The prognosis depends on the following:

• Type of injury
• Location of the fracture
• Cause of the nonunion
• Presence of any associated risk factors

RECOMMENDED READING

Buckwalter JA, Einhorn TA, Bolander ME, Cruess RL. Healing of the musculoskeletal tissues. In: Rockwood CA, Green DP, eds. *Fractures in adults*. Philadelphia: Lippincott–Raven 1996:261–299.

Ostrum RF, Reddi AH, Friedlander, et al. Bone injury, regeneration, and repair. In: Sheldon S, ed. *Orthopaedic basic science*. Rosemont, IL: American Academy of Orthopaedic Surgeons, 1994:472–477.

Nursemaid's Elbow

 Basics

DESCRIPTION

Nursemaid's elbow results from injury to the annular ligament that surrounds the radial head at the elbow in a young child (Fig. 1). The injury causes guarding and failure to use the elbow. It is not a subluxation or dislocation, however. It usually affects children between 1 and 5 years of age. Boys and girls are equally affected.

SYNONYMS

- Pulled elbow
- Annular ligament entrapment

GENETICS

No genetic predisposition is known.

INCIDENCE

This is one of the most common elbow injuries in young children.

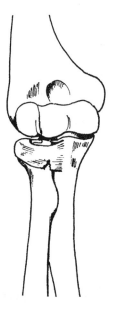

Fig. 1. Nursemaid's elbow is a strain or a tear in the annular ligament around the radial neck.

CAUSES

With traction, a small part of the annular ligament that surrounds the radial head is pulled into the joint and may be partially torn, causing painful rotation of the radius. This injury does not usually result from a fall onto the arm, which more typically produces a buckle fracture of the arm.

RISK FACTORS

- Age between 1 and 5 years
- Stubborn behavior (pulling away)

ICD-9-CM

832.0 Annular ligament disruption

 Diagnosis

SIGNS AND SYMPTOMS

- Pain in the elbow after a traction injury, such as pulling on the arm by a parent or sibling (Fig. 2)
- Usually, minimal pain to palpation
- No significant swelling
- Resistance by the patient to use of the elbow

The response to reduction of the displaced ligament is the most diagnostic feature of all. The child starts using the elbow again shortly, and there is no residual tenderness.

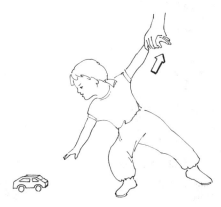

Fig. 2. The mechanism of nursemaid's elbow is traction, not a fall.

DIFFERENTIAL DIAGNOSIS

- Buckle or greenstick fracture of the distal humerus
- Growth plate injury of the distal humerus or proximal radius
- Infection, juvenile rheumatoid arthritis, and Lyme disease, which are all possibilities but occur much less frequently than nursemaid's elbow

PHYSICAL EXAMINATION

The child usually holds the elbow at the side and refuses to use the extremity.

LABORATORY TESTS

There are no laboratory tests to aid in the diagnosis.

PATHOLOGIC FINDINGS

- The ligament surrounding the radial head is partially, but not totally, torn.
- Few specimens have actually been examined, because the natural history of the condition is benign.

IMAGING PROCEDURES

- Radiographs are not required if the diagnosis is clear.
- If in doubt, order anteroposterior and lateral films of the elbow to rule out fracture.

Management

SURGICAL TREATMENT

- Not needed
- Closed manipulation always successful

PHYSICAL THERAPY

In this age group, children hardly ever need physical therapy for this injury.

MEDICAL TREATMENT

- Rule out other conditions (usually by physical examination).
- Reduce the displaced annular ligament by flexing the child's elbow fully and bringing the child's hand up to touch the shoulder, while supinating the forearm (Fig. 3). A slight "pop" is usually felt. The maneuver may initially be resisted by the child, but then the child begins to use the arm again.

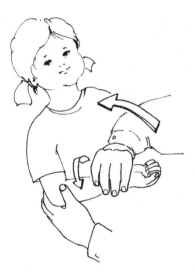

Fig. 3. Nursemaid's elbow is usually reduced by flexion and supination.

- A sling or splint is not usually needed, unless the episode is a recurrence.
- The child should be allowed to return to activities as tolerated.
- Medications are not usually needed once the injury is reduced, but acetaminophen may be given.
- If stronger medication is needed, suspect another diagnosis.

PATIENT EDUCATION

Educate parents about the traction mechanism of the injury and the need to avoid pulling on the child's elbow.

MONITORING

Monitoring is not needed, unless problems persist.

COMPLICATIONS

- None are known, except misdiagnosis, such as missing a fracture about the elbow.
- This can be distinguished by a different mechanism and greater swelling and tenderness.

PROGNOSIS

The prognosis is generally excellent; there should be no sequelae. A few children suffer a recurrence, which can be reduced and splinted for 1 to 2 weeks.

RECOMMENDED READING

Sponseller PD. Disorders of bone, joint and muscle. In: Oski FA, ed. *Principles of practice of pediatrics*. Philadelphia: Lippincott–Raven, 1993:1037–1038.

Olecranon Fracture

Basics

DESCRIPTION

The olecranon represents the proximal articulating unit of the ulna for the elbow joint. It articulates with the trochlea of the distal humerus and is responsible for flexion and extension of the elbow joint. It is also the insertion site of the triceps tendon expansion. This fracture can occur in any age group, and males and females are affected equally.

INCIDENCE

It may occur in the younger patient after a fall or sports injury or in the older patients after a fall.

CAUSES

The most common mechanisms of injury are as follows:

- Direct blow to the elbow
- Fall on the outstretched hand with the elbow in flexion

CLASSIFICATION

Olceranon fractures may be nondisplaced or displaced. They may be pure tension injuries with a single fracture, or they may be highly comminuted if the fractures occur from direct force in a fall.

ASSOCIATED CONDITIONS

- Elbow dislocation
- Radial head fracture
- Triceps avulsion
- Elbow instability

ICD-9-CM

813.01 Closed olecranon fracture
813.11 Open olecranon fracture

Diagnosis

SIGNS AND SYMPTOMS

- Pain, swelling, ecchymosis, and deformity generally occur after a direct blow or fall on an outstretched hand with the elbow in flexion.
- These injuries are often associated with radial head fractures and elbow dislocations (Fig. 1).

DIFFERENTIAL DIAGNOSIS

- Distal humerus fracture
- Elbow dislocation
- Radial head fracture

PHYSICAL EXAMINATION

- Comprehensive neurologic examination, concentrating on the ulnar nerve
- Palpable defect often detected on posterior elbow

LABORATORY TESTS

Before surgery, routine preoperative laboratory tests are performed, depending on the age and medical condition of the patient.

IMAGING PROCEDURES

- Obtain routine anteroposterior and lateral radiographs of the elbow.
- Radiocapitellar view may be helpful if there appears to be an associated radial head injury. Severely comminuted fractures may require a computed tomography scan for identification of fracture fragments and preoperative planning.

Management

GENERAL MEASURES

Initial evaluation should include particular attention to the function of the triceps muscle, radial and ulnar nerves, and vascular status of the upper extremity.

SURGICAL TREATMENT

- Avulsion fractures must be operatively repaired because of the associated triceps insertion disruption. The triceps tendon is simply sutured back to the olecranon.
- Transverse fractures are repaired using two Kirschner wires that are fixed in the bony fragments and a tension band wire to resist the pull of the triceps muscle.
- Oblique fractures are repaired using interfragmentary screw fixation and an accompanying tension band wire.
- Severely comminuted fractures are not amena-

ble to tension wiring and generally require more extensive fixation with compression plating.

PHYSICAL THERAPY

Decreased range of motion and muscle strength are common sequelae of elbow immobilization after olecranon fractures. These conditions are addressed with strengthening and gentle passive range-of-motion exercises, which are gradually progressed to active range-of-motion exercises when there is radiographic evidence of callus formation and fracture healing.

MEDICAL TREATMENT

- Nondisplaced fractures are treated with immobilization in a long arm splint or cast with the elbow in 90 degrees of flexion for 4 weeks.
- Follow-up radiography is necessary 7 to 10 days after injury to make sure that the fracture has not displaced.

PATIENT EDUCATION

Even with a perfect reduction, patients may still have decreased range of motion. Patients often lose 5 to 10 degrees of extension.

PREVENTION

Elbow pads should be used for contact sports and skating.

MONITORING

Document preoperative and postoperative neurovascular status, specifically for radial and ulnar nerve function.

COMPLICATIONS

- Radial neuropathy
- Ulnar neuropathy
- Flexion contracture
- Elbow arthritis
- Malunion
- Nonunion

PROGNOSIS

- Prognosis is good for patients with nondisplaced fractures.
- Outcomes vary with the severity of injury in patients with displaced fractures.

RECOMMENDED READING

Browner BD, Jupiter JB, Levine AM, et al., eds. *Skeletal trauma.* Philadelphia: WB Saunders, 1992:1134–1141.

Clark CR, Bonfiglio M. *Orthopaedics.* New York: Churchill Livingstone, 1994:176–177.

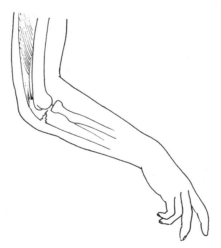

Fig. 1. Olecranon fracture involves the proximal ulna and most often enters the elbow joint.

Basics

DESCRIPTION

Osteoarthritis may occur in virtually all the joints of the body, and the end result is loss of the articular cartilage with secondary bone changes: osteophytes, subchondral sclerosis, and subchondral cysts.

SYNONYMS

- Degenerative joint disease
- Wear-and-tear arthritis

GENETICS

Most cases do not have a clear-cut genetic predisposition.

INCIDENCE

Osteoarthritis, the most common form of arthritis, affects males and females equally, and in contrast to inflammatory arthritis, it occurs principally in older patients.

CAUSES

There is no known cause of osteoarthritis (idiopathic osteoarthritis). The common pathway is loss of the articular cartilage with progressive overloading of the joint.
Many conditions that injure the joint may lead to secondary arthritis:

- Trauma: posttraumatic arthritis
- Infection: postinfectious arthritis
- Avascular necrosis: arthritis associated with the condition

RISK FACTORS

- Obesity
- Risk factors for avascular necrosis: steroid use, hip dislocations, displaced femoral neck fractures
- Septic arthritis

CLASSIFICATION

Classification is by single or multiple joint involvement.

ASSOCIATED CONDITIONS

No conditions are associated with osteoarthritis.

ICD-9-CM

715.9 Osteoarthritis, unspecified whether generalized or localized

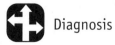 Diagnosis

SIGNS AND SYMPTOMS

- Discomfort with weight bearing and joint motion
- Stiffness
- Loss of function
- —Inability to do heavy work
- —Inability to tie or put on shoes
- —Limitation to short distance walking

DIFFERENTIAL DIAGNOSIS

The diagnosis of osteoarthritis is not difficult when the disease is in the moderate or advanced stages. Early arthritis can be confused with the following conditions:

- Tendinitis or bursitis
- Stress fractures
- Synovial proliferative disorders
- —Pigmented villonodular synovitis
- —Synovial chondromatosis

PHYSICAL EXAMINATION

The principal features are as follows:

- Loss of range of motion (especially internal rotation of the hip)
- Joint effusions
- Osteophytes
- Deformity

LABORATORY TESTS

There are no specific laboratory features.

PATHOLOGIC FINDINGS

Loss of the thickness and organization of the articular cartilage is noted.

IMAGING PROCEDURES

- Anteroposterior and lateral radiographs are the main imaging modalities. In the knee, foot, and ankle, weight-bearing radiographs are performed.
- Magnetic resonance imaging can be used to exclude other diagnoses such as avascular necrosis, stress fractures, and neoplasms.

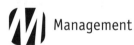 Management

GENERAL MEASURES

General measures include rest, activity modification, and antiinflammatory medication.

SURGICAL TREATMENT

The two main types of surgery are realignment osteotomy and joint replacement.

Realignment Osteotomies

The joint surfaces are repositioned by cutting the bone and changing the axis of weight bearing. This is done to allow the healthiest articular cartilage to bear the most weight.

Arthroplasty

The arthritic joint surfaces are removed, and a new joint surface is implanted. The bearing surface is typically metal on high-density polyethylene. Examples are total hip arthroplasty, total knee arthroplasty, and total shoulder arthroplasty.

PHYSICAL THERAPY

Physical therapy is useful to place patients on a program to preserve muscle strength and range of motion and to avoid contractures. Activity modification is an important component of therapy.
Heavy-impact activity such as running, contact sports, and heavy work exacerbates patients' symptoms. Using a cane in the opposite hand significantly reduces the forces across the hip joint and will both relieve discomfort and improve gait.

MEDICAL TREATMENT

Nonsteroidal antiinflammatory medications are the mainstays in the nonoperative treatment of arthritis. Sometimes, it is necessary to try up to three or four different classes of nonsteroidal drugs before finding one that works well for the patient.

PATIENT EDUCATION

Patients are taught to avoid activities that worsen their pain and are shown how to prevent contractures.

MONITORING

Patients are followed at 3- to 12-month intervals depending on the severity of their symptoms. Plain radiographs are taken every 6 to 12 months

COMPLICATIONS

The two major complications of nonoperative treatment are the side effects of nonsteroidal antiinflammatory medications and contractures with loss of the ability to walk. Gastrointestinal bleeding is the most common and serious complication of the nonsteroidal antiinflammatory agents.

PROGNOSIS

The prognosis is excellent with modern methods of joint replacements, which are durable and provide excellent function.

RECOMMENDED READING

Moskowitz RW. Clinical and laboratory findings in osteoarthritis. In: McCarthy DJ, Koopman WJ, eds. *Arthritis and allied conditions*, 12th ed. Malvern, PA: Lea & Febiger, 1993:1735–1760.

Osteoarthritis. In: Klippel JH, ed. *Primer on the rheumatic diseases*, 11th ed. Atlanta, GA: Arthritis Foundation, 1997:104–107.

Osteochondritis Dissecans

 Basics

DESCRIPTION

This is a pathologic joint entity of localized bone necrosis with overlying cartilage injury. Osteochondritis primarily affects the knee, but it is also seen in the hip (in late Legg-Calvé-Perthes disease) the elbow, and the ankle. Osteochondritis dissecans occurs primarily in the second decade of life, although it is also seen in children and older adults. It is more common in males. Older adolescents, after physeal closure, have less ability to heal these lesions with conservative treatment.

Several forms of "Little League elbow" are types of osteochondritis dissecans: osteochondritis of the radial head and that of the capitellum.

SYNONYM

Osteochondral fracture

GENETICS

- Increased predilection in some families
- No known mendelian pattern

INCIDENCE

This condition is more frequent in active sports participants, both children and young adults.

CAUSES

Multiple reported causes exist, usually including trauma and ischemia to the articular surface in a skeletally immature patient.

RISK FACTORS

- Certain persons may be more susceptible to trauma, such as those with joint laxity, genu valgum, obesity, or intraosseous vascular anomalies.
- Sports-active children and adolescents are more commonly affected.

CLASSIFICATION

Based on Arthroscopic Stages of the Lesion

1. Subchondral bone only, with the cartilage intact
2. Partial separation of the fragment
3. Complete separation of the fragment but remaining in its fracture bed
4. Complete separation of the fragment out of the fracture bed (free-floating fragment)

Based on Scintigraphy

- Lesion present radiographically but a normal scan
- Increased uptake over the lesion
- Increased uptake over the lesion and the femoral condyle
- As above, with increased uptake over the tibial plateau as well
- Increased activity a sign of reparative process and of favorable prognostic value

ICD-9-CM

732.7 Osteochondritis dissecans

 Diagnosis

SIGNS AND SYMPTOMS

- Knee pain
- Effusion (often hemarthrosis)
- Thigh atrophy
- Tenderness over the lesion
- Occasionally, locking or catching of the knee if the fragment has become a loose body in the joint
- Pain often insidious and activity related
- Lesion in one of four places in the knee

—Lateral aspect of the medial femoral condyle
—Posterior part of the lateral femoral condyle
—Joint surface of the patella
—Trochlear groove

DIFFERENTIAL DIAGNOSIS

- Stress fracture: usually with acute onset of pain
- Anterior cruciate ligamentous injury: knee instability by clinical examination
- Physiologic ossific irregularities: multiple small centers of ossification possibly normal in the young child's knee
- Meniscal injury: usually more locking or clicking of the knee
- Spontaneous osteonecrosis of the knee: lesion often larger

PHYSICAL EXAMINATION

- Note the presence or absence of an effusion.
- Grade the effusion as minimal, moderate, or tense.
- Determine the location of tenderness.
- Perform range of motion and McMurray's and Lachman's tests.
- Observe the patient's gait.
- Flex the knee to 90 degrees, by internally rotating the tibia and slowly bringing it into extension. Symptoms are often elicited at about 30 degrees and are relieved by external rotation.

PATHOLOGIC FINDINGS

- A separated articular chondral fragment with attached necrotic bone is noted.
- Many believe that the lesion is secondary to repetitive microtrauma to the area.

IMAGING PROCEDURES

- Anteroposterior, lateral, and tunnel radiographs are helpful.
- Tunnel radiographs are taken with the knee in 45 degrees of flexion. This view allows improved visualization of the most common sites of osteochondritis dissecans.
- Bilateral radiographs are obtained help to rule out ossification irregularities.
- Four stages are noted based on bone scan, varying by how much of the femur and tibia demonstrates uptake (see Classification).
- Magnetic resonance imaging may better show the size of the lesion, but it is not always indicated. It shows osteochondritis dissecans before plain films show it.
- Arthrography demonstrates whether the articular cartilage is intact.

Management

GENERAL MEASURES

Treatment based on the following:

- Age of the patient
- Stage of disease
- Size and location of the lesion: Lesions presenting before physeal closure have the best prognosis; conservative treatment is usually tried first, consisting of decreasing impact and movement of the affected joint.

—Small lesions (less than 5 mm) can often be observed or excised, if completely separated.
—Larger lesions should be replaced and surgically fixed whenever possible.

- Knee pain after 6 weeks of conservative management is an indication for surgical intervention.

SURGICAL TREATMENT

- Many lesions can be treated by arthroscopy.
- Open arthrotomy is an alternative means of gaining exposure.
- Fixation may be with wires, screws, or resorbable pins.
- Drilling of the fragment bed is often warranted to aid in healing.
- Cartilage transplantation and repair are newer techniques that will likely have applicability to this lesion.

PHYSICAL THERAPY

- This is rarely needed.
- Quadriceps strengthening exercises may decrease symptoms.

MEDICAL TREATMENT

Small lesions presenting before physeal closure that are undisplaced from the surrounding subchondral bone should be managed with immobilization for 6 to 12 weeks with the knee flexed appropriately to unload the affected area. Displaced fragments should be treated with surgical intervention, either arthroscopic or open fixation or excision.
The patient may weight bear on leg as tolerated by pain, preferably with the knee immobilized at an angle to unload the affected area. Patients with tender lesions should have the offending activities, or sporting events, limited for 6 weeks.

PATIENT EDUCATION

Stress the importance of avoiding the offending activities and the risk of early osteoarthritis.

MONITORING

Undisplaced fragments treated conservatively should be followed closely for any evidence of displacement. Plain radiographs are usually sufficient, but magnetic resonance imaging may be needed.

COMPLICATIONS

- Nonunion of the reduced fragment may occur.
- Displacement of a nondisplaced lesion causes locking and increased pain in the knee.
- Large fragments may lead to early osteoarthritis, especially if presentation occurs at an older age.

PROGNOSIS

Small, nondisplaced fragments or those in patients presenting before physeal closure do well and often have no long-term sequelae. Larger fragments may lead to early osteoarthritis.

RECOMMENDED READING

Cahill B. Treatment of juvenile osteochondritis dissecans and osteochondritis dissecans of the knee. *Clin Sports Med* 1985;4:367–375.

Guhl JF. Arthroscopic treatment of osteochondritis dissecans. *Clin Orthop* 1982;167:65–75.

Kasser JR, ed. *Orthopaedic knowledge update 5.* Rosemont, IL: American Academy of Orthopaedic Surgeons, 1996:438–439.

Morrissy RT, Weinstein SL, eds. *Lovell and Winter's pediatric orthopaedics,* 4th ed. Philadelphia: JB Lippincott, 1996:761–763.

Osteochondroma

 Basics

DESCRIPTION

An osteochondroma is a common developmental dysplasia of the peripheral growth plate that results in a lobulated outgrowth of cartilage and bone from the metaphysis. This appears as a cartilage-capped bony projection from the metaphysis of long bones. It can occur in any bone that develops from enchondral ossification.

Osteochondroma most commonly occurs in long bones. The most usual locations include the proximal or distal femur, proximal tibia, pelvis, or scapula.

The lesion most often occurs in 10- to 25-year-old persons and stops growing at skeletal maturity. Growth of the lesions parallels that of the patient after about age 4 years. There is no significant difference in frequency between males and females.

SYNONYMS

- Osteocartilaginous exostosis
- Osteochondromatosis
- Diaphyseal aclasis

GENETICS

Multiple osteochondromatosis is often inherited in an autosomal dominant manner. To date, three different genetic mutations have been isolated.

INCIDENCE

This most common benign bone lesion makes up 40% of all benign bone tumors.

CAUSES

The cause of osteochondroma is unknown. However, the pathogenesis of many of the symptoms and deformity is understood. The symptoms result from pressure on adjacent nerves and muscle and local irritation. The skeletal deformity is due to undergrowth of the affected bones, with narrower bones more seriously affected. Therefore, the tibia and radius grow longer than the ulna and fibula. This phenomenon produces valgus at the knee, ankle, and elbow in some patients.

ASSOCIATED CONDITION

Multiple hereditary exostosis

CLASSIFICATION

- Solitary osteochondroma (nonheritable)
- Multiple osteochondromas (autosomal dominant)

ICD-9-CM

756.4 Osteochondroma

 Diagnosis

SIGNS AND SYMPTOMS

- Hard, painless, fixed mass
- Associated symptoms of tissue or nerve irritation

DIFFERENTIAL DIAGNOSIS

- Chondrosarcoma
- Parosteal osteosarcoma
- Periosteal chondroma

PHYSICAL EXAMINATION

- Note any hard, painless, fixed mass in the metaphyseal region of the fastest growing bones; the region around the knee is most common.
- Height in most patients falls in the low-normal range.
- Group findings occur in four major categories:

—Local impingement, which may include peroneal palsy and soreness of the muscles about the knee
—Valgus at knee, ankle, elbow and wrist (variable)
—Limb length inequality
—Malignant degeneration, occurring in later adulthood

- Physical examination and radiography should be able to confirm the diagnosis.

LABORATORY TESTS

Blood tests are not altered by this condition.

PATHOLOGIC FINDINGS

One sees normal hyaline cartilage undergoing normal enchondral ossification, occurring on the end of a stalk or ridge of bone.

IMAGING PROCEDURES

- Plain film typically depicts a compact pedunculated or sessile protuberance of bone, often with a stalk and a cartilaginous cap. It is a well-defined lesion projecting from the metaphysis.
- Computed tomograms are helpful in locations that are difficult to image, such as the scapula, pelvis, and proximal femur.
- Magnetic resonance imaging scans can be used when there is a suspicion of malignancy. The size of the cartilage cap can be measured (a cap smaller than 1 cm is worrisome for malignancy). Symptomatic bursae can be detected with magnetic resonance imaging.

 Management

GENERAL MEASURES

Local measures or analgesics are indicated for minor aches.

SURGICAL TREATMENT

- Surgical resection of symptomatic lesions is successful with minimal mobility.
- In patients with the multiple osteochondroma form of the disorder, new lesions may form in multiple areas with growth.
- Osteotomies and physeal stapling may be done for angular disturbances.

PHYSICAL THERAPY

This is not commonly necessary.

MEDICAL TREATMENT

- The lesion may be left untreated unless symptomatic. It should be followed clinically, because there is a 1% to 10% risk of malignant transformation to chondrosarcoma in persons with multiple osteochondromas.
- The analgesic of choice for aches caused by the lesions is recommended.
- Activity is allowed as tolerated.

PATIENT EDUCATION

- Reassure the patient about the benign nature of the lesions.
- Teach adults to be alert for growth or new onset of pain in osteochondroma, which may be a sign of malignant transformation.

MONITORING

Patients should be followed regularly (1 to 2 years) for angular disturbances, limb length inequality, or serious problems from pressure of lesion, so they can be treated in a timely fashion before more complex intervention is needed.

COMPLICATIONS

- Less than 1% of these lesions may undergo malignant transformation to chondrosarcoma.
- Enlarging, painful lesion in an adult may indicate malignant transformation.

PROGNOSIS

- The prognosis is good.
- The chance of recurrence after excision of a solitary lesion is less than 5%.
- The risk of malignant transformation of isolated osteochondromas is less than 1%.
- Patients with multiple hereditary exostosis have a 1% to 10% risk of malignant transformation.

RECOMMENDED READING

Bullough PG, Vigorita VJ. *Atlas of orthopaedic pathology with clinical and radiologic correlations.* Baltimore: University Park Press, 1984.

Netter FH. *CIBA collection of medical illustrations,* vol 8, part II. Summit, NJ: CIBA-Geigy, 1990:123–126.

Basics

DESCRIPTION

Osteogenesis imperfecta (OI) is a diverse group of inherited connective tissue disorders. The bones, teeth, eyes, hearing, and soft tissue may be affected.

SYNONYMS

- Lobstein's disease
- Vrolik's disease
- Van der Hoeve's disease
- Fragilitas ossium
- Osteomalacia congenita
- Osteoporosis fetalis

GENETICS

- Type I. Autosomal dominant with variable penetrance and expressivity
- Type II. Autosomal recessive or dominant
- Type III. Autosomal recessive
- Type IV. Autosomal dominant with variable penetrance and expressivity

All types have a moderately high rate of spontaneous mutation.

INCIDENCE

- The incidence ranges from 1 per 20,000 births to 1 per 50,000 births.
- Less severe forms, which may not be diagnosed at birth, have reported an incidence of 4 to 5 cases per 100,000 births.
- Overall, this disease probably affects 1 per 10,000 persons.
- No preferential gender distribution is seen.

Age-Related Factors

- Types II and III are diagnosed at birth with perinatal death or intrauterine fractures, respectively.
- Types I and IV may be diagnosed after birth, but generally in early childhood.
- In the milder forms, the incidence of fractures decreases with age.

CAUSES

Defects in type I collagen are the cause.

RISK FACTORS

No known risk factors exist other than heredity.

CLASSIFICATION

The Sillence classification is the most widely accepted:

- Type I. This is the common mild form. Fractures occur in later childhood and decrease toward adolescence. Patients with type IA do not have dentinogenesis imperfecta, whereas those with type IB do.

- Type II. This is lethal in the perinatal period, with many of the mutations occurring in the glycine residues of type I collagen.
- Type III. This is a severe form.
- Type IV. This is a moderately severe form, with glycine point mutations in type I collagen; clinically, this type has great variation, overlapping types I and III.

In 1906, Looser proposed a classification of OI based on the chronologic appearance of fractures. Patients with numerous fractures at birth exhibited the "congenita" form of the disease, whereas those in whom fractures occurred after the perinatal period exhibited the "tarda" form of the disease.

ASSOCIATED CONDITIONS

- Platybasia and potential neurologic sequelae
- Dentinogenesis imperfecta
- Hypermobile joints with increased incidence of joint dislocation
- Inguinal, umbilical, and diaphragmatic hernias

ICD-9-CM

756.51 Osteogenesis imperfecta

 Diagnosis

SIGNS AND SYMPTOMS

- Fragility of bone
- Short stature
- Scoliosis
- Defective dentinogenesis of deciduous teeth, permanent teeth, or both, resulting in soft, translucent, and brownish teeth
- Middle ear deafness
- Laxity of ligaments, which results in hypermobile joints and an increased incidence of joint dislocation
- Blue sclerae and tympanic membranes
- Skull: patients possibly having misshapen skulls with a wide intertemporal measurement and small, triangular faces

DIFFERENTIAL DIAGNOSIS

- Very-low-birth-weight infant
- Primary hyperparathyroidism
- Scurvy
- Hypophosphatasia
- Achondrogenesis
- Chondroectodermal dysplasia
- Juvenile osteoporosis
- Nonaccidental injury (child abuse)
- Spina bifida
- Thanatophoric dwarfism
- Congenital syphilis
- Malignancy (e.g., leukemia)

It may be difficult to discern child abuse from OI. Fractures from child abuse occur most frequently in children younger than 3 years of age. A single fracture may occur in either situation; however, multiple fractures at different stages of healing, posterior rib fractures, and metaphyseal corner fractures are highly specific for nonaccidental injury. A positive family history and signs such as abnormal dentition, blue sclerae, or systemic osteopenia revealed by radiographs may be helpful in the diagnosis of OI.

PHYSICAL EXAMINATION

- OI is diagnosed by fractures of unusual frequency or mechanism.
- A thorough history and physical examination are most important in the diagnosis of OI. A positive family history and signs such as abnormal dentition, blue sclerae, laxity of ligaments, scoliosis, or bowing and fragility of bone are helpful.

LABORATORY TESTS

- There are no specific serum laboratory tests.
- Cultures of dermal fibroblasts for characterization of type I collagen may be part of the workup. The matching of a child's type I collagen with a previously described molecular abnormality may establish the diagnosis of OI, but the absence of matching does not necessarily exclude the diagnosis.

PATHOLOGIC FINDINGS

- The bone often appears woven and only occasionally has a lamellar pattern.
- The cortices are thin, and the trabeculae in the metaphyses are markedly attenuated.
- The collagen fibers of the cornea and skin share in the disturbance and have a looser arrangement and thinner fibers.

SPECIAL TESTS

Dermal punch biopsy is used when routine diagnostic criteria are inconclusive. The synthesis and structure of type I collagen produced by the cultured fibroblasts obtained from biopsy can then be analyzed.

IMAGING PROCEDURES

- Plain radiography may reveal systemic osteopenia.
- Other radiographic findings may include long bones with narrow diaphyses and bowing, protrusio acetabuli, vertebral or other fractures, scoliosis, "concertina" femur, and cystic-appearing metaphyses.
- Bones are gracile and osteopenic, with thin cortices and an attenuated trabecular pattern.
- The pelvis may have a trefoil shape, and protrusio acetabuli is common, presumably because of repeated fractures.
- The osteopenic vertebrae may fracture easily, resulting in a flattened or biconcave shape. Severe scoliosis and kyphosis may eventually develop.

Osteogenesis Imperfecta

- The head is misshapen, and the skull exhibits wormian bones, a salient feature of OI.
- In severe cases, the metaphyses may appear cystic, a finding occasionally present at birth but more often developing during infancy or childhood. Popcorn calcifications in the metaphyseal and epiphyseal regions have been described. Flaring of the metaphyseal regions indicates impaired bone modeling.

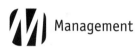 Management

GENERAL MEASURES

Treatment depends on the type of OI.

Type I

Type I may have little impact on the patient.

Type II

Type II, lethal perinatal OI, has some degree of variability. In the most severe cases, early death occurs before orthopaedic intervention.

Types III and IV

Types III and IV are the greatest therapeutic challenges. Several systemic treatment modalities have been attempted, but medical management remains ineffective, experimental, or theoretic. Theoretically, molecular treatments for specific types of OI should cure the disease, but this remains a goal for the future.

Exercise

Initiate an aggressive program of exercises, starting with bracing, working to develop ambulatory potential, and proceeding with appropriate seating, including a wheelchair if required.

Fractures

- Closed treatment methods usually are employed for fractures. Fractures heal readily, but the callus formed in response to the fracture is identical in structure to the rest of the skeleton (i.e., it is easily deformed by forces associated with weight bearing or the action of muscles across the fracture site). Use of lightweight splints or braces may be helpful in getting the child to bear weight soon and avoid the compounding problems of immobilization. Devices such as a parapodium may help a child to acquire an upright posture.
- Internal fixation may be pursued if management by closed treatment proves difficult. Intramedullary fixation is superior to plates and screws because these devices tend to dislodge from the weakened bone.

SURGICAL TREATMENT

Anesthesia

- Patients with OI are at high risk for a variety of reasons: Restricted neck and jaw mobility, pulmonary function abnormalities from thoracic cage distortion, dentinogenesis imperfecta, and valvular heart disease are present in many patients.
- Succinylcholine should be avoided because it can cause fractures resulting from muscle fasciculations.
- Anticholinergic agents should be avoided because these can cause malignant hyperthermia.

Osteotomy

- At about 5 years of age, corrective osteotomies of larger bones with intramedullary fixation for the lower and upper extremities can be performed.
- These procedures have been done with solid rods, by employing exchanges as the child grows.
- The Bailey-Dubow elongating rod is an option that diminishes the rate of reoperation.
- Intramedullary rod placement is believed to be optimal for children with the potential to stand.
- There is no absolute rule about when intramedullary rod placement should be performed. Risk-to-benefit analysis should consider recurrent fracture and deformity versus infection, pain, and the need for repeat rod placement.
- In patients with mild forms of OI, customary fracture management may apply. In more severe forms, recurrent fracture and subsequent bowing may be seen.

Scoliosis

- Scoliosis is one of the most difficult disorders to treat in OI.
- The curves tend to advance relentlessly, and bracing is ineffective in controlling the progression of the deformity.
- Spinal fixation is not always effective because of the poor quality of the bone.
- Newer methods of instrumentation are changing the approach to scoliosis in OI.
- Curves may be fused early (at 40%) to halt the relentless progression. This is important in maintaining function and in preventing respiratory complications.
- A less common area of spinal involvement is at the craniocervical junction: Basilar invagination may result and present with neurologic signs resulting from brainstem compression. Once the condition is diagnosed, decompression and spinal stabilization are recommended.

PHYSICAL THERAPY

Physical therapy is an important component of the treatment plan to help maximize age-appropriate activities and skills, as follows:

- Goals for physical therapy include muscle and bone strengthening, standing, and often ambulation.

- Hydrotherapy is a relatively safe form of exercise and allows active motion of extremities, aids in development of head and trunk control, and strengthens extremity musculature.
- Orthotics are an important adjunct and may be applied to maintain alignment or to prevent bowing of long bones.
- Braces should be lightweight and total contact in design with joint hinges.

PATIENT EDUCATION

- Understanding the necessity of muscle strengthening and range-of-motion exercises is important.
- Family members must monitor the skin around braces and casts.
- They must also try to recognize when fractures occur and be compliant with frequent follow-up.

MONITORING

- Scoliosis: Patients with OI must be followed closely from an early age for the development and progression of scoliosis (starting at age 6 years). They must also continue to be monitored as adults.
- Neurologic signs: Patients must be followed for neurologic signs of brainstem compression that may be caused by basilar invagination.
- Dentinogenesis imperfecta: Affected patients should be seen by their dentists every 3 to 6 months.
- Activity: This is allowed as tolerated, except in patients with recent fractures or surgery.

COMPLICATIONS

A softened base of the skull may lead to platybasia and potential neurologic sequelae.

PROGNOSIS

- Type II disease is lethal in the perinatal period.
- Type III is the next most severe form, and these patients often require multiple orthopaedic procedures.
- Types I and IV are milder forms of OI, with type I the mildest. The fracture rate in Type IV decreases around puberty. Presenile hearing loss may be the most significant long-term handicap in patients with type I disease.

RECOMMENDED READING

King JR, Bobechko WP. Osteogenesis imperfecta: an orthopaedic description and surgical review. *J Bone Joint Surg Br* 1971;53:72–89.

Zaleske DJ. Metabolic and endocrine abnormalities. In: Morrissy RT, Weinstein SC, eds. *Lovell and Winter's pediatric orthopaedics*, vol 1, 4th ed. Philadelphia: Lippincott–Raven, 1996:137–202.

Basics

DESCRIPTION

Osteogenic sarcoma (OGS) is a malignant primary sarcoma of bone. Histologic criteria include a malignant spindle cell stroma directly producing osteoid. The tumor usually affects the long bones and extends into the soft tissues and may metastasize. Bones most commonly affected include those that grow most rapidly:

- Femur (41.5%)
- Tibia (16.5%)
- Humerus (15%)

Adolescents in their second decade are the most commonly affected group. The median age range at presentation is 13 to 17 years. Some authors report a slight male predominance (1.3:1). Both the age of onset and the location of the lesion correspond to the time and region of the greatest longitudinal growth of the axial skeleton.

SYNONYM

Osteosarcoma

GENETICS

This disease is not genetically transmitted.

INCIDENCE

Primary sarcomas of bone are rare, with only approximately 2,000 new cases per year in the United States. OGS is one of the most common primary bone sarcomas, representing up to 40%.

CAUSES

- The cause of classic high-grade OGS is unknown.
- A relationship between incidence and high rates of growth has been noted.
- OGS occasionally develops in areas of preexisting bone lesions such as Paget's disease, fibrous dysplasia, bone infarcts, or osteogenesis imperfecta.

RISK FACTORS

Whereas patients with classic OGS tend to be taller than age-matched control subjects, no increased risk with unusual height has been documented. Chronic bone lesions in older patients (e.g., those with Paget's disease) have a slight, but definite, increased risk of developing OGS.

CLASSIFICATION

- Many subtypes exist, classified according to histologic criteria.
- The most common type is high-grade intramedullary OGS.
- Lesions are usually staged according to the Enneking staging system.

ASSOCIATED CONDITION

Retinoblastoma (high incidence of osteosarcoma)

ICD-9-CM

170.9 Osteogenic sarcoma

 Diagnosis

SIGNS AND SYMPTOMS

- Pain and swelling are the most consistent symptoms of OGS.
- Onset is usually gradual and progressive.
- Pain is aching and persistent.
- Significantly, many patients report night pain, which awakens them. Laboratory analysis shows elevated alkaline phosphatase levels in 50% of cases.

DIFFERENTIAL DIAGNOSIS

- Infection
- Ewing's sarcoma
- Giant cell tumor
- Metastatic disease
- Eosinophilic granuloma

PHYSICAL EXAMINATION

- A soft tissue mass is often palpable and tender.
- The mass is frequently warm and may limit range of motion of the adjacent joint.
- Patients, once diagnosed, usually undergo a staging workup including chest and abdomen computed tomography and computed tomography or magnetic resonance imaging of the lesion; a staging biopsy should be done.

LABORATORY TESTS

Alkaline phosphatase is elevated in 50% of cases. In patients with a high pretherapeutic alkaline phosphatase level, serial measurements may be used to monitor therapeutic response and tumor recurrence.

Osteogenic Sarcoma

PATHOLOGIC FINDINGS

Many subtypes of OGS have been identified. All OGS types have a malignant fibrous stroma forming bone as a least common denominator. Broad histologic subtypes are as follows:

- Fibrogenic
- Chondrogenic
- Osteogenic

IMAGING PROCEDURES

- The location of OGS is usually the metaphysis of a long bone.
- Lesions typically demonstrate features of bone destruction, bone formation, periosteal reaction, and a mineralized soft tissue mass.
- The classic radiographic appearance is that of a destructive lesion of bone that is itself forming bone.
- Rapid cortical destruction and periosteal reaction at the proximal or distal margin may produce the classic "Codman's triangle." Alternatively, radial reactive trabeculation may produce a sunburst appearance.
- Lesions rarely involve the joint.

Management

GENERAL MEASURES

Any destructive lesion of a long bone that is forming bone should immediately be referred to an experienced musculoskeletal oncologist.

SURGICAL TREATMENT

- Historically, treatment generally consisted of amputation.
- Newer surgical techniques and chemotherapeutic regimens allow limb salvage in the majority of cases.
- Resected bone segments may be replaced by allografts or large segment metal prosthesis endoprosthesis, depending on the situation.

PHYSICAL THERAPY

Most patients with local extremity lesions begin gait training and physical conditioning. In the upper extremity, function of the hand and elbow must be maintained.

MEDICAL TREATMENT

- See General Measures.
- Once the diagnosis has been made, activity should be restricted to prevent fracture, which could necessitate an amputation. Patients with lower extremity tumors are placed on crutches.
- Multiple chemotherapy regimens are being developed, refined, and evaluated. Current regimens include three to six different cytotoxic agents given for 10 to 12 weeks preoperatively and 6 months postoperatively (see Prognosis).

PATIENT EDUCATION

Patients who have been successfully treated must be alert for any new areas of bone pain that could herald a bone metastasis.

MONITORING

After definitive treatment, patients should be followed to detect recurrence or metastasis. Patients are monitored closely for the first 2 years with computed tomography scans of the chest every 3 to 4 months to detect pulmonary metastases. Plain radiographs of the limb are performed to detect local recurrences.

COMPLICATIONS

- Recurrence of the tumor is the most feared complication. Metastasis may occur years after diagnosis and treatment.
- Other complications secondary to limb salvage surgery are relatively common and include the following:

—Local recurrence occurs in about 5% to 10% of patients, usually within 2 years. Pulmonary metastases occur in about one-third of patients and generally are found within 3 years.
—Infection
—Pathologic fracture
—Loosening of prosthetic components
—Wound breakdown

PROGNOSIS

Historically, patients with primary OGS had a 5-year survival rate of only 20% to 30%. Newer chemotherapeutic regimens are effective in killing occult metastases. With preoperative and postoperative multiagent chemotherapy and wide resection, more recent series report a 70% survival rate at 5 years.

RECOMMENDED READING

Goorin AM, Frei E III, Abelson, HT. Adjuvant chemotherapy for osteosarcoma: a decade of experience. *Surg Clin North Am* 1981;61:1379–1389.

McCarthy E, Frassica FJ eds: Bone Pathology. New York: pps 205–220

Spjut HJ, Dorfman HD, Fechner RE, et al. *Tumors of bone and cartilage.* Washington, DC: Armed Forces Institute of Pathology, 1971:141–194.

Basics

DESCRIPTION

This is a small (nidus 0.5 to 1.5 cm), solitary, benign, painful lesion most commonly seen in the bones of the lower extremities. The proximal femur is the most common site, followed by the tibia. However, almost any bone may be affected, including the phalanges.

GENETICS

No genetic predisposition is known.

INCIDENCE

- Comprising 10% of all benign bone tumors
- Primarily in the age group of 5 to 25 years
- More common in men than women at a ratio of 3:1 (reason unknown)

CAUSES

The cause is unknown.

CLASSIFICATION

It is a benign bone tumor, less than 1.5 cm in diameter and not locally aggressive. Lesions similar to this histologically but greater than 1.5 cm are called osteoblastomas.

ASSOCIATED CONDITION

Osteoblastoma is a similar lesion, but somewhat larger. It has a greater predilection for the spine.

ICD-9-CM

213.9 Osteoid osteoma

Diagnosis

SIGNS AND SYMPTOMS

- Pain is more severe at night and is often specifically relieved by aspirin or other nonsteroidal antiinflammatory agents.
- A limp is common.
- There may be mild atrophy or wasting of muscles in the area.
- The region is tender to palpation.
- If the osteoid osteoma is near a joint, it may cause stiffness; if it involves the spine, scoliosis may be seen.
- The presence of osteoid osteoma in more than one site in a patient has not been reported.

DIFFERENTIAL DIAGNOSIS

- Osteomyelitis
- Stress fracture
- Buckle fracture

PHYSICAL EXAMINATION

- Mild swelling, erythema, and occasional muscle wasting in the involved area
- Absence of fever
- Tenderness and stiffness in the region of the osteoid osteoma

LABORATORY TESTS

No laboratory findings aid in the diagnosis.

PATHOLOGIC FINDINGS

On cross section, the nidus appears as a haphazard arrangement of osteoblasts and trabeculae, which is then surrounded by a dense shell of cortical bone. On microscopic examination, the nidus is composed of dense normal woven bone with osteoblastic rimming, and the reactive shell around it is composed of dense cortical bone. The cells all have a normal, benign appearance.

IMAGING PROCEDURES

- Computed tomography (CT) scans are the best imaging modality and show an oval radiolucent nidus of approximately 5 to 10 mm surrounded by a dense reactive zone. The nidus is often visible in the cortex of bone.
- In many areas, because the bone is not seen in cross section, the diagnosis may not be apparent with plain films.
- CT is best for confirming the lesion, by the presence of the characteristic "target" appearance of the nidus and its sclerotic rim. However, the location must be known, to obtain the correct position on the CT scan.
- Bone scanning is useful to confirm or localize an osteoid osteoma if the lesion's location cannot be determined by plain radiographs. The bone scan is always focally positive.

Management

GENERAL MEASURES

Osteoid osteomas may resolve spontaneously in 2 to 6 years. Nonsteroidal antiinflammatory agents may be used during this time to control the pain. Because of pain or intolerance to analgesics, many patients request excision of the lesion. This may be done by curettage of the central nidus or by en bloc excision of the nidus and its shell. If the nidus is completely removed, recurrence is unlikely. Other, more experimental minimally invasive therapies include drilling and radiofrequency ablation using CT guidance.

For patients treated nonoperatively, activity may be allowed as tolerated. After surgical excision, partial weight bearing should be recommended for 6 to 8 weeks until the bone has had time to remodel and gain strength.

SURGICAL TREATMENT

- Accurate localization of the lesion preoperatively is of paramount importance.

- En bloc excision is least likely to be followed by recurrence, but it weakens the bone temporarily by removing the hard cortical shell.
- Curettage is usually adequate as long as the surgeon is positive that the entire nidus has been removed.
- Return to function is excellent in the majority of cases.
- Recurrence of symptoms is seen in 5% to 10% of cases, probably resulting from the inability to visualize and excise the osteoid osteoma completely.

MEDICAL TREATMENT

- Aspirin, regular or enteric-coated
- Ibuprofen
- Naproxen
- Salicylsalicylic acid (salsalate), for patients with bleeding disorder or anticoagulation (does not affect platelet function)

PATIENT EDUCATION

- Patients should be counseled about the benign nature of the lesion and its tendency to resolve spontaneously over the years.
- Patients may be offered medical or surgical treatment and allowed to choose between the two.
- For intensely painful or disabling lesions, or in patients unable to tolerate nonsteroidal antiinflammatory agents, surgery is often selected.

MONITORING

Frequent monitoring is not needed because these lesions have no malignant potential.

COMPLICATIONS

- Fracture through excision site recurrence
- Gastritis or ulcers from nonsteroidal antiinflammatory treatment

PROGNOSIS

The prognosis is excellent. No risk of malignant transformation exists.

RECOMMENDED READING

Bullough PG, Vigorita VJ. Atlas of orthopaedic pathology with clinical and radiologic correlations. Baltimore: University Park Press, 1984:197–204.

Kneisel JS, Simon MA. Medical management compared with operative treatment for osteoid osteoma. J Bone Joint Surg Am 1992;74:179–185.

Lichtenstein L. Osteoid osteoma. In: Lichtenstein L, ed. Bone tumors, 2nd ed. St. Louis: CV Mosby, 1959:202–204.

Netter FH. CIBA collection of medical illustrations, vol 8, part II. Summit, NJ: CIBA-Geigy, 1990:120.

Spjut H, Dorfman H, Fechner R, et al. Tumors of bone and cartilage. Washington, DC: Armed Forces Institute of Pathology, 1970:120–133.

Osteomyelitis

 Basics

DESCRIPTION

Osteomyelitis is inflammation or infection of bone.

SYNONYM

Bone infection

INCIDENCE

- The incidence is higher in childhood, with a peak occurring in the later years of the first decade.
- It affects fewer than 1% of children.
- A seasonal variation in acute hematogenous osteomyelitis may occur, with more cases in late summer and early autumn.

CAUSES

Although the causes remain unknown, factors suspected as having an association with infection include trauma and an altered immune system (especially in adults). Most children who develop osteomyelitis are otherwise completely healthy.

RISK FACTORS

There appears to be a predilection toward males that is not clearly understood. Deficient immune systems as a result of viral illness, trauma, anesthesia, or malnutrition may also play a role in the development of osteomyelitis.

CLASSIFICATION

Most commonly, this classification is based on the nature of onset: acute, subacute, or chronic.

- Acute: This is most often from hematogenous spread. The most common organism is *Staphylococcus aureus,* followed by *Streptococcus* or gram-negative organisms in neonates; it is usually *S. aureus* in infants and children.

- Subacute: This accounts for one-third of primary bone infections and is characterized by insidious onset, mild symptoms, longer duration of infection, and inconclusive laboratory data. The most common organism is *Staphylococcus* species. It usually requires longer duration of antibiotic treatment than the acute condition.
- Chronic: *S. aureus* is the most common organism. Usually, these patients have sequestra and multiple cavities that require curettage and occasionally bone grafting.

Other schemes present are focused on factors such as patient age (neonatal, child, or adult), causative organism (pyogenic or granulomatous), or route of infection (hematogenous, direct inoculation, or contiguous spread).

ASSOCIATED CONDITIONS

Nearly half of these patients have a history of a recent or a concurrent infection such as a viral or upper respiratory infection. Clinically, trauma to the affected part is noted in 30% to 50% of these patients with acute hematogenous osteomyelitis.

ICD-9-CM

730.0 Acute or subacute osteomyelitis
730.1 Chronic osteomyelitis

 Diagnosis

SIGNS AND SYMPTOMS

Pain is the most common symptom, followed by swelling, erythema, warmth and limited range of motion of the adjacent joints. Fever is not always present. Children may not be able to verbalize symptoms; therefore, refusal to bear weight, inability to walk or move a limb, and development of a limp all suggest infection. The index of suspicion must be highest in the neonate.

DIFFERENTIAL DIAGNOSIS

- Trauma
- Septic arthritis
- Cellulitis
- Malignancy (leukemia or Ewing's sarcoma)
- Thrombophlebitis
- Sickle cell crisis
- Toxic synovitis
- Eosinophilic granuloma
- Osteoid osteoma

Consider a firm diagnosis when two of the four criteria are present:

- Pus aspirated from bone
- Positive bone or blood culture
- Symptoms of pain, swelling, warmth, and decreased range of motion
- Typical radiographic changes consistent with osteomyelitis

PHYSICAL EXAMINATION

The goal of the examination is to localize the area of involvement and to identify any possible source. The appearance of the child may vary from cranky to lethargic, depending on the extent and duration of infection. Before palpation, visually assess the amount of limb movement or usage. Tenderness to palpation may need to be elicited by the parent, with instructions to differentiate the cry of a frightened child from a cry of true pain. Tenderness, warmth, and erythema are usually present in the metaphyseal region of the bone.

LABORATORY TESTS

- The white blood cell count is not a reliable indicator of infection, but if it is, it elevated may be helpful.
- Blood cultures should also be obtained with the initial diagnostic blood sample. These are positive in 40% to 50% of cases, and if so, they may eliminate the need to aspirate bone to obtain the organism.

• The erythrocyte sedimentation rate is a nonspecific acute-phase reactant that is elevated in more than 90% of cases and is a reliable indicator of infection. It begins to elevate at 48 to 72 hours and returns to normal after 2 to 3 weeks if the infection has resolved. Because of the lag time of the sedimentation rate, it is not helpful in assessing resolution of infection.

• An elevated level of C-reactive protein resulting from inflammation is also useful. This test is more reliable in assessing infection because it not only peaks earlier (50 hours versus 3 to 5 days) but also returns to normal earlier (7 days).

• Aspiration of the site may be performed to identify the causative organism. The specimen should be sent for Gram stain, aerobic and anaerobic cultures, acid-fast bacilli, and tests for fungi. Bone cultures are positive in 80% of acute cases. Some clinicians suggest fine-needle biopsy with an 11-gauge bone biopsy (or bone marrow) needle for histologic examination. This usually requires heavy sedation to allow the patient to be comfortable and to obtain a specimen from the proper area reliably. The site of involvement is usually metaphyseal bone rather than hard cortical bone, so it is possible to penetrate the bone for a sample. If the site of involvement is not clear, it should be localized using bone scanning or magnetic resonance imaging. All cultures and laboratory tests should be obtained before starting antibiotic treatment.

PATHOLOGIC FINDINGS

• Infection begins in the sinusoids of the metaphysis, usually near the end of a long bone.

• As the infection spreads, the medullary vessels thrombose and cause a mechanical blockage of inflammatory cells. This results in inflammatory cell migration into the medullary cavity, with consequent intraosseous pressure buildup and development of pus. The pus then takes the path of least resistance and exits through the metaphyseal cortex, thereby elevating the periosteum. A subperiosteal abscess subsequently forms under the elevated periosteum.

• The elevated periosteum is manifest approximately 10 to 14 days later as a periosteal reaction.

IMAGING PROCEDURES

Radiographs

Soft tissue swelling is the earliest radiographic sign of osteomyelitis. Classic radiographic bony changes such as osteopenia, bone resorption, and new periosteal bone formation may not occur until 5 to 7 days after the onset of symptoms.

Bone Scan

This technique may be used to localize the area of involvement. Results may be falsely negative in the first month of life. Bone aspiration will not affect bone scan results if the scan is performed within 48 hours of aspiration. Bone scanning has a sensitivity of 89%, a specificity of 94%, and an overall accuracy of 92%. A bone scan is not needed if the area of involvement is already known.

Computed Tomography

This method is not useful in diagnosing acute osteomyelitis, but it may assist in differentiating other lucent lesions such as osteoid osteoma or chondroblastoma.

Magnetic Resonance Imaging

This technique may be useful in differentiating between acute and chronic osteomyelitis.

Ultrasound

Ultrasound may help to identify a subperiosteal fluid collection, but it does not penetrate bone well. Therefore, it is not useful in assessing metaphyseal fluid collections.

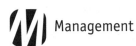 Management

GENERAL MEASURES

Principles of treatment include identification of the organism, selection of an appropriate antibiotic, surgical débridement if necessary, and sufficient duration of treatment to allow complete resolution. Surgery is not indicated if the condition is detected early and no dead bone is present.

SURGICAL TREATMENT

Indications

Indications for surgery are controversial but usually include the following:

• Aspiration of frank pus initially
• Presence of significant bone resorption
• Failure of symptom resolution after 36 to 48 hours of antibiotic treatment

Procedure

Surgical treatment consists of opening the periosteum, drilling the cortex, and débriding any devascularized bone.

MEDICAL TREATMENT

Antibiotic selection consists of oxacillin in combination with cefotaxime or gentamicin in neonates and oxacillin alone in infants and children. Cefazolin is recommended in patients allergic to penicillin. Clindamycin or vancomycin is recommended in patients allergic to both penicillin and cephalosporin. The duration of antibiotic treatment is debatable, but it typically involves intravenous antibiotics for 5 days until symptoms resolve and antibiotic sensitivities are identified. After this, a regimen of 4 to 6 weeks of oral therapy is indicated, provided an appropriate oral antibiotic is available.

COMPLICATIONS/PROGNOSIS

Most children do extremely well with appropriate treatment, and they suffer no long-term effects. Problems arise usually when infection is not recognized or treated in a timely manner, with the possible development of chronic osteomyelitis. Growth plate arrest may occur, if the infection crosses the growth plate. Pathologic fracture may develop if the bone is stressed too early.

RECOMMENDED READING

Morrisy RT, Weinstein SL, eds. *Lovell and Winter's pediatric orthopaedics*, 4th ed. Philadelphia: JB Lippincott, 1996:579–612.

Osteonecrosis (Avascular Necrosis)

 Basics

DESCRIPTION

Avascular necrosis (AVN) is the *in situ* death of a segment of cancellous bone from lack of circulation, secondary to traumatic or atraumatic causes. The most common sites are the femoral head, scaphoid, talus, and humeral head; however, avascular necrosis can occur in any bone. It is most common in the 30- to 40-year age group, and it affects males and females equally. Legg-Calvé-Perthes disease is a type of AVN which occurs in patients 4 to 12 years of age.

CAUSES

Osteonecrosis can have either a traumatic or a nontraumatic origin. Traumatic osteonecrosis is most commonly associated with femoral neck fractures, dislocations of the femoral head, displaced fractures of the scaphoid and talar neck, and four-part fractures of the humeral head. Atraumatic osteonecrosis is thought to be secondary to occlusion of the arterial vessels, injury or pressure on the arterial wall, or occlusion to the venous outflow vessels. The exact cause of these vascular insults is unknown, but it is currently thought to be the result of increased intramedullary pressure.

RISK FACTORS

- Trauma
- Corticosteroids
- Ethanol use
- Blood dyscrasias (e.g., sickle cell disease, hypercoagulable states
- Dysbarism (e.g., caisson disease [exposure to hyperbaric oxygen])
- Excessive radiation therapy
- Gaucher's disease

CLASSIFICATION

0. No pain, normal physical examination, normal radiographs, normal bone scan, normal magnetic resonance imaging (MRI) scan, increased intraosseous pressure
I. Minimal pain, decreased internal rotation, normal radiographs, nondiagnostic bone scan, early nuclear medicine changes, increased intraosseous pressures
II. Moderate pain, decreased range of motion, radiographic sclerosis, positive bone scan, positive MRI scan, increased intraosseous pressure
III. Advanced pain, decreased range of motion, radiographic crescent sign and femoral head flattening, positive bone scan, positive MRI scan, increased intraosseous pressure

IV. Severe pain, pain with any range of motion, radiographic femoral flattening and crescent sign with acetabular degeneration, positive bone scan, positive MRI scan, increased intraosseous pressure

Specific Sites and Eponyms

- Legg-Calvé-Perthes disease: femoral head
- Sever's disease: calcaneus
- Köhler's disease: tarsal navicular
- Freiberg's infarction: second metatarsal head
- Panner's disease: capitellum
- Kienböck's disease: lunate

ICD-9-CM

733.40 Aseptic bone necrosis (osteonecrosis)

 Diagnosis

SIGNS AND SYMPTOMS

Pain is often insidious in onset, is described as aching, and is minimally relieved by antiinflammatory medications. Pain increases with time and is worsened by weight bearing.

DIFFERENTIAL DIAGNOSIS

- Initial symptoms can mimic primary or metastatic bone tumors.
- Late stages of the disease are difficult to differentiate from osteoarthritis.

PHYSICAL EXAMINATION

Physical examination varies according to the stage of the disease.

- Early: There may be only subtle findings such as muscle atrophy or loss of range of motion.
- Late: In patients with arthritis, there may be severe loss of range of motion and pain on positioning of the joint.

LABORATORY TESTS

Patients with atraumatic osteonecrosis should have a complete blood count, peripheral blood smear, and coagulation studies to rule out blood dyscrasias.

PATHOLOGIC FINDINGS

Grossly necrotic bone, fibrous tissue, and subchondral collapse may be seen. Histologically, early changes involve autolysis of osteocytes, followed by inflammatory cell invasion. If the infarct is large enough and the blood supply can be reestablished, new woven bone forms, which eventually remodels through creeping substitution.

IMAGING PROCEDURES

Radiographs are diagnostic in later stages of the disease. MRI and a bone scan are often required for diagnosis of earlier disease stages.

 Management

GENERAL MEASURES

The treatment of osteonecrosis remains controversial. Many centers have had success with core decompression (drilling a 5- to 10-mm tract through the area of osteonecrosis) in the early stages of the disease. Later stages often require total joint replacement for disease in the hip, knee, or shoulder or fusion for disease in the ankle or wrist. There is some evidence that anticoagulation therapy may be helpful.

SURGICAL TREATMENT

Core decompression is a procedure in which a large-bore needle is inserted into the necrotic bone and a core of bone and medullary cavity is removed. It is thought to decompress the increased intraosseous pressure and to restore blood flow to the affected segment. Many centers report up to a 90% success rate using this procedure in stage I and II disease.

PHYSICAL THERAPY

This is not helpful.

PATIENT EDUCATION

Outcomes depend on the stage of the disease and are sometimes unpredictable. Many patients ultimately require joint reconstructive procedures.

PREVENTION

Prevention includes avoidance of prolonged high-dose steroid use or alcohol abuse.

MONITORING

Serial radiographs and repeat MRI scans are helpful to follow the progression of the disease.

COMPLICATIONS

- Collapse of the joint surface
- Ankylosis

PROGNOSIS

The prognosis depends on the age group and bone affected and is much better for children than adults. Prognosis is also improved if the disease is diagnosed in its earlier stages.

RECOMMENDED READING

Brashear HR, Raney RB. *Handbook of orthopaedic surgery*, 10th ed. St. Louis: CV Mosby, 1986:378–379.

Miller MD. *Review of orthopaedics*. Philadelphia: WB Saunders, 1992:70–72.

Simon SR. *Orthopaedic basic science*. Rosemont, IL: American Academy of Orthopaedic Surgeons, 1994:279–283.

Basics

DESCRIPTION

Osteoporosis is a disease characterized by a low bone mass and the subsequent development of nontraumatic or traumatic fractures. It affects all bones. Most commonly, fractures occur in the distal forearm (wrist), the thoracic and lumbar vertebrae, and the proximal femur (hip).

GENETICS

The genetic component of this disease is unknown.

INCIDENCE

• Osteoporosis is responsible for more than 1 million fractures yearly, and fractures of the vertebral body are the most common.
• There are roughly 275,000 new osteoporotic hip fractures each year in the United States.
• The fracture rate increases with age, especially over 75 years.
• Osteoporotic fractures are more common in women than in men, with the following ratios at different sites:

—5:1 for distal forearm fractures
—7:1 for vertebral fractures
—2:1 for hip fractures

RISK FACTORS

• White (Northern European descent) and Asian ethnicity
• Female gender
• Late menarche, nulliparity, early menopause, excessive exercise (producing amenorrhea)
• Increasing age
• Positive family history
• Small body frame (less than 127 lb)

CAUSES

• Idiopathic secondary
• Nutritional: milk intolerance, vegetarian dieting, low dietary calcium, excessive alcohol intake

• Lifestyle: smoking, inactivity
• Medical: type I diabetes, Cushing's syndrome, hyperparathyroidism, thyrotoxicosis, anorexia nervosa
• Medications: glucocorticoid drugs, long-term lithium therapy, chemotherapy, anticonvulsants (phenytoin impairs vitamin D metabolism), long-term phosphate-binding antacid use, thyroid replacement drugs

CLASSIFICATION

Primary

Postmenopausal: Associated with Loss of Estrogen

Type I.   Excess loss of cancellous bone with relative sparing of cortical bone: wrist, and vertebral fractures
Type II. More concordant loss of both cortical and cancellous bone: hip fractures

Senile

Associated with poor calcium absorption, seen in patients more than 75 years of age

Secondary

When a clearly identifiable etiologic mechanism is recognized

ICD-9-CM

733.0 Generalized osteoporosis
733.01 Senile osteoporosis
733.7 Posttraumatic osteoporosis

 Diagnosis

SIGNS AND SYMPTOMS

• Patients have pain during weight bearing, with lower extremity fractures (femoral neck and pelvis), and midline pain secondary to vertebral compression fractures.
• Clinical features include kyphosis and vertebral fractures (compression fractures especially of T-11–L-1), hip fractures, pelvic fractures, and distal radius (wrist) fractures.

DIFFERENTIAL DIAGNOSIS

• Osteomalacia
• Hyperparathyroidism
• Hyperthyroidism
• Cushing's syndrome
• Neoplasm (myeloma, leukemia)

PHYSICAL EXAMINATION

• Vertebral fractures are associated with loss of stature. In the thoracic spine, this is associated with a progressive increase in the degree of kyphosis, and in the lumbar spine, it is associated with progressive flattening of the lordotic curve.
• Tenderness is often not over the spinous processes themselves, but rather it is paraspinal from actively contracting paraspinal muscles. This is the major cause of chronic back pain in spinal osteoporosis.

LABORATORY TESTS

• Urinary calcium, hydroxyproline, free cortisol, and serum alkaline phosphatase levels are helpful in evaluating osteopenic conditions, although they are usually unremarkable in osteoporosis.
• In most cases, there is no indication to measure the calcitropic hormones (parathyroid hormone, calcitriol, or calcitonin) unless a specific indication exists based on history, examination, and biochemical screening.

PATHOLOGIC FINDINGS

Excessive bone loss results from abnormalities in the bone remodeling cycle. The cycle is initiated by resorption of old bone, recruitment of osteoblasts, deposition of new matrix, and mineralization of that newly deposited matrix. In osteoporosis, there is a loss of a small amount of bone mass with each cycle.

High-Turnover Osteoporosis

Conditions that increase the rate of activation of the bone remodeling process increase the proportion of the skeleton that undergoes remodeling at any one time and speed the rate of bone loss. This is the pattern most associated with secondary causes of osteoporosis.

Osteoporosis

Low-Turnover Osteoporosis

In normal aging, there appears to be a progressive impairment of the signaling between bone resorption and bone formation, such that with every cycle of remodeling, there is an increase in the deficit between resorption and formation because osteoblast recruitment is inefficient.

SPECIAL TESTS

Special studies used for the workup of osteoporosis include single-photon (appendicular) and double-photon (axial) absorptiometry, quantitative computed tomography, and dual-energy x-ray absorptiometry. This last test is the most accurate, with less radiation. Biopsy (after tetracycline labeling) may be used to evaluate the severity of osteoporosis and to identify osteomalacia.

IMAGING PROCEDURES

- Plain radiographs are often unremarkable until bone loss has reached 30%.
- Moderate osteoporosis of the thoracic and lumbar spine often causes signs of overall loss of bone density (osteopenia).
- The vertebral bodies have a striated appearance from the loss of secondary trabeculae and reinforcement of sharply defined primary trabeculae.
- Because of the loss of trabecular bone, there is accentuation of the cortices, resulting in the appearance of "picture framing."
- The vertebral bodies become weakened, and the intervertebral disc may protrude into the adjacent vertebral body.
- Changes can range from bending and buckling of the end plates to complete compression fractures.

- Bone loss in the appendicular skeleton (extremities) is initially most readily apparent at the ends of long and tubular bones because of the predominance of cancellous bone in these regions.
- Widening of the medullary canal with thinning of the cortices can be seen.
- Occasionally, osteoporotic fractures are not identified on initial radiographs, but are identified by radionuclide bone scan, computed tomography scans, magnetic resonance imaging scans, or repeat plain radiographs as healing occurs.

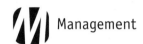 Management

GENERAL MEASURES

- Physical activity: weight-bearing exercise regimens
- Calcium supplements: 1,000 to 1,500 mg per day (more effective in senile osteoporosis)
- Estrogen: effective in postmenopausal osteoporosis when treatment is initiated within 6 years of menopause
- Calcitonin (Calcimar, Miacalcin): like estrogen, inhibits bone resorption and slows down the rate of bone loss; doses usually starting as low as 25 U subcutaneously 3 times per week and gradually increasing over a period of 2 to 3 months if needed
- Bisphosphonates (etidronate): used to stabilize or increase bone mass and possibly to reduce the vertebral fracture rate; 2 (1,25 dihydroxy)
- Calcitriol (Rocaltrol): the most potent metabolite of vitamin (1,25 dihydroxy)D; increases intestinal calcium absorption; some studies showing a reduction in vertebral fracture rate over calcium alone; daily dose commonly 0.25 μg

SURGICAL TREATMENT

Surgical treatment is related to management of impending or completed fractures. Vertebroplasty, the percutaneous injection of methacrylate into osteoporotic vertebrae which have collapsed, shows promise but awaits long-term study.

PATIENT EDUCATION

Prevention of bone loss in asymptomatic women is generally achieved through behavior modification and pharmacologic intervention. The initial approach is based on lowering risk factors through alterations in nutrition and lifestyle. Any weight-bearing activity suffices, and exercise programs should focus on compliance through recreational therapy.

COMPLICATIONS

Fractures may occur.

PROGNOSIS

The earlier therapy is instituted, the better is the prognosis.

RECOMMENDED READING

Favus MJ. *Primer on the metabolic bone diseases and disorders of mineral metabolism,* 2nd ed. New York: Raven, 1993:223–263.

Miller M. *Review of orthopaedics,* 2nd ed. Philadelphia: WB Saunders, 1996:28–32.

Basics

DESCRIPTION

First described by Sir James Paget in 1877, Paget's disease (osteitis deformans) is a bone disorder commonly seen in the geriatric population. It is a chronic and slowly progressive disease of disorganized bone remodeling. As implied by the name, osteitis deformans, the involved bone may be severely deformed and enlarged, features that suggest an inflammatory origin. Paget's disease can affect any bone. The process is often asymmetric and may involve one bone (monostotic) or multiple bones (polyostotic).

GENETICS

Ample evidence exists to suggest that first-degree relatives of affected persons carry a higher risk (up to seven times higher) of developing the disease than those without any family history of the disease.

INCIDENCE

• This disease of late adulthood is rarely seen before the fourth decade of life.
• It affects 3% to 4% of the population older than 50 years of age and is slightly more common in men.
• Its prevalence increases with advancing age, up to 15% by the ninth decade.

CAUSES

• Genetic associations have been identified.
• Infectious (one of the paramyxoviruses): Some investigators believe that the cause is a slow virus because of the long incubation periods, absence of fevers, and involvement of a single organ system.

RISK FACTORS

• First-degree relatives of affected persons
• Advancing age

CLASSIFICATION

Active Phase

• Early (lytic) phase (purely bone destruction)
• Mixed phase (both bone destruction and formation)
• Late (sclerotic) phase, when bone formation predominates

Inactive Phase

• Many older patients have inactive disease with no radiographic progression, symptoms, or laboratory abnormalities.

ICD-9-CM

731.0 Paget's disease of bone

Diagnosis

History and physical examination (the involved area is warm to the touch because of the increased vascularity of the underlying bone), laboratory tests, plain radiographs, and bone scan to evaluate the extent of skeletal involvement are the basic components of the diagnostic evaluation.

SIGNS AND SYMPTOMS

Clinical manifestations depend on the severity of the disease and the site of involvement. They include the following:

• Pain: Many patients are asymptomatic, whereas others experience mild to severe bone pain. Acute bone pain suggests pathologic fracture or malignant degeneration. Pain is usually constant and unrelated to activity.
• Frontal bossing and conductive hearing loss may be present.
• Spine: If the spine is involved, the patient may develop spinal stenosis with or without radiculopathy.
• Arthritis: Pagetic arthritis is common in the hip and knee. Patients have severe pain and difficulty in ambulating.

DIFFERENTIAL DIAGNOSIS

• Metastatic cancer
• Fibrous dysplasia
• Paget's sarcoma

PHYSICAL EXAMINATION

The most common findings are bowing of the extremity and local warmth if the bone is subcutaneous, such as the tibia. Restricted range of motion is common in the hip in patients with pagetic arthritis.

LABORATORY TESTS

• Increased serum alkaline phosphatase levels are noted (normal in 6% of patients).
• The 24-hour hydroxyproline determination is performed (normal in 5% of patients).
• Serum calcium is determined. Unless there is concurrent generalized inactivity, hyperparathyroidism, hyperthyroidism, or malignancy, serum calcium levels are usually normal.
• Determination of urine pyridinoline cross-links is now the most sensitive test.

Paget's Disease

PATHOLOGIC FINDINGS

- Highly vascular bone resulting from high turnover rate
- Multiple pathologic fractures resulting from structurally weaker bone
- Histologically, more numerous osteoclasts and less mature (but fully mineralized) bone

SPECIAL TESTS

Increased urinary excretion of pyridinoline is well associated with the extent of the disease.

IMAGING PROCEDURES

- Plain films demonstrate enlarged bone with thick, coarsened trabeculae, as well as both sclerotic and lytic changes in the affected bone.
- A flamed-shaped area of radiolucency strongly suggests an advancing edge of a pagetic lesion.
- A "hot" technetium-99m methylene diphosphonate bone scan is also observed.

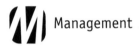 Management

GENERAL MEASURES

- Therapy depends on severity of the disease: Not all patients require treatment.
- Indications for treatment include bone pain, high-output cardiac failure, and prevention of pathologic fracture.
- Pain from associated arthritis can be treated with nonsteroidal antiinflammatory drugs; narcotics should be avoided.
- A cane or walker may be used for gait stabilization.
- Surgery is indicated in patients with severe arthritis who are refractory to medical management or in patients with impending pathologic fractures; preoperatively, medical therapy should be initiated to reduce disease activity, to minimize blood loss, and to optimize surgical outcome.

SURGICAL TREATMENT

Surgery is generally done for three reasons:

1. Replacement of an arthritic joint
2. Internal fixation of a long bone fracture
3. Correction of a long bone deformity

Total hip arthroplasty is extremely effective in relieving pain and improving function. Intramedullary rods are the main modality for fixing long bone diaphyseal fractures (multiple osteotomies may be necessary to correct the deformities). Single or multiple osteotomies with internal fixation can be used to correct long bone deformities.

PHYSICAL THERAPY

Physical therapy may be used to improve the patient's ambulatory ability before or after surgery.

MEDICAL TREATMENT

Medical treatment should be initiated in symptomatic patients or in preparation for orthopaedic surgery to prevent perioperative hypercalcemia or excessive bleeding. Calcitonin and biphosphonates are commonly used.

Calcitonin

- Calcitonin inhibits bone resorption by direct action on osteoclasts.
- Side effects include nausea, facial flushing, and polyuria.

Biphosphonates

- These are potent inhibitors of bone resorption.
- They bind to hydroxyapatite crystals in bone and thereby prevent osteolysis.
- They may also function as metabolic poisons for osteoclasts.
- Common side effects include nausea, vomiting, and loose bowel movements.

PATIENT EDUCATION

- Patients should be well informed about their disease and the goals of treatment.
- Treatment should be aimed at slowing or arresting disease progression, providing pain relief, or restoring function.
- Appropriate consultations should be made to address any extraskeletal abnormalities (e.g., deafness).
- The need for long-term follow-up should be emphasized.
- Resources for patient education in the United States can be obtained from the Paget Foundation, 200 Varick Street, New York, NY 10014 (tel. 212-229-1502).

MONITORING

Patients are generally followed once a year. Usually, plain radiographs are obtained.

COMPLICATIONS

- Pathologic fractures
- High-output cardiac failure
- Malignant degeneration (Paget's sarcoma)

PROGNOSIS

- Most patients with Paget's disease are asymptomatic and have a normal life expectancy.
- Long-term survival for patients with Paget's sarcoma (less than 1% of patients with Paget's disease) is poor, about 20% survival in 5 years.

RECOMMENDED READING

Bockman RS, Weinerman SA. Medical treatment for paget's disease of bone. Rosemont, ILL: Am. Acad. Orthop. Surg. *Instr Course Lect* 1993;42:425–435.

Kaplan FS, Singer FR. Paget's disease of bone: pathophysiology, diagnosis, and management. *J Am Acad Orthop Surg* 1995;3:336.

McCarthy EF and Frassica FJ. Pathology of Bone & Joint Disorder. Philadelphia: WB Saunders, 1998:165–172.

Basics

DESCRIPTION

This is an infection of the radial or ulnar margins of the nails (lateral fold) of the hand (Fig. 1).

INCIDENCE

- Common
- Affecting all ages

CAUSES

- Typically secondary to the introduction of *Staphylococcus aureus* under the nail fold
- May be related to a hangnail, biting the nail edge, or manicure instrumentation

ASSOCIATED CONDITIONS

Eponychia

- This is an infection of the periungual tissue at the proximal nail bed (Fig. 2).
- Treatment is similar to that of paronychia: After incision with a scalpel, a small clamp is inserted into the abscess and the inflammatory pocket is opened (Gram stain, culture, and antibiotics as in paronychia).

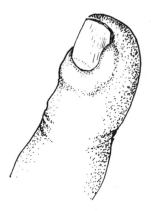

Fig. 1. Swelling along the nail. There may or may not be pus coming from the involved area.

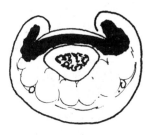

Fig. 2. Infection spreading along the nail bed.

Felons

- The infection is in the pulp of the finger.
- Treatment: Incision and drainage are performed with a lateral incision down to the bone, then spreading with a clamp to disrupt the fibrous septa (Gram stain, culture, and antibiotics as in paronychia).

Subungual Abscess

- This is an infection beneath the nail.
- Treatment: After administering an adequate digital block, remove the nail plate and the nail. Obtain a specimen for Gram stain and culture. Irrigate and gently débride any purulent material. Replace nonadherent gauze. One dose of intravenous antistaphylococcal antibiotics should be given, followed by a 10- to 14-day course of penicillin or erythromycin. Follow-up as in paronychia is indicated.

ICD-9-CM

681.02 Paronychia (finger)
681.9 Paronychia with lymphangitis
757.5 Eponychia
681.9 Subungual abscess

 Diagnosis

SIGNS AND SYMPTOMS

- Redness and swelling on the side of the nail fold with pain
- Possibly becoming fluctuant with discharge

DIFFERENTIAL DIAGNOSIS

- Eponychia
- Felons
- Subungual abscess

LABORATORY TESTS

These tests are not needed unless the infection is aggressive and is spreading.

PATHOLOGIC FINDINGS

Typically, these infections are caused by *S. aureus*. Changes consistent with acute inflammation are noted.

IMAGING PROCEDURES

Imaging is not necessary unless the nail infection is chronic, aggressive, unresponsive to treatment, or related to trauma.

Management

GENERAL MEASURES

Early Diagnosis

If there is erythema without an abscess, then treat with oral antibiotics and warm, soapy soaks.

Abscess

If an abscess has formed, then it needs immediate drainage with a scalpel, and the purulent material must be sent for Gram stain and culture. A digital block with local anesthetic can be used. The lateral fifth of the nail can be removed. The wound should be irrigated copiously with saline solution through an angiocatheter or needle and subsequently packed with nonadherent sterile gauze. A 10- to 14-day course of empiric antibiotics should be initiated. A synthetic penicillin is the drug of choice, or erythromycin for penicillin-allergic patients, because *S. aureus* is the most common causative organism.

Chronic Paronychia

Chronic paronychia often occurs in patient populations exposed to water. These patients have often concomitant fungal infections and should have a topical antifungal ointment added to the regimen.

MEDICAL TREATMENT

Synthetic penicillins are the drugs of choice.

MONITORING

Reevaluate within 48 hours of initial treatment to ensure that treatment is effective.

PREVENTION

- Keep the nail clean and appropriately trimmed.
- Use gloves for work and washing.
- Avoid nail biting.

COMPLICATIONS

Progressive infection may require more aggressive treatment if it involves the pulp of the finger or extends into the bone.

PROGNOSIS

The prognosis is good, with appropriate care.

RECOMMENDED READING

Neveaser RJ. Infections. In: Green DP ed. *Operative hand surgery.* NY: Churchill Livingstone, 1993:1022–1024.

Patellar Dislocation

 Basics

DESCRIPTION

Patellar dislocation usually refers to lateral displacement of the patella out of its normal alignment in the trochlear groove of the femur.

- It is seen primarily in young patients (16 to 20 years old).
- The risk of recurrence varies with age: 60% in children 11 to 14 years old, 30% in young adults 19 to 28 years old, and rarely in adults older than 28 years.
- It occurs more often in females than in males.

GENETICS

A congenital predisposition is thought to exist for most patellar dislocations, especially those arising from a twisting event.

INCIDENCE

The incidence is difficult to quantitate because many knees relocate spontaneously and are misdiagnosed. There is a 24% incidence of a positive family history. Up to 73% of patients with instability demonstrate at least one of the following structural abnormalities:

- Shallow patellofemoral groove
- Patella alta
- Excessive Q angle
- Ligamentous laxity
- Excessive femoral anteversion
- Vastus medialis dysplasia
- Excessive genu valgus
- Pes planus

CAUSES

- Ten percent of these injuries: a direct blow to the medial aspect of the patella
- Severe valgus injury to the knee
- Twisting injury or other minor trauma, usually associated with congenital deficiencies

RISK FACTORS

- Positive family history
- Congenital deficiencies
- Participation in football, basketball, baseball, gymnastics, or dancing
- Osteochondral fragments
- Age younger than 14 years
- High level of activity or competition in a youth
- Mechanism other than a direct blow
- Palpable medial defect
- Contralateral evidence of dysplasia
- Hypermobility of the patella
- Multiple prior dislocations
- Patella alta

CLASSIFICATION

- Subluxation: The patella sits on the edge of the femoral groove, but not out of the track.
- Dislocation: The patella is completely displaced out of the patellofemoral groove, usually laterally.

ASSOCIATED CONDITIONS

- Connective tissue disease with ligamentous laxity, such as Ehlers-Danlos and Marfan's syndromes
- Femoral anteversion and pes planus

ICD-9-CM

836.3 Patellar dislocation

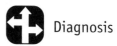 Diagnosis

SIGNS AND SYMPTOMS

- Patients with acute dislocation may present with the knee held in a flexed position, as a result of hamstring spasms.
- The femoral condyles may be prominent medially.
- Often, the patella has spontaneously reduced, with findings of the following:

—Diffuse parapatellar tenderness
—Positive apprehension test
—Palpable defect at the insertion of the vastus medialis muscle
—Hemarthrosis

DIFFERENTIAL DIAGNOSIS

- Cruciate ligament injury
- Patellar fracture
- Patellofemoral pain syndrome
- Osteochondral fracture

PHYSICAL EXAMINATION

After the acute symptoms subside, examine the knee for the following:

- Effusion
- Apprehension, with patellar translation both medially and laterally
- Lateral tracking of the patella (in the shape of a "J") with the knee extended from a flexed position (Fig. 1)
- Injury to the medial, collateral, or cruciate knee ligaments
- Lateral tilt

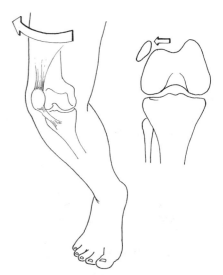

Fig. 1. Patellofemoral dislocation is almost always lateral.

PATHOLOGIC FINDINGS

Abnormalities in the patellofemoral articulation allow the pull of the vastus lateralis and lateral retinaculum muscles to overcome that of the vastus medialis, even during minor trauma. This unbalanced pulling often tears the medial retinaculum and vastus medialis insertion.

IMAGING PROCEDURES

- Postreduction plain radiographs are obtained for evidence of osteochondral fragments.
- Axial views of the bilateral patella may show significant lateral tracking.
- Magnetic resonance imaging or computed tomography is rarely helpful.

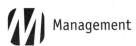 Management

GENERAL MEASURES

Reduce acute dislocations and then immobilize the knee. Surgical stabilization is recommended for the following:

- Recurrent dislocations
- Dislocations in carefully selected, highly active, competitive athletes
- Acute dislocations with avulsive detachment of the vastus medialis muscle by bony fragment seen on radiography

SURGICAL TREATMENT

- Lateral release with advancement of the medial retinaculum is the most effective method for preventing recurrence.
- Patients with excessive Q angles (more than 150 degrees) may also benefit from distal realignment, using the Hauser, Elmslie-Trillat, or Fulkerson procedure.
- To prevent distal migration of the tibial tubercle, procedures that involve tibial physis should be avoided in children with open physeal plates.
- Arthroscopy does not have a place in treatment of patellar dislocation other than for intraarticular assessment of patellofemoral tracking.

PHYSICAL THERAPY

- The main goal of therapy is to strengthen the injured extensor mechanism and to improve patellofemoral tracking. Straight leg raises may begin immediately with appropriate support.
- Recurrent dislocations often advance more quickly with physical therapy to strengthen the quadriceps.

MEDICAL TREATMENT

- Reduce acute dislocation by gentle, steady extension of the knee, facilitated with the patient prone and the patient's hip extended to relax the hamstrings.
- Avoid forceful manipulation.
- Once the knee is reduced, immobilize it in extension with a compression dressing.
- Evaluate the medial retinacular structure for tenderness every 2 weeks for up to 6 weeks.
- When the patient is comfortable, apply a Neoprene sleeve with a laterally based felt pad.
- Advise the patient that analgesics may be taken in the acute phase.

PATIENT EDUCATION

Discuss the risk factors for recurrent dislocation with a possible recommendation that the patient avoid high-risk activities or sports.

MONITORING

Patients are followed at 2- to 4-week intervals to monitor the progress of quadriceps rehabilitation.

COMPLICATIONS

- Recurrent dislocations
- Reflex sympathetic dystrophy
- Hemarthrosis with a lateral release
- Patellofemoral arthritis
- Osteochondral fractures

PROGNOSIS

Overall, 75% of patients are treated successfully with conservative means. The key is to identify patients at risk for recurrence and to treat them more aggressively early in the course.

RECOMMENDED READING

Cash JD, Hughston JC. Treatment of acute patellar dislocation. *Am J Sports Med* 1988;16:(2)44–50.

Morrissy RT, ed. *Lovell and Winter's pediatric orthopaedics,* vol 2, 3rd ed. Philadelphia: JB Lippincott, 1990:1117–1120.

Patellar Fracture

 Basics

DESCRIPTION

• Fracture of the kneecap, the largest sesamoid bone in the body
• Possibly also involving injury to the quadriceps tendon or patellar ligament
• Affecting all ages and both sexes

SYNONYM

Broken kneecap

GENETICS

The incidence of congenital bipartite and tripartite patella is 8% in the general population.

INCIDENCE

Patellar fractures and other extensor mechanism injuries represent 1% of fractures diagnosed each year.

CAUSES

• Direct blow to the patella from a fall or traffic accident injury in which the knee hits the dashboard
• Sudden powerful quadriceps muscle contracture

RISK FACTORS

A traumatic incident is a risk factor.

CLASSIFICATION

These injuries are classified by the pattern of the fracture:

• Vertical
• Transverse
• Stellate
• Polar

ASSOCIATED CONDITIONS

• Other long bone fractures
• Quadriceps tendon rupture
• Patellar ligament rupture
• Knee ligament
• Meniscus injuries

ICD-9-CM

822.2 Patellar fracture

 Diagnosis

SIGNS AND SYMPTOMS

• Acute knee pain and swelling after a traumatic incident
• Inability to extend or straighten the affected knee
• Possible visible or palpable defect of the extensor mechanism

DIFFERENTIAL DIAGNOSIS

• Distal femoral or tibial plateau fracture
• Collateral ligament tear
• Anterior cruciate ligament tear
• Quadriceps tendon or patellar ligament rupture

PHYSICAL EXAMINATION

• Check for pain or swelling in the affected knee.
• Perform an active knee extension test to identify the loss of integrity to the extensor mechanism.

LABORATORY TESTS

No laboratory tests are indicated.

PATHOLOGIC FINDINGS

• Fracture hematoma
• Variable amounts of cartilage damage
• Bony comminution

IMAGING PROCEDURES

Plain Radiographs

• Plain radiographs (anteroposterior, lateral, and "sunrise" views) are most useful for diagnosing a patellar fracture and for surgical planning.
• On the lateral view, the presence of patella alta (high-riding patella) with no fracture is consistent with a rupture of the patellar ligament.
• The presence of patella baja (low-riding patella or location closer to the tibia than expected) without fracture is consistent with a quadriceps tendon rupture.

Computed Tomography

This technique is helpful in planning surgical treatment of comminuted fractures.

⚡ Management

GENERAL MEASURES

• The diagnosis of patellar fracture is confirmed with the skin intact (closed fracture).
• An open patellar fracture is a surgical emergency requiring urgent irrigation and débridement.

SURGICAL TREATMENT

An orthopaedic surgeon should determine whether an open wound represents an open fracture requiring urgent surgery. If surgery is required, the knee should be splinted in extension until the patient can be taken to the operating room for open reduction of the fracture fragments and internal fixation.

Surgery is required for the following:

• A greater than 3-mm separation of the fragments
• A greater than 2-mm stepoff of the articular surface
• An open fracture

Surgical treatment of fractures falls into the following categories:

• Vertical fractures: Open reduction and internal fixation are performed with 3.5- or 4.0-mm screws. Once the wound is healed at 2 weeks, early controlled range of motion can begin.

• Transverse fractures: Open reduction and internal fixation are performed using a tension band technique (tension bands are used to resist the concentration of the quadriceps muscle, which will displace the fracture) including wires and pins. Patients are typically in a cast for 4 to 6 weeks with controlled range of motion afterward.
• Stellate or comminuted fractures: Pins, screws, and wires are used to hold the pieces together until healing occurs. Longer cast immobilization is usually needed. If the patella is too comminuted to be reconstructed, a patellectomy can be performed by removing the bone under the extensor mechanism and suturing the tendon.

PHYSICAL THERAPY

• Knee stiffness is common after these injuries; progressive range-of-motion exercises are required.
• Avoid overzealous passive motion, however, to reduce the risk of refracture or displacement until healing is complete.
• Nonsurgical patients may bear weight as tolerated in the cast or splint.
• Patients may resume active range-of-motion exercises once the cast is removed.

MEDICAL TREATMENT

• If the fracture is minimally displaced and the patient is able to extend the leg actively, the knee should be placed in a cylinder cast or a locked brace for 6 to 8 weeks.
• Analgesics may be taken as needed.

PATIENT EDUCATION

• Injury to the cartilage and bone is typical in patellar fractures.
• The risk of future knee pain and arthritis exists.
• The risk of decreased motion after a patellar fracture is present.
• Full recovery can take up to 1 year.
• Protective knee pads may prevent recurrence in situations in which knee strikes are common (e.g., basketball, in-line skating)

MONITORING

Serial radiographs are obtained at 1-month intervals to evaluate healing.

COMPLICATIONS

• Fracture nonunion
• Malunion
• Refracture
• Need for hardware removal
• Arthritis

PROGNOSIS

• Nondisplaced patellar fractures: 95% good to excellent results
• Patients with transverse or vertical fractures after open reduction and internal fixation: 60% to 80% good to excellent results
• Stellate fractures: worst prognosis

RECOMMENDED READING

Johnson EE. Fractures of the patella. In: Rockwood CA, Green DP, Bucholz RW, et al., eds. *Rockwood and Green's fractures in adults,* vol 2, 5th ed. Philadelphia: Lippincott–Raven, 1996:1956–1972.

Patellar Tendon Rupture

 Basics

DESCRIPTION

Patellar tendon rupture is a disruption of the segment of the quadriceps extensor mechanism extending from the inferior aspect of the patella to the tibial tubercle.

- Patients generally younger than 40 years
- Affecting men and women equally

CAUSES

Ruptures generally result from trauma in which a violent quadriceps muscle contraction occurs against resistance in the extended knee, such as a fall.

RISK FACTORS

- History of patellar tendinitis
- Steroid injections around the patellar tendon

ICD-9-CM

844.8 Patellar tendon rupture

 Diagnosis

SIGNS AND SYMPTOMS

- Defect in the patellar tendon
- Inability to extend the knee from the flexed position
- Injured patella possibly resting more proximally than the uninjured knee and migrating proximally with active quadriceps contraction
- Acute injuries generally associated with significant knee effusion and pain on active or passive range of motion

DIFFERENTIAL DIAGNOSIS

Extensor Mechanism Injuries

- Quadriceps tendon rupture
- Patellar dislocation
- Patellar fracture

Intraarticular Disorders

- Ligament tears
- Occult tibial plateau fractures
- With these last two, extensor mechanism function remains intact.

PHYSICAL EXAMINATION

- Check for pain or swelling in the affected knee.
- Perform an active knee extension test to identify loss of integrity to the extensor mechanism.
- Palpate for a defect at the patellar tendon.

PATHOLOGIC FINDINGS

Complete rupture of the patellar tendon is noted.

IMAGING PROCEDURES

- Obtain plain anteroposterior and lateral radiographs of the knee to rule out patellar fracture and tibial plateau fractures.
- Most commonly, the patella ruptures from the inferior pole of the patella and may be accompanied by a small, avulsed fragment of bone.

 Management

GENERAL MEASURES

Patellar tendon ruptures require operative repair. Patients with acute ruptures should be placed in a knee immobilizer for comfort and referred to an orthopaedist for surgical treatment.

SURGICAL TREATMENT

- Acute ruptures need to be surgically fixed.
- Earlier repair allows for maintenance of patellar tendon length and better functional results in the long term.
- Chronic patellar tendon tears generally require some type of reconstructive procedure.
- Patients are generally treated using a long leg cast or a knee brace locked in extension for approximately 6 weeks after surgery.

PHYSICAL THERAPY

- Initiate knee flexion exercises 6 to 8 weeks after surgery (after the cast or brace is removed).
- Some patients may require physical therapy for quadriceps strengthening and range-of-motion exercises.
- Many patients can perform much of their rehabilitation on their own.

MEDICAL TREATMENT

- Most patients with acute ruptures require some type of knee immobilizer for comfort until surgery can be performed.
- Patients may bear weight as tolerated.
- Patellar tendon ruptures require operative repair.
- Analgesics can be given for pain management during acute ruptures and after surgery.

MONITORING

- See patients 7 to 10 days after surgery for removal of stitches.
- Remove the cast or unlock the brace 6 to 8 weeks after surgery.

COMPLICATIONS

- Poor postoperative wound healing
- Knee stiffness

PROGNOSIS

- Most patients treated with early patellar tendon repair have good or excellent results.
- Chronic tendon ruptures are more difficult to manage and often have only fair to good results.

RECOMMENDED READING

An HS. *Synopsis of orthopaedics*. New York: Thieme, 1991:246–249.

Clark CR, Bonfiglio M, eds. *Orthopaedics: essentials of diagnosis and treatment*. New York: Churchill Livingstone, 1994:242–244.

Fu FH, Stone DA, eds. *Sports injuries: mechanisms, prevention, treatment*. Baltimore: Williams & Wilkins, 1994:302–304.

Basics

DESCRIPTION

Patellofemoral syndrome is characterized by diffuse anterior knee pain, usually of insidious onset, that is worsened by activities involving flexion of the knee.

SYNONYM

Moviegoer's knee

GENETICS

No known mendelian pattern exists.

INCIDENCE

• The incidence is unknown.
• It often occurs during adolescence, but any age may be affected, especially if patient has begun a new sport or activity that increases stress on the knee.
• It is more common in females.

CAUSES

• Habitual overloading of the patellofemoral joint related to

—Overuse
—Lower extremity malalignments
—Poorly developed quadriceps muscles
—Dysplastic changes about the patellofemoral articulation

• Subset of these cases appears in adolescent girls with

—Increased femoral anteversion
—External tibial torsion
—Genu varum
—Excessive Q angle
—Heel cord contractures
—Pronated feet

RISK FACTORS

Sports involving repetitive motion, such as cycling and running, as risk factors.

ICD-9-CM

719.46 Knee pain

Diagnosis

SIGNS AND SYMPTOMS

• Diffuse anterior knee pain aggravated by stair climbing, prolonged sitting, and other bent-knee activities
• In young athletes, possible history of increased activity, but frequently no identifiable predisposing event
• Parapatellar tenderness and swelling (location important to ruling out other causes of pain, such as quadriceps or patellar tendinitis)
• Lateral retinaculum frequently contracted, demonstrated by lack of lateral patellar translation and a positive tilt test
• Apprehension sign (pain with compression of the patellofemoral joint) (Fig. 1)
• Generalized ligamentous laxity
• Abnormal Q angle (angle made by patellar and quadriceps tendons, usually less than 100 degrees) (Fig. 2)
• Signs of patellar maltracking

DIFFERENTIAL DIAGNOSIS

• Quadriceps tendinitis
• Distal patellar tendinitis
• Patellofemoral arthrosis
• Symptomatic plica syndrome
• Osteochondritis diseccans
• Patellofemoral instability
• Reflex sympathetic dystrophy, especially if the patient has had previous patellofemoral surgery

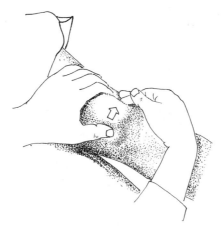

Fig. 1. Patients who previously experienced patellofemoral subluxation or dislocation exhibit a positive apprehension sign when the patella is pushed laterally.

PHYSICAL EXAMINATION

• Check for pain or swelling in the affected knee.
• Check the Q angle of the affected knee.
• Look for the apprehension sign and for signs of patellar maltracking.
• Perform the patellar tilt test (elevating the lateral margin of the patella).

LABORATORY TESTS

There are no serum laboratory tests to identify this disease.

PATHOLOGIC FINDINGS

• Malalignment
• Arthroscopically demonstrated lateral tracking or subluxation of patella
• Contracted lateral retinaculum (unclear whether this is a cause or an effect)
• Q angle abnormalities (may be altered by tibial or femoral torsion)

IMAGING PROCEDURES

• A lateral radiograph (30 degrees of flexion) may be helpful in diagnosing patella alta or patella baja, as well as degenerative changes.
• Axial views (Merchant's view) with the knee flexed at 30 and 45 degrees are helpful in determining the congruence angle and any evidence of subluxation.
• Bilateral views should be obtained for comparison.
• Computed tomography and magnetic resonance imaging are rarely useful in evaluating this disorder.

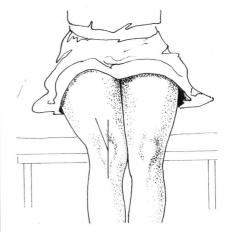

Fig. 2. The Q angle is the angle formed between the tibial tubercle, the patella, and the femur. The greater the angle, the more likely the development of patellofemoral syndrome.

Patellofemoral Syndrome

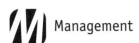 Management

GENERAL MEASURES

- Physical therapy is the first line of treatment for this disorder. Patients must be motivated to improve strength.
- Surgical correction is an option if conservative measures fail, but patients must realize that these results depend on intensive postoperative physical therapy.
- Distal realignment may be performed if there is evidence of subluxation or dislocation of the patella.
- Reflex sympathetic dystrophy may complicate the clinical picture and should be ruled out before undertaking surgical repair.

SURGICAL TREATMENT

- Lateral retinacular release is often the first surgical option and has a 75% to 85% rate of favorable results; it can be done as an open procedure or arthroscopically.
- Distal realignment of the tibial tubercle using Fulkerson's procedure or a tubercle anteriorization procedure may be considered in patients with malalignment.
- Chondral shaving to decrease synovitis may have a limited effect.
- Patellectomy should be used only as a salvage procedure and only after alignment has been corrected.

Contraindications for Surgery

- Severe patellofemoral arthritis is a contraindication for surgery.
- Overzealous release of the lateral side may lead to medial subluxation.

PHYSICAL THERAPY

- Aimed at strengthening the quadriceps and improving patellar tracking
- Straight leg lifts and terminal arc motion exercises with or without ankle weights
- Closed kinetic chain exercises, squats, lunges, and step downs used instead of open kinetic chain and isometric exercises
- General aerobic exercise and occasionally bracing with a patellar cutout
- Transcutaneous electrical nerve stimulation possibly helpful early on to reduce pain

MEDICAL TREATMENT

Most patients (50% to 80%) are successfully treated without surgery. Conservative management consists of the following:

- Reduction of symptoms using nonsteroidal antiinflammatory drugs
- Avoidance of offending activities
- Reconditioning aimed at strengthening the quadriceps tendon and improving patellar tracking without increasing the load on the patellofemoral joint
- Taping of the patella to counter the abnormal mechanics while the patient performs reconditioning exercises
- Gradual return to normal activities
- Maintenance of improved strength

PATIENT EDUCATION

- Nothing reduces patellofemoral crepitus.
- Any improvement strongly depends on participation in physical therapy.
- Optimization and maintenance of knee extensor mechanism function are key to preventing recurrence.
- Open kinetic chain exercises often worsen the symptoms, and leg extension machines should be avoided.

COMPLICATIONS

Hemarthrosis is the most common complication of a lateral release, so great care must be taken for hemostasis at the time of the operation. Other complications include the following:

- Reflex sympathetic dystrophy
- Recurrent medial subluxation
- Synovitis
- Saphenous neuritis
- Thrombophlebitis
- Patellofemoral osteoarthritis

PROGNOSIS

- Most patients note an improvement of symptoms with physical therapy, but they must maintain the strength of the quadriceps to avoid recurrence.
- Patients who require surgical intervention do not fare as well, unless a specific cause for the pain, such as subluxation or malalignment, is found.

RECOMMENDED READING

DeHaven KE, Dolan WA, Mayer PJ. Chondromalacia patella in athlete: clinical presentation and conservative management. *Am J Sports Med* 1979;7:5–12.

Henry JH, Craven PR. Surgical treatment of patellar instability: indications and results. *Am J Sports Med* 1981;9:82–91.

Morrissy RT, ed. *Lovell and Winter's pediatric orthopaedics*, vol 2, 3rd ed. Philadelphia: JB Lippincott, 1990:1114–1117.

Basics

DESCRIPTION

Peroneal tendon subluxation is an increased and abnormal motion of the peroneal tendon out of its groove behind the fibula. The tendons snap in and out of their correct positions with ankle motion (Fig. 1).

GENETICS

No known mendelian predisposition exists.

INCIDENCE

- Rare
- Most common between ages 10 and 25 years

CAUSES

- Usually traumatic, classically occurring as a result of skiing injuries in which the ligaments of the peroneal retinaculum are torn
- May develop spontaneously in predisposed persons, probably resulting from an underlying shallow groove behind the fibula or ligamentous laxity

RISK FACTORS

Athletic patients are at risk.

ASSOCIATED CONDITION

Ligamentous laxity

ICD-9-CM

718.3 Peroneal tendon subluxation

 Diagnosis

SIGNS AND SYMPTOMS

- Lateral ankle pain with activity that does not resolve
- Snapping of the peroneal tendons over the fibula
- Tenderness behind the lateral malleolus along the peroneus brevis muscle; subluxation

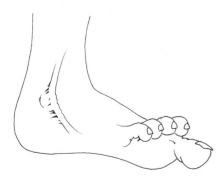

Fig. 1. The peroneal tendons may subluxate anteriorly over the fibular head if the retinaculum is torn or stretched.

elicited with the patient attempting to dorsiflex the affected foot from a plantar flexed, everted position

DIFFERENTIAL DIAGNOSIS

- Ankle sprain
- Lateral malleolar fracture
- Lateral ligament disruption
- Osteochondral talar dome fracture

PHYSICAL EXAMINATION

- Have the patient attempt to dorsiflex the ankle from a plantar flexed, everted position to reproduce the symptoms.
- Have the patient sit facing you and ask the patient to rotate the foot in a circular fashion while you palpate behind the lateral malleolus muscle. If a disorder is present, the peroneal tendons may glide or move out of their groove and over the fibula.
- Peroneal tendons normally snap in place within their sheath. Only a movement out of the sheath with reproduction of symptoms is diagnostic.

LABORATORY TESTS

There are no laboratory tests for this condition.

PATHOLOGIC FINDINGS

- Possible shallow groove for the peroneal tendons behind the fibula
- Attenuated superior or inferior peroneal retinaculum

IMAGING PROCEDURES

- Computed tomography demonstrates the shape of the peroneal groove.
- Magnetic resonance imaging may demonstrate a longitudinal tear of the peroneus brevis.
- Plain films are needed to rule out any other ankle disorder because this is a rare entity and subjective symptoms are nonspecific.

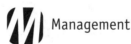 Management

GENERAL MEASURES

- Activity modification may reduce the occurrence of subluxation in certain patients if it is activity specific.
- An ankle brace may limit the excursion of the foot and may decrease the episodes.
- Conservative treatment should be employed initially.
- Surgery is commonly necessary to resolve the patient's symptoms of conservative treatment fails.
- Cast treatment is unlikely to be successful in chronic cases.

SURGICAL PROCEDURE

- Subluxating tendons require a peroneal groove-deepening procedure to locate the tendons more securely in their recess behind the fibula or a repair of the peroneal retinaculum (or both).

PHYSICAL THERAPY

Physical therapy has not been proven effective.

MEDICAL TREATMENT

- After an acute, initial episode, cast immobilization may help to relieve the patient's symptoms and to reduce inflammation.
- Patients with recurrent subluxation and resistant cases may require surgery.
- Nonsteroidal antiinflammatory agents can be used both acutely and during rehabilitation to relieve pain and to facilitate physical therapy.

PATIENT EDUCATION

- Educate the patient about the anatomy of the lower limb and which positions of eversion and dorsiflexion of the ankle are most likely to reproduce the subluxation.
- The condition does not lead to degenerative joint disease or permanent sequelae, but it may cause the ankle to give way unexpectedly.

MONITORING

Reeducation in ankle strengthening exercises is sometimes necessary.

COMPLICATIONS

- Complications of surgery include recurrence and sural neuroma.
- If symptomatic recurrence develops, other surgical procedures may be employed to treat symptoms.

PROGNOSIS

- Some cases are managed conservatively.
- Results are best when nonoperative measures are employed.
- The surgical success rate is 80% to 90%.

RECOMMENDED READING

Zoellner G, Clancy WG: Recurrent dislocation of the peroneal tendon. *J Bone Joint Surg* 1979:61-A; 292–294, 1979.

Perthes' Disease

 Basics

DESCRIPTION

Perthes' disease is a disorder of the hip in young children in which idiopathic juvenile avascular necrosis of the femoral head leads to a cascade of complicating factors and subchondral fracture of the head. Bone resorption begins and can result in collapse of the femoral head. This irregularity may evolve, much later, into subsequent degenerative joint disease.

SYNONYMS

- Legg-Calvé-Perthes disease
- Coxa plana
- Osteochondritis (or arthritis) deformans juvenilis

GENETICS

A positive family history is noted in only 2% to 10% of cases.

INCIDENCE

- Less than 1% of the population affected
- Most common in children 4 to 8 years old, but reported from 2 years of age to the late teens
- Males affected four to five times more often than females

CAUSES

The cause is unknown, but most current theories are based on vascular embarrassment of the femoral head. Various proposed causes of the limited blood supply include the following:

- Trauma
- Intraosseous venous hypertension or obstruction
- Hypercoagulable disorders

Minor trauma may have role in initiating events in any of these theories.

RISK FACTORS

- Small stature
- Lower socioeconomic level
- Increased parental age
- Living in urban areas
- Ethnicity (Asian, Inuit, Central European)

CLASSIFICATION

Classification systems all based on radiographs showing the extent of involvement of the femoral head

Catterall Staging System

Stage I. Anterior femoral head involvement only
Stage II. Entire medial dome involvement
Stage III. Progression into the lateral column of the head
Stage IV. Whole-head involvement

Stulberg Classification System

This system describes the end result after healing of Perthes' disease, in terms of sphericity and congruity of the femoral head with the acetabulum.

ASSOCIATED CONDITIONS

- Short stature
- Avascular necrosis of the tarsal navicular vessels (Köhler's disease)

ICD-9-CM

732.1 Perthes disease

 Diagnosis

SIGNS AND SYMPTOMS

- Insidious onset of a limp (most common presentation)
- Pain either absent or mild
- When pain present, usually related to activity and relieved by rest
- Pain usually in the groin area, but can be referred to the anteromedial thigh or knee
- Limited abduction and internal rotation
- Child often leaning the trunk over the affected limb while walking (Trendelenburg's sign)
- Mild atrophy of the thigh, calf, and buttock, in long-standing disease
- Leg length inequality (late finding)

DIFFERENTIAL DIAGNOSIS

- Septic arthritis
- Toxic synovitis
- Juvenile rheumatoid arthritis
- Traumatic avascular necrosis node
- Sickle cell disease
- Multiple or spondyloepiphyseal dysplasia
- Glycogen storage diseases
- Hypothyroidism
- Tumors

PHYSICAL EXAMINATION

- Observe the child's gait for indications of pain: short, quick steps or shift of the shoulders with each stride.
- Check for limitation of internal or external rotation compared with the other side.
- Check abduction while holding the child's pelvis still.

LABORATORY TESTS

There are no tests to rule in Perthes' disease. On occasion, laboratory studies may be indicated to rule out hyperthyroidism, septic arthritis, or sickle cell disease.

PATHOLOGIC FINDINGS

- The physeal plate shows the formation of histologic clefts.
- Cartilage clusters are present, extending into the metaphysis.

IMAGING PROCEDURES

Radiographs show several stages of the disease.

Initial Phase

- The epiphysis is smaller than the contralateral side, with widening of the medial joint space.
- Physeal irregularity and subchondral radiolucency are also possibly present.

Fragmentation Phase

- The bony epiphysis begins to fragment.
- Mixed lucent and dense areas appear in the epiphysis.

Reparative Phase

• Normal bone density returns.
• Alterations in the shape of the femoral head and neck become obvious.

Healed Phase

• Residual deformity is revealed.
• A bone scan shows increased uptake, a helpful feature before radiographs show changes.
• Magnetic resonance imaging detects infarction but does not give information on the stage of the disease (no specific indication for this test).
• Arthrography is useful for assessing femoral head deformity and congruency.

Management

GENERAL MEASURES

• The position of best containment is determined by plain radiographs or arthrography.
• If the femoral head is containable, maintain it in this position by abduction orthosis or casts or by femoral or acetabular osteotomy. If the femoral head is not containable, salvage procedures can reduce pain, equalize leg length, and improve movement.
• Surgery is not recommended for children younger than 6 years old unless significant subluxation is shown.

SURGICAL TREATMENT

Osteotomy of the femur or acetabulum (or both) repositions the femoral head into a contained place within the acetabulum and allows further growth and remodeling to occur in a spheric, congruous fashion. The osteotomy is usually fixed internally, so early motion may be started.

PHYSICAL THERAPY

• Physical therapy may be helpful for maintaining range of motion of the hip.
• Therapy is most critical to maintain abduction motion.

MEDICAL TREATMENT

• Restoration of joint motion is critical to maintaining synovial and, therefore, cartilage nutrition.
• Containment of the femoral head in the acetabulum prevents deformity.
• A cast or brace must be worn full time, but weight bearing is allowed.
• If weight bearing is painful, protect the child with the use of crutches.
• If marked stiffness occurs, put the patient at rest until stiffness resolves.

PATIENT EDUCATION

• Maintaining range of motion is important; therefore, encourage the child to participate in physical therapy.
• The family must monitor the skin around the child's braces or casts.
• Parents should be told that the disease often takes approximately 2 years to heal.
• Patients usually have a largely pain-free childhood, even though problems may develop later in adulthood.
• Healing of the disorder cannot be accelerated.
• No effective means of prevention exists.
• Early detection is important, so containment can be achieved before significant deformity of the femoral head occurs.

MONITORING

• Brace or cast containment usually averages 6 to 18 months or until the reossification stage occurs and the risk of femoral head collapse has passed.
• Examine the child out of the brace to check range of motion.
• Take radiographs with the child in the brace.
• See the patient every 4 to 8 weeks until reossification occurs.

COMPLICATIONS

Loss of sphericity or collapse causes the following:

• Early degenerative joint disease
• Leg length discrepancy
• Loss of range of motion with flexion and adduction contractures

PROGNOSIS

Good Prognosis

• The younger the physis is at healing stage, the better the potential will be for remodeling of the femoral head.
• Poor results are rare in children younger than 6 years old.
• Almost always, symptoms resolve after the healing phase, and patients have freedom from pain during the teenage years.

Poor Prognosis

• Child older than 8 years at presentation
• Involvement of the lateral column of the femoral head
• Poor range of motion
• Nonconcentric or noncontained femoral head after healing
• Approximately 50% of patients with Perthes' disease as a child will need hip replacement by later adulthood (50 to 60 years old).

RECOMMENDED READING

Herring JA. The treatment of Legg-Calvé-Perthes disease. *J Bone Joint Surg Am* 1994;76:448–460.

McAndrew MP, Weinstein SL. A long-term follow-up of Legg-Perthes disease. *J Bone Joint Surg Am* 1984;66:860–868.

Stulberg SD, Cooperman DR, Wallensten R. The natural history of Legg-Calvé-Perthes disease. *J Bone Joint Surg Am* 1981;63:1095–1104.

Weinstein SL. Legg-Calvé-Perthes disease. In: Morrissy RT, Weinstein SL, eds. *Lovell and Winter's pediatric orthopaedics*, 4th ed. Philadelphia: JB Lippincott, 1996, p 951–992.

Phalangeal Joint Arthritis

 Basics

DESCRIPTION

Phalangeal joint arthritis is a degenerative "wear and tear" process involving articular tissues that leads to the destruction of cartilage, local bone loss, and the formation of osteophytes.
Most commonly affected joints are as follows:

- Distal interphalangeal joints of the hand
- Proximal interphalangeal joints of the fingers
- Carpometacarpal joint of the thumb

GENETICS

A single gene mutation is implicated in the development of osteoarthritis. For example, primary generalized osteoarthritis, a disease commonly affecting middle-aged women and characterized by nodular arthritis involving the distal interphalangeal foint of the hand and occasionally the knees and other joints, is thought to be the result of a single gene mutation that substitutes cysteine for arginine in position 519 of the type II procollagen gene.

INCIDENCE

- This condition occurs in 37.4% of people between the ages of 18 and 79 years.
- It increases sharply to include 85% of persons older than 70 years of age.
- Osteoarthritis of the hand increases in prevalence with advancing age, with the average age of onset being 58 years.
- It is more common in men younger than 45 years old.
- Women predominate beyond 45 years of age.

CAUSES

- Genetic changes in cartilage
- Mechanical changes in cartilage
- Chemical changes in cartilage

RISK FACTORS

- Increasing age
- Trauma

CLASSIFICATION

- Primary: no preexisting joint problem
- Secondary: previous history of trauma or other joint conditions

—Infection
—Hemophilia

ASSOCIATED CONDITION

Arthritis of the hip and knee

ICD-9-CM

716.94 Arthritis of hand/fingers

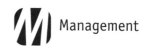 Diagnosis

SIGNS AND SYMPTOMS

- Rapid onset of pain in the digital joints with no specific history of trauma
- Progressive deformity of the distal and proximal interphalangeal joints of the hand
- Rare involvement of the MCP joints
- Most common complaints: pain and morning stiffness
- Finger deformity in osteoarthritis in a lateral deviation pattern shown during physical examination and on radiography
- Decrease in range of motion and stiffness from joint space incongruity and osteophytes that block flexion and extension
- Eventual periarticular soft tissue contracture further limiting joint motion

DIFFERENTIAL DIAGNOSIS

- Rheumatoid arthritis
- Inflammatory arthropathies
- Gout
- Pseudogout
- Trauma
- Septic arthritis

PHYSICAL EXAMINATION

- Reduced range of motion
- Ankylosis
- Osteophytes

LABORATORY TESTS

When appropriate:

- Rheumatoid factor
- HLA-B27
- Antinuclear antibody
- Erythrocyte sedimentation rate

PATHOLOGIC FINDINGS

Early Disease

- Increased water content in the cartilage
- Increased proteoglycan level

Progressive Disease

- Decrease in both cartilaginous water and proteoglycan levels
- Increased friction with motion
- Decreased shock-absorbing capability of cartilage
- Eventual progressive cartilage fissuring and destruction

End-Stage Disease

- Abnormal joint loading
- Subchondral microfractures
- Cyst formation

IMAGING PROCEDURES

Plain film radiographs demonstrate the following:

- Narrowing of joint spaces
- Subchondral sclerosis
- Osteophyte formation
- Cyst formation

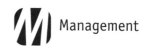 Management

GENERAL MEASURES

- Rest
- Avoidance of aggravating activity

SURGICAL TREATMENT

- Proximal interphalangeal joints: arthrodesis or arthroplasty
- Distal interphalangeal joints: arthrodesis
- Carpometacarpal joint: Arthroplasty with tendon interposition

PHYSICAL THERAPY

- Active isometric and passive range-of-motion exercises to maintain motion
- Ultrasound and diathermy therapy to decrease the inflammation

MEDICAL TREATMENT

- Splinting of the involved joints with well-padded splints to decrease pain and swelling
- Analgesics (acetaminophen, aspirin)
- Antiinflammatory medications
- Local steroid injections

PATIENT EDUCATION

- Reassure patients about the relatively benign natural course of the disease.
- Treatments are effective in relieving pain and in preventing progressive deformity.
- Control further articular damage by minimizing joint loading.

MONITORING

Patients are checked at 6- to 12-month intervals.

COMPLICATIONS

- Articular deformity
- Nonunion in attempted joint fusion
- Malunion in attempted joint fusion
- Prosthetic dislocation
- Wearing of prosthesis
- Infection

PROGNOSIS

Excellent pain control and restoration of function are achieved in the majority of patients with analgesics, exercise, and arthroplasty.

RECOMMENDED READING

Mankin H. Form and function of articular cartilage. In: Simon SR, ed. *Orthopaedic basic science*. Rosemont, IL: American Academy of Orthopaedic Surgeons, 1994:252–262.

Swanson AB, Swanson G. Osteoarthritis in the hand. *J Hand Surg* 1983;8:669–675.

Basics

DESCRIPTION

These dislocations involve the following joints of the hand:

- Metacarpophalangeal (MCP)
- Proximal interphalangeal (PIP)
- Distal interphalangeal (DIP)

SYNONYMS

Gamekeeper's thumb (MCP joint dislocation)

GENETICS

No known mendelian pattern exists.

INCIDENCE

- Common
- Joint dislocation generally occurs in skeletally mature patients.
- In the pediatric population, the physes are weaker than the capsular structures. Consequently, physeal fractures or separations are more common in children than joint dislocations.
- PIP dislocations are common in basketball and baseball players.

CAUSE

Trauma is the cause of these dislocations.

RISK FACTORS

None are known.

CLASSIFICATIONS

Proximal Interphalangeal Joint Dislocations

1. Dorsal (most common, resulting from volar plate injury)
2. Volar (rare, associated with central slip disruption)
3. Rotatory (rare, from "buttonholing" of one condyle of the head of proximal phalanx through the space between the central slip and the lateral band)

Metacarpophalangeal Joint Dislocations

1. Lateral (collateral ligament injuries)
2. Dorsal

Distal Interphalangeal Dislocation

1. Simple (reducible)
2. Complex (irreducible because of entrapment of the volar plate between two dislocated middle and proximal phalanges)

ASSOCIATED CONDITIONS

- Injuries of the periarticular structures of the involved joints
- Phalangeal fractures or neurovascular or other soft tissues injuries
- Associated avulsion fractures of the phalanx

ICD-9-CM

834.0 Dislocation, phalanx

 Diagnosis

SIGNS AND SYMPTOMS

- Pain
- Deformity (Fig. 1)
- Instability from ligamentous disruption
- Loss of motion
- Altered sensation or perfusion (or both) from neurovascular compression

DIFFERENTIAL DIAGNOSIS

- Fracture dislocation
- Chronic dislocation
- Collateral ligament injury
- Associated volar plate injury

PHYSICAL EXAMINATION

- Examine the hand to determine whether the point of maximal tenderness is over the collateral ligaments, central slips, volar plate, or bony structures.
- Evaluate the stability of the joint to radial and ulnar stresses.
- Order appropriate radiographic studies.

PATHOLOGIC FINDINGS

- Dislocations of the phalangeal joints often result in injuries to surrounding soft tissue structures.
- Lateral dislocations of these joints lead to collateral ligament tears.
- The palmar plate is at risk in hyperextension injuries and dorsal dislocations.
- In gamekeeper's thumb (dislocation of the thumb MCP joint with or without avulsion fracture of the metacarpal base), both the collateral ligament and the palmar plate are torn.

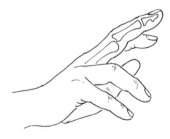

Fig. 1. Interphalangeal joint dislocations are almost always dorsal, owing to hyperextension injuries.

Phalanx Dislocation

IMAGING PROCEDURES

• Initial radiographs include true lateral, anteroposterior, and oblique views of the hand, to evaluate the phalangeal bones and joints adequately.
• Stress views are important in assessing dislocations when ligamentous disruptions are possible.
• Arthrography is helpful in identifying the nature and location of a ligamentous injury.

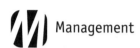 Management

GENERAL MEASURES

• Phalangeal dislocations: Attempt closed reduction, unless the injury is chronic (Fig. 2). Minimize swelling with rest, ice, and elevation.
• Ligamentous tears: Use protective immobilization with either "buddy" taping for collateral injuries or extension block splinting for volar plate disruption.
• Central slips ruptures: Splint the injured joint in extension, followed by serial casting.
• Irreducible dislocation or open dislocation: Surgical intervention is needed.

SURGICAL TREATMENT

The phalangeal joint can be approached by a dorsal or volar incision, depending on the type of dislocation and the anticipated associated injuries requiring surgical repairs.

PHYSICAL THERAPY

Active and gentle passive range-of-motion exercises are begun once stability of the joint is confirmed.

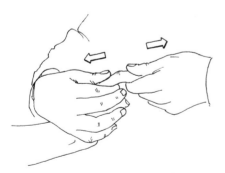

Fig. 2. Interphalangeal dislocation is reduced by longitudinal traction and gentle flexion.

MEDICAL TREATMENT

• Most complete ruptures of the collateral ligaments, volar plates, or central slips: Immobilize for 3 to 6 weeks.
• PIP joints: Splint in 15 degrees of flexion after reduction of dorsal dislocations. Not all complete disruptions of collateral ligament in PIP dislocations require surgery.
• MCP joints: Immobilize in 50 to 70 degrees degrees of flexion.
• Central slip disruptions: Use an extension splint for 3 weeks, followed by dynamic splinting.
• Dislocations of the DIP and IP joints: Traction is indicated.
• MCP joint dislocation reduction: Gentle traction and hyperextension of the proximal phalanx are indicated. Push the joint into flexion while maintaining contact with the metacarpal head to avoid entrapment of periarticular soft tissues. Entrapment of periarticular structures likely when the range of motion of the joint decreases after reduction or if the dislocation is irreducible.
• Analgesics or nonsteroidal antiinflammatory drugs are used as needed.

PATIENT EDUCATION

• Advise patients regarding cause of the injury.
• Prescribe strict immobilization of the involved joint to achieve stability and healing.
• Urge the use of proper warm-up exercises to help prepare the muscles for stress.
• Advise patients to use protective handwear during contact sports.

MONITORING

Patients are followed at 3- to 6-week intervals to ensure that they maintain adequate range of motion.

COMPLICATIONS

• Complex dislocations
• Recurrent displacement
• Angulation
• Flexion contractures
• Stiffness
• Associated neurovascular injuries

PROGNOSIS

Most patients regain normal function with proper treatment. Some loss of motion (approximately 10%) can be expected.

RECOMMENDED READING

Dray G, Eaton R. Dislocations and ligament injuries in the digits. In: Green DP, ed. *Operative hand surgery,* vol 1, 3rd ed. New York: Churchill Livingstone, 1993:767–798.

Green DP, Rowland SA. Fractures and dislocations in the hand. In: Morrissy RT, ed. *Rockwood and Green's fractures in adults,* 3rd ed. Philadelphia: JB Lippincott, 1991:675–744.

Basics

DESCRIPTION

A phalanx fracture is a break in of one or more phalanges in the fingers.

SYNONYM

Finger fractures

INCIDENCE

- The reported incidence varies because patients with phalanx fractures present to a variety of medical practitioners.
- Fractures of the distal phalanx constitute more than 50% of all hand fractures.
- Fractures of the metacarpals and the phalanges are probably the most common fractures in the skeletal system.
- These fractures occur among all ages.
- Common causes vary significantly with age.
- These fractures are more common in people younger than 20 or older than 70 years.
- Both sexes are affected equally.

CAUSES

Crush injury is causative. The specific cause depends on age:

- Children younger than 10 years: compression
- Adolescents and young adults 10 to 39 years old: sports-related injuries
- Adults 30 to 69 years old: machinery-related injuries
- Elderly persons (60 years and older): accidental falls

Other causes include crush injury and motor vehicle accidents.

RISK FACTORS

Involvement in a sport or in a job or hobby that involves power tools or machinery is a risk factor.

CLASSIFICATION

The Jupiter and Belsky system classifies fractures according to the following:

- Phalanx involved
- Location of fracture within the phalanx
- Pattern of fracture
- Fracture complexity
- Whether fracture is open or closed
- Whether fracture is stable or unstable to motion

ASSOCIATED CONDITIONS

These conditions include other possible fractures in the hand and upper extremity.

ICD-9-CM

816.00 Phalanx fracture

Diagnosis

SIGNS AND SYMPTOMS

- Pain, swelling, or deformity after some trauma to the finger
- Laceration
- Decreased range of motion
- Numbness of the affected digit

DIFFERENTIAL DIAGNOSIS

Pathologic fracture, most commonly with an enchondroma (benign cartilage tumor)

PHYSICAL EXAMINATION

- Determine the mechanism of injury and where it occurred (whether in a clean or dirty environment).
- Determine how much time has elapsed since the injury.
- Ascertain the patient's age, hand dominance, occupation, and hobbies.
- Assess and document the patient's neurovascular status.
- Examine the hand to determine the precise area of tenderness and whether there are any lacerations and possible open fractures.
- Evaluate the hand for any significant injury to soft tissues, including tendons, ligaments, nerves, and blood vessels.
- Evaluate the digit for length, rotation, and angular alignment, attributes that allow for normal functions of pinch, grasp, and hook grasp.
- Determine the angulation and rotational alignment by comparing the appearance of the injured digit with that of adjacent digits.
- Assess the plane of the nail plate by comparing nail plate alignment, in digital extension and full flexion, with that of surrounding digits.

PATHOLOGIC FINDINGS

- Crush injury is the most common cause of distal phalanx fractures.
- Most such fractures are comminuted.
- A direct blow is more likely to cause a transverse or comminuted fracture.
- Twisting injury more often results in an oblique or spiral fracture.
- Digital function is impaired not only by fracture stability or deformity, but also by concomitant injury to soft tissues, including tendons, ligaments, blood vessels, and nerves.
- Injury to soft tissue structures is common.

IMAGING PROCEDURES

Radiography

- Oblique view to assess intraarticular fractures
- True lateral view to evaluate injuries involving a finger
- Low-kilovolt mammography film recommended as initial screening test for foreign body (e.g., wood splinter, most glass) because many foreign bodies are not visible on plain film

Other Techniques

- Computed tomogaphy preferred method for detecting wood and thorns
- Magnetic resonance imaging final backup for all types of foreign bodies except gravel

Phalanx Fracture

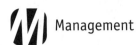 Management

GENERAL MEASURES

- Immobilize unstable closed fractures for 3 to 4 weeks.
- Surgery is indicated for all intraarticular fractures and for unstable fractures associated with significant soft tissue injury or when a fracture remains unstable after closed reduction

SURGICAL TREATMENT

Indications

- Failure of closed reduction to maintain rotation, length, or angular alignment
- Intraarticular fracture in which joint congruity is lost, resulting in small joint dysfunction
- Unstable fractures associated with significant soft tissue injury in which fracture instability precludes a normal soft tissue rehabilitation program

Closed Reduction With External Fixation

Percutaneous pin or screw fixation may be used with closed reduction if acceptable reduction can be achieved.

Indications

- No more than 10 to 15 degrees of angular deformity
- Gross comminution with accompanying soft tissue envelope injury
- Soft tissue injury in which further open dissection may compromise bone or digit viability
- Segmental defect in which digital length needs to be preserved and formal open reduction and internal fixation delayed

Open Reduction and Internal Fixation

- Open reduction and internal fixation are indicated if adequate closed reduction cannot be achieved.
- These techniques are also preferred even when closed reduction is possible but high-force demands occur during soft tissue rehabilitation.

Indications

- Periarticular and intraarticular fractures
- Segmental defects

Internal fixation may be done with plates, lag screws, wire, or intramedullary devices other than Kirschner wires. The direct visualization afforded by an open approach permits more accurate reduction and adequate implant application.

PHYSICAL THERAPY

- The patient is encouraged to perform range of motion for all fingers not included in the splint, to prevent stiffness.
- Digital performance deteriorates when active range of motion is delayed longer than 3 weeks.
- Soft tissue mobilization with active motion is initiated once clinical healing is achieved (evidenced by minimally tender fracture site that is not painful when manipulated), usually at 3 to 4 weeks.
- The radiographic appearance of union lags behind clinical union. Postoperatively, range-of-motion exercises are usually initiated at 2 to 4 weeks.

MEDICAL TREATMENT

Treatment must always include management of any soft tissue injuries and must allow these injuries them to be rehabilitated as fracture stability improves.

Buddy Taping

- Certain nondisplaced and impacted transverse fractures of the phalanges are ideally managed with "buddy" taping in which two fingers are taped together so one acts as a splint for the other.
- The fracture must truly be stable with minimal angulation in any plane.

Closed Reduction and Splinting

- Manage phalangeal fractures by closed reduction and external immobilization with a splint.
- Use digital nerve block for anesthesia.
- Manipulate the distal fragment to align with the proximal fragment.
- Place the splint.
- The fracture must be stable after reduction for the splint to maintain reduction.
- Splint the hand in the "intrinsic plus" position with the metacarpophalangeal joints at 90 degrees of flexion and the interphalangeal joints in full extension.
- Use a gutter splint, depending on the fingers involved.
- Children tolerate immobilization better than adults, and adults will likely have more joint stiffness.

PATIENT EDUCATION

- Underscore the importance of performing range-of-motion exercises to prevent stiffness in affected and surrounding digits.
- Emphasize the significance of maintaining therapy and range-of-motion exercises to ensure functional outcome.

MONITORING

- Obtain postreduction radiographs immediately and again in 3 to 7 days to check for displacement.
- Obtain subsequent radiographs to monitor for displacement and to assess for healing.
- Monitor the patient until the fracture has clinically healed and finger function is acceptable.

COMPLICATIONS

Malunion

This most common complication of phalangeal fracture may result in the following:

- Malrotation requiring rotational osteotomy
- Lateral deviation requiring closing wedge osteotomy
- Volar angulation requiring volar closing wedge osteotomy
- Intraarticular realignment osteotomy

Tendon Adherence

- This is common, especially in crush injuries.
- Intensive hand rehabilitation is needed.
- Only after maximum passive joint motion is regained, consider surgical treatment.

Nonunion

This is rare, but it is more common in open fractures.

Soft Tissue Interposition

This is rare.

Infections

Infections are more common in open fractures.

PROGNOSIS

A poor prognosis is more likely in the following:

- Age older than 50 years
- Associated tendon injuries (especially extension)
- Associated joint injury
- More than one fracture in a finger
- Crush injury
- Skin loss

RECOMMENDED READING

Fisher TJ. Phalangeal fractures. In: *Hand surgery update*. Rosemont, IL: American Academy of Orthopaedic Surgeons, 1996:3–10.

Green DP, Butler TE. Fractures and dislocations in the hand. In: Rockwood CA, Green DP, Bucholz RW, et al., eds. *Rockwood and Green's fractures in adults*, vol 1, 4th ed. Philadelphia: Lippincott–Raven, 1996:607–743.

Basics

DESCRIPTION

Pigmented villonodular synovitis (PVNS) is an uncommon lesion characterized by diffuse proliferation of the synovium to form yellow-brown villous projections. The knee is the most commonly affected joint, followed by the hip and shoulders. Lesions are almost always unilateral.

SYNONYMS

• Giant cell tumor of the tendon sheaths and joints
• Hemorrhagic villous synovitis

GENETICS

No known correlation exists.

INCIDENCE

• Uncommon
• Usually found in young to middle-aged adults
• No definite gender correlation; may have slight female predominance

CAUSES

• The cause is unknown.
• Studies in animals have produced similar lesions in response to recurrent hemarthroses, but lesions resolve when the inciting stimulus is removed.
• In humans, slow progression of PVNS is the rule.

RISK FACTORS

PVNS may have a slight association with recurrent hemarthrosis, but this is not definitely established.

ASSOCIATED CONDITIONS

None are known.

ICD-9-CM

215.3 Benign neoplasm, knee

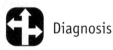 Diagnosis

SIGNS AND SYMPTOMS

• Insidious onset
• Slow progression
• Recurrent nontraumatic effusions
• Symptoms: pain, swelling, and limitation of range of motion
• Joint possibly warm to the touch
• Mild to moderate effusion
• Tender mass occasionally palpated (especially in the suprapatellar pouch of the knee)

DIFFERENTIAL DIAGNOSIS

• Inflammatory arthritis
• Traumatic effusions
• Infection
• Synovial sarcoma
• Hemosiderosis
• Hemochromatosis

PHYSICAL EXAMINATION

• Perform a complete examination of the knee, looking for the following:

—Ligamentous and meniscal status
—Possible effusion
—Warmth at the joint
—Pain
—Swelling
—Tender mass

• Determine the range of motion of the affected joint.
Assess for muscle atrophy.
• With shoulder, ankle, and hip involvement, there may be no physical finds or only subtle findings such as decreased range of motion or muscle atrophy.

LABORATORY TESTS

Joint aspiration reveals murky reddish brown fluid.

PATHOLOGIC FINDINGS

• Lesions may be large and diffuse or more discrete.
• Grossly, PVNS is characterized by villous projections or matted nodules stained with hemosiderin.
• Microscopically, elongated villi or nodules contain inflammatory infiltrates, foamy histiocytes, and hemosiderin deposits.

IMAGING PROCEDURES

Radiography

• Early findings

—Frequently no abnormalities
—Subtle erosions or periosteal reaction in non–weight-bearing actions
—Late findings

—Erosive lesions on both sides of the joint
—Possible diffuse joint space narrowing seen in late cases

Magnetic Resonance Imaging

This is increasingly helpful in both establishing diagnosis and directing treatment. Areas of extremely low signal are seen in the synovial lining on both T_1- and T_2-weighted images ("signal dropout"). Characteristically, one sees joint effusion and irregularity of the synovial lining.

Management

GENERAL MEASURES

• PVNS is a benign lesion. The potential for malignant degeneration has been reported but is extremely rare.
• In diffuse lesions, it is almost impossible to remove the entire lesion without injuring important ligaments and capsular structure; therefore, the recurrence rate is high.
• In severe or recurrent cases, radiotherapy has been effective.

SURGICAL TREATMENT

Lesions are removed by complete synovectomy, either open or arthroscopic, depending on the nature and location of the lesion.

MEDICAL TREATMENT

• Make appropriate referrals to establish the diagnosis and consider treatment options.
• Treat patients symptomatically with the following:

—Immobilization
—Splinting
—Antiinflammatory medication
—Analgesics

PATIENT EDUCATION

Even with appropriate care, the recurrence rate is high.

MONITORING

Magnetic resonance imaging is effective in detecting early local recurrences. Patients with asymptomatic local recurrences are treated with observation.

COMPLICATIONS

• Recurrence is common.
• Articular damage and bone loss may occur in long-standing disease.

PROGNOSIS

The prognosis is good.

RECOMMENDED READING

Cotten A, Flipo RM, Chastanet P, et al. Pigmented villonodular synovitis of the hip: review of radiologic features in 58 patients. *Skeletal Radiol* 1995;24:1–6.

O'Sullivan B, Cummings B, Catton C, et al. Outcome following radiation treatment for high-risk pigmented villonodular synovitis. *Int J Radiat Oncol Biol Phys* 1995;32:777–786.

Spjut HJ, Dorfman HD, Fechner RE, et al. *Tumors of bone and cartilage.* Washington, DC: Armed Forces Institute of Pathology, 1971:405–410.

Polydactyly

 Basics

DESCRIPTION

Polydactyly is a duplication of the fingers or toes that is detected at birth (Fig. 1).

SYNONYM

Accessory digits

GENETICS

Polydactyly of the index finger and polysyndactyly of the ring and long fingers are probably autosomal dominant conditions.

INCIDENCE

- Occurs in 1 in 150 blacks, versus 1 in 1,500 whites
- No significant difference between the sexes

CAUSES

The cause is unknown, unless the condition is associated with a syndrome.

RISK FACTORS

African heritage is a risk factor.

CLASSIFICATION

Preaxial (Involving Thumb or Great Toe) (Fig. 2): Wassel Classification

  I. Bifid distal phalanx
 II. Duplicated distal phalanx
III. Bifid proximal phalanx
 IV. Duplicated proximal phalanx
  V. Bifid metacarpal
 VI. Duplicated metacarpal

Central

Postaxial (Involving Small Finger or Toe): Stelling and Turek Classification

Type A. Complete duplication with bony attachment to an adjacent digit
Type B. Rudimentary, incomplete duplication of the phalanges

ASSOCIATED CONDITIONS

- Holt-Oram syndrome
- Fanconi's syndrome
- Trisomy 13
- Ellis–van Creveld syndrome

ICD-9-CM

755.0 Polydactyly (general)
755.01 Polydactyly (fingers)
755.20 Polydactyly (toes)

 Diagnosis

SIGNS AND SYMPTOMS

Duplicated fingers or toes are the signs of this condition.

PHYSICAL EXAMINATION

- Check for active and passive movement at each joint.
- Assess the stability of the digit.
- Look for an angular deformity at each joint.
- Look at the skin coverage and webbing.
- All these factors are important in determining surgical treatment.

PATHOLOGIC FINDINGS

The digits may vary in the extent of development of the phalanges and tendons.

IMAGING PROCEDURES

Plain film radiography of hand is indicated.

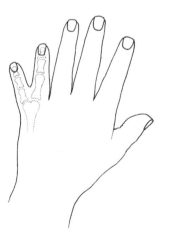
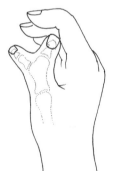

Fig. 1. Polydactyly involves variable skeletal duplications.

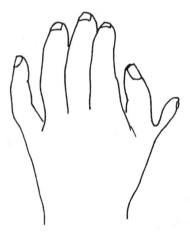

Fig. 2. Polydactyly is termed preaxial if it involves the thumb.

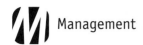 Management

GENERAL MEASURES

Mild, Type B Postaxial Polydactyly

This is treated in the newborn period by tying off the digit if it has no underlying skeletal connection. This method is

- Safe
- Not associated with bleeding complications
- Associated with a satisfactory appearance

The rudimentary digit falls off in about 10 days.

Type A

- Cosmetic concerns: Surgery is indicated to restore a normal appearance.
- Polydactyly of the foot: Surgery is often needed to make normal shoe wear possible.

SURGICAL TREATMENT

- Excision of the least developed digit with preservation of the ulnar collateral ligament
- Combination of the split portion

PATIENT EDUCATION

Inform patients with complex or preaxial polydactyly about the possibility of angular deformity of the thumb during growth.

MONITORING

For complex polydactyly, follow periodically with yearly checkups during growth.

COMPLICATIONS

- Small skin tag at the site of the polydactyly removal (rare)
- Angular deformity possible after complex polydactyly reconstructions

PROGNOSIS

Prognosis is good for patients with rudimentary, type B postaxial polydactyly. In other types of polydactyly, there may be a risk of angular growth of the adjoining digit or stiffness. In this case, however, problems are rarely symptomatic.

RECOMMENDED READING

Watson BT, Hennrikus WL. Postaxial type-B polydactyly: prevalence and treatment. *J Bone Joint Surg Am* 1997;79:65–69.

Popliteal Cyst in a Child

 Basics

DESCRIPTION

Popliteal cyst is a painless soft tissue mass in the medial popliteal fossa behind the knee.

GENETICS

No mendelian pattern is known.

INCIDENCE

• Most common soft tissue lesion about the knee in children
• Affecting children 2 to 14 years of age
• Incidence decreasing after age 9 years
• Twice as common in males

CAUSES

• Possibly resulting from weakness in the posterior knee joint capsule between the semimembranosus muscle and the medial head of the gastrocnemius
• Rarely related to intraarticular lesions

RISK FACTORS

• Juvenile rheumatoid arthritis
• Other chronic inflammation of the knee

ICD-9-CM

727.51 Popliteal cyst

 Diagnosis

SIGNS AND SYMPTOMS

• Protrusion between the medial head of the gastrocnemius and semimembranosus muscles
• Swelling of medial side of popliteal space just lateral to the semitendinosus muscle
• Usually asymptomatic, but can cause discomfort and restrict range of motion of knee if excessively enlarged
• Usually waxing and waning in size depending on the child's activity level
• Typically present for some time before child is brought to physician

DIFFERENTIAL DIAGNOSIS

• Malignant disease
• Vascular anomaly
• Soft tissue abscess

PHYSICAL EXAMINATION

• Examine the affected lower limb for swelling of the medial side of the popliteal space just medial to the semimembranosus muscle.
• Compress the cyst to check for pain; it is usually painless, but it may cause discomfort or decreased range of motion if it is excessively large.

• The remainder of the knee examination is usually normal.
• Examine the gait; no limp should be evident.
• Transilluminate the cyst in a darkened room with a point light source (e.g., strong penlight) (Fig. 1):
—With the patient prone, place the light source on the skin next to the area of swelling.
—If the mass illuminates more strongly and evenly than the surrounding fatty tissue, the fluid-filled nature of cyst will be confirmed, and a diagnosis of solid tumor is excluded.

LABORATORY TESTS

Most of the time, if the cyst is aspirated, the cyst fluid is clear and gelatinous. However, if it is not, send the aspirate for the following:

• Cell count
• Gram stain
• Culture

These tests are used to rule out septic arthritis or soft tissue abscess.

PATHOLOGIC FINDINGS

• Synovial fluid-filled sac in the semimembranosus-gastrocnemius interval
• Rarely related to intraarticular lesions

IMAGING PROCEDURES

• Plain-film radiography: to rule out bony disease
• Duplex ultrasound and magnetic resonance imaging (rarely indicated): to characterize the cyst further and to rule out malignancy

Fig. 1. A diagnosis of popliteal cyst in a child may be confirmed by transillumination.

Management

GENERAL MEASURES

• The patient's activity is restricted when the cyst is large.
• Surgical excision may be necessary if the cyst is symptomatic; the recurrence rate after surgical excision is 4%.

SURGICAL TREATMENT

• Excision of the cyst through a transverse incision in the posterior popliteal region; may be done as an outpatient procedure
• Immobilization for several weeks postoperatively

MEDICAL TREATMENT

• No treatment is required if no intraarticular lesion is present. Left untreated, 70% of cysts disappear spontaneously after months to years.
• If it is desired to confirm the diagnosis and increase the chance of resolution, one may aspirate the cyst with a large-bore needle followed by immobilization for immediate decompression; there is a high recurrence rate, however.

PATIENT EDUCATION

• Inform parents about the benign nature of the condition.
• Explain the similarity of the pathologic process to that of Baker's cyst in adults.
• Mention the lack of underlying knee disease and the absence of increased synovial fluid production.

MONITORING

• No routine follow-up is needed.
• Instruct the parent to return if the lesion changes in symptoms or in character.

COMPLICATIONS

The rate of recurrence of the cyst after surgical treatment is about 40%.

PROGNOSIS

Of these cysts, 70% resolve spontaneously within 2 months to 5 years.

RECOMMENDED READING

Morrissy RT, Weinstein SL, eds. *Lovell and Winter's pediatric orthopaedics*, 4th ed. Philadelphia: JB Lippincott, 1996:1065–1066.

Scott WN, ed. *The knee*. St. Louis: CV Mosby, 1994:267–268.

Szer IS, Klein-Gitelman M, DeNardo BA, et al. Ultrasonography in the study of prevalence and clinical evolution of popliteal cysts in children with knee effusions. *J Rheumatol* 1992;19:458–462.

Basics

DESCRIPTION

Popliteal cyst in an adult is a distended bursa in the posterior fossa of the knee that is often directly connected to the joint space.

SYNONYM

Baker's cyst

GENETICS

No known mendelian pattern exists.

INCIDENCE

- Unknown
- Bimodal distribution: one subset in children, the other in older adults
- In adults, cysts are usually the result of articular abnormalities; in children, the primary disorder
- Males and females affected equally

CAUSES

This intrinsic problem of the knee increases intraarticular pressure and forces fluid into the medial gastrocnemius bursa or causes a synovial herniation through a weak spot in the posterior capsule.

RISK FACTORS

These include a previous history of intraarticular knee disease (i.e., history of meniscus tear or arthritis).

ASSOCIATED CONDITIONS

- Rheumatoid arthritis
- Reiter's syndrome and other spondyloarthropathies
- Osteoarthritis
- Gout
- Chronic anterior cruciate ligament tear
- Medial or lateral meniscal tears

ICD-9-CM

727.51 Popliteal cyst

Diagnosis

SIGNS AND SYMPTOMS

- Mass in the popliteal fossa of the knee, usually on the medial side
- Possible knee effusion and tenderness
- Instability or catching (locking during range of motion) (rare)
- History of trauma (uncommon)
- Possible ruptured cyst with swollen, tender calf; could be confused with deep venous thrombosis

DIFFERENTIAL DIAGNOSIS

- Lipoma in the posterior fossa
- Pseudoaneurysm (usually pulsatile)
- Primary bone malignancy (i.e., parosteal osteosarcoma)
- Deep venous thrombosis
- Soft tissue tumor

PHYSICAL EXAMINATION

- Range of motion
- Ligament stability

—Anterior cruciate
—Posterior cruciate
—Medial collateral
—Lateral collateral

- Joint tenderness
- Presence or absence of an effusion
- Point tenderness

LABORATORY TESTS

- HLA-B27 (spondyloarthropathies)
- Rheumatoid factor

PATHOLOGIC FINDINGS

- Multiple bursae in popliteal fossa, swelling usually secondary to intraarticular disease
- Posteromedial meniscal tear

IMAGING PROCEDURES

- Anteroposterior and lateral radiographs
- Magnetic resonance imaging to evaluate the size of the cyst and differentiate the cyst from a soft tissue tumor

Management

GENERAL MEASURES

- Conservative treatment is the mainstay.
- The patient may continue all activities, limited only by pain.
- The examiner evaluates the joint space after failed treatment and addresses any pathologic features.
- Excised cysts often recur if joint disease is not corrected.
- Cysts often resolve spontaneously after treatment of articular abnormality.

SURGICAL TREATMENT

- Arthroscopic evaluation and treatment of any articular disease are indicated.
- A cyst that persists after treatment of the joint disorder should be removed through a posteromedial incision.

PHYSICAL THERAPY

Goals

- Strengthening quadriceps
- Stretching hamstrings
- Correcting atrophy and atonia of the quadriceps femoris muscle

Postoperative Therapy

A knee immobilizer is used for 48 hours before the patient resumes physical therapy.

MEDICAL TREATMENT

- Symptomatic care, including analgesics, nonsteroidal antiinflammatory drugs
- Resolution of most cysts with conservative care and reassurance
- Rehabilitation with elastic wraps for support
- Observation
- Aspiration is possible if diagnosis is confirmed and pain is severe; cyst usually recurs (Ensure that the mass to be aspirated is not a pseudoaneurysm.)
- Intraarticular cortisone injections are often beneficial
- Treatment of the underlying internal knee disease is the best treatment

PATIENT EDUCATION

Reassure the patient that the cyst is benign and will not damage the knee.

MONITORING

Patients are followed at 1-month intervals until range of motion returns.

COMPLICATIONS

- Recurrence
- Rupture, causing a painful, swollen calf and lower extremity (possibly simulating deep venous thrombosis)

PROGNOSIS

- Most cysts resolve once the intraarticular disorder is corrected.
- Untreated cysts may increase in size, but they often reach a stable, constant size.

RECOMMENDED READING

Childress HM. Popliteal cysts associated with undiagnosed posterior lesions of the medial meniscus. *J Bone Joint Surg Am* 1954;36:1233–1237.

Gristina AG, Wilson PD. Popliteal cysts in adults and children: a review of 90 cases. *Arch Surg* 1964;88:357–363.

Hughston JC, Baker CL, Mello W. Popliteal cysts: a surgical approach. *Orthopedics* 1991;14:147–150.

Posterior Cruciate Ligament Injury

 Basics

DESCRIPTION

Injury to the posterior cruciate ligament (PCL), the primary stabilizer to posterior translation of the tibia on the femur at the knee, may occur.

GENETICS

No mendelian pattern is known.

INCIDENCE

- Uncommon
- Young adults affected
- Males affected more than females

CAUSES

- Direct blow to the anterior tibia with the knee flexed and the foot planted
- Hyperflexion without a blow
- Hyperextension

RISK FACTORS

- Motor vehicle accident
- Participation in high-contact sports
- Hyperextension injury to the knee

ASSOCIATED CONDITIONS

Popliteal artery injuries

ICD-9-CM

717.84 Disruption of the posterior cruciate ligament

 Diagnosis

SIGNS AND SYMPTOMS

- Knee pain and swelling after the injury with improvement in generalized pain symptoms at several weeks
- Symptomatic instability, especially when climbing stairs
- Recurrent effusion
- Possible posterior knee pain
- Knee recurvatum (late finding)

DIFFERENTIAL DIAGNOSIS

- Anterior cruciate ligament injury
- Tibial plateau fracture
- Meniscal tear

PHYSICAL EXAMINATION

Perform a complete neurovascular examination.

Involved Drawer Test

- Position the patient supine with the knee flexed 90 degrees and the foot stabilized on the examining table.
- Apply posterior force directed on the anterior tibia.
- Note the excursion of the tibia underneath the femoral condyles.
- Note the quality of the end point.
- Compare with the contralateral side.

The position of the affected knee can reveal a posterior sag of the tibia when the patient is supine with both hips flexed 45 degrees and both knees flexed at 90 degrees and the patient's feet are flat on the table.

Lachman's Test

- Anterior drawer test at 30 degrees of flexion
- To rule out associated anterior cruciate ligament rupture

LABORATORY TESTS

None are indicated.

PATHOLOGIC FINDINGS

Either midsubstance rupture or proximal or distal bony avulsion is noted.

IMAGING PROCEDURES

Plain Film Radiography

- Anteroposterior and lateral views of the knee are obtained to evaluate for fracture about the knee.
- A possible avulsion fracture is excluded.

Magnetic Resonance Imaging

This technique is used to evaluate for a PCL tear.

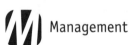 Management

GENERAL MEASURES

- Assess for associated injuries to the knee.
- Patients may be weight bearing as tolerated.

SURGICAL TREATMENT

- Surgical reconstruction is reserved for patients with symptomatic swelling and activity-related pain.
- The procedure entails reconstruction of the ligament with an autograft or allograft.
- Arthroscopically assisted repairs are technically demanding but avoid wide surgical exposure.

Relative Indications for Surgery

- Posterior drawer greater than 15 mm, decreasing with internal rotation of the tibia
- Associated ligamentous, meniscal, or articular surface injuries
- Giving way of knee
- Pain
- Progressive articular deterioration on radiography

PHYSICAL THERAPY

A specific PCL-insufficient knee program is initiated.

MEDICAL TREATMENT

- History and physical examination for a provisional diagnosis
- Radiography and magnetic resonance imaging to confirm the diagnosis
- Initial treatment nonoperative, except in high-performance athletes
- Knee immobilizer and crutch ambulation as tolerated until comfortable
- Early range of motion and strengthening
- Knee braces of questionable utility
- Analgesics in the acute phase of the injury

PATIENT EDUCATION

Isolated PCL injuries are often treated nonoperatively.

MONITORING

Patients are followed at 3- to 6-month intervals to check on their prognosis with range of motion and muscle strength.

COMPLICATIONS

- Recurrent symptomatic giving way of the knee
- Failure of reconstruction
- Flexion contractures
- Degenerative joint disease

PROGNOSIS

The prognosis is extremely good. Many patients do not require surgery.

RECOMMENDED READING

Feagin JA Jr. Isolated posterior cruciate ligament injury. In: Feagin JA Jr, ed. *The crucial ligaments.* New York: Churchill Livingstone, 1994:91–97.

Basics

DESCRIPTION

Posterior interosseous nerve syndrome (PINS) is pain on the lateral side of the elbow caused by entrapment of the posterior interosseous nerve by one of several structures (Fig. 1)

SYNONYM

Radial tunnel syndrome

GENETICS

No mendelian pattern is known.

INCIDENCE

- Uncommon
- Most common from age 20 to 50 years
- Affects males and females approximately equally

CAUSES

One of the following structures is involved:
- Fibrous edge of the supinator muscle (most common cause)
- Fibrous band over the radial head
- Radial recurrent vessels to the elbow
- Edge of the extensor radialis brevis muscle

RISK FACTORS

Repetitive supinating or gripping motions are risk factors.

CLASSIFICATION

No classification system is used.

ASSOCIATED CONDITION

Lateral epicondylitis

ICD-9-CM

723.4 Brachial neuritis or radiculitis not otherwise specified

Diagnosis

SIGNS AND SYMPTOMS

- Aching pain in the muscles of the lateral forearm, just distal to the elbow (the extensor-supinator mass)
- Symptoms usually following muscular effort
- Numbness rare, because course of sensory nerve separate from that of motor nerve

DIFFERENTIAL DIAGNOSIS

- Lateral epicondylitis (tennis elbow): usually a more proximal pain, directly over the lateral epicondyle or radial head (i.e., over the elbow itself)
- Cervical radiculopathy (nerve compression in the neck): usually associated with a more radiating pain
- Cheiralgia paresthetica (Wartenberg's symptom): entrapment of the radial sensory nerve, producing numbness

PHYSICAL EXAMINATION

Complete Neurovascular Examination of the Affected Limb

- The aching region in PINS is about four fingerbreadths distal to the lateral epicondyle of the elbow.

- Pain is worsened by active supination of the forearm (turning the palm up) or extension of the wrist.
- Pain is worsened by pressing down on the extended long finger.
- Sensation of the forearm and hand is normal.
- Motor strength may be diminished in chronic cases, owing to long-standing compression.

Local Anesthetic Injection

Inject local anesthetic into the extensor-supinator mass and lateral side of the elbow, on separate days, to determine where pain relief occurs.

LABORATORY TESTS

These are not helpful in diagnosis.

PATHOLOGICAL FINDINGS

- On surgical exploration: compression of the radial nerve
- Nerve possibly having constricted area from long-standing pressure

IMAGING PROCEDURES

These need not be carried out unless an unusual mass is felt in the area.

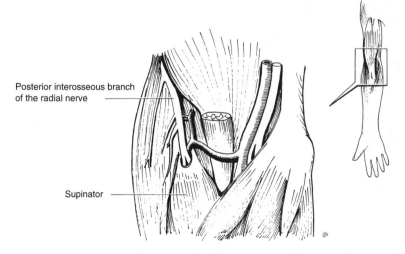

Posterior interosseous branch of the radial nerve

Supinator

Fig. 1. The posterior interosseous branch of the radial nerve may become entrapped in the arcade around the supinator muscle.

Posterior Interosseous Nerve Entrapment

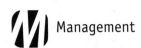 Management

GENERAL MEASURES

- Rest from aggravating activity
- Splinting
- Surgery if conservative measures are not successful
- After conservative or surgical cure, slow resumption of activity
- Repetitive supination or gripping activities limited to the extent that they do not cause discomfort

SURGICAL TREATMENT

- Surgical exploration of path of posterior interosseous nerve in this region; may be done as an outpatient procedure
- Release of constricting structures
- Results usually satisfactory
- No permanent deficit resulting from release

PHYSICAL THERAPY

- Occupational therapy is begun when the splint is removed, for gradual mobilization and strengthening of the elbow.
- This should be done by an experienced hand therapist.

MEDICAL TREATMENT

- Rest from the causative activity, if one can be identified.
- If no cause identified, immobilization of the elbow and forearm in a splint
- Nonsteroidal antiinflammatory agents

PATIENT EDUCATION

- Demonstrate motions that constrict the nerve.
- Explain the dosing and side effects of analgesics.
- Explain that changing manual jobs or repetitive motions may prevent the development of full-blown PINS.

MONITORING

Patients are followed every 3 months until the symptoms resolve.

COMPLICATIONS

Recurrence is possible.

PROGNOSIS

- Most patients have a good result after conservative or surgical cure.
- Causative activities should be modified or eliminated, if possible.

RECOMMENDED READING

Lister GD, Belsole RB, Kleinert HE. The radial tunnel syndrome. *J Hand Surg* 1979;4:52–59.

Basics

DESCRIPTION

The posterior tibial tendon inverts the subtalar joint during the heel rise of the gait. The posterior tibial tendon also locks the transverse tarsal joint so the weight of the body can be transferred along the lateral border of the foot.

- Posterior tibial tendon rupture is posttraumatic pain in the medial aspect of foot, with increasing flatfoot deformity.
- Most patients recall a specific traumatic episode.
- Some cases present in an insidious manner.
- History can be confusing in many patients with a simple complaint of a painful foot.

SYNONYM

Acquired flatfoot

GENETICS

No mendelian pattern is known.

INCIDENCE

- Most common cause of adult acquired flatfoot
- Common in patients with seronegative spondyloarthropathies
- Affecting adults 40 to 60 years of age
- More common in women

CAUSES

- Tenuous blood supply to the tendon
- Chronic tendinitis around the posterior tibial tendon leading to attenuation
- Eventual rupture

RISK FACTORS

- Hypertension
- Obesity
- Diabetes
- Previous medial foot trauma
- Seronegative spondyloarthropathies

CLASSIFICATION

Stage I. Pain and weakness without deformity
Stage II. Flexible flatfoot deformity
Stage III. Rigid flatfoot

ASSOCIATED CONDITIONS

No other conditions are associated with this disorder.

ICD-9-CM

727.68 Posterior tibial tendon rupture

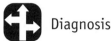 Diagnosis

SIGNS AND SYMPTOMS

- Increasingly painful foot medially with progressive flatfoot deformity
- "Too many toes" sign: visualizing three or more toes lateral to the lateral malleolus when viewed from posterior

DIFFERENTIAL DIAGNOSIS

- Flatfeet
- Posterior tibial tendinitis
- Tarsal tunnel syndrome
- Neuropathy
- Charcot's joints

PHYSICAL EXAMINATION

- Conduct a neurovascular examination of the affected foot.
- Watch the patient's gait.
- The patient should be unable to invert the foot from a plantar flexed, everted position (a position that isolates the posterior tibial tendon). There is tenderness at the medial insertion of the posterior tibial tendon into the navicular bone, or along the tendon itself as it curves around the medial malleolus (most posterior tibial tendon ruptures occur between the medial malleolus and the navicular insertion).

LABORATORY TESTS

None are needed.

PATHOLOGIC FINDINGS

- Progressive attenuation of the tendon
- Eventual rupture
- Subtalar joint then falling into progressive valgus

IMAGING PROCEDURES

- Weight-bearing radiographs to demonstrate the foot deformity
- Anteroposterior views to assess lateral subluxation of the talonavicular joint or divergence of the talus and calcaneous bones
- Magnetic resonance imaging to demonstrate a posterior tibial tendon tear if the diagnosis is in question

Management

GENERAL MEASURES

- Immobilization is needed until the pain resolves.
- The patient may bear weight as tolerated with immobilization.
- Patients with incomplete tears may benefit from nonsteroidal antiinflammatory drugs (NSAIDs) and cast immobilization. Complete tears with a flexible flatfoot usually require surgical reconstruction of the posterior tibial tendon with flexor digitorum longus tendon.
- Patients who decline surgery may obtain support from a hind foot stabilizing orthosis.
- Rigid flatfoot deformities may require arthrodesis (joint fusion).

SURGICAL TREATMENT

Stage I. Tenosynovectomy
Stage II. Tendon transfer
Stage III. Subtalar fusion

PHYSICAL THERAPY

Physical therapy is used for muscle strengthening and range of motion.

MEDICAL TREATMENT

Stage I. Rest, NSAIDs, immobilization
Stage II. Medial heel wedge with longitudinal arch support and medial outward flare
Stage III. NSAIDs, analgesics

PATIENT EDUCATION

Inform the patient that disorder can be difficult to treat and requires prolonged immobilization.

MONITORING

Patients are followed every 3 months until their symptoms resolve.

COMPLICATIONS

Progressive acquired flatfoot deformity with midfoot collapse may occur.

PROGNOSIS

The prognosis is good with subtalar arthrodesis for late reconstruction. Nonoperative treatment is successful early in the disease.

RECOMMENDED READING

Anderson RB, Davis WH. Management of adult flatfoot deformity. In: Myerson M, ed. *Foot and ankle deformities*. Philadelphia: WB Saunders, 2000:1024–1038.

Posteromedial Bow of Tibia

Basics

DESCRIPTION

Posteromedial bowing of the tibia is an angulation of the lower leg noticed at birth (Fig. 1).

- The foot is typically in a calcaneovalgus position.
- The angulation of leg is due to a bend in the tibia.
- The angle gradually corrects itself during growth.
- The limb length discrepancy persists.

GENETICS

No mendelian pattern is known.

INCIDENCE

- This condition is rare.
- Noticed at birth
- Occurs equally in males and females

CAUSES

- Unknown but thought to be due to intrauterine positioning
- May also represent an inborn error in physeal growth
- Unlikely to be due to a fracture because of the proportionate shortening that follows

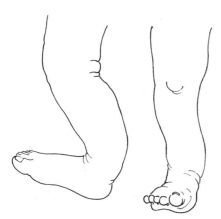

Fig. 1. Posteromedial bow of the tibia occurs just above the ankle of infants.

RISK FACTORS

No risk factors are known.

ASSOCIATED CONDITIONS

No conditions are known to be associated with posteromedial bow.

ICD-9-CM

736.89 Posteromedial bowing of the tibia

Diagnosis

SIGNS AND SYMPTOMS

- At birth, the foot and lower leg are not in their appropriate positions.
- The ankle is dorsiflexed, and the foot is in the calcaneovalgus position. There is an obvious bow in the distal part of the tibia posteromedially.
- The condition is painless.
- The condition is almost always unilateral.

DIFFERENTIAL DIAGNOSIS

- Tibial fracture
- Fibular hemimelia
- Calcaneovalgus foot (similar foot position)
- Congenital pseudarthrosis and neurofibromatosis, which are associated with an anterolateral bow

PHYSICAL EXAMINATION

- Perform a complete examination of the lower extremity.
- The leg appears shortened below the knee.
- Measure the leg length bilaterally.
- Measure the range of foot dorsiflexion, plantar flexion, inversion, and eversion.
- The foot is calcaneovalgus.
- Check for active function of all ankle muscles.

PATHOLOGIC FINDINGS

All muscles, tendons, and tissues are within normal limits, although the anterolateral muscles are light. Only the bone is abnormal, with thickening and bowing.

IMAGING PROCEDURES

- Plain radiographs reveal the deformity.
- Angulation of the tibia may be up to 60 degrees.
- Tibial bone may be normal or thickened.
- No internal cystic change is seen.

Management

GENERAL MEASURES

• This often resolves spontaneously with growth. Initial treatment is therefore watchful waiting.
• Residual deformity may be up to 6 to 8 degrees of angulation and limb length inequality of up to 5 cm at maturity. Usually, it is much less.
• Patients with limb length inequality projected to be greater than 2 cm at skeletal maturity should be candidates for epiphysiodesis or limb lengthening, depending on the degree of discrepancy and their preference for a major versus a minor procedure.

SURGICAL TREATMENT

• Epiphysiodesis of the contralateral tibial epiphysis is the most common procedure. This is performed near adolesence, long after the bow has straightened.
• Residual angulation of the tibia is sometimes problematic (5% to 10% of patients).
• Osteotomy of the tibia is used to correct the angulation.
• Tibial lengthening procedures are also rarely used.

PHYSICAL THERAPY

Physical therapy is not indicated.

MEDICAL TREATMENT

• Casting, bracing, and stretching give no benefit in the majority of cases. In some extreme cases, a splint may be helpful in placing the foot flat to allow walking.
• The condition corrects itself during growth and must only be watched.
• No activity restrictions are necessary.
• A heel lift may benefit some patients with larger limb length inequalities.

PATIENT EDUCATION

• Educate the family about the benign course of the disease.
• Bowing should correct itself over the first few years.
• Impress on the family that the patient will need to be followed throughout growth to assess limb lengths and angulation and to assess the need for surgical procedures.

MONITORING

• Obtain radiographic measurement of limb lengths (scanogram) by age 5 years, so these can be plotted onto a growth curve.
• Usually, growth inhibition remains proportionate.
• Radiographic measurement allows for prediction of final discrepancy and determination of the need for future surgery.

COMPLICATIONS

• Limb length inequality is the main complication
• Thought to be due to damage to physis by asymmetric forces as a result of bowing
• Limb length inequality correctable by surgery

PROGNOSIS

• Prognosis is generally good.
• No long-term sequelae occur as long as lengths are corrected.

RECOMMENDED READING

Hoffman A, Wenger DR. Posteromedial bowing of the tibia: progression of discrepancy in leg lengths. *J Bone Joint Surg Am* 1981;63:384–390.

Morrissy RT, Weinstein SL, eds. *Lovell and Winter's pediatric orthopaedics,* 4th ed. Philadelphia: JB Lippincott, 1996:1070–1071.

Pappas AM. Congenital posteromedial bowing of the tibia and fibula. *J Pediatr Orthop* 1984;4:525–535.

Prepatellar Bursitis

Basics

DESCRIPTION

Prepatellar bursitis is an inflammation of the fluid-filled sac in front of the kneecap that lubricates the motion of the tendons, ligaments, muscle, and skin of the knee. Bursae develop wherever friction occurs between structures, such as over a bunion or an osteochondroma. These sacs are lined with a membranous synovium that produces and absorbs fluid, and they are subject to the same pathologic processes: acute or chronic trauma or infection, as well as low-grade inflammatory conditions, such as gout, syphilis, tuberculosis, and rheumatoid arthritis.

SYNONYMS

- Housemaid's knee
- Carpenter's knee
- Carpet-layer's knee

GENETICS

No known mendelian pattern exists.

INCIDENCE

- Common
- Particularly common in middle and old age
- Both men and women equally affected

CAUSES

- Acute injury such as from a fall or motor vehicle accident
- Repetitive minor trauma

RISK FACTORS

Occupations that create repetitive pressure and trauma to the anterior aspect of the knee are risk factors.

CLASSIFICATION

- Traumatic
- Septic
- Inflammatory

ICD-9-CM

726.65 Prepatellar bursitis

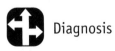

Diagnosis

SIGNS AND SYMPTOMS

- Pain, worse with motion of and pressure over the knee
- Erythema
- Obvious swelling over the inferior patella (Fig. 1)

DIFFERENTIAL DIAGNOSIS

- Intraarticular disorders of similar nature
—Septic
—Low-grade inflammatory
—Traumatic
- Cellulitis

PHYSICAL EXAMINATION

- Examine the knee carefully and compare the normal with the abnormal side.
- Check for joint effusion.
- Palpate the quadriceps and patellar tendons and check for knee extension with the knee flexed 90°
- Palpate the patella for tenderness.
- Check for erythema and local warmth.

LABORATORY TESTS

Routine Tests

- Cell count and differential
- Crystal analysis
- Gram stain
- Culture

Secondary Tests (If Joint Is Aspirated)

- Glucose
- Total protein
- Mucin clot test

PATHOLOGIC FINDINGS

Usually, gram-positive organisms (*Staphylococcus aureus*) are found.

IMAGING PROCEDURES

Anteroposterior and lateral radiographs are obtained to rule out an intraarticular or bony process.

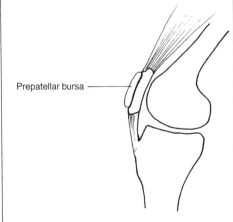

Prepatellar bursa

Fig. 1. Prepatellar bursitis produces swelling in the bursa directly over the kneecap.

Management

GENERAL MEASURES

- Immobilize the joint in extension (knee immobilization).
- Treat traumatic bursitis symptomatically with nonsteroidal antiinflammatory agents.
- Perform excision for cases that do not resolve.

SURGICAL TREATMENT

- Indicated for fibrosis or synovial thickening with painful nodules that fails to respond to medical treatment
- Indicated for septic prepatellar bursitis that does not respond to antibiotics

PHYSICAL THERAPY

- Therapy is given as needed to regain range of motion lost as a result of immobilization and to restore quadriceps strength.
- A change of occupation or duties may decrease the risk of recurrence resulting from repeated minor trauma.

MEDICAL TREATMENT

Traumatic

This often heals spontaneously with immobilization, nonsteroidal antiinflammatory agents, and heat or ice for symptomatic relief.

Septic

- Immobilize the joint.
- Administer parenteral antibiotics.
- Perform incision and drainage of bursa indicated if no improvement occurs within 36 to 48 hours.

PATIENT EDUCATION

Patients are instructed to avoid provocative activities such as prolonged kneeling. Protective coverings over the knee are helpful for patients with occupational exposures.

MONITORING

Magnetic resonance imaging can be used if it is necessary to determine the extent of the process: joint infection versus prepatellar bursal involvement.

COMPLICATIONS

Infection and chronic drainage may occur after repeated aspirations.

PROGNOSIS

Most patients do well with immobilization and nonsteroidal antiinflammatory medications.

RECOMMENDED READING

Crenshaw, AH. In: *Campbell's operative orthopaedics, S. T. Canale, ed 9th ed. St. Louis: CV Mosby, 1997:777–782.*

Basics

DESCRIPTION

Puncture injuries of the foot often occur on the plantar surface of the forefoot. The object is usually a nail, needle, or pin, but it can be any object that punctures the soft tissue (rather than only lacerating it). Other objects include thorns, glass, and splinters. Although it may sound like a simple injury, there is controversy regarding therapy.

INCIDENCE

- Puncture wounds of the foot constitute 0.5% to 1% of all emergency room visits by children.
- Only 0.6% of children with puncture wounds develop late, deep infection.
- Anecdotally, this injury is more common in children.
- Males are more often affected than females.

CAUSES

- The penetrating object carries with it organisms from the skin and from the sock or shoe sole if socks and shoes are worn. *Pseudomonas* and other atypical infections are common.
- Many times, the flora is polymicrobial.
- Usually, the site developing infection is a synovial-lined space such as tendon sheath, joint, or plantar bursa, or else it is bone.

RISK FACTORS

- Walking barefoot
- Construction work

CLASSIFICATION

- Early presentation: day of injury
- Late presentation: at least 3 to 5 days after puncture, when deep infection develops

ICD-9-CM

681 Cellulitis
See codes for other specific diagnoses

 Diagnosis

SIGNS AND SYMPTOMS

- Acute phase: pain, swelling, and bleeding
- Late presentation: redness, tenderness, cellulitis, fluctuance or drainage (purulent or serous); patient usually limping, refusing to bear weight, or walking on the heel

DIFFERENTIAL DIAGNOSIS

- Osteomyelitis (metatarsal or cuneiform)
- Septic arthritis
- Tenosynovitis, including gonococcal
- Septic bursitis of the foot
- Cellulitis

PHYSICAL EXAMINATION

Early Presentation

- Assess the depth, severity, and contamination of the soft tissue as well as evidence of a retained foreign body.
- Evaluate for joint involvement both by proximity and examination of joint motion.
- Examine shoe wear and alert the caretaker to the presence of a retained foreign body (i.e., material from the sock or shoe).

Late Presentation

- Evaluate for local and systemic evidence of infection: erythema, swelling, cellulitis, fluctuance, and changes in lymph nodes (popliteal, inguinal).
- Evaluate the joint for sepsis.
- Check for pain with range of motion of the adjacent joints: metatarsophalangeal joint, interphalangeal joint, or midfoot joint.
- Circumferential or dorsal swelling is more likely to indicate a deep infection.

LABORATORY TESTS

- Early presentation: usually none
- Late presentation (infection suspected): white blood count with differential and an erythrocyte sedimentation rate can be helpful although nonspecific

SPECIAL TESTS

Late presentation: area of infection (joint, bursa or tendon sheath) may be aspirated to confirm diagnosis and to obtain an organism, which may guide treatment

IMAGING PROCEDURES

- Plain radiography: to rule out bony involvement or retained foreign body; in late presentations, may also evaluate for osteomyelitis or gas in tissue
- Magnetic resonance imaging: may be reserved for difficult cases with deep involvement
- Bone scan: Alternative to magnetic resonance imaging, but does not offer the same anatomic details and soft tissue visualization and not as informative overall

Puncture Wounds of the Foot

⚠ Management

GENERAL MEASURES

Acute Presentation

- Local irrigation and débridement are indicated.
- There is debate whether prophylactic antibiotics are necessary in patients with acute puncture.
- Tetanus prophylaxis should be updated, and a booster should be given.
- Instruct the patient to return if signs of deep infection develop.

Late Presentation

Deep infections require irrigation and débridement, and tissue cultures should be obtained. Soft tissue infections are often gram positive (*Staphylococcus* or *Streptococcus*), and joint or bony involvement is believed to result from *Pseudomonas aeruginosa*.

If the patient presents with cellulitis, aspiration should be attempted, and the patient should be treated empirically with oral or intravenous therapy for 24 hours with clinical evaluation. If the condition is improved, the patient should complete a 5-day course of oral antibiotics. If the patient is not improved, or if *Pseudomonas* is recovered from the aspirate, surgical drainage is preferred.

In patients with a small, localized abscess that has been adequately drained with no other evidence of infection, oral antibiotic coverage is probably adequate (this should be changed to culture-specific treatment as soon as possible). Weight-bearing activity may be resumed as tenderness disappears.

SURGICAL TREATMENT

- If needed, the site of infection should be localized by either physical examination or plain radiography; occasionally, magnetic resonance imaging is needed.
- The approach should be the most direct to the pathologic features and should follow the tract of the puncture wound, if possible.
- Plantar incisions are acceptable.
- Thorough débridement should be performed.
- Cultures should be sent for identification, including *Mycobacterium* if clinically indicated.

MEDICAL TREATMENT

- Acute puncture: No drugs are indicated.
- Late presentation: After aspiration, administer antibiotics that cover gram-positive organisms; add coverage of *Pseudomonas* if this organism is recovered or if symptoms do not resolve.

PATIENT EDUCATION

After an acute puncture wound, patients should be instructed about the signs and symptoms of infection and told to return if these occur.

MONITORING

Follow-up examination is performed by a primary care physician or a specialist if symptoms persist.

COMPLICATIONS

- Osteomyelitis
- Septic arthritis

PROGNOSIS

- Prognosis is generally good, once the underlying problem is treated.
- Complication rates vary, depending on the source.
- Total complication rates have been stated to be as high as 15%.
- Rates for osteomyelitis are about 0.8% to 1.6%.
- Septic arthritis and osteochondritis are excessively rare.
- Complications include cellulitis, abscess, osteomyelitis, osteochondritis, and septic arthritis.

RECOMMENDED READING

Fischer MC, Goldsmith JF, Gilligan PH. Sneakers as a source of *Pseudomonas aeruginosa* in children with osteomyelitis following puncture wounds. *Pediatrics* 1978;62:535–540.

Fitzgerald RH, Cowan JDE. Puncture wounds of the foot. *Orthop Clin North Am* 1975;6:965–974.

Johanson PH. *Pseudomonas* infections of the foot following puncture wounds. *JAMA* 1968;204:170–176.

Reichl M. Septic arthritis following puncture wound of the foot. *Arch Emerg Med* 1989;6:277–281.

Basics

DESCRIPTION

Rupture of the quadriceps tendon (knee extensor mechanism) causes a loss of extension of the leg. It can occur in any age group and affects males and females equally. In patients older than 40 years of age, rupture may be due to tendon degeneration.

CAUSES

- Direct trauma to the knee
- Forced flexion of the knee that is resisted by maximal quadriceps contraction

RISK FACTORS

- Age more than 40 years
- Collagen vascular disease
- Hemodialysis

Classification

Complete versus incomplete

ICD-9-CM

844.8 Quadriceps tendon rupture

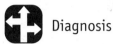 Diagnosis

SIGNS AND SYMPTOMS

- Inability to extend the knee actively
- Pain
- Knee effusion
- Ecchymosis about the knee
- Palpable defect in the quadriceps tendon (Fig. 1)
- If partial rupture, ability to extend leg weakly

DIFFERENTIAL DIAGNOSIS

- Patellar fracture
- Patellar ligament or tendon rupture
- Knee ligament injury
- Tibial plateau fracture
- Femoral condyle fracture
- Quadriceps rupture distant from the tendon
- Acute hemarthrosis with pseudoparalysis

PHYSICAL EXAMINATION

- The patient's inability to extend the leg actively is an important factor.
- The patient may be able to hold the knee in an extended position because of the intact retinacular structure. Patients should be asked to extend the knee from the flexed position (at least 90° of flexion).
- Nearly full range of passive movement is possible.
- The examiner palpates 1 to 2 cm proximal to the superior patella for a defect. One should compare to the opposite side.
- Routine knee ligament examination is performed to ensure that no other damage has occurred.

PATHOLOGIC FINDINGS

Degenerative changes are seen in the quadriceps tendon in patients with collagen vascular disease and in persons older than 40 years.

SPECIAL TESTS

Aspiration of the knee can relieve the hemarthrosis but is not routinely needed. If small fat globules are noted in the aspirate, fracture should be suspected.

IMAGING PROCEDURES

- Routine anteroposterior and lateral radiographs are needed to rule out fracture.
- Occasionally, computed tomography and magnetic resonance imaging are required to assess the quadriceps tendon if the physical examination is indeterminant.

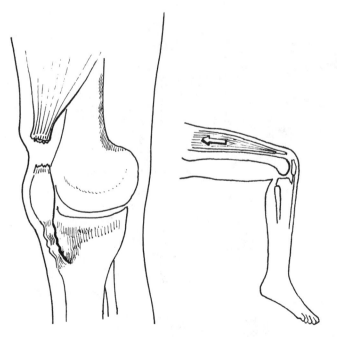

Fig. 1. Quadriceps tendon rupture produces a palpable defect above a low-riding pattella.

Quadriceps Tendon Rupture

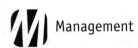 Management

GENERAL MEASURES

Partial Tears With an Intact Extensor Mechanism

These tears are treated nonoperatively with knee immobilization and partial weight bearing. The knee is kept in full extension with a cylinder cast or knee immobilizer, and toe-touch or partial weight bearing with crutches is allowed for 6 weeks. The patient then undergoes physical therapy for range of motion and strengthening.

Partial Tears With Weakened Extensor Mechanisms and Complete Tears

These tears are treated with surgical repair. Ideally, operative repair should be performed within 1 week.

Quadriceps Ruptures of More Than 2 Weeks' Duration

Muscle retraction can occur with adherence of the quadriceps muscle to the femur. Delay in treatment may require quadriceps lengthening or tendon or muscle transfers.

SURGICAL TREATMENT

Primary End-to-End Repair

Most authors advocate this procedure, and 90% of patients regain full range of motion and quadriceps strength.

Overlapping Technique

Similar results have been seen using an overlapping technique in which the ruptured ends are freshened and then sutured together with a 5-cm area of tendon overlap. Postoperatively, patients are maintained in a knee immobilizer or a cylinder cast for 3 to 5 weeks.

PHYSICAL THERAPY

- After 6 weeks, a brace is occasionally used to protect against extremes of motion.
- Therapy includes passive range of motion with active flexion and passive extension.
- Strengthening of the quadriceps is also begun.

MEDICAL TREATMENT

Analgesics are indicated.

PATIENT EDUCATION

Advise patients that they may have decreased range of motion after successful treatment of quadriceps tendon ruptures. Some patients also have decreased extension power (5- to 10-degree lack of extension).

MONITORING

Patients are followed at 1-month intervals until they attain a full range of motion and a smooth gait.

COMPLICATIONS

- Rerupture of the tendon
- Knee stiffness
- Leg weakness

PROGNOSIS

Ninety percent of patients regain full range of motion and quadriceps strength.

RECOMMENDED READING

Brashear HR, Raney RB. *Handbook of orthopaedic surgery,* 10th ed. St. Louis: CV Mosby, 1986:419–421.

Browner BD, Jupiter JB, Levine AM, et al. *Skeletal trauma.* Philadelphia: WB Saunders, 1992:1710–1716.

Basics

DESCRIPTION

Radial head fractures occur in the proximal 2 to 3 cm of the radius. The radial head articulates with capitellum, so these fractures are intraarticular. Radial head fractures account for 20% of all elbow fractures and can occur in any age group.

CAUSES

This fracture generally results from a fall on the outstretched hand with the forearm in pronation.

CLASSIFICATION

Many different radiographic classification have been proposed. However, the Schatzkcer and Tile classification is the only system that incorporates treatment and prognosis.

ASSOCIATED CONDITIONS

- Elbow dislocation
- Carpal fractures
- Wrist fractures
- Monteggia's fractures
- Radial head dislocation
- Elbow instability secondary to extensive damage to soft tissue restraints

ICD-9-CM

813.07 Radial head fracture

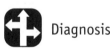

Diagnosis

SIGNS AND SYMPTOMS

- Tenderness or swelling over the lateral surface of the elbow
- Painful range of motion of the elbow

DIFFERENTIAL DIAGNOSIS

- Distal humerus fracture
- Radial head dislocation

PHYSICAL EXAMINATION

- The physician should examine for range of supination and pronation and for elbow flexion and extension.

- Because of the mechanism of injury, the examiner must rule out wrist, hand, and other fractures in the elbow.
- It is also important to palpate the entire forearm to rule out interosseous membrane rupture.
- The neurovascular status of the forearm and hand should be examined closely.

IMAGING PROCEDURES

- Routine anteroposterior and lateral radiographs of the elbow are obtained.
- A radiocapitellar view may be necessary to identify nondisplaced fractures or to characterize displaced or comminuted fractures further.
- Severely comminuted fractures may require a computed tomography scan for identification of fracture fragments and preoperative planning.

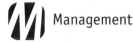

Management

GENERAL MEASURES

- For nondisplaced or minimally displaced fractures: Early mobilization should be initiated for stable fractures that involve less than one-third of the articular surface.
- Fractures involving more than one-third of the articular surface: Treat with a splint for 1 to 2 weeks, followed by protected range of motion for 7 to 10 days.
- Moderately displaced fractures or those with fragments blocking range of motion at the elbow: Treat with surgical repair (open reduction with internal fixation or excision of the radial head).
- Comminuted radial head fractures: Treat with excision of the radial head alone or excision with placement of a silicone radial head prosthesis.

Activity

For nondisplaced or minimally displaced fractures, active and passive range of motion should be initiated 2 weeks after injury. Patients with moderately displaced and severely comminuted fractures should begin active and passive range of motion as soon as deemed possible by the operative surgeon.

SURGICAL TREATMENT

- Fixation of moderately displaced fractures is generally accomplished with the use of small-diameter screws.
- Comminuted fractures are treated with excision of the radial head; a prosthetic head may or may not be placed.

PHYSICAL THERAPY

Decreased range of motion and decreased muscle strength are common sequelae of elbow immobilization after radial head fractures. Therefore, it is important to begin active and passive range-of-motion exercises as soon as possible.

MEDICAL TREATMENT

Analgesics are indicated.

PATIENT EDUCATION

Elbow stiffness can occur even with a perfect surgical result.

MONITORING

It is important to document preoperative and postoperative neurovascular status, specifically radial and ulnar nerve function.

COMPLICATIONS

- Radial neuropathy
- Ulnar neuropathy
- Decreased elbow range of motion
- Elbow arthritis
- Malunion
- Nonunion
- Elbow instability

PROGNOSIS

- Nondisplaced fractures: good prognosis
- Displaced fractures: outcomes varying with the severity of injury

The prognosis for recovery of full elbow function is inversely proportional to the degree of comminution and the extent of associated ligamentous injuries.

RECOMMENDED READING

Browner BD, Jupiter JB, Levine AM, et al., eds. Skeletal trauma. Philadelphia: WB Saunders, 1992:1128–1134.

Clark CR, Bonfiglio M. Orthopaedics. New York: Churchhill Livingstone, 1994:176–177.

Reiter's Syndrome

 Basics

DESCRIPTION

First described by Hans Reiter in 1916, Reiter's syndrome is a form of reactive, inflammatory arthritis that is associated with urogenital, ocular, mucocutaneous, and musculoskeletal involvement.

Because of the often variable presentation of the disease and the similarities with other seronegative arthritides as well as with gonococcal arthritis, diagnosis is often difficult or is missed by the primary care physician. Furthermore, the classic triad of symptoms—urethritis (or cervicitis in females), conjunctivitis, and arthritis—is often not present. Conversely, the symptoms of the urethritis or conjunctivitis are so mild they are missed. Cervicitis is often asymptomatic, thus making the probability of missing the diagnosis in women even greater.

GENETICS

HLA-B27 gene: Persons with this gene are thought to be more susceptible to the disease; 70% to 90% of affected individuals have this haplotype.

INCIDENCE

- The incidence of Reiter's syndrome is not known and appears to depend on the population studied.
- In Rochester, Minnesota, the incidence in men less than 50 years of age was found to be 3.5 per 100,000; another large study in a different population found the incidence in men less than 50 years old to be 33 in 100,000.
- Reiter's syndrome typically affects men 20 to 40 years of age, with a peak onset in the 20- to 29-year age group.
- Male-to-female ratios are generally in the range of 5:1. Sexually transmitted Reiter's syndrome affects men more than women.

CAUSES

The cause of the disease is generally thought to be an immune response to a sexually transmitted bacterial infection or to bacterial gastroenteritis. Most cases are sexually transmitted, as opposed to enteric. Organisms that have been associated with the disease include the following:

- *Chlamydia trachomatis* (serotypes D to K)
- *Chlamydia psittaci*
- *Campylobacter fetus*
- *Campylobacter jejuni*
- *Salmonella enteritidis*
- *Salmonella heidelberg*
- *Salmonella paratyphi*

- *Shigella flexneri*
- *Ureaplasma urealyticum*
- *Yersinia enterocolitica*
- *Yersinia pseudotuberculosis*
- *Giardia lamblia*
- *Cryptosporidium*

RISK FACTORS

- Human immunodeficiency virus: Some studies have linked Reiter's syndrome to infection with this virus, but this association requires further study.
- HLA-B27 haplotype
- Poor hygienic conditions and thus wider exposure to enteric pathogens
- Increased sexual activity and thus wider exposure to sexually transmitted pathogens
- Geographic location, although this may be related to hygienic conditions and sexual behavior of the population

CLASSIFICATION

This syndrome is categorized with the group of seronegative arthritides along with ankylosing spondylitis, psoriatic arthritis, and enteropathic arthritis.

ASSOCIATED CONDITIONS

Human immunodeficiency virus syndromes

ICD-9-CM

099.3 Reiter's syndrome

 Diagnosis

SIGNS AND SYMPTOMS

The onset of the disease process generally occurs 1 to 4 weeks after enteric or sexually transmitted infection.

Classic Presentation

The triad of urethritis, conjunctivitis, and arthritis is present in fewer than one-third of affected persons.

- From 30% to 50% of patients demonstrate conjunctivitis; it is usually bilateral, mild, and noninfectious appearing (small amounts of sterile discharge) and is often unnoticed by both patient and physician; it lasts only a few days.
- Less commonly seen but much more serious is unilateral, acute uveitis, which requires ophthalmologic evaluation.
- Urethritis or cervicitis (or vaginitis) occurs early in the course of the disease.
- Genitourinary symptoms may evolve after sexual or enteric exposure.

- Up to 80% of men have symptoms of dysuria and prostatitis; a mild, nonpurulent discharge may also be noted.
- Pyuria may be seen, but it is rare.
- Cervicitis in women is usually mild and often goes unnoticed; thus, persons in whom Reiter's syndrome is suspected should undergo close examination of the genital areas.

Most Common Presentation

This includes acute oligoarticular arthritis with effusion, marked tenderness, and overlying erythema.

- This is typically asymmetric and involves both the large and small joints of the lower extremities, although upper extremity involvement may also be present.
- Usually, one or two joints demonstrate more severe involvement than do other involved joints.
- Axial involvement, with spondylitis or sacroiliitis, is seen in 10% of affected persons with the acute disease; such involvement is much more common in the chronic form of the disease.

Enthesopathies

An enthesis is an insertion of a tendon or ligament into the bone to which it attaches.

- Usually, it is the insertion of the Achilles tendon into the calcaneus, the plantar fascia, and the tendons of the extensor hallucis longus and extensor digitorum longus, giving rise to so-called "sausage toes."
- The finding of a sausage toe (or finger) is significant because it suggests Reiter's syndrome or psoriatic arthritis.
- Although severe, the condition usually lasts only days to weeks before resolving.

Skin and Mucous Membrane Involvement

This usually occurs weeks after the inciting infection. It is generally manifested in one of several typical lesions: keratoderma blennorrhagica, circinate balanitis, buccal erosions, or nail dystrophy.

- Keratoderma blennorrhagica is seen in up to 15% of affected individuals and is marked by clear vesicles that crust, form hyperkeratotic lesions, and finally heal in the course of months. The palms and soles are most typically affected.
- Circinate balanitis, present in 20% to 50% of affected men, is marked by small vesicles about the margins of the glans penis that are painless and are also self-limited.
- Small, painless, shallow erosions in the buccal mucosa are also seen in approximately 10% of patients.

DIFFERENTIAL DIAGNOSIS

The differential diagnosis must include the other seronegative spondyloarthropathies:

- Psoriatic arthritis
- Ankylosing spondylitis
- Enteropathic arthritis
- Löfgren's syndrome

Psoriatic arthritis often presents with sausage digits, and enteropathic arthritis may be associated with gastrointestinal symptoms mimicking enteric Reiter's syndrome. The differential diagnosis must also include gonococcal arthritis, which may also present with urethritis and may be associated with a positive sexual history.

PHYSICAL EXAMINATION

Results of the physical examination can vary. Findings include the following:

Asymmetric Oligoarticular Arthritis

- This involves predominately the lower extremities.
- It may also involve the upper extremities, particularly the elbow and the joints distal to the elbow.
- Usually, one or two joints demonstrate more severe involvement than do other involved joints.
- All involved joints should be examined for the presence of effusion, surrounding erythema, tenderness, and range of motion.

Axial Involvement with Spondylitis or Sacroiliitis

Range of motion of the lumbar spine and Patrick's test are essential.

Enthesopathies

Physical examination reveals a markedly tender, swollen, erythematous digit with a decreased range of motion.

Profile

Because of the variable, often mild presentation of the disease, Reiter's syndrome must be suspected in young persons, particularly men aged 20 to 40 years, with symptoms of oligoarticular arthritis.

LABORATORY TESTS

- Positive HLA-B27 haplotype
- Elevated erythrocyte sedimentation rate
- Elevated C-reactive protein
- Elevated C3 and C4 complement levels
- Moderate leukocytosis with left shift
- Mild anemia
- Negative antinuclear antibody and rheumatoid factor
- Joint fluid aspirate generally revealing an elevated white blood cell count with values from 500 to 50,000 with predominantly neutrophils

- Normal glucose and negative cultures, despite increased protein levels in the synovial fluid
- Urethral swabs or cervical brushings as well as fecal samples, to be sent enzyme-linked immunoassay, direct fluorescent antibody tests, or DNA probe for chlamydial RNA

IMAGING PROCEDURES

Radiographs are essential for documenting joint destruction. In most cases, however, there are no radiographic changes unless the patient has chronic Reiter's syndrome. Thus, the diagnosis should be based on the physical examination.

Anteroposterior and Lateral Radiographs of the Involved Joints

Look for joint destruction, which may manifest as decrease in joint space, degenerative changes on either side of the involved joint, and deformity of the joint. Radiographs may also point to earlier changes, such as effusion, although this should be noted on the physical examination.

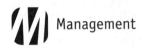 Management

GENERAL MEASURES AND MEDICAL TREATMENT

Goals

Treatment is generally twofold, aimed at relieving the symptoms and eradicating the infection to prevent chronic Reiter's syndrome.

Nonsteroidal Antiinflammatory Drugs

Nonsteroidal antiinflammatory drugs, such as indomethacin (25 to 50 mg orally four times daily) are generally used.

Physical Therapy

Prolonged bed rest should be avoided, to prevent muscle atrophy or contractures; rather, a gradual physical therapy program aimed at maintaining range of motion should be instituted.

Steroids

- Intraarticular injection of steroids may be helpful.
- Cutaneous lesions can be controlled with topical corticosteroids.

Long-Term Antibiotics

There is limited scientific evidence that long-term treatment with antibiotics is effective in shortening the acute course of the disease or in preventing chronic disease. However, a prolonged course of doxycycline (100 mg orally

twice daily) is generally recommended for patients with *Chlamydia trachomatis*—induced disease. Because cases of enteric form of Reiter's syndrome are fewer, appropriate antibiotic treatment for these patients is less well defined. Some studies have demonstrated that administration of sulfasalazine (2 g per day) has been associated with good results.

Immunosuppressive Agents

Drugs such as methotrexate should be reserved only for patients with severe, unremitting symptoms.

SURGICAL TREATMENT

Occasionally, arthroplasty is necessary.

PHYSICAL THERAPY

Physical therapy is useful to maintain joint conditioning.

MONITORING

Patients are followed-up at 3- to 6-month intervals, depending on the severity of their symptoms.

COMPLICATIONS

Chronic arthritis may occur.

PROGNOSIS

The arthritis typically resolves over several months to a year and leaves no disability, but up to 40% to 60% of untreated persons may go on to develop chronic, recurrent disease. This is typically marked by chronic joint discomfort with occasional exacerbations that are less severe than the initial presentation. However, in 20% of patients with chronic arthritis, the continued joint inflammation may eventually lead to permanent joint destruction and deformity. Sacroiliitis and spondylitis are present in up to 70% of patients with chronic disease, and they may also be affected by joint destruction or ankylosis.

RECOMMENDED READING

Dieppe PA, Doherty M, Macfarlane D, et al. *Rheumatological medicine.* New York: Churchill Livingstone, 1985:80–86.

Kasser JR, ed. *Orthopaedic knowledge update 5.* Rosemont, IL: American Academy of Orthopaedic Surgeons, 1996:172–173.

Kirchner JT. Reiter's syndrome: a possibility in patients with reactive arthritis. *Postgrad Med* 1995;97:111–122.

Schumacher HR, ed. *Primer on the rheumatic diseases,* 10th ed. Atlanta: Arthritis Foundation, 1993:158–161.

Rheumatoid Arthritis

 Basics

DESCRIPTION

Rheumatoid arthritis is a chronic, systemic, autoimmune inflammatory disease affecting synovial joints as well extraarticular systems, including the skin, eyes, cardiovascular system, bronchopulmonary system, spleen, and nervous system.

GENETICS

- Family studies indicate a genetic predisposition.
- An association with the class II major histocompatibility complex is reported.

INCIDENCE

- Affecting 0.3% to 2.1% of the population
- Variable onset, but most frequently between the ages of 35 and 50 years
- Females affected two to three times more than males

CAUSES

- Unknown
- Probably a combination of genetic predisposition and environmental factors causing a systemic autoimmune disorder

RISK FACTORS

Genetic predisposition is a risk factor.

CLASSIFICATION

- Classic rheumatoid arthritis
- Definite rheumatoid arthritis
- Probable rheumatoid arthritis
- Possible rheumatoid arthritis based on clinical criteria

ASSOCIATED CONDITIONS

Felty's syndrome: chronic rheumatoid arthritis, splenomegaly, neutropenia, and, on occasion, anemia and thrombocytopenia

ICD-9-CM

714.0 Rheumatoid arthritis

 Diagnosis

SIGNS AND SYMPTOMS

Rheumatoid arthritis is characteristically bilateral and symmetric. Initial symptoms include morning stiffness and swelling in the hands and wrists. Typically, the wrist and metacarpophalangeal joints are affected first, followed by proximal interphalangeal and then distal interphalangeal involvement. Deformities of the wrists and hand occur late, after the hypertrophic synovium has destroyed the capsuloligamentous structures. Tendon ruptures can occur dorsally at the distal ulna or scaphoid. Chronic, progressive deformities of ulnar subluxation occur at the metacarpophalangeal joints. The deformities in the digits are caused by displacement or rupture of the normal tendon anatomy (swan neck or bouttonière deformities).

- In two-thirds of patients, symptoms begin with fatigue, anorexia, generalized weakness, and vague musculoskeletal symptoms until the appearance of synovitis becomes apparent.
- Pain, swelling, and tenderness are localized to the joints; pain is aggravated by movement.
- Morning stiffness lasts more than 1 hour.
- Synovitis of the wrist is an almost uniform feature.
- Symmetric joint involvement occurs.
- An isolated foot problem, such as nonspecific inflammation of forefoot or hind foot, may be the only symptom in early stages of the disease.
- Extraarticular manifestations include rheumatoid nodules (20% to 30%), rheumatoid vasculitis, pleuropulmonary disease, neuropathy, pericarditis, and osteoporosis.

DIFFERENTIAL DIAGNOSIS

- Osteoarthritis
- Acute rheumatic fever
- Ochronosis
- Systemic lupus erythematosus
- Polymyalgia rheumatica
- Juvenile rheumatoid arthritis
- Spondyloarthropathies
- Reiter's syndrome
- Psoriatic arthritis
- Infectious arthritis

PHYSICAL EXAMINATION

The presentation of patients with rheumatoid arthritis and other inflammatory arthropathies is variable and subtle. Important aspects on the physical examination include the following:

General Findings

- Joint effusion
- Boggy synovium
- Subluxation

Hand (Fig. 1)

- Ulnar drift of the fingers
- Subluxation of the metacarpaphalangeal joint
- Boggy synovium of the joints

Large Joints (Knee, Elbow): Effusion Easily Palpable

- Effusion
- Restricted range of motion
- Pain on range of motion

Large Joints (Hip, Shoulder): Effusion Not Palpable

- Loss of motion
- Painful arc of motion

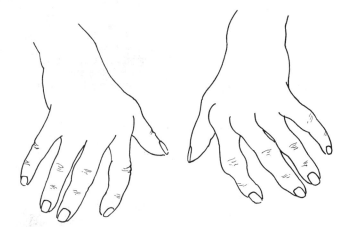

Fig. 1. The hand in rheumatoid arthritis is characterized by metacarpophalangeal fullness and ulnar deviation.

LABORATORY TESTS

• No test is specific for the diagnosis, although serum rheumatoid factor is present in two-thirds of patients.
• Normochromic, normocytic anemia occurs.
• Increased erythrocyte sedimentation rate is seen in nearly all patients.

PATHOLOGIC FINDINGS

Chronic inflammation of the synovial tissue occurs, with subsequent bone and cartilage destruction.

SPECIAL TESTS

Synovial fluid analysis confirms an inflammatory arthritis, but it is nonspecific regarding which of the various inflammatory arthropathies (e.g., rheumatoid arthritis, systemic lupus erythematosus, psoriasis, Reiter's syndrome) is present.

IMAGING PROCEDURES

Imaging is not helpful early in the disease, but, as disease progresses, loss of articular cartilage, bone erosions, and juxtaarticular osteopenia are seen in roentgenograms of the affected joints.
Plain radiographs demonstrate subluxed or dislocated metacarpophalangeal or proximal interphalangeal joints. The articular surfaces are eroded in these joints as well.

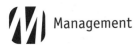 Management

GENERAL MEASURES

Early involvement of a rheumatologist can be helpful to make the diagnosis and to manage the patient. The patient should understand early on that this is chronic inflammatory disorder and many effective palliative treatments are available.

Management of patients with rheumatoid arthritis involves an interdisciplinary approach. The goals of treatments are to relieve pain, to reduce inflammation, and to maintain function. Various medications are used to relieve pain and to reduce inflammation. Surgical treatment should be considered at any time to maximize the treatment. Any patient who may need surgery must have a thorough examination of the cervical spine. (The cervical spine is involved in up to 90% of patients with rheumatoid arthritis.) The instability of the cervical spine, including atlantoaxial subluxation and basilar invagination, is a common result of pannus formation with bone erosion and ligament attenuation. The patient's activities should be as tolerated, and patients are encouraged to have as active a lifestyle as possible.

SURGICAL TREATMENT

Synovectomy has been useful in some patients with persistent pain secondary to severe synovitis while no significant joint destruction is present. In addition, early tenosynovectomy of certain joints prevents tendon rupture. In patients with severely destroyed joints, arthroplasties and total joint replacements have been successful in relieving pain in many joints, especially the hips and knees. Selected fusion in the foot and ankle also is effective in relieving pain and in improving walking ability.

PHYSICAL THERAPY

• It is used to maintain strength and range of motion of affected joints.
• It does not modify the natural history of the disease process.

MEDICAL TREATMENT

Aspirin and nonsteroidal antiinflammatory drugs are the first-line medications. Patients

taking disease-modifying drugs, such as gold compounds, D-penicillamine, antimalarial agents, and sulfasalazine, need close monitoring. Other medications include glucocorticoid therapy and immunosuppressive medications, such as azathioprine and cyclophosphamide.

PATIENT EDUCATION

It is important for the patient to understand the nature of this disease and the treatment options.

MONITORING

Monitoring occurs on an individual basis and also depends on treatment.

COMPLICATIONS

These are variable, depending on the treatment chosen.

PROGNOSIS

• No medical or surgical treatment exists for cure; however, the disease is treatable.
• Some surgical treatment (e.g., synovectomy in upper extremity) can actually slow the progression of disease.
• The fluctuating disease activity makes prediction of disease behavior difficult.
• Ten to 12 years after diagnosis, fewer than 20% of patients have no evidence of disability or deformity.
• Median life expectancy is shortened by 3 to 7 years.

RECOMMENDED READING

Wilson JD, Braunwald E, Isselbacher KJ, et al., eds. *Harrison's principles of internal medicine*, 12th ed. New York: McGraw-Hill, 1991:1880–1887.

Rotator Cuff Injuries

 Basics

DESCRIPTION

Rotator cuff disorders include acute and chronic degenerative injuries to the musculotendinous structures making up the shoulder rotator cuff (supraspinatus, infraspinatus, subscapularis, and teres minor muscles) (Fig. 1).

- These injuries can occur at any age, but older patients tend to have chronic degenerative tears, whereas injuries in the younger group usually follow trauma.
- These injuries affect males and females equally.
- They are most common in young athletes (20 to 30 years) and older arthritic patients (50 to 70 years).
- Classic full-thickness tears are more common in the older population.

GENETICS

No known genetic inheritance pattern exists.

INCIDENCE

- Tears were found in 39% in a cadaveric study, but many of these may have been asymptomatic.
- These injuries are more common in persons involved in sports involving overhead motion and in swimmers.

CAUSES

- Eccentric overload of surrounding muscles
- Primary or secondary impingement
- Acute traumatic injury
- Instability

RISK FACTORS

Risk factors include participation in overhead sports and work.

CLASSIFICATION

- Acute or macrotraumatic presentation: Identify the mechanism of injury.

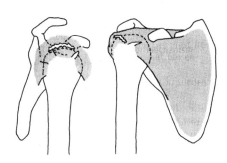

Fig. 1. A rotator cuff tear. **A:** Lateral view. **B:** Anterior view. (From Steinberg GG, Akins CM, Baran DT. *Orthopaedics in primary care,* 3rd ed. Philadelphia: Lippincott Williams & Wilkins, 1999, with permission.)

- Overuse or microtraumatic presentation: Analyze the pattern of training and competition.

ASSOCIATED CONDITIONS

- Impingement syndrome
- Biceps tendinitis

ICD-9-CM

840.4 Rotator cuff tear
726.11 Cuff tendinitis

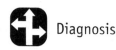 Diagnosis

SIGNS AND SYMPTOMS

- Shoulder pain, the most common presenting symptom, which may increase at night
- Fatigue
- "Catching" in the shoulder during use
- Stiffness
- Weakness
- Symptoms of instability
- Occasionally, deterioration in athletic performance
- Pain in the region of upper deltoid that can radiate down the arm but must be distinguished from sciatica
- Night pain (common)
- Older athletes (older than 40 years) more likely to have an acute tear from a fall, owing to a deteriorated cuff
- Instability to be ruled out as a source of pain

DIFFERENTIAL DIAGNOSIS

- Glenohumeral instability
- Biceps tendinitis
- Impingement syndrome
- Cervical spine disease
- Thoracic outlet syndrome
- Adhesive capsulitis
- Suprascapular neuropathy
- Calcific tendinitis

PHYSICAL EXAMINATION

Evaluate the arm for the following:

- Muscle wasting
- Points of tenderness
- Muscle strength
- Active range of motion (forward flexion, abduction, internal and external rotation)

A discrepancy in active and passive range of motion suggests a rotator cuff tear, as does any objective weakness beyond pain or neurologic deficit.

- Test for instability

—Load and shift test
—Anterior apprehension sign (a feeling of apprehension of impending instability when the abducted arm is extended backward)
—Relocation test (Fowler's sign)

- Impingement tests: Hawkins', Neer's tests.
- Gerber's sign: test for motor weakness

PATHOLOGIC FINDINGS

- Often, thinning and degeneration of the cuff lead to ease of tearing.
- The patient may have superior migration of the humeral head with impingement under the acromion.
- Biceps tendinitis or subacromial bursitis often accompanies cuff tears.

IMAGING PROCEDURES

Radiography

- Plain radiographs often normal
- Sclerosis and cystic changes in greater tuberosity or acromion (eyebrow sign) possible
- Narrowed acromiohumeral distance

Arthrography

- Single or double contrast: the current standard, with almost 100% sensitivity for full-thickness tears
- Not as helpful with partial-thickness tears

Ultrasonography

- 91% sensitivity and specificity for cuff tears
- Helpful in diagnosing bicipital disease (operator-dependent)

Magnetic Resonance Imaging

- 90% to 95% sensitivity and specificity
- Can detect size, location, and characteristics of a cuff problem
- Can be used to determine the size of partial tears

◢◢ Management

GENERAL MEASURES

In older athletes, acute trauma could represent a disruption of the rotator cuff. Athletes can have a combination of underlying causes, and a nonoperative approach is indicated until the components can be determined.

SURGICAL TREATMENT

• This involves repair of rotator cuff tears

—By direct suture of tendons
—By tendon-to-bone repair

• Treatment is nearly always accompanied by subacromial decompression to avoid further cuff injury.
• Many repairs are done arthroscopically with good results, but most are done with an open technique.

PHYSICAL THERAPY

• Strengthening focuses on the rotator cuff muscles, biceps, and scapular stabilizers.
• Rubber tubing and free weights are most practical.
• Therapy is advanced as symptoms warrant.

MEDICAL TREATMENT

• Most cuff problems (approximately 80%) are treated nonoperatively.
• Initially, treat acute injuries with rest until symptoms resolve.

—Nonsteroidal antiinflammatory drugs are useful if chronic injury and tendinitis are suspected.
—Corticosteroid injection into the subacromial space is helpful if impingement is a major contributor to symptoms.
—Avoid immobilization.

• The rehabilitation program involves an increasing regimen of stretching and strengthening of cuff, once the patient is asymptomatic.
• Patients should avoid overhead activities.
• Patients may have to modify their work or sports to avoid reinjuring the shoulder, such as changing their swimming stroke.
• The clinicians should investigate further if pain and weakness persist.
• One should consider surgery if the injury fails to respond to 6 to 12 months of conservative treatment.

PATIENT EDUCATION

• Stress the importance of regaining strength through training protocols.
• Patients can often compensate for small tears and do not require treatment after acute symptoms resolve.

PREVENTION

Preparation with attention to overall body conditioning, flexibility, strengthening and correct technique can avoid many shoulder injuries associated with sports.

COMPLICATIONS

Failure of repair may occur, especially if the patient begins active motion exercises before 6 weeks after surgery. Deltoid avulsion is a difficult complication; care must be taken when releasing the deltoid from its anterior acromial attachment.
Stiff shoulder may result, but rarely is a frozen shoulder the outcome of isolated rotator cuff repair.

PROGNOSIS

• More than 80% of patients' symptoms resolve with nonoperative management.
• Patients requiring surgical intervention also do well, especially if the disease is addressed in the first 2 months.
• Elderly patients with large, chronic cuff tears rarely obtain significant relief from operative or nonoperative treatment.

RECOMMENDED READING

Cofield RH. Current concepts review: rotator cuff disease of the shoulder. *J Bone Joint Surg Am* 1985;67:974–979.

DeLee JC, Drez D Jr, eds. *Orthopaedic sports medicine: principles and practice,* vol 2. Philadelphia: WB Saunders, 1994:623–656.

Hawkins RJ, Kunkel SS. Rotator cuff tears. In: Torg JS, ed. *Current therapy in sports medicine.* St. Louis: CV Mosby, 1990:316–340.

Hawkins RJ, Misamore GW, Hobeika PE. Surgery for full-thickness rotator cuff tears. *J Bone Joint Surg Am* 1985;67:1349–1355.

Scaphoid Fracture

 Basics

DESCRIPTION

- Fracture of the most radial (on the side of the thumb) bone in the wrist, just distal to the articular surface of the radius
- Most common fracture of the carpal bone
- Frequent problems: delayed diagnosis and non-union
- Usually, an injury of young adults (males more commonly than females, probably because of activity level) after a fall, athletic injury, or motor vehicle accident
- Rare in children

SYNONYM

Navicular fracture

INCIDENCE

This is the most common fracture of the wrist after distal radius fracture.

CAUSES

- A fall on an outstretched hand causes this injury.
- The scaphoid is a critical link, spanning the proximal and distal rows of carpal bones, a situation that renders it vulnerable to fracture with a compressive load.

RISK FACTORS

For fracture, the following are risk factors:

- Significant wrist impact
- Young male patient
- Presence of snuffbox tenderness

Risk factors for nonunion are as follows:

- Proximal pole fracture
- Distal oblique or vertical fracture
- Displacement of the fracture

CLASSIFICATION

- Chronologically: acute or chronic
- Anatomically: in proximal pole, waist (mid-portion), or distally
- Displaced or nondisplaced
- Direction: transverse or oblique

ICD-9-CM

814.01 Scaphoid fracture

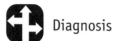 Diagnosis

SIGNS AND SYMPTOMS

- Tenderness in the snuffbox region of the wrist (Fig. 1)
- Pain or clicking with motion of the wrist
- Minimum swelling or ecchymosis
- High index of suspicion to avoid missing the diagnosis
- Patients occasionally presenting late, months or years after the injury, with persistent ache, weakness, or clicking

DIFFERENTIAL DIAGNOSIS

- Ligament injury or sprain
- Distal radius fracture
- Wrist instability

PHYSICAL EXAMINATION

- Pain with wrist motion is common.
- Swelling is variable, because the fracture may or may not produce much bleeding.
- Tenderness is noted on the dorsoradial side of the wrist.
- Typically, palpate the snuffbox region, between the short and long extensor tendons to the thumb, which becomes prominent when the patient is asked to point the thumb upward like a hitchhiker.
- If tenderness is found here, presume that the patient has a fracture until proven otherwise.

LABORATORY TESTS

There are no laboratory tests to aid in the diagnosis.

PATHOLOGIC FINDINGS

The scaphoid is vulnerable to nonunion because it is mostly covered by articular cartilage, its blood supply travels from distal to proximal, and the bone is bathed in synovial fluid.

IMAGING PROCEDURES

- Posteroanterior and lateral radiographs of the wrist
- Best to place the patient's fingers flexed into a fist
- Displacement of the normal fat plane on the volar surface of the navicular, a finding suggestive of injury
- Scaphoid view (anteroposterior view with 30 degrees of supination and ulnar deviation)
- Bone scan (in acute phase)
- Plain tomograms, which can be helpful if the diagnosis is in doubt, or a computed tomography scan with three-dimensional reconstruction

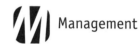 Management

GENERAL MEASURES

Patients who are immobilized should be in well padded casts to allow for swelling. Ice, elevation, and analgesics should be used as needed. Patients should be admonished not to attempt pushing or lifting while they are wearing the cast.

SURGICAL TREATMENT

- Treat acute fractures by reduction and fixation with Kirschner wires or screws.
- Treat chronic fractures by bone grafting, with or without additional fixation.
- If there is extensive degenerative arthritis because of late treatment of the fracture, perform a salvage procedure, consisting of excision of the proximal row of carpal bones or partial wrist fusion.

PHYSICAL THERAPY

Physical therapy is often useful to maintain finger range of motion during immobilization and to regain wrist motion postoperatively.

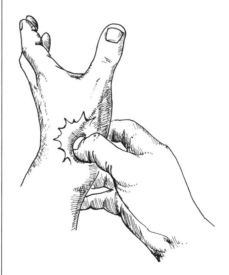

Fig. 1. Tenderness in the snuffbox should produce suspicion of a scaphoid fracture.

MEDICAL TREATMENT

- Acutely, protect and elevate the wrist.
- Immobilize the wrist in a thumb spica case for 2 weeks if the patient has snuffbox tenderness, even though a fracture is not seen initially.
- Repeat radiographs should be repeated at 10 to 14 days, at which time the fracture edges may be better seen.
- For nondisplaced fracture, the patient should be placed in a long arm thumb spica cast for 6 weeks, followed by a short arm thumb spica cast for 6 weeks.
- The patient should not be allowed active use of the wrist until union of fracture is ensured.
- Displaced fractures require surgery.

PATIENT EDUCATION

- Patients should be informed of the difficulty of making the diagnosis of an acute fracture and the need for prophylactic immobilization if there is snuffbox tenderness.
- Discuss the tenuous blood supply and the risk of delayed union or nonunion from the start, so the patient understands seriousness of the injury and the need to plan for any necessary work modifications.
- Stress the risk of wrist arthritis if the fracture is untreated.

MONITORING

Patients with acute fractures are followed every 2 to 4 weeks until the fracture is healed and rehabilitation has been completed.

COMPLICATIONS

- Nonunion
- Reflex sympathetic dystrophy
- Arthritis
- Wrist instability

PROGNOSIS

- Nondisplaced fractures heal more than 90% of time.
- Displaced fractures have a higher nonunion rate unless they are internally fixed.

RECOMMENDED READING

Cooney WP, Linscheid RL, Dobyns JH. Fractures and dislocations of the wrist. In: Rockwood CA, Green DP, Bucholz RW, et al., eds. *Rockwood and Green's fractures in adults,* 4th ed. Philadelphia: Lippincott–Raven, 1996:745–861.

Herbert TJ, Fisher WE. Management of the fractured scaphoid using a new bone screw. *J Bone Joint Surg Br* 1984;66:114–123.

Russe O. Fracture of the carpal navicular. *J Bone Joint Surg Am* 1960;42:759–768.

Schmorl's Nodes

Basics

DESCRIPTION

Schmorl's nodes are intraosseous vertebral lesions that are common incidental findings on plain radiographs as well as computed tomographic and magnetic resonance images (MRI) of the spine. They represent disc material that has herniated through weak areas in the adjacent vertebral end plates and into the vertebral body. These weak areas may in some cases be the physiologic sequelae of the regression of vascular canals near the end of vertebral growth (particularly in young patients), whereas in other cases they represent a weakened end plate or subchondral bone. Such herniations may also occur through pathologically weakened bone. They are usually found in the thoracic or lumbar spine, although there have been reports of Schmorl's nodes of the cervical spine.

These lesions were first described in 1930 by Christian Georg Schmorl as the cause of Scheuermann's kyphosis, a condition caused by decreased growth of the anterior portion of the end plates of at least three adjacent vertebral bodies. Although the origin of Scheuermann's kyphosis remains unclear, Schmorl's nodes are unlikely to be the cause because they are not universally present. One study showed them to be present in only 41% of 54 patients.

SYNONYMS

• Vertebral end plate irregularities
• Intraosseous disc herniations

GENETICS

• No specific genetic correlation has been made.
• Those metabolic bone diseases with genetic predispositions may predispose persons to an increased incidence of intraosseous disc herniation secondary to decreased bone density or defective bony matrix of the vertebral bodies.

INCIDENCE

• Approximately 10% in the general population
• No sex predilection
• Age ranging from childhood to old age, depending on the predisposing condition

CAUSES

• Degenerative or acute rupture of the disc end plate and extrusion of the nucleus pulposus occur with sufficient force to penetrate the vertebral body superior or inferior to it.
• Penetration may be secondary to acute trauma in the case of a normal vertebra and disc.

• In the degenerative setting, penetration may occur slowly over time because of a weakened vertebral body.
• Often, there is no obvious cause.

ASSOCIATED CONDITIONS

• Scheuermann's (juvenile) kyphosis
• Trauma
• Osteoporosis and other metabolic disorders
• Neoplastic disorders
• Degenerative disc disease

ICD-9-CM

722.30 Schmorl's node

Diagnosis

SIGNS AND SYMPTOMS

• Patients may be asymptomatic or may have pain secondary to Schmorl's nodes.
• Symptoms prompting radiographs may not necessarily be caused by this lesion.
• Symptoms usually relate to the degenerative change or insufficiency of the particular disc and consist of axial backache or back pain.
• Pain may radiate laterally around the trunk, but not distally down the extremities.

DIFFERENTIAL DIAGNOSIS

• Degenerative subchondral cyst
• Bone neoplasm: osteoid osteoma, metastatic cancer to bone, aneurysmal bone cyst, early eosinophilic granuloma, lymphoma, multiple myeloma

PHYSICAL EXAMINATION

• Tenderness may or may not be elicited by deep palpation or percussion over the spine.
• The degree of kyphosis in the spine should be estimated.
• A complete neurologic exam should be performed, but a neurologic deficit is unlikely. If present, other causes should be sought.

IMAGING PROCEDURES

• Plain radiographs show indentation into the vertebral body with radiolucencies within the body surrounded by varying degrees of sclerosis. Variable degrees of disc thinning may be present as a result of the displaced nucleus. These are benign-appearing lesions.
• MRI may demonstrate low signal on T_1-weighted and high signal on T_2-weighted images in the setting of acute intraosseous herniation, which is more likely to be symptomatic. Old, usually asymptomatic lesions show the opposite findings on T_1-weighted and T_2-weighted images. MRI is more sensitive than plain radiographs in detecting the lesion.
• Bone scanning may be useful in differentiating an acute lesion from an older lesion, although MRI is the standard.

Management

GENERAL MEASURES

Treatment is symptomatic. In the setting of an acute intraosseous herniation, nonsteroidal antiinflammatory drugs and rest are the mainstay of care until the patient is able to resume normal activity. Bracing may be initiated for comfort if needed.

SURGICAL TREATMENT

This is not a surgical entity.

PHYSICAL THERAPY

Physical therapy may help with persistent backaches. It should consist of extensor strengthening and flexibility and endurance training.

MONITORING

If the diagnosis is unclear or if pain does not resolve within 6 to 8 weeks, serial radiographs should be taken to ensure that the lesion does not grow or change in character. An MRI scan may also help to rule out a malignant disease.

PROGNOSIS

Prognosis is generally good. In the setting of loss of significant disc space, degenerative joint disease of the facet joints may result, with additional symptoms.

RECOMMENDED READING

Hamanishi C, Kawabata T, Yosii T, et al. Schmorl's nodes on magnetic resonance imaging: their incidence and clinical relevance. *Spine* 1994;19:450–453.

Hurxthal LM. Schmorl's nodes in identical twins: their probable genetic origin. *Lahey Clin Found Bull* 1966;15:89–92.

Murray PM, Weinstein SL, Spratt K. The natural history and long-term follow-up of Scheuermann kyphosis. *J Bone Joint Surg Am* 1993;75:236–248.

Seymour R, Williams LA, Rees JI, et al. Magnetic resonance imaging of acute intraosseous disc herniation. *Clin Radiol* 1998;53:363–368.

Warner WC. Kyphosis. In: Morrissy RT, Weinstein SL, eds. *Lovell and Winter's pediatric orthopaedics*, 4th ed. Philadelphia: Lippincott–Raven, 1996:687–715.

Basics

DESCRIPTION

Sciatica is pain referred down the leg in a distribution of the sciatic nerve. The sciatic nerve is from lumbosacral plexus L-2 to S-3.

• Five different areas of pain are noted:

—Back pain: midline lumbosacral, radicular radiation pattern
—Buttock pain: deep-seated, "crampy" pain in younger patients
—Thigh: sharpest type of pain
—Posterior or lateral thigh, or both (L-5, S-1)
—Anterior thigh pain (high lumbar root L-2, L-3, L-4)

INCIDENCE

This occurs in 2% to 3% of the general public.

CAUSES

Most sciatica is from the intervertebral disc (L4-5 most common) and mechanical compression of the lumbosacral nerve roots.

ICD-9-CM

722.10 Displacement of herniated disc

Diagnosis

SIGNS AND SYMPTOMS

Back

• Most patients have previous back pain, and 50% of these have a history of trauma.
• Pain lateralizes to the hip or leg, gradually or suddenly.
• There may be a precipitating event, such as bending over or straining.

Leg

• Leg pain usually is more significant than back pain.
• L-5 to S-1 root compression: cramp or a vise-like feeling in the gastric belly or peroneals
• L-4: medial shin or lateral thigh
• L-5: lateral calf
• S-1: back of calf
• L-1: groin; L-2: medial thigh; L-3: anterior thigh
• Most adults have pain below the knee.

Foot

• The most common symptom is paresthesia.

—L-5: foot dorsum; S-1: lateral foot
—Actual foot pain is unusual.

• Rarely, motor symptoms predominate; consider spinal tumor or peripheral neuropathy.
• Aggravating or relieving factors

—Bending, stooping, lifting, coughing, sneezing, straining, and sitting worsen pain.
—Standing, walking, and resting are more tolerable.
—Lying with knee or hip flexed and sleeping with a pillow under the knees give some relief.

DIFFERENTIAL DIAGNOSIS

• Sciatica, the possible result of any painful lesion in the lumbosacral region
• Diabetic neuropathy
• Disc space infection or epidural abscess
• Spondylogenic: disc rupture, spinal stenosis, muscle sprain
• Psychogenic: vague and stocking glove type pain
• Neurogenic: spinal cord tumor or cysts

PHYSICAL EXAMINATION

Spine

• Variable examination: most physical findings in legs, not back
• Lumbar spine flattened and flexed
• Limited spine extension, forward flexion, and lateral flexion toward affected side
• "Sciatic scoliosis": patient leans away from side of pain

Extremities

• Test all muscle groups and make a chart to document baseline hip flexion/extension/adduction/abduction, knee flexion/extension/adduction/abduction, ankle dorsiflexion/plantar flexion/eversion/inversion/flexor hallucis longus/extensor hallucis longus.
• Test sensation with pinprick in all dermatomes; compare in the contralateral limb.
• Test reflexes (see later).
• Trendelenburg's sign: A lurch or pelvic tilt is noted with ambulation, as is weakness of the hip adductors (gluteus medius and minimus).

• Root tension sign: A limited straight leg raise (with a small amount of hip internal rotation and adduction—slowly raise leg) reproduces leg pain at less than 60 degrees of flexion (Fig. 1)
• Lasgue's sign: Pain is increased on forced dorsiflexion of the ankle with straight leg raising and is relieved with hip or knee flexion (Fig. 2)
• Bowstring sign: Perform straight leg raising to the point of sciatica. Allow the knee to flex, then place the foot on the shoulder. Apply popliteal fossa pressure to the nerve, to reproduce leg pain.
• Well leg raising sign: Lift the well leg; the opposite symptomatic side has a painful axilla or midline disc.
• Femoral nerve stretch test: Unilateral thigh pain is produced by knee flexion, tension on the second to the fourth roots.
• The diagnosis also suggested by motor weakness or by sensory or reflex changes.
• Muscle wasting is rare unless the lesion is present for more than 3 weeks; marked wasting suggests a tumor.

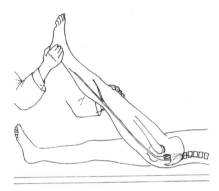

Fig. 1. The straight leg raising test is used to detect nerve root stretch. The knee is kept straight while the hip is flexed.

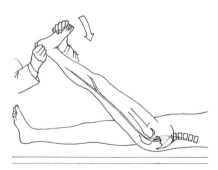

Fig. 2. The Lasgue maneuver confirms nerve tension, with increased pain as the ankle is dorsiflexed.

Sciatica

LABORATORY TESTS

In patients more than 50 years of age, one should exclude the diagnosis of multiple myeloma with a complete blood count, erythrocyte sedimentation rate, and serum protein electrophoresis.

PATHOLOGIC FINDINGS

Nuclear pulposus extruded through a weakened annular fibrosis.

IMAGING PROCEDURES

Plain Radiography

- Anteroposterior view of the lumbosacral spine
- Anteroposterior view of the pelvis

Screening Radiography

- Compression fractures (lateral view)
- Spondylolisthesis (lateral view)
- Pedicle destruction in metastatic bone disease (anteroposterior view)
- Scoliosis (anteroposterior view)
- Tumors of the pelvis (anteroposterior view of the pelvis)

Magnetic Resonance Imaging

These scans are the procedure of choice to detect and define anatomy of the following:

- Herniated discs (false-positive results, 20%)
- Compression from vertebral body fractures
- Marrow involvement from neoplastic processes spinal cord tumors

Computed Tomography

These scans are also effective and are primarily used in patients who cannot undergo magnetic resonance imaging and in patients with previous surgery with metal implants (secondary to the metal artifacts on magnetic resonance imaging scans) (false-positive rate of herniated discs, 36%).

SURGICAL TREATMENT

- If conservative treatment fails after 6 weeks
- If neurologic deficit, cauda equina (see later)
- Microdiscectomy: may miss associated disease
- Percutaneous discectomy for contained, sequestered discs
- Current standard: laminotomy and discectomy

PHYSICAL THERAPY

Physical therapy can be useful for back exercises, healthy back educational programs, and aerobic conditioning.

MEDICAL TREATMENT

Conservative Treatment

This is highly successful.

- Patient education (limited bending, heavy lifting; back school, back and cardiovascular exercise, weight loss)
- Limited bed rest (1 to 3 days), then gradual increase in activity
- Drugs

—Muscle relaxants
—Nonsteroidal antiinflammatory drugs
—Avoidance of narcotics

Management

GENERAL MEASURES

A systematic approach is necessary to arrive at the correct diagnosis and to minimize disability.

Invasive Treatment

- Epidural steroids not proven acutely
- Chemonucleolysis (dissolving disc chemically) risky

PATIENT EDUCATION

Patients are instructed on care of the back, to minimize disability.

MONITORING

The patient should be seen at 2–4-week intervals to document strength and recovery.

COMPLICATIONS

- Cauda equina syndrome. Large central disc herniation causing bowel/bladder problems
- Persistent pain
- Progressive spondylosis (disc degeneration)

PROGNOSIS

Good, Eighty percent of patients recover spontaneously.

RECOMMENDED READING

McCulloch JA, Transfeldt EE, eds. *MacNab's backache,* 3rd ed. Philadelphia: Williams & Wilkins, 1997:513.

Basics

DESCRIPTION

• Scoliosis is a three-dimensional curvature of the spine, best appreciated on an anteroposterior radiograph and physical examination. Both thoracic and lumbar segments of the spine may be affected.
• It is most commonly defined as a curve greater than 10 degrees.
• The most common type is idiopathic scoliosis.
• Scoliosis may occur at any age. The most common age at diagnosis of idiopathic scoliosis is 11 to 13 years.
• Small curves of idiopathic scoliosis are almost equally prevalent in males and females. Females, however, are three to four times more likely to develop progression of the curve. In other types of scoliosis besides idiopathic, there is less difference in prevalence between male and female patients.

GENETICS

Idiopathic scoliosis is transmitted as autosomal dominant with incomplete penetrance and variable expressivity.

INCIDENCE

• Prevalence of curves greater than 10 degrees is about 2% to 3%.
• Prevalence of curves requiring bracing (more than 25 degrees) is about 0.3%.
• Prevalence of curves requiring surgery is about 1 in 1,000.

CAUSES

Idiopathic Scoliosis

• Theories about cause of idiopathic scoliosis include a subtle connective tissue abnormality or neurohormonal defect.
• Causes of congenital scoliosis include hemivertebrae and fusions between vertebrae.

Neuromuscular Scoliosis

• Cerebral palsy
• Traumatic paralysis
• Spina bifida
• Poliomyelitis
• Friedreich's ataxia
• Virtually any systemic neurologic condition that affects the trunk

Connective Tissue—Associated Scoliosis

• Marfan's syndrome
• Ehlers-Danlos syndrome
• Neurofibromatosis

RISK FACTORS

• Progressive idiopathic scoliosis
• Positive family history
• Female gender
• Premenarchal status
• Paralytic scoliosis
• Severe spinal cord injury before adolescence
• Scoliosis in cerebral palsy including total involvement

CLASSIFICATION

Etiology

• Idiopathic
• Congenital
• Neuromuscular
• Connective tissue
• Degenerative

Location (of the Apex or Middle of the Curve)

• Thoracic
• Thoracolumbar
• Lumbar

Subclassification of Idiopathic Scoliosis by Age

• Infantile (less then 3 years)
• Juvenile (3 to 10 years)
• Adolescent (11 years or older)

ASSOCIATED CONDITIONS

• Almost any systemic neurologic disorder
• Most connective tissue disorders

ICD-9-CM

737.30 Idiopathic scoliosis
754.2 Congenital scoliosis

 Diagnosis

SIGNS AND SYMPTOMS

• They vary, depending on the location of the spine affected.
• For thoracic curves, the ribs are rotated on the convex side, producing a "rib hump."
• The scapula on the same side becomes more prominent.
• With thoracolumbar and lumbar curves, one side of the pelvis becomes more prominent, giving the appearance of a "high hip."
• Symptoms are few until adulthood, when back pain and nerve root pain may develop.

DIFFERENTIAL DIAGNOSIS

• Isolated rib rotation may occur without scoliosis
• Kyphosis: a curvature in the sagittal plane only, which may be confused with scoliosis, clavicle fracture, or Sprengel's, deformity may give the appearance of a "high shoulder."
• Leg length inequality may cause the appearance of a "high hip."

PHYSICAL EXAMINATION

• Examine the patient while he or she is standing, to see shoulder, rib, and hip asymmetry.
• Measure leg lengths.
• Do the forward bend test with the patient's legs straight and observe the entire spine for asymmetry between the right and left sides (Fig. 1). This test is most useful and highly sensitive, and it is used in school screening programs. If there is asymmetry, measure the slope between the right and left sides of the rib cage.
• Some patients with a positive forward bend test do not have significant scoliosis. Follow-up a positive test with a radiograph if the rib slope is more than 6 degrees.
• Repeat the test if an abnormality is found.
• Quantify rib prominence or a hump by a scoliometer.
• Observe any kyphosis and lordosis.
• Inspect the skin over the entire spine for dimples, hair, or vascular markings, which may signal an underlying congenital anomaly.
• Rule out ligamentous laxity.

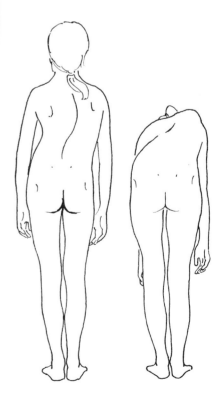

Fig. 1. The forward bend test exaggerates the rib deformity in scoliosis and allows sensitive diagnoses.

Scoliosis

- Examine for café-au-lait spots or neurofi-bromas.
- Perform a careful neurologic examination.

LABORATORY TESTS

None are needed for diagnosis or nonoperative treatment.

PATHOLOGIC FINDINGS

The vertebrae are rotated toward the convexity of the curve. In addition, individual vertebrae are misshapen because of growth while curved.

IMAGING PROCEDURES

- Standing posteroanterior radiography of the entire spine is indicated.
- Lateral films should be obtained if associated abnormal kyphosis is present.
- Magnetic resonance imaging is indicated only if there is possible spinal cord disease.
- Spine films usually show the iliac crests and allow determination of the Risser stage for skeletal maturity. The Risser stage is the amount of ossification of the iliac growth cartilage. Risser 0 is unossified, skeletally immature, whereas Risser V is fully ossified, mature.

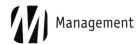 Management

GENERAL MEASURES

- Observation for curves greater than 25 degrees in growing patients
- Bracing for curves between 25 and 40 degrees in growing patients
- Surgery for curves greater than 45 degrees
- Physical therapy and exercise if there is pain or stiffness

SURGICAL TREATMENT

If a curve is to be fused, a rod is used to correct the curve, and a bone graft is placed along this to cause the vertebrae to fuse together. Only the curved region is fused. The neurologic risk is currently less than 1%.

PHYSICAL THERAPY

- Strengthening and stretching of abdominal and extensor muscles if pain exists
- Not indicated for routine cases of scoliosis
- Does not help correct the curves

MEDICAL TREATMENT

- Patients with larger curves (greater than 45 degrees) should see an orthopaedic surgeon to see whether correction is indicated. Patients with moderate curves (25 to 40 degrees) should be braced if significant growth remains.
- Patients with minor curves (less than 25 degrees) should be observed if they are still growing, but they can be discharged if skeletal maturity has been reached.
- Encourage patients to be as active as possible.
- The spine in patients with scoliosis is not unstable.

PATIENT EDUCATION

- Instruct patients in the general guidelines and treatment options.
- Remind parents of the genetic nature of the condition, so relatives and young siblings with scoliosis may be detected while bracing is still an option.

PREVENTION

Curve worsening may be effectively prevented in growing children by use of a brace. It must be worn 18 to 23 hours per day.

MONITORING

- Growing children should be seen every 4 to 6 months, usually with radiographs.
- Adults should be seen every 1 to 5 years.
- Patients with congenital scoliosis should be monitored for associated anomalies.

COMPLICATIONS

- Severe curves (greater than 70 degrees) may compromise pulmonary function.
- Curves greater than 40 degrees pose an increased risk of back pain in adulthood.
- Surgical complications include neurologic injury (less than 1%), infection, and failure of the vertebrae to fuse.

PROGNOSIS

Pulmonary compromise occurs mainly in patients with curves greater than 130 degrees. This may include cor pulmonale in congenital or neuromuscular curves. Most untreated curves greater than 40 to 50 degrees in adulthood slowly become worse.

RECOMMENDED READING

Loustien J, Ogilive JS, eds. *Mais textbook of scoliosis*. Philadelphia: WB Saunders, 1993:219–257.

Weinstien SL. The natural history of untreated idiopathic scoliosis. *J Bone Joint Surg Am* 1981;63:702–803.

Basics

DESCRIPTION

Septic arthritis is an infection of the joint space. It can affect any joint, at any age, although it is believed to be more common in children. There is no gender preference in monarticular septic arthritis. Gonococcal septic arthritis is four times more common in females. In infants, the fetal vascular arrangement with capillaries penetrating the physeal plate into the epiphysis persists until age 18 months, so there may be spread of infection from the metaphysis indirectly to the epiphysis and then to the joint. Severe, irreparable damage to the epiphyseal plate can occur.

INCIDENCE

- Occurring in 0.4% of live births
- Variable in children and adults

CAUSES

- *Staphylococcus aureus* causes 80% of cases of septic arthritis in the first 6 months of life.
- Neonatal septic arthritis is also caused by group B streptococci, *Candida,* and gram-negative enteric bacteria.
- In children less than 2 years old, *Haemophilus influenzae* is a cause. (Since 1989, vaccination against *H. influenzae* has become nearly universal and is protective against this source.)
- In children, gram-negative bacilli, *Streptococcus,* or *Neisseria meningitidis* is the cause.
- Young adults

—*N. gonorrhoeae* is the most common cause.
—*S. aureus* is the next most common cause.
—Other causes include gram-negative bacilli, *Pseudomonas,* and *Streptococcus.*

- In patients with sickle cell anemia, *Salmonella* is the cause in approximately 50% of infections.
- Lyme disease is not a cause of septic arthritis; it is a reactive arthritis.

RISK FACTORS

- Neonates with multiple potential sources of infection
- Concurrent rheumatologic disease, joint prostheses, human immunodeficiency virus infection, diabetes mellitus, hemophilia, sickle cell anemia (*S. aureus* or *Salmonella*), or intravenous drug abuse (gram-negative organisms)

CLASSIFICATION

- Monarticular septic arthritis often affects the knee and is frequently associated with nongonococcal bacterial arthritis.

- Polyarticular septic arthritis is seen in approximately 5% of all patients with septic arthritis. Three to four joints are usually affected, and 40% of patients have extraarticular septic foci.
- The greatest risk factor for development of polyarticular septic arthritis is the presence of a concurrent rheumatologic disease. More than 50% of patients with polyarticular septic arthritis have some form of rheumatologic disorder, most commonly rheumatoid arthritis.

ASSOCIATED CONDITION

Osteomyelitis

ICD-9-CM

711.00 Septic arthritis

Diagnosis

SIGNS AND SYMPTOMS

- Children generally are febrile, irritable, apprehensive, and lethargic and have decreased appetite including nausea, vomiting, or headaches. However, some children may appear healthy with fever of unknown origin and perhaps findings localized to a given extremity.
- In the neonate, 75% of patients may not be acutely sick, but symptoms may include failure to eat or to gain weight, and 25% may have signs of sepsis.
- Tenderness to palpation or joint motion is the earliest physical sign in children and adults.
- Swelling, erythema, warmth, muscular spasm, and decreased range of motion may appear later.
- Joint effusion is usually present.

DIFFERENTIAL DIAGNOSIS

- Osteomyelitis
- Rheumatologic disease
- Inflammatory arthropathy

PHYSICAL EXAMINATION

Tenderness to palpation is usually the earliest physical sign. Other signs include fevers, irritability, swelling, warmth, erythema, muscle spasm and limited range of motion, and joint effusion.

LABORATORY TESTS

- Gram stain
- Cell count and differential
- Culture of the synovial fluid aspirate
- Erythrocyte sedimentation rate (ESR)
- White blood cell count
- Urate crystal determination
- Culture and sensitivity

Gram stain is positive in only 30% to 40% of patients. A white blood cell count in the aspirate higher than 100,000 cells/mL in an immune-competent patient strongly suggests the presence of infection. In addition, more than 90% of the cells will be polymorphonuclear cells. Infected synovial fluid also has a low pH. The ESR is useful when it is elevated to 50 to 100 mm per hour unless the patient has had previous antibiotic therapy. This test may be helpful to assess patient's response to treatment because a return to normal values correlates with clinical improvement. The ESR is unreliable in neonates, in children with sickle cell disease, and in patients taking steroids. A high systemic white blood cell count with left shift is relatively nonspecific. Forty to 75% of patients with septic arthritis have a normal white blood cell count at the time of initial diagnosis.

Blood culture should always be obtained before treatment is started because, in 40% of cases, the organism can be identified with blood cultures. Fewer cultures are positive if antibiotics have already been administered.

PATHOLOGIC FINDINGS

These are characterized by purulent synovial fluid, often with more than 90% polymorphonuclear cells. The synovium becomes thickened. If the infection persists for more than a few days without treatment, destruction of joint cartilage may begin.

IMAGING PROCEDURES

Radiographs may show periarticular soft tissue swelling and distention of the joint capsule. In neonates, a lateral shift of the femoral neck with respect to the acetabulum is strong evidence of septic arthritis of the hip.

Neither magnetic resonance imaging nor computed tomography is useful in diagnosis of joint infection within the first 24 to 36 hours. Bone scintigraphy can detect alterations in bone much earlier than plain radiographs, but these scans are usually unnecessary because of greater reliability of aspiration. Bone scanning is recommended only when there is poor localization of clinical findings.

Management

GENERAL MEASURES

- Consider septic arthritis an orthopaedic emergency.
- Begin intravenous antibiotics immediately after obtaining samples for culture.
- Aspiration and intravenous antibiotics may be sufficient to treat some organisms in superficial joints.
- Surgical drainage is necessary for all infections that do not respond to aspiration or antibiotics within 72 hours, have loculated synovial fluid, or involve the hip.

Septic Arthritis

- Arthroscopic drainage may be the best treatment option for certain joints such as the knee, elbow, ankle, and shoulder.
- Splint in a position of comfort until clinical improvement and then begin muscle strengthening and range-of-motion exercises.

SURGICAL TREATMENT

- Open irrigation and débridement are needed to sterilize the joint and to remove all inflamed cells, enzymes, and debris. Leave an opening in the joint capsule to allow drainage.
- Consider arthroscopic irrigation and débridement in the knee, shoulder, elbow, and ankle.
- Gonococcal arthritis is a special exception in that it does not usually need surgical drainage.

PHYSICAL THERAPY

Once clinical improvement is noted, deformity should be prevented and function gradually reestablished. Muscle strengthening exercises using isometric regimens should be instituted, and active range-of-motion exercises are started, guided by the patient's discomfort. Some studies have shown benefit from continuous passive motion in inhibiting the formation of adhesions and pannus and in promoting better nutrition of the cartilage during healing phase.

MEDICAL TREATMENT

Septic arthritis is an orthopaedic emergency. Principles of treatment include adequate administration of bactericidal antibiotics, drainage, and early immobilization.
Antibiotics must be started immediately after aspiration and blood cultures have been obtained. Antibiotics may be divided into initial and definitive. Initial diagnosis usually applies a combination of agents administered parentally until the identity and susceptibility of the bacteria are known. Initial antibiotic choices are based on broad coverage and knowledge of common causative organisms.
There is debate about the best methods for drainage, decompression, and cleansing of the joint. When septic arthritis is diagnosed early in a superficial joint, such as the ankle or elbow, it is reasonable to aspirate the joint, begin appropriate antibiotics, and carefully monitor the patient for 24 to 48 hours. Joint aspiration may be repeated as necessary. Surgical drainage is indicated for all joints that do not respond to antibiotics and aspiration within 72 hours, for those in which the synovial fluid appears to be loculated, and for infections involving the hip.

Splint the joint in the position of comfort until clinical signs show a decrease in swelling and tenderness and the patient has a comfortable range of motion. A regimen of 3 to 6 weeks of antibiotic treatment is usually needed.
Oral antibiotics may be used if the following apply:

- The patient demonstrates a clinical response to intravenous antibiotics.
- The organism causing infection is known.
- The organism is susceptible to orally administered antibiotics.
- Adequate serum bactericidal concentrations with oral administration can be reached.
- The patient tolerates oral antibiotics.

Medications

Initial treatment for gonococcal arthritis should include hospitalization. The most common causative organism is *Staphylococcus*, except in children less than 4 years of age. Because most infections are caused by penicillin-resistant strains, a beta-lactamase–resistant cephalosporin, such as ceftriaxone or cefazolin, is usually a first-line drug. After local signs of infection have subsided, an oral antibiotic such as amoxicillin with clavulanic acid may be substituted. Duration of intravenous antibiotic treatment should be at least 7 days. Open drainage is rarely necessary, except with hip involvement.

PATIENT EDUCATION

- Patients must understand the need for compliance with antibiotics and the necessity of preventing deformity and reestablishing function through physical therapy.
- Key in prevention of recurrence if the organism is gonococcal is patient education and treatment of sexual partners.

PREVENTION

- Treatment of systemic infections and prevention of gonorrhea may decrease the risk of septic arthritis.
- Most important is to recognize and treat the condition early, to avoid complications.

MONITORING

The patient should be monitored in a hospital setting initially until the following occur:

- The patient is clinically stable.
- Appropriate antibiotics are instituted.
- Response to tests is noted (patient afebrile in 48 to 72 hours, decreased swelling and tenderness, return of white blood cell count to normal, and decreasing ESR).

- Once a response to tests is noted, the patient may be sent home and improvement may be monitored by physical examination, ESR, and possibly C-reactive protein and radiographs.
- Worsening clinical status may indicate a need for repeat aspiration.

COMPLICATIONS

- Delay in diagnosis and treatment beyond 5 days from the onset of symptoms play a significant role in the incidence of complications.
- Pathologic dislocation associated with septic arthritis of the hip occurs predominantly in children who are treated late and is rarely seen in adults.
- Destruction of articular cartilage can lead to restricted joint motion or ankylosis of the joint. Damage to the cartilaginous epiphysis and growth plate in children leads to joint deformity and leg length discrepancy. Septic necrosis of the femoral head, in hip infections, can cause growth disturbance and lead to later degenerative joint disease.
- Patients with prostheses in joints other than site of principal infection may seed the prosthetic joints hematogenously, thus causing a generalized septic picture. Patients with prosthetic heart valves must be evaluated for seeding of the prosthesis.

PROGNOSIS

- If diagnosis is made promptly and appropriate treatment is begun, the prognosis is usually good for complete recovery. Prognosis is worse in immunocompromised or premature patients.
- Patients with prosthetic joint involvement frequently need the prosthesis to be removed to clear the infection.
- Delay in diagnosis in patients with a generalized septic condition is associated with a poor prognosis, and aggressive surgical débridement and antibiotic therapy to address the joint infection are critical.

RECOMMENDED READING

Goldenberg DL, Reed JI. Bacterial arthritis. *N Engl J Med* 1985;312(12):764–771.

Morcuende JA, Weinstein SL. Common pediatric problems: orthopaedic urgencies and emergencies. In: Clark CR, Bonfiglio M, eds. *Orthopaedics*. New York: Churchill Livingstone, 1994:269–284.

Warner WC. Infectious arthritis. In: Crenshaw AH, ed. *Campbell's operative orthopedics*, 8th ed. St. Louis: Mosby–Year Book, 1992:151–176.

Basics

DESCRIPTION

Septic arthritis is a bacterial or fungal infection of the joints of the foot.

CAUSES

In immunocompetent patients, the most common causes are trauma, puncture wounds, and hematogenous seeding from systemic infections.

Patients with diabetes and those with peripheral vascular disease may develop septic arthritis from direct extension of infected foot ulcers.

RISK FACTORS

- Diabetes
- Peripheral vascular disease
- Immunocompromise
- Previous foot trauma

ASSOCIATED CONDITION

Osteomyelitis

ICD-9-CM

741.00 Septic arthritis

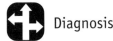 Diagnosis

SIGNS AND SYMPTOMS

- Pain and erythema are usually present at the infection site.
- The patient may complain of difficulty in bearing weight on the affected extremity.
- Areas of fluctuance may be palpable.
- Depending on the severity and aggressiveness of infection, systemic symptoms such as fever, chills, and sepsis may be present.

DIFFERENTIAL DIAGNOSIS

- Fracture
- Soft tissue abscess
- Osteomyelitis
- Gout
- Tumor
- Reiter's syndrome
- Charcot's joint

PHYSICAL EXAMINATION

- Try to localize affected joint by careful palpation.
- Note erythema, swelling, and tenderness of the involved joint.
- Patients may be unable to bear weight on the affected extremity.
- Aspirate the affected joint and send the aspirate for culture, cell count, Gram stain, urate crystals, and glucose determinations.

LABORATORY TESTS

Examine synovial fluid from the affected joint for cell count, Gram stain, glucose, and urate crystals. Culture synovial fluid and blood.

PATHOLOGIC FINDINGS

- Infections of the foot joints can arise by adjacent spread, direct inoculation, or hematogenous seeding. The most common organism infecting the joints is *Staphylococcus aureus*.
- *Haemophilus influenzae* infection is seen in children less than 6 years of age.
- *Neisseria gonorrhoeae* is the most common cause of septic arthritis in adults.
- Patients with diabetes and those with peripheral vascular disease are more likely to have polymicrobial infections with gram-negative organisms and anaerobes.

IMAGING PROCEDURES

- Radiographs may show adjacent osteomyelitis or soft tissue swelling.
- Computed tomography and magnetic resonance imaging show fluid in the joint.

Management

GENERAL MEASURES

- Acute joint infections can be treated with parenteral antibiotics and repeated aspiration of the affected joint.
- If purulence does not improve, if effusions continue to form beyond 5 to 6 days, or if the infection is chronic, the joint should be opened surgically and be irrigated and débrided.
- In both acute and chronic infections, the patient should be splinted to immobilize the infected joint and should be non-weight bearing on the affected extremity.

SURGICAL TREATMENT

If medical treatment fails, then the patient requires débridement of all devitalized soft tissue and bone.

MEDICAL TREATMENT

- The patient should be non-weight bearing on the affected extremity until the pain subsides, and the joint should be immobilized.
- Antibiotics are selected on the basis of culture results.

MONITORING

The patient should be followed closely, and the joint should be reaspirated as the effusion reaccumulates.

COMPLICATIONS

Progressive infections can require amputation.

PROGNOSIS

Most infections resolve with aggressive treatment, including antibiotics and surgical débridement.

RECOMMENDED READING

Mann R, Coughlin M, eds. *Surgery of the foot and ankle*. St. Louis: CV Mosby, 1993:859–875.

Septic Knee

 Basics

DESCRIPTION

A septic knee is an infection of the synovial lining of the knee joint. This condition is common and may occur in infants, children, adults, and the geriatric population. Predisposing factors include arthritis, intravenous drug abuse and alcoholism, steroid use, and any form of immunosuppression.

INCIDENCE

This is fairly common.

CAUSES

- *Staphylococcus aureus* is the most common cause.
- Other common organisms:

—Hemolytic *Streptococcus*
—*Pneumococcus*
—*Gonococcus*
—*Meningococcus*
—*Salmonella*
—*Brucella*
—*Haemophilus influenzae*

RISK FACTORS

- Intravenous drug abuse and alcoholism
- Trauma
- Human immunodeficiency virus disease
- Steroids
- Immunocompromised hosts

ICD-9-CM

711.96 Septic arthritis, knee

 Diagnosis

SIGNS AND SYMPTOMS

- Monarticular erythema
- Swelling
- Fluctuant joint capsule
- Pain on range of motion or weight bearing
- Possible fever and leukocytosis

DIFFERENTIAL DIAGNOSIS

- Acute osteomyelitis
- Periarticular cellulitis
- Prepatellar bursitis
- Gout
- Pseudogout
- Acute rheumatoid arthritis
- Hemophilia

PHYSICAL EXAMINATION

The key findings are as follows:

- Joint effusion
- Painful range of motion
- Possible erythema

LABORATORY TESTS

- The complete blood count may show leukocytosis with a left shift, and the erythrocyte sedimentation rate is almost always elevated.
- The primary test is analysis of fluid aspirated from the knee joint. Opinions vary on the leukocyte count that is diagnostic of a septic joint; however, most authors agree that an aspirate with greater than 100,000 white cells with greater than 90% polymorphonuclear cells is strongly suggestive. The fluid will have low glucose and high protein levels. The aspirate should be sent for Gram stain and culture.
- The fluid should also be sent for crystal evaluation to rule out gout or pseudogout.
- Any patient suspected of having septic arthritis should have two to three blood cultures drawn before the administration of antibiotics.
- The erythrocyte sedimentation rate is also elevated and may be helpful in following the disease course.

PATHOLOGIC FINDINGS

- If the infection is not recognized and treated early, rapid destruction of articular cartilage will take place.
- Cartilage erosion leads to inflammatory changes in the underlying bone and later to frank osteomyelitis. The amount of destruction depends on virulence of the organism and the length of time infection has been present.
- Long-standing septic arthritis can progress to fibrous or bony ankylosis and septicemia.

IMAGING PROCEDURES

Chronic, low-grade septic arthritis can be difficult to diagnose. Magnetic resonance imaging scans always show a large effusion and hypertrophy of the synovium.

 Management

GENERAL MEASURES

In general, management is usually surgical: open arthroscopic débridement. If the infection is discovered early, one may try nonoperative treatment with intravenous antibiotics and serial aspirations.

SURGICAL TREATMENT

Irrigation and débridement consist of opening the knee either arthroscopically or through a standard knee approach and washing the joint with multiple liters of normal saline. All loculations are found and are broken to allow complete drainage.

PHYSICAL THERAPY

Gentle active and passive range of motion of the knee should be initiated after the acute episode has cleared.

MEDICAL TREATMENT

- Early diagnosis and prompt treatment are indicated to prevent severe and permanent damage.
- Institute antibiotic therapy as soon as appropriate specimens are obtained for culture.
- Empiric antibiotic therapy should cover gram-positive organisms.
- Antibiotic coverage should be appropriately modified when Gram stain and culture results are available.
- The joint should be irrigated and débrided urgently. Multiple débridements may be necessary.
- Immobilization of the leg in a knee immobilizer is also recommended throughout the acute episode. Once the infection has subsided, gentle active and passive range-of-motion exercises can be begun.

PATIENT EDUCATION

Patients are encouraged to work on early range of motion. Stiffness will occur and can be permanent without range-of-motion exercises.

COMPLICATIONS

- Fibrous or bony ankylosis of the knee
- Osteomyelitis
- Septicemia
- Degenerative joint disease

PROGNOSIS

When treatment is instituted early, prognosis is generally good. Outcomes are poor if diagnosis is significantly delayed.

RECOMMENDED READING

Brashear HR, Raney RB. *Handbook of orthopaedic surgery*, 10th ed. St. Louis: CV Mosby, 1986:125–127

Clark CR, Bonfiglio M. *Orthopaedics*. New York: Churchill Livingstone, New York, 1994:176–177

Basics

DESCRIPTION

Also called enthesopathies, these are inflammatory diseases associated with a negative rheumatoid factor or antinuclear antibody titer that affect the spine and multiple peripheral joints. Included in the seronegative spondyloarthropathies are ankylosing spondylitis (AS), Reiter's syndrome, psoriatic arthritis, and enteropathic arthritis. Onset is usually before 40 years of age and may occur during adolescence. Men are affected more than women.

SYNONYMS

- Reiter's syndrome
- Reactive arthritis

GENETICS

More than 50% to 90% are HLA-B27 positive (AS, 90%; other enthesopathies, 50% to 70%), although, as in AS, only 2% of HLA-B27–positive persons develop AS.

INCIDENCE

HLA-B27 gene frequency varies with race: up to 10% of whites, 3% of African-Americans, 0.1% of black Africans, and up to 25% of some groups of Native Americans.

CAUSES

Patients have a genetic predisposition with an environmental influence. Many of these patients develop high levels of antibodies directed against *Chlamydia, Yersenia, Salmonella,* and *Campylobacter.* Triggering bacteria may share a similar antigenic amino acid sequence with a sequence on the B27 molecules, rendering these "self" proteins foreign in appearance and therefore vulnerable to immunogenic attacks.

RISK FACTORS

- Male sex
- HLA-B27 positive (relative risk)
- Jewish descent (enteropathic arthritis)

ASSOCIATED CONDITIONS

- Iritis
- Aortitis
- Colitis
- Arachnoiditis
- Amyloidosis
- Pulmonary fibrosis
- Sarcoidosis

ICD-9-CM

721.90 Ankylosing spondylitis

 Diagnosis

SIGNS AND SYMPTOMS

- AS: Findings include bilateral sacroiliitis with acute uveitis, insidious onset of back or hip pain, and enthesitis.
- Reiter's syndrome: The classic clinical picture is a young man presenting with the triad of urethritis, conjunctivitis, and arthritis. Other common presenting symptoms include plantar heel pain, oral ulcers, and genital lesions.
- Psoriatic arthropathies: These affect up to 10% of patients with psoriasis. Small joints of the hands (distal interphalangeal) and feet are most commonly involved with nail pitting, sausage-like digits, and "pencil in cup" deformity of these small joints on radiographs.
- Enteropathic arthritis: This affects up to 20% of patients with Crohn's disease or ulcerative colitis. Presentation can be similar to that of AS. Asymmetric involvement of large, weight-bearing joints (hips and knees) is common. Abdominal manifestations include stomatitis, cramping, abdominal pain, bloody diarrhea (ulcerative colitis), and dehydration.

DIFFERENTIAL DIAGNOSIS

- AS
- Reiter's syndrome
- Psoriatic arthritis
- Enteropathic arthritis
- Rheumatoid arthritis (seropositive)
- Infection (Lyme disease)

LABORATORY TESTS

- Rheumatoid factor and antinuclear antibody titers
- HLA-B27 (poor yield because less than 2% of HLA-B27–positive patients develop seronegative spondyloarthropathies)
- Erythrocyte sedimentation rate

PATHOLOGIC FINDINGS

- Enthesopathy (inflammation at ligament-bone insertion sites)
- Synovitis
- Pulmonary fibrosis
- Colitis
- Aortitis

IMAGING PROCEDURES

- Obtain plain radiographs.
- AS: Findings include symmetric sacroiliac joint narrowing, squaring of the vertebral bodies, ascending spinal syndesmophytes seen with time, and protrusio acetabuli.
- Reiter's syndrome: Findings include sacroiliac joint narrowing (can be asymmetric) skipping areas of spinal involvement.
- Psoriatic arthritis: Findings include small joint involvement, commonly the distal interphalangeal joints of the hands, with a "pencil in cup" deformity and autofusion of the joints; bony resorption in the hand can be severe.
- Enteropathic arthritis: Findings are similar to those of AS.

Seronegative Spondyloarthropathies

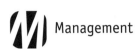 Management

GENERAL MEASURES

- Postural training
- Strengthening and range-of-motion exercises
- Sleeping on a firm mattress (AS)

SURGICAL TREATMENT

Hip arthritis may be severe, resulting in the need for hip replacement. Cervical spine deformities may occur, necessitating a corrective osteotomy.

PHYSICAL THERAPY

Physical therapy is often necessary to maintain joint range of motion and to prevent contractures.

MEDICAL TREATMENT

- Avoidance of contact sports (AS)
- Low impact exercises
- No dietary restrictions
- Drugs: nonsteroidal antiinflammatory drugs, disease-modifying agents such as sulfasalazine or methotrexate, and eye drops for uveitis

PATIENT EDUCATION

- Genetic aspects of the disease should be explained.
- Patients with AS with a sudden onset of neck or back pain need to be evaluated for acute fractures.

MONITORING

Close follow-up with rheumatologists and orthopaedic surgeons is indicated. Depending on the severity of the disease, patients are seen every 3 to 6 months.

PREVENTION

Although the disease cannot be prevented, careful treatment and follow-up can prevent contractures, as well as pulmonary and cardiac complications.

COMPLICATIONS

Cardiac involvement such as aortic insufficiency, pulmonary fibrosis, gastrointestinal complications such as perforations or fistulas, and vertebral (cervical) fractures (AS) may occur.

PROGNOSIS

In general, prognosis is better for pediatric-onset than for adult-onset spondyloarthropathies. In patients with AS, the prognosis is determined by the rate of disease progression.

RECOMMENDED READING

Brinker MR, Miller MD. Basic sciences. In: Miller MD, ed. *Review of orthopaedics*. Philadelphia: WB Saunders, 1996:1–122.

Brown CR. Medical treatment of arthritis. In: Callaghan, JJ, Dennis, DA, Paprosky WG, et al., eds. *Callaghan's orthopaedic knowledge update: hip and knee reconstruction*. Rosemont, IL: American Academy of Orthopaedic Surgeons, 1995:69–78.

Kredich D, Patrone NA. Pediatric spondyloarthropathies. *Clin Orthop* 1990;169:18–22.

Miller-Blair DJ, Tsuchiga N, Yamaguchi A, et al. Immunologic mechanisms in common rheumatologic diseases. *Clin Orthop* 1996;326:43–54.

Basics

DESCRIPTION

Shin splints comprise pain and discomfort in the leg from repetitive running on hard surfaces or forceful excessive use of foot dorsiflexors. They occur commonly, especially in patients from the teen years to the early thirties.

SYNONYMS

- Medial tibia stress syndrome
- Periostitis of the tibia
- Runner's leg

CAUSE

Periostitis at the origin of the posterior tibialis muscle is the cause.

RISK FACTORS

- Running or jogging, especially a recent increase in distance
- Pronated feet

ASSOCIATED CONDITIONS

- It usually affects healthy athletes.
- Any deformity of the leg that increases stress on the leg may predispose.

ICD-9-CM

844.9 Shin splints

Diagnosis

SIGNS AND SYMPTOMS

- Exercise-induced pain occurs along the medial-posteromedial distal two-thirds of the tibia (rarely anterolateral).
- Pain is usually dull or intense and is present at the onset of the workout.
- Pain may persist after the workout and may eventually dissipate.

DIFFERENTIAL DIAGNOSIS

- Stress fractures
- Chronic exertional compartment syndrome
- Tendinitis

PHYSICAL EXAMINATION

- Localize tenderness by palpation in a long region of the crest of the tibia (Fig. 1).
- Local tenderness with pain is noted on resisted plantar flexion and inversion.

- The clinical presentation of medial tibia stress syndrome may closely resemble that of stress fractures and compartment syndrome, which can carry a far worse prognosis if undiagnosed.
- Exertional compartment syndrome has characteristic physical findings of pain with passive stretch of the muscles and fullness of the leg compartments to palpation. It may even cause weakness and numbness of the leg and foot. Intracompartmental pressure measurements are diagnostic of compartment syndrome.

LABORATORY TESTS

- Erythrocyte sedimentation rate is in the normal range and is elevated for osteomyelitis.
- Compartment measurement after exercise may be needed to diagnose exertional compartment syndrome.

PATHOLOGIC FINDINGS

Inflammation at the origin of the soleus or flexor digitorum longus is noted.

IMAGING PROCEDURES

- Serial plain radiographs are needed to rule out stress fracture.
- Periosteal change is seen radiographically several weeks after the onset of symptoms.
- A bone scan reveals a diffuse area in the posterior tibial cortex of increased uptake, in contrast to a focal area of reuptake in stress fracture.

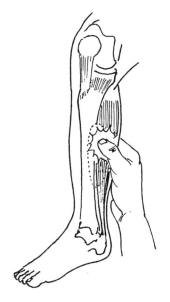

Fig. 1. Shin splints produce pain in the anterior or posterior border of the tibia over a long segment.

Management

GENERAL MEASURES

Ensure adequate nutrition and vitamin C intake.

SURGICAL TREATMENT

Only after maximal nonoperative treatment has failed should posterior medial fascia release be considered.

PHYSICAL THERAPY

Avoid running on uneven surfaces.

MEDICAL TREATMENT

- Decrease in training activity until symptoms resolve
- Nonsteroidal antiinflammatory drugs
- Analgesics
- Ice on the area of injury
- Orthotic or shoe modification to decrease pronation
- Diagnostic lidocaine (Xylocaine) injection into adjacent soft tissues to provide relief
- Strengthening and stretching exercises after acute symptoms disappear

PATIENT EDUCATION

- Emphasize the importance of rest initially, followed by stretching and strengthening exercises.
- Running should be done only slowly and gradually.

COMPLICATIONS

Undiagnosed stress fracture can lead to complete fracture and displacement.

PROGNOSIS

- Most cases respond well to nonoperative treatment.
- Gradual return to activity can be expected.
- Variation of the causative regimen of training will help to prevent recurrence.

RECOMMENDED READING

Eisele SA, Sammarco, GJ, et al. Chronic exertional compartment syndrome. *Instruct Course Lect* 1992;42:213–217.

Michael RH, Holder LE. The soleus syndrome: a cause of medial tibial stress (shin splints). *Am J Sports Med* 1985;13:87–94.

Rettig AC, Shelbourne KD, McCarroll JR, et al. The natural history and treatment of delayed union stress fractures of the anterior cortex of the tibia. *Am J Sports Med* 1988;16:250–255.

Basics

DESCRIPTION

Short stature is defined as height under third percentile for age of general population. There are many causes for short stature; orthopaedic causes are discussed here. The most common orthopaedic cause is osteochondrodysplasia, a group of skeletal disorders characterized by an intrinsic abnormality in the growth and remodeling of cartilage and bone. More than 600 types are identified. Diagnosis is usually apparent from birth or early childhood.

SYNONYM

Dwarfism, defined as disproportionate short stature

GENETICS

Most dysplasias are transmitted autosomally as either dominant or recessive traits. However, many affected persons acquire the disorder as a new mutation and may pass it on to their children.
Genetic testing is becoming available for many disorders and may be useful in family planning when the history is positive.

INCIDENCE

The incidence is approximately 1 in 3,000 to 1 in 5,000 live births.

CAUSES

• A defect in the locus for the fibroblast growth factor receptor accounts for achondroplasia.
• The gene for the cellular sulfate transporter accounts for diastrophic dysplasia.
• Mucopolysaccharidoses are due to enzyme deficiencies in the pathway of mucopolysaccharide metabolism.
• Not all causes are identified.

RISK FACTORS

• Family history
• Consanguinity
• Regionally concentrated dysplasias (e.g., diastrophic dysplasia in Finland, metaphyseal dysplasia in Amish communities)

CLASSIFICATION

• International Classification of Osteochondrodysplasia most widely accepted
• According to body segment most severely affected: short limb, short trunk
• According to area of extremity involved: epiphyseal, metaphyseal, diaphyseal
• Patients with epiphyseal involvement most likely to have contractures and arthritis because of involved joint surfaces
• The term "rhizomelic" often used when extremity shortening is greatest in proximal segments, as in achondroplasia

ASSOCIATED CONDITIONS

• Neurologic and respiratory symptoms, owing to spinal deformity
• Mental retardation in Hurler's syndrome
• Hip dysplasia
• Clubfeet in diastrophic dysplasia and spondyloepiphyseal dysplasia
• Scoliosis

ICD-9-CM

259.4 Dwarfism, nonspecific
756.4 Achondroplasia
756.56 Multiple epiphyseal dysplasia
756.59 Spondyloepiphyseal dysplasia
756.4 Metatropic dysplasia

Diagnosis

SIGNS AND SYMPTOMS

Achondroplasia

• Most common skeletal dysplasia
• Midface hypoplasia
• Rhizomelic dwarfism
• Frontal bossing
• Delay in motor milestones
• Thoracolumbar kyphosis
• Spinal stenosis (mostly lumbar)
• Overweight
• Narrowed foramen magnum
• Height usually less than 50 inches

Hypochondroplasia: Autosomal Dominant Mild Short Limb Dwarfism

• Severe cases share many features with achondroplasia.
• Mild frontal bossing

• No midface hypoplasia
• Symmetric shortening of extremities
• Mild kyphosis and lordosis

Diastrophic Dysplasia: Rhizomelic Dwarfism

• Autosomal recessive transmission
• Cauliflower ear
• Major joint contracture
• Hitchhiker (abducted) thumb
• Foot deformity
• Scoliosis
• Cervical spina bifida with kyphosis

Multiple Epiphyseal Dysplasia: Autosomal Dominant

• Mild short stature
• Short limbs
• Irregular epiphyseal ossification with deformity
• Hips, knees, and ankles most severely involved

Mucopolysaccharidoses

• Joint contractures
• Organomegaly
• Often cataracts
• Sometimes developmental delay

Multiple Epiphyseal Dysplasia: One of Most Common Dysplasias

• Autosomal dominant with disturbed ossification in many epiphyses
• Joint pain
• Decreased range of motion
• Prominent joints
• Extremity angular deformities
• May not present until later in childhood, because only mild short stature
• Final height 57 to 67 inches

Multiple Osteocartilaginous Exostoses

• Autosomal dominant
• Mild short stature
• Local impingement on tendons, nerves, spinal canal
• Deformity of extremities
• Leg length discrepancy
• Risk of malignant degeneration in 1%

Spondyloepiphyseal Dysplasia

• Cervical spine instability
• Scoliosis
• Joint contractures
• Stiffness at hip and knee

DIFFERENTIAL DIAGNOSIS

- Consult with a geneticist or endocrinologist.
- Consider other alternatives:

—Constitutional short stature
—Malnutrition
—Hormonal disorder
—Chronic illness
—Chronic steroid use

PHYSICAL EXAMINATION

To make the diagnosis of skeletal dysplasia, it is important to know the following information about the patient:

- Length at birth
- Current height and percentile
- Body proportion by comparing limb and trunk length ratio
- Dysmorphism (morphologic variations of bone and soft tissue that may characterize disorder)
- Complete neurologic examination to rule out stenosis or instability
- Quantitated range of motion and contractures
- Examination for angular disturbances of the limbs and for scoliosis and kyphosis of the spine

LABORATORY TESTS

These tests are usually not indicated, but they can be useful. They include the following:

- Chemistry profile
- Endocrine evaluation
- Urine workup for storage disorder

PATHOLOGIC FINDINGS

- They vary with the different types of disorder.
- Most dysplasias show alterations in cartilage, ligament, and tendon.

IMAGING PROCEDURES

Radiographic evaluation should include the following:

- Lateral skull and cervical spine
- Lateral lumbar spine
- Anteroposterior film of the pelvis
- Anteroposterior film of the hand and wrist

Management

GENERAL MEASURES

Orthopaedic management of patients with osteochondrodysplasia is mainly symptomatic treatment, correcting and achieving alignment and stability.

SURGICAL TREATMENT

- Spinal fusion, decompression, and instrumentation are used to correct spinal disorders.
- Osteotomy is used to correct extremity deformities.
- Patients with early osteoarthritis from epiphyseal deformity may benefit from joint replacement.

PHYSICAL THERAPY

Skeletal deformity is not corrected with physical therapy; however, it may improve the function of a patient.

MEDICAL TREATMENT

- Evaluate and treat cervical spine instability with collar or fusion, if indicated.
- Decompress neurologic claudication from spinal stenosis if indicated.
- Document and follow scoliosis and kyphosis.
- No medications are available for skeletal dysplasia at this time.
- Accurate genetic counseling is indicated.
- Recognition and treatment of musculoskeletal abnormalities and intrinsic medical problems are needed.
- With age, many patients need powered devices for transport because arthritis or spinal disorder decreases mobility.
- Growth hormone is not useful to increase stature.
- Limb lengthening may gain up to 1 additional foot of height in achondroplasia.

PATIENT EDUCATION

- Genetic counseling is indicated.
- Refer families when a positive history becomes known.

MONITORING

Patients should be followed approximately every 6 months to monitor developmental milestones and skeletal deformities.

COMPLICATIONS

- Degenerative disease of the hips and knees is common. Cervical instability is seen in spondyloepiphyseal dysplasia and mucopolysaccharidoses.
- Complications vary with the different types of disorder.

PROGNOSIS

Spinal instability, stenosis, and arthritis are frequent in many of the dysplasias.

RECOMMENDED READING

Bassett GS. The osteochondrodysplasias. In: Morrissy RT, Weinstein SL. *Lovell and Winter's pediatric orthopaedics*, 4th ed. Philadelphia: Lippincott–Raven, 1996:203–255.

Beighton, P, Giedion ZA, Gorlin R, et al. International classification of osteochondrodysplasia. *Ann Intern Med* 1992;44(2) 223–229.

Kopits SE. Orthopaedic complications of dwarfism. *Clin Orthop* 1976;114:153–179.

Basics

DESCRIPTION

Glenohumeral arthritis, although not as common as that affecting the hip and knee, results in substantial disability, especially in tasks of daily living such as personal hygiene and meal preparation. It is more common in the elderly population.

GENETICS

No known genetic component exists.

INCIDENCE

An equal incidence is noted in men and women.

CAUSES

• Rheumatoid arthritis or osteoarthritis (most common)
• Repetitive trauma
• Humeral head fracture
• Recurrent dislocation

RISK FACTORS

Professional throwing athletes and manual laborers are at higher risk for later degenerative disease.

CLASSIFICATION

Outerbridge's classification, although originally developed for cartilaginous lesions of the knee, can be used to classify any cartilage lesion during arthroscopy.

 Stage I. Softening of the articular cartilage
 Stage II. Fibrillation of the cartilage surface
 Stage III. Partial-thickness loss
 Stage IV. Full-thickness loss with exposed bone

ASSOCIATED CONDITIONS

• Rotator cuff tear
• Inflammatory arthritis
• Collagen vascular disease

ICD-9-CM

716.91 Glenohumeral arthritis

 Diagnosis

SIGNS AND SYMPTOMS

• Pain in the shoulder joint, especially with activity
• Decreased range of motion

DIFFERENTIAL DIAGNOSIS

• Rotator cuff and acromioclavicular disorders can mimic glenohumeral arthritis.
• Metastatic tumor and cervical radiculopathy can cause similar symptoms.
• Rarely, Lyme disease, pigmented villonodular synovitis, or other inflammatory arthropathies can result in shoulder pain.

PHYSICAL EXAMINATION

• Assess range of motion of the shoulder, with attention to scapulothoracic motion, because patients compensate with motion of the scapula.
• Test strength, especially of the rotator cuff and the biceps tendon, because these may be ruptures.
• A full neurologic examination of the upper extremity helps to differentiate cervical or brachial plexus disease.
• Injection of the subacromial space or joint with lidocaine may help in the diagnosis.

LABORATORY TESTS

Workup for rheumatoid arthritis and Lyme disease may be indicated if they are suspected clinically.

PATHOLOGIC FINDINGS

• Typical degeneration of the articular cartilage and hypertrophy and inflammation of the synovium
• Degeneration or rupture of the rotator cuff or biceps tendons

IMAGING PROCEDURES

• Anteroposterior and lateral radiographs of the affected shoulder should be obtained before other imaging modalities. Subchondral sclerosis, cyst formation, narrowing of the joint space, and peripheral osteophytes all may be seen. Superior subluxation of the humeral head may be present and in severe cases may articulate with the acromion.
• Magnetic resonance imaging or computed tomography may be valuable to assess the rotator cuff or any bone or soft tissue lesions.
• Arthrography of the affected joint may help to assess the rotator cuff.
• Ultrasound is employed in some institutions for this indication.

Management

GENERAL MEASURES

Avoidance of exacerbating activity is important.

SURGICAL TREATMENT

• Arthroscopy may be useful to assess and débride the joint.
• Synovectomy has been performed in patients with rheumatoid arthritis, mostly in Europe, with inconsistent results. Prosthetic replacement of the joint with either a hemiarthroplasty (limited to the humeral side) or a total shoulder procedure (which also replaces the glenoid) is highly reliable in relieving pain.
—These procedures often do not restore range of motion, and patients can lose overhead motion.
—Total shoulder replacement is less common because of the complication of glenoid component loosening. An intact rotator cuff gives better, more consistent results.

PHYSICAL THERAPY

• A short course of physical therapy to learn appropriate exercises is helpful.
• Patients should be started on an exercise program to maintain range of motion and to strengthen the rotator cuff.

MEDICAL TREATMENT

• Activity modification, nonsteroidal antiinflammatory drugs, and analgesics: first line of treatment
—Acetaminophen, aspirin
• Physical therapy for range of motion and strengthening exercises
• Steroid injection into the glenohumeral joint

PATIENT EDUCATION

• Arthroplasty can significantly improve symptoms of pain.
• Motion and strength are less predictably improved.
• An exercise program is indicated for strength and range of motion.

MONITORING

Patients are followed at 3 to 4 months with nonoperative treatment. Patients are followed at 1-month intervals after arthroplasty until they regain their range of motion and strength.

COMPLICATIONS

Complications of surgery include the following:

• Loosening of the components
• Infection
• Dislocation

PROGNOSIS

Chronic arthritic pain is unlikely to improve with time. Long-term follow-up is excellent after shoulder arthroplasty.

RECOMMENDED READING

Barrett WP, Franklin JL Jackins SE. Total shoulder arthroplasty. *J Bone Joint Surg Am* 1987;69:865–872.

Basics

DESCRIPTION

The proximal humerus consists of the articular surface of the shoulder joint and the attachments of the rotator cuff on the greater tuberosity and lesser tuberosities. Fractures often occur after a fall directly onto the shoulder. Patients with osteoporotic bone are at the highest risk.

This injury is more common in the elderly with osteoporotic bone but can be seen in all age groups. Osteoporosis may contribute to comminution in these fractures. Seventy percent of these fractures occur in women.

GENETICS

No known genetic association exists.

INCIDENCE

- The proximal humerus is involved in 5% to 7% of all fractures and in 76% of all humeral fractures in patients older than 40 years.
- The incidence is 3.7 per 1,000 per year in patients more than 50 years old.

CAUSES

- In elderly patients: a fall onto an outstretched arm or directly onto the shoulder
- In younger patients: similar mechanism or high-energy injury such as a motor vehicle accident

RISK FACTORS

- Poor vision and balance
- Reduced muscle mass in the elderly that provides less energy absorption in direct blows and less dynamic support to absorb the impact

CLASSIFICATION

Neer's classification divides the proximal humerus into four parts:

- Articular surface
- Greater tuberosity
- Lesser tuberosity
- Surgical neck, which is the border between the round proximal metaphysis and the diaphyseal portion of the bone

Fractures are classified as having one to four parts, based on the number of fragments. For a fragment to be a part, it must be displaced at least 1 cm and or angulated 45 degrees.

ICD-9-CM

812.00 Fracture, upper end humerus

 Diagnosis

SIGNS AND SYMPTOMS

- Pain and swelling around shoulder joint, often with ecchymosis that may extend to the elbow or chest wall and neck
- Pain with range of motion
- Patient possibly supporting the affected arm

DIFFERENTIAL DIAGNOSIS

- Acute rotator cuff tear or strain
- Anterior or posterior shoulder dislocation (similar presentation)
- Pain in the proximal shoulder (may be from acromioclavicular joint dislocation or biceps tendon rupture)

PHYSICAL EXAMINATION

- Examine the skin to check its integrity.
- Palpate the humerus, clavicle, and scapula.
- Perform a neurovascular examination of the entire upper extremity to rule out an associated injury.

LABORATORY TESTS

No routine tests are indicated unless surgery is anticipated.

PATHOLOGIC FINDINGS

- Fractures involving the tuberosities may result in rotator cuff tear.
- Anterior dislocation of the shoulder may also be concurrent.

IMAGING PROCEDURES

- Three views of the proximal humerus should be obtained in all fractures:

—Anteroposterior
—Lateral
—Axillary (Scapular Y-view may be adequate in patients who cannot tolerate abduction for the axillary view.)

- Computed tomography may be helpful in comminuted fractures when surgery is planned.

 Management

GENERAL MEASURES

Many fractures, especially minimally displaced surgical neck fractures, may be amenable to reduction. These fractures may be made more stable by impacting the shaft into the humeral head.

SURGICAL TREATMENT

Displaced fractures according to Neer's criteria may require surgical fixation. The weak metaphyseal bone of the proximal humerus and the need to preserve the rotator cuff make fixation difficult. Trends are toward minimal fixation with sutures, wires, or smooth pins. Four-part fractures may require prosthetic replacement.

PHYSICAL THERAPY

Early passive motion is imperative to prevent a frozen shoulder, especially in operated shoulders. Active motion should not begin until 4 to 6 weeks after surgery.

MEDICAL TREATMENT

- Oral narcotic analgesics are appropriate in the acute setting.
- A sling or swath is appropriate treatment in the emergency setting. Some authors recommend a coaptation splint, which is U-shaped and extends from the axilla, around the elbow, and up over the lateral shoulder. In minimally displaced fractures, this may represent definitive treatment.
- Patients may be ambulatory in a sling.

PATIENT EDUCATION

Emphasize that fractures may take 6 to 10 weeks to heal and that compliance with physical therapy is important. Shoulder stiffness is common, and patients must work hard to regain their range of motion. Many patients become discouraged with the long recovery period.

MONITORING

Follow-up radiographs are taken every 1 to 4 weeks to assess reduction of the fracture and bony healing.

COMPLICATIONS

- Osteonecrosis of the humeral head
- Nonunion
- Malunion
- Shoulder stiffness
- Axial nerve injury in up to 31% of patients

Operative Complications

- Loss of fixation
- Neurovascular injury
- Axillary artery injury

PROGNOSIS

- Most fractures go on to union without operative treatment.
- Some shoulder motion may be lost.

RECOMMENDED READING

Kristiansen B, Barfod G, Bredesem J, et al. Epidemiology of proximal humerus fractures. *Acta Orthop Scand* 1987;58:75–77.

Slipped Capital Femoral Epiphysis

 Basics

DESCRIPTION

Slipped capital femoral epiphysis (SCFE) is a disorder of the hips of adolescents or preadolescents in which the femoral head is displaced and moves (through the growth plate) relative to the rest of the femur (Fig. 1). The femoral head remains in the acetabulum but moves relatively posteroinferiorly, as can be seen on a radiograph. From an external perspective, the most notable features are the outward rotation of the lower femur and leg and a limp.
Eighty percent of cases occur during the growth phase of adolescence (boys, 10 to 16 years; girls, 10 to 14 years). More males are affected than females; the male-to-female ratio is 2.4:1.

SYNONYM

Epiphyseolysis

GENETICS

A 5% to 7% incidence is noted in family members of patients who have SCFE as compared with 2 to 10 per 100,000 in the general population.

INCIDENCE

The incidence is 2 to 10 per 100,0000 in the general population per year.

CAUSES

• It is likely multifactorial, resulting in a weakened growth plate (physis) with higher-than-normal stresses placed across it.
• Endocrine factors such as hypothyroidism, panhypopituitarism, hypogonadal conditions, and renal osteodystrophy may weaken the physis, but these are rare.
• During the preadolescent or adolescent age, the growth plate is weaker.
• Increased shear stress may be generated by obesity, decreased femoral anteversion, or trauma.

RISK FACTORS

• Adolescence: 80% of cases during the growth spurt
• Male sex: 2.4:1
• Obesity: weight-to-height ratio greater than

the ninetieth percentile in 50% to 75% of patients
• Black race
• Contralateral SCFE: 50% of patients eventually having a bilateral slip (25% at initial presentation)
• Delayed skeletal maturity

CLASSIFICATION

Stable versus Unstable

• Stable: Weight bearing without crutches is possible; 95% of patients have satisfactory results with proper treatment.
• Unstable: Weight bearing without crutches is not possible. This type has a higher rate of avascular necrosis and severe slip, so only 50% will have satisfactory results with treatment.

Chronologic Classification

• Acute (less than 3 weeks)
• Chronic (more than 3 weeks)

Anatomic Classification

Grade 0. Preslip: impending slip with no discernible displacement
Grade I. Mild: 1% to 33% slip
Grade II. Moderate: 33% to 50% slip
Grade III. Severe: more than a 50% slip

ASSOCIATED CONDITIONS

• Hypothyroidism
• Hyperparathyroidism
• Chronic renal failure

ICD-9-CM

732.2 Slipped capital femoral epiphysis

 Diagnosis

SIGNS AND SYMPTOMS

Symptoms

• Pain may be acute (less 3 weeks) or chronic (more than 3 weeks) and may vary in severity.
• Pain occurs in the groin, medial thigh, or knee.

Signs

• Decreased internal rotation of the hip as compared with the contralateral side
• Gait abnormality
• Trendelenburg's gait (during stance, the upper body leans toward the affected side)
• Antalgic gait (the patient bears weight on the affected side as little as possible)
• Externally rotated gait
• Symptoms and signs of hypothyroidism including cold intolerance, delayed bone age, lethargy, coarse hair

DIFFERENTIAL DIAGNOSIS

• Perthes' disease: usually presenting as a painless limp at a younger age (4 to 8 years) and distinguishable on radiographs
• Proximal femoral fractures: 90% with high-energy trauma
• Stress fracture of proximal femur: more common after skeletal maturity

PHYSICAL EXAMINATION

• Pain on palpation of groin or proximal femur
• Pain greatest with internal rotation or abduction
• Hip external rotation greater than internal rotation
• Most patients having little or no internal rotation of the hip
• The affected limb resting in more external rotation than the contralateral limb
• Rule out endocrine disorders, such as hypothyroidism, panhypopituitarism, hypogonadal conditions, and renal osteodystrophy by history.

LABORATORY TESTS

An endocrine workup is indicated for patients with significant delay in skeletal maturity or with symptoms suggesting an endocrine problem.

PATHOLOGIC FINDINGS

An abnormally wide growth plate is caused by an increase in the size of the zone of hypertrophy. The slip runs through this zone. The femoral neck is retroverted (rotated back) in most affected patients, a finding suggesting a long-standing period of abnormal force on the femur.

IMAGING PROCEDURES

• Plain anteroposterior and lateral films are usually adequate for diagnosis. Findings are most pronounced on the lateral film.
• There is apparent varus angulation of the epiphysis on the femoral neck. The appearance of the epiphysis has been likened to "ice cream falling off of its cone."
• "Kline's line": This loss of the intersection of the epiphysis by the lateral cortical line of the femoral neck is best seen on a lateral view.
• Widening and blurring of the physis (growth plate) are seen.
• A relative decrease in the height of the epiphysis (compared with the contralateral side) is noted.
• "Pistol-grip deformity": In chronic stages, reactive bone forms along the inferomedial portions of the femoral neck.
• Computed tomography or magnetic resonance imaging will usually demonstrate an impending slip (also called a "preslip"), if the diagnosis is suspected or radiographs do not show it.

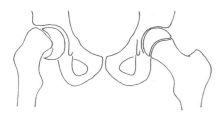

Fig. 1. Slipped capital femoral epiphysis occurs through the growth plate, as seen in the right hip here.

Management

GENERAL MEASURES

Complete avoidance of weight bearing is needed until the slip is stabilized.

SURGICAL TREATMENT

• The goal is to prevent further slippage by inducing closure of the physis. Under fluoroscopic control, a single guide pin is percutaneously placed from the anterior neck, across the physis, into the center of the femoral epiphysis. Because the neck slips anteriorly on the ephiphysis, the starting point is on the anterior femoral neck rather than on the lateral cortex of the proximal femur. An appropriate-length 6.5- or 7.2-mm cannulated screw is then placed over the guidewire. Extreme care is taken to avoid leaving a screw that penetrates the chondral surface of the epiphysis because this will likely lead to chondrolysis.
• In severe unstable slips, some surgeons advocate attempted reduction of the slip by traction or gentle closed manipulation.
• Osteotomies for severe slips may be performed at a later date to correct severe deformity. Although controversial, prophylactic pinning of the contralateral hip is generally not recommended, except in patients with known metabolic or endocrine disorders or patients in whom appropriate follow-up is unlikely.
• For patients with degenerative joint disease, options are hip fusion in the young patient and total hip replacement in the older patient.

PHYSICAL THERAPY

Postoperative instruction in ambulation with crutches or a walker is indicated, with partial weight bearing if the slip is stable.

MEDICAL TREATMENT

• Prevention of further slip is the cornerstone of therapy.
• Place the child immediately at bed rest and admit for surgery, usually done through a single, percutaneously placed screw to close the physis.

PATIENT EDUCATION

• The child and parent must understand the need for immediate non–weight bearing and early (usually the same day) surgery to prevent further slip, as well as the need for careful postoperative monitoring for osteonecrosis, chondrolysis, degenerative joint disease, and, most important, SCFE of the contralateral hip.
• Any pain in the contralateral thigh should be reported immediately.
• After surgery, maintain partial weight bearing to non–weight bearing for 6 weeks. Vigorous sports are not allowed until the physis has closed (usually at around 6 months postoperatively).

PREVENTION

Although controversial, prophylactic pinning of the contralateral hip is generally not recommended, except in patients in whom communication is impaired or appropriate follow-up is unlikely.

MONITORING

Obtain anteroposterior and lateral radiographs to monitor every 3 to 4 weeks for physeal closure, osteonecrosis, chondrolysis, degenerative joint disease, and contralateral SCFE.

COMPLICATIONS

• Osteonecrosis: This is a devastating complication in which blood supply to the femoral head is lost, leading to collapse and severe degenerative joint disease. It is most strongly associated with unstable slip. The risk is 40% for unstable slips and 5% for stable slips.
• Chondrolysis: Acute dissolution of articular cartilage with subsequent pain and stiffness of the joint is thought to be a complication of penetration of the screw through the chondral surface.
• Degenerative joint disease: Undiagnosed or untreated SCFE leading to degenerative joint disease is believed by some authors to be the leading cause of total hip replacement in the United States.

PROGNOSIS

Prognosis depends on the severity of the slip and the presence of complications. Even without complications, there is still an increased incidence of degenerative joint disease. If the patient is able to lose weight, this will help to decrease the risk of degeneration and to increase the success of total hip replacement.

RECOMMENDED READING

Canale ST. Slipped capital femoral epiphyis. In: Crenshaw AH, ed. *Campbell's operative orthopaedics,* 8th ed. St. Louis: Mosby–Year Book, 1992:1149–1181.

Carney BT, Weinstein SL, Noble J. Long-term follow-up of slipped capital femoral epiphysis. *J Bone Joint Surg Am* 1991;73:667.

Kehl DK. Slipped capital femoral epiphysis. In: Morrissy RT, Weinstein SL, eds. *Lovell and Winter's pediatric orthopaedics,* 4th ed. Philadelphia: Lippincott–Raven, 1996:993–1022.

Snapping Hip

 Basics

DESCRIPTION

Snapping of the hip is a sensation that is normally felt on an infrequent basis by many people. If it becomes frequent or painful, patients may seek attention and treatment. The causes may include structures outside or inside the joint.

Snapping of the hip is most common in young adults, but it may occur at any age, including the elderly. One of the causes is related to snapping after total joint replacement. It is slightly more common in females than in males.

SYNONYMS

- Popping hip
- Tendinitis
- Coxa saltans

GENETICS

No known genetic predisposition exists.

INCIDENCE

This is an uncommon clinical problem.

CAUSES

- Internal: This refers to a structure in front of the joint, such as the psoas tendon, which is causing the snapping by riding over the front of the femoral head or the pubic ramus.
- External: This refers to the snapping of the iliotibial band or the anterior fibers of the gluteus maximus riding over the greater trochanter. This type may also follow multiple intramuscular injections into the buttock that render the gluteus and iliotibial band fibrotic and contracted.
- Intraarticular: This includes loose bodies or a tear in the acetabular labrum, which may cause sensation of snapping or clicking. Rarely, snapping may occur after total hip arthroplasty, owing to malposition or loosening of the femoral component.

RISK FACTORS

- Coxa vara, or decreased angle of the femoral neck, renders the greater trochanter more prominent and increases the risk of snapping.
- Another risk factor is a history of multiple intramuscular injections into the buttock, which may cause fibrosis of the gluteus and may, in turn, may predispose to snapping.

ASSOCIATED CONDITIONS

Snapping hip usually occurs in isolation and is not related to any systemic conditions or other skeletal problems.

ICD-9-CM

726.0 Bursitis
719.65 Snapping hip

 Diagnosis

SIGNS AND SYMPTOMS

- The patient has a sensation of muscle jumping over the front or the side of the hip. The patient may be able to point to the location of snapping, thus aiding in diagnosis.
- The patient may have difficulty getting into or arising from a squat.
- The diagnosis may be confirmed by blocking the movement of the psoas or the iliotibial band during flexion and extension of hip.

DIFFERENTIAL DIAGNOSIS

- Snapping of the meniscus may masquerade as snapping hip, because the hip and knee usually flex together.
- Exostosis around the hip may contribute to snapping.
- Habitual hip subluxation in children and adolescents is an uncommon phenomenon, which may be confused with a snapping hip.

PATHOLOGIC FINDINGS

In the internal type, the psoas and iliacus tendons ride in a groove between the iliopectineal eminence and the anterior inferior iliac spine. They may cause snapping by riding over each other, over the psoas bursa, or over the bone during flexion and extension. The iliotibial band attaches to the tensor fasciae latae and the gluteus maximus and minimus. It remains taut during flexion and extension, and it rides over the trochanteric bursa. Any thickening of this bursa, or increasing tension of the tendon, may contribute to the snapping.

IMAGING PROCEDURES

- Plain radiography of the pelvis is indicated to rule out any bony abnormality of the pelvis or joint. A computed tomography scan may be helpful if a structural abnormality is found.
- Ultrasound has been shown to document the snapping, but it is rarely clear or easy to interpret.
- Iliopsoas bursography is done under fluoroscopy, with contrast medium injected anteriorly into the bursa. The psoas tendon may be seen to flip over the front of the hip corresponding with the symptoms, if it is the cause.
- A hip arthrogram combined with a computed tomography scan may be helpful in diagnosing a torn acetabular labrum.
- Magnetic resonance imaging is not routinely helpful.

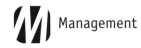 Management

GENERAL MEASURES

Injection into the appropriate region is an intermittent step between physical therapy and surgery. It may be done using a mixture of local anesthetics (e.g., lidocaine, to confirm the diagnosis) and steroid, to interrupt the inflammatory cycle and perhaps to provide permanent relief.

SURGICAL TREATMENT

If other measures do not help, surgery may be offered, depending on the underlying cause. If it is the iliotibial band, this can be incised over the greater trochanter to relieve the pressure. If it is the psoas tendon, it may be lengthened at the pelvic brim. Surgery is reserved for the most recalcitrant cases because the results are unpredictable when no structure abnormalities have been identified. Intraarticular factors, such as a loose body or a torn acetabular labrum, may be dealt with appropriately.

PHYSICAL THERAPY

Stretching the iliotibial band or psoas tendon may alleviate the problem.

MEDICAL TREATMENT

• Make diagnosis by physical examination and imaging.
• The extent of treatment depends on how much snapping bothers the patient. If it is significant, the following are advised:

—Avoidance of provocative activities
—Stretching exercises
—Antiinflammatory medications
—Injection with steroids
—Surgery

• Activities involving flexion and extension, or adduction (such as running on the side of an incline) may predispose to snapping.
• The patient should refrain from these activities.

Drugs

• Nonsteroidal antiinflammatory agents

—Dosing schedules vary from quick-onset, short duration, to once-a-day agents, which are less effective for acute pain.
—Gastrointestinal upset is a possible side effect, and these drugs are to be used cautiously in patients with a history of gastric ulcer disease.

• Avoidance of narcotic.

PATIENT EDUCATION

The phenomenon of a snapping tendon or other structure should be explained to the patient, including the rationale for rest and stretching.

PREVENTION

• Perform adequate stretching before and after sports.
• Avoid frequent intramuscular injections into the gluteal muscles.

MONITORING

Because this is a benign condition, patients may be allowed to self-monitor and return for follow-up if symptoms warrant.

PROGNOSIS

• Usually not a long-standing problem
• Does not lead to arthritis

RECOMMENDED READING

Lyons JC, Peterson LFA. The snapping iliopsoas tendon. *Mayo Clin Proc* 1984;59:327–329.

Schaberg JE, Harper MC, Allen WC. The snapping hip syndrome. *Am J Sports Med* 1984;12:361–365.

Soft Tissue Tumors

 Basics

DESCRIPTION

Soft tissue tumors may occur in any area of the skeleton and at any age. They may be composed of tissue originating from muscle, fat, vessels, nerves, or fibrous tissue. Benign tumors far outnumber malignant ones. Reactive lesions also cause soft tissue tumors. The difficulty arises in differentiating the malignant from the benign. These tumors can affect any area of the body, trunk, or extremities.

- Only 15% of sarcomas occur in children.
- More than 40% of sarcomas occur in patients more than 55 years old.
- Soft tissue tumors may occur at any age; however, types may vary.
- In childhood, most common types include the following:

—Popliteal cyst
—Ganglion of wrist or ankle
—Neuroblastoma
—Neurectodermal tumor
—Rhabdomyosarcoma

- No difference in gender risk is noted overall. However, sarcomas are more common in males.

GENETICS

Most soft tissue tumors are not inherited. A notable exception is neurofibromatosis, which is associated with multiple soft tissue tumors and is inherited in an autosomal dominant manner.

INCIDENCE

Soft tissue tumors in the aggregate are common. However, the ratio of benign to malignant types is 100:1. Nevertheless, vigilance must be maintained to avoid missing malignant tumors.

CAUSES

- The cause is largely unknown.
- Myositis ossificans may occur with trauma.
- Reactive granuloma may occur with implantation or retention of a foreign body.

CLASSIFICATION

The Musculoskeletal Tumor Society classifies benign and malignant tumors separately.

Benign Lesions

Stage 1. Inactive
Stage 2. Active
Stage 3. Aggressive

Malignant Tumors

Stage I. Low grade
Stage II. High grade
Stage III. Metastatic

A tissue type may be assigned to each tumor.

ICD-9-CM

238.1 Neoplasm, connective tissue, uncertain behavior

 Diagnosis

SIGNS AND SYMPTOMS

- Presence of a mass
- Possible loss of range of motion of the adjacent joint
- Usually painless or minimally painful
- Absence of pain not a reason to ignore the lesion

DIFFERENTIAL DIAGNOSIS

- Intramedullary bone tumor with soft tissue extension
- Bone tumor arising from the surface of the bone

PHYSICAL EXAMINATION

- Inspect the lesion for size, depth, and mobility.
- Obtain a history of recent growth.
- Note consistency and fixation to surrounding structures.
- It is more likely to be benign if small (less than 5 cm), soft, and superficial.
- It is more likely to be malignant if large (more than 5 cm), hard, and deep.

- Assess the effect on adjacent parts:
—Presence of limp
—Restricted joint motion
—Palpatation of lymph nodes
—Examination of abdomen

LABORATORY TESTS

These are largely not helpful, but screening tests may be helpful if a workup for malignant disease is undertaken.

PATHOLOGIC FINDINGS

Careful histologic evaluation is necessary, taking into account cell features, matrix production, and tissue organization. Incorrect histologic diagnosis is not uncommon.

IMAGING PROCEDURES

- Plain radiographs should be obtained first to look for phleboliths (indicating hemangioma) or rings and stipples (indicating chondroma). A lesion may appear radiodense if it is sandwiched between two tissues of lower density or radiolucent, as in deep lipomas in which the fat is contrasted between bone and muscle. Spotty calcifications occur in 20% to 30% of synovial sarcomas.
- Ultrasound is used to look for homogeneity and size, but it has largely been replaced by magnetic resonance imaging (MRI).
- MRI is superior in its ability to provide excellent soft tissue definition and to characterize some tissues. Many new signal combinations are now available. The technique may need to be discussed with the radiologist beforehand.

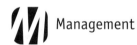 Management

GENERAL MEASURES

Observation is chosen for inactive benign lesions (e.g., lipomas, ganglions) if they are not causing symptoms.

SURGICAL TREATMENT

- The extent of surgery depends on the degree of malignancy.

- Benign tumors may be excised at their margins.
- Malignant tumors (sarcomas) should be excised with a layer of normal tissue around them. Approximately 95% of patients are treated with limb-sparing surgery.
- Attachment to nerves or major vessels may prevent effective resection of malignant tumors.
- If the lesion cannot be safely removed leaving a functional limb, amputation may be recommended.
- Radiation therapy is often used to decrease the risk of local recurrence.

PHYSICAL THERAPY

Physical therapy is often used postoperatively to restore function.

MEDICAL TREATMENT

- Lesions that are clearly benign may be observed if they are not causing symptoms, such as popliteal cysts and ganglions in children, which often resolve with time, and myositis ossificans, which may diminish with time.
- If the nature of lesion is not clear, it is important not to fall into the trap of complacency.
- Initiate a diagnostic workup under the direction of an orthopaedist knowledgeable about the diagnoses.
- Activity may increase the symptoms of some tumor types, such as popliteal cyst or ganglion or myositis ossificans.

Drugs of Choice

Chemotherapy is an effective adjuvant for a few of the malignant tumors of soft tissue (such as rhabdomyosarcoma and Ewing's tumor). Protocols vary from type to type and may be used before surgery in some types to shrink the tumor and to make resection more feasible.

PATIENT EDUCATION

- The patient should be given a general understanding of the behavior of his or her tumor type.
- Discuss the importance of follow-up and the risk of recurrence.

MONITORING

- Follow the patient at suitable intervals with physical examination or, in some cases, serial MRI.
- After the resection of malignant tumors patients, are followed at 3-month intervals for 2 years to look for pulmonary metastases (computed tomography scans) and then every 4 to 6 months for 5 more years. MRI scans are used to check for local recurrence 6 months after surgery and then once a year.

COMPLICATIONS

- Infection
- Recurrence
- Misdiagnosis
- Injury to local nerves and vessels

PROGNOSIS

Prognosis depends on the following:

- Grade of malignancy
- Anatomic extent
- Treatment given
- Superficial sarcomas (located above the fascia) have an excellent prognosis (more than 80%), whereas deep, large, high-grade lesions have the worst prognosis (only 50% to 60% long-term survival).

RECOMMENDED READING

Bullough P, Vigorita V. *Atlas of orthopaedic pathology*. New York: Churchill Livingstone, 1984:10.1–13.20

Enzinger F, Weiss S. *Soft tissue tumors*, 3rd ed. St Louis: Mosby–Year Book, 1995.

Frassica F, Chang B, Ma L, et al. Soft tissue sarcomas: general features, evaluation, imaging, biopsy, and treatment. *Curr Orthop* 1997;11:105–113.

Sim F, Frassica F, Frassica D. Soft tissue tumors: evaluation, diagnosis and management. *J Am Acad Orthop Surg* 1994;2:211.

Spina Bifida

 Basics

DESCRIPTION

Occult spina bifida refers to incomplete closure of the posterior elements (laminar arches) of the spine. The defect occurs at birth, but it may not be detected until later. Males and females are affected equally (Fig. 1).
Spina bifida may be a benign finding of no clinical consequence, such as when it occurs at the fifth lumbar or first sacral vertebra with no neurologic deficit. It may be a clinically significant problem if it is associated with congenital neurologic deficit at the same levels. It may occur at any level of the spine or at multiple levels, although it is most common at the caudal end. Secondary problems may develop in the kidneys and lower limbs if there is a neurologic deficit.

SYNONYMS

- Spinal dysraphism
- Rachischisis
- Myelomeningocele

GENETICS

- It is not inherited in a mendelian fashion.
- A genetic defect is not known.
- The risk of occurrence in first-degree relatives is slightly increased (3.2%).

INCIDENCE

- The incidence of spina bifida occulta is 2% to 3% of general population.
- The overall incidence of neural tube defects in the United States is about 1 per 1,000.
- It is slightly higher in whites and lower in African-Americans.
- The rate varies throughout the world from country to country.

CAUSES

- Unknown
- Failure of closure of the neural tube or its late rupture

RISK FACTORS

- Affected first-degree relative
- White race
- Poor perinatal nutrition

CLASSIFICATION

- Spina bifida occulta: inconsequential, skin-covered defect in the lower lumbar spine with no neurologic deficit; slightly increased risk of spondylolisthesis the only associated problem
- Myelomeningocele: bony defect, usually involving several missing laminae, with exposed meninges and usually some neurologic deficit at the same level
- Lipomeningocele: caudal fatty mass arising from the spinal canal, palpable under the skin, with an associated neurologic deficit but no significant risk of hydrocephalus

ASSOCIATED CONDITIONS

- Hydrocephalus
- Chiari's malformation
- Kyphosis
- Scoliosis
- Renal problems
- Latex allergies
- Sprengel's deformity
- Fracture

ICD-9-CM

741.93 Lumbar spina bifida
756.17 Spina bifida occulta

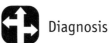 Diagnosis

SIGNS AND SYMPTOMS

Local Signs

- Abnormality in the skin of the back over site of lesion, ranging from a dimple to a hairy or vascular marking
- Fatty mass (lipomeningocele)
- Exposure of the meninges (myelomeningocele)
- Spina bifida occulta has no physical signs.

Distant Signs

- Motor weakness
- Atrophy of the calf or thigh
- Neurogenic bladder

Symptoms

None are directly attributable to the spina bifida, except it predisposes to an increased incidence of spondylolisthesis, which may cause backache.

DIFFERENTIAL DIAGNOSIS

- Defect from prior laminectomy
- Radiographic delay in ossification of an intact arch

PHYSICAL EXAMINATION

- Examine the patient for scoliosis and kyphosis.
- Note the quality of skin covering, because this predicts the late risk of breakdown.
- Record the motor level of the lesion on each limb as the lowest that has contraction against resistance.
- Record strength in the major muscle groups for future comparison.
- Record the lowest level of sensation, because this predicts pressure sores.
- Note the presence of contractures or deformities of each joint.
- Observe the patient's gait, if possible.
- Look for signs of hydrocephalus or Chiari's malformation (Fig. 2).

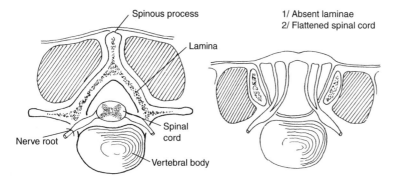

Fig. 1. Normal posterior spinal elements (*left*) are disrupted in spina bifida (*right*).

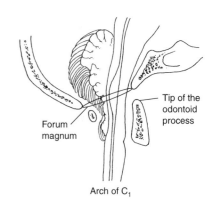

Fig. 2. Chiari's malformation with cerebellar compression may cause brainstem symptoms in spina bifida.

LABORATORY TESTS

Prenatal screening using amniocentesis and determination of alpha-fetoprotein and acetylcholinesterase are available for those at increased risk of a neural tube defect. Ultrasound may be used as a prenatal imaging test, with about 80% sensitivity.

PATHOLOGIC FINDINGS

The pathologic features of a typical myelomeningocele include a flattened spinal cord with scarring and abnormal neural elements. Often there is associated hydrocephalus or Chiari's malformation with herniation of the cerebellar tonsils through the foramen magnum.

IMAGING PROCEDURES

• Baseline radiography of the spine early in infancy, to rule out congenital anomalies such as hemivertebrae and bars of bone between vertebrae, which are present in up to 20% of children with true spina bifida
• Baseline imaging for hydrocephalus in the first few days of life, to make treatment decisions about shunting
• Magnetic resonance imaging of the neuraxis, if needed, to determine the presence of a syrinx, Chiari's malformation, or tether of the spinal cord

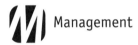 Management

GENERAL MEASURES

• At birth, child should be seen by an experienced neurologist, with consultation with neurosurgeon, orthopaedic surgeon, and urologist.
• Avoid latex exposure.
• Offer genetic counseling to family.

SURGICAL TREATMENT

• Clubfoot surgery: to lengthen tendons and realign bones to create a foot that will be flat on the ground
• Spine surgery: indicated for patients with unbalanced and impairing sitting, to straighten and fuse the spine using implanted rods

PHYSICAL THERAPY

• Patients should be followed throughout growth to maximize mobility, to monitor use of equipment (wheelchair or braces), and to monitor muscle strength.
• Therapist may also help the patient to prevent weight gain.

MEDICAL TREATMENT

• Prescribe long-term, low-dose prophylactic antibiotic therapy for patients with recurrent urinary tract infections.
• Monitor motor strength and sensory level and record throughout the patient's life to detect tethering or other complications.
• Treat clubfoot deformities by casting initially.
• Treat other deformities by stretching or bracing or surgery.
• Teach the family how to protect insensate skin.
• Involve the family in a support group such as Spina Bifida Association of America.
• Some instances of hip subluxation do not need surgery, especially if the condition is high and bilateral in a nonambulator.
• Encourage patients to maximize activity by the most efficient means, either by using a wheelchair or by walking with braces.
• Offer wheelchair sports to those athletically inclined, as a means of building social skills and self-image.

PATIENT EDUCATION

• Teach which products contain latex and how to avoid them.
• Discuss signs and symptoms of shunt failure, if applicable.
• Teach prevention of skin pressure sores.
• Teach bowel and bladder continence.
• Encourage weight control early in childhood.

PREVENTION

• Folate, 0.4 mg daily, used periconceptually, may prevent spina bifida.
• Folate supplementation in the first part of pregnancy can dramatically decrease the rate of this birth defect.

MONITORING

• Follow patients with myelomeningocele every 4 to 6 months to detect new deformities and to monitor the fit of braces and equipment.
• Follow every 3 to 6 months for signs of neurologic deterioration, which may be due to shunt failure, syrinx (cyst in the cord), tethering of the cord, or Chiari's malformation.

COMPLICATIONS

• Shunt failure
• Cord tethering at the site of opening, causing weakness with growth
• Fracture: risk higher with higher neurologic deficit. Signs include the following:

—Low-grade fever
—Swelling
—Warmth without much pain

• Pressure sore over insensate skin, especially of the ischium, foot, or trochanter
• Renal failure, owing to poor self-care

PROGNOSIS

• Infant mortality is only slightly increased now with excellent neonatal care.
• Long-term independence is not possible in some patients with central nervous system complications.

RECOMMENDED READING

Asher M, Olson J. Factors affecting the ambulatory status of patients with spina bifida. *J Bone Joint Surg Am* 1983;65:350–6.

Lindseth RE. Myelomeningocele. In: Morrissy RT, Weinstein SL, eds. *Lovell and Winter's pediatric orthopaedics,* 4th ed. Philadelphia: Lippincott–Raven, 1996:503–540.

McLone DG, Herman JM, Gabrieli AP, et al. Tethered cord as a cause of scoliosis in myelomeningocele. *Pediatr Neurosurg* 1990;16:8–13.

Tosi LL, Slater JE, Shaer C, et al. Latex allergy in spina bifida patients-prevalence and implications. *J Pediatr Orthop* 1993;13:709–712.

Spinal Stenosis

 Basics

DESCRIPTION

Spinal stenosis occurs when bony or other structures cause chronic compression of a nerve root laterally or the cauda equina or spinal cord centrally. The most common sources of the compression are osteophytes that form as a result of osteoarthritis or other degenerative changes in the facet or intervertebral joints.
Lower extremities are the most often affected, with pain and claudication-type symptoms. These are often present in the gluteal region. Severe stenosis may result in bowel or bladder dysfunction.
Spinal stenosis is most common in the elderly population, and there is no known predilection for either sex.

SYNONYM

Neurogenic claudication

GENETICS

No known genetic association exists.

INCIDENCE

• Up to 90% of the adult population will suffer from back pain at some point in their lives.
• The number suffering from spinal stenosis is less than 5%.

CAUSES

• Compression of nerve roots or spinal cord most often results from joint-narrowing osteophytes, resulting from degenerative joint disease.
• Compression may also be due to space-filling tumors or other lesions.
• Metastatic disease may cause nerve compression.
• Degenerative spondylolithesis and scoliosis may also contribute to symptoms.

RISK FACTORS

Increasing age is the only known correlating factor.

CLASSIFICATION

This is not widely used.

ICD-9-CM

724.00 Spinal stenosis
724.02 Lumbar spinal stenosis
723.0 Cervical spinal stenosis

 Diagnosis

SIGNS AND SYMPTOMS

• The clinical spectrum is wide.
• Lumbar stenosis can affect one nerve root laterally or multiple root levels simultaneously. Central compression can cause a more widespread syndrome.
• Complaints include sciatica or claudication-type symptoms, especially in the gluteal region.
• Pain may increase with sitting and may lessen with ambulation, features that differentiate this condition from vascular claudication.
• Extension of the spine may worsen symptoms.
• Flexion may relieve symptoms by widening the spinal canal.
• Patients may walk in a stooped-over position.
• Motor and sensory changes are often absent, but weakness of extensor hallucis longus is common.
• Symptoms may be vague; these patients may be labeled hysterical by other physicians.

DIFFERENTIAL DIAGNOSIS

• Vascular claudication is the most common mimicking syndrome.
• Herniated lumbar disc may also cause similar symptoms.
• Spinal stenosis more proximally in the spine may cause more distal symptoms and should be sought.

PHYSICAL EXAMINATION

• Perform a complete motor and sensory examination of affected extremities.
• Range of motion of spine activities will demonstrate positions that increase or decrease symptoms.
• Straight leg raising may demonstrate increased leg pain by stretching the affected nerve.
• Perform a rectal examination to rule out cauda equina syndrome.
• Perform a full vascular examination to rule out vascular claudication.

PATHOLOGIC FINDINGS

Degenerative changes with osteophytes and thickening of the ligaments and joint capsules account for the compression.

SPECIAL TESTS

Myelography and computed tomography myelography have been used to outline the nerve roots and spinal cord and to quantitate the severity of the stenosis. These tests are often bypassed in favor of magnetic resonance imaging. Injections of facet joints or discograms may help in identifying the source of the pain.

IMAGING PROCEDURES

Plain radiographs of the lumbar or cervical spine help to exclude other processes and show the degenerative changes. Many adults have signs of degenerative disease of the spine either without symptoms or in areas that do not correlate to their pain.
Radiographs are obtained if pain fails to improve or the clinical course is not progressing as expected.

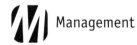 Management

GENERAL MEASURES

A brace or corset may help for short periods but is not recommended for long-term use, owing to possible weakening of paraspinous muscles.

SURGICAL TREATMENT

• This is indicated when pain causes significant reduction in quality of life and when symptoms are not relieved by conservative treatment.
• Patients with radicular symptoms benefit from decompression of affected nerve roots. Patients with central stenosis require laminectomy for decompression.
• Patients with instability, spondylolisthesis, or previous surgery may require decompression and fusion of affected segments.
• Back pain without radicular symptoms is a less favorable indication, and surgery will give unpredictable results.

PHYSICAL THERAPY

Range of motion of the spine and strengthening of the paraspinous and abdominal muscles may help reduce symptoms.

MEDICAL TREATMENT

Occasionally Helpful

- Rest
- Isometric abdominal exercises
- Pelvic tilt
- Weight reduction

Short-Term Relief

- Lumbar epidural steroids
- Nonsteroidal antiinflammatory drugs or acetaminophen

Patients should remain active and should avoid positions and activities that exacerbate their symptoms.

PATIENT EDUCATION

Patients should be informed that this condition will rarely lead to paralysis or the need for a wheelchair. Patients with progressive symptoms and severe disability should consider decompression.

MONITORING

Follow-up of 6 to 12 weeks to a few months is appropriate until symptoms begin to improve.

COMPLICATIONS

After surgery, the following may occur:

- Instability
- Arachnoiditis (scarring of the nerve roots)
- Failure to improve

PROGNOSIS

- Most improve without surgery.
- Patients with well-defined radicular symptoms have an 85% success rate with surgery.

RECOMMENDED READING

Baratz ME, Watson AD, Imriglia JE. *Orthopaedic surgery: the essentials*. New York: Thieme, 1999:223–225.

Johnsson KS, Rosen I, Cloen A. The natural course of lumbar spinal stenosis. *Clin Orthop* 1992;270:82–86.

Spine Fusion

 Basics

DESCRIPTION

Spine fusion is a procedure that causes two or more vertebral levels to be joined with solid bony healing in the spine. It is performed to correct spinal instability from traumatic, degenerative, or iatrogenic causes and in cases of spinal deformity to prevent progression of the deformity.

Spinal fusion can be performed in all decades of life. More spinal fusions are performed in females, owing to the association of scoliosis (adolescent and adult) with female gender.

INCIDENCE

Over the last 2 decades, the incidence of spinal fusion in the United States has more than doubled in the adult population. In general, approximately 1% of the population have had spine fusions for a variety of reasons.

CAUSES

Spinal fusions are performed for various reasons, including the following:

- Congenital scoliosis
- Idiopathic scoliosis
- Spondylolisthesis
- Degenerative scoliosis
- Spinal fractures
- Postsurgical instability

RISK FACTORS

Patients who smoke or have diabetes have a higher risk of failure of their spine fusion.

IMAGING PROCEDURES

Plain radiographs are used to assess adequacy and maturation of a spinal fusion. The presence of continuous bridging bone over the fusion site is the best evidence of a well-healed fusion.

When a failure to heal (pseudarthrosis) is suspected, the following are indicated:

- Computed tomography scan
- Three-dimensional computed tomography scan
- Plain tomography

Management

GENERAL MEASURES

Success of an individual fusion depends on the following factors:

- Patient age
- Surgical technique
- Use of bone graft
- Patient's nutritional status
- Patient's smoking status. Some series have shown that cigarette smoking can increase the rate of pseudarthrosis by up to eightfold.

SURGICAL TREATMENT

Spinal fusions can be performed in different ways, depending on individual case requirements:

- Anterior surgical approach
- Posterior surgical approach

Combined surgical approach depending on the requirements of an individual case. Spinal instrumentation can be used anteriorly or posteriorly to facilitate fusion rates. Localized bone graft, iliac crest bone graft, rib graft, fibular graft, or allograft can be used to facilitate spinal fusion.

PHYSICAL THERAPY

- Physical therapy is useful to increase walking ability and to improve aerobic conditioning.
- It is not required after spinal fusion.
- Its use varies from surgeon to surgeon.

PATIENT EDUCATION

- Spinal fusion predisposes to further spinal difficulties in life.
- Generalized total body fitness, avoiding smoking, and preventing osteoporosis are important factors to minimize these problems.

MONITORING

Activity

During healing and maturation of a spinal fusion, patients are often required to limit their physical activity. For 6 weeks after fusion, patients often have activity restrictions, which vary from surgeon to surgeon. By 6 months postoperatively, most patients are released to unlimited activities; however, most physicians advise against high-impact activities such as running, downhill skiing, and lifting heavy weights.

Follow-Up Care

In general, bone is the slowest healing tissue in the human body, but it has the ability to heal completely without a scar. Healing of spinal fusion is similar to fracture healing. Both spinal instrumentation and appropriate immobilization limit the local motion that allows a fusion to heal. In adults, it takes up to 6 months for a fusion to become solid and up to 2 years for it to attain full strength. In children, bone heals more rapidly, and full fusion strength can occur within 6 to 12 months.

During first 2 years after spinal fusion surgery, patients require follow-up with their treating surgeon to monitor the healing of the fusion every 2 to 3 months.

Once solidly healed, patients should be followed every few years to see whether they are developing problems related to early degenerative changes at levels adjacent to the fused levels.

COMPLICATIONS

Depending on the Indications for Surgery

- Failure to return to normal function
- Pseudarthrosis

Depending on the Surgical Technique

- Pseudarthrosis rates of 10% are not uncommon in the literature. Fortunately, not all pseudarthroses are painful or require treatment.
- Spinal fusion increases load and stresses at levels adjacent to the fusion, a situation that can lead to a significant rate of early generation at the junctional levels.
- Neurologic injury may occur.

PROGNOSIS

The prognosis varies greatly, depending on the following:

- Diagnosis
- Smoking status
- Surgical technique
- Patients with impending litigation and patients who were injured at work tend to have less favorable results than patients without these preexisting conditions.

RECOMMENDED READING

Aaron AD. Bone healing and grafting. In: Kasser JR, ed. *Orthopaedic knowledge update 5*. Rosemont, IL: American Academy of Orthopaedic Surgeons, 1996:573–679.

Hanley EN Jr, David SM. Who should be fused? Lumbar spine. In: Frymoyer JW, ed. *The adult spine*. Philadelphia: Lippincott–Raven, 1997:2157–2174.

Zdeblick TA. Spinal instrumentation. In: Kasser JR, ed. *Orthopaedic knowledge update 5*. Rosemont, IL: American Academy of Orthopaedic Surgeons, 1996:675–679.

Basics

DESCRIPTION

Spondylolisthesis is an abnormal anteroposterior translation of two vertebral bodies relative to each other. This translation is due to a defect in either the pars interarticularis (spondylolysis) or the posterior ligamentous-bony restraints. It affects the spine and sometimes the nervous system (Fig. 1).
Isthmic spondylolisthesis usually begins in childhood, but there is a slight increase in incidence in adolescence up to 6% in males. Degenerative spondylolisthesis occurs mainly in older adults.
Spondylolisthesis is more often associated with the female gender. Females develop more pronounced slips at a younger age.

GENETICS

• An increased risk is associated with a positive family history.
• About one-fourth of affected patients have a positive family history of spondylolisthesis.

INCIDENCE

• Five percent of the general population have either spondylolysis or spondylolisthesis.
• The prevalence is 0% at birth, 3% to 4% at 6 years, and 5% to 6% in adulthood.
• It does not occur until 5 to 6 years of age, when the incidence is 3.3%.

CAUSES

• The cause of isthmic spondylolisthesis is a stress fracture through a thin part of the posterior elements (pars interarticularis).
• The causes of degenerative spondylolisthesis are degeneration and instability of the disc.

RISK FACTORS

• A family history of spondylolisthesis is a risk factor.
• Particular physical activities in adolescence, such as playing the lineman position in football and participating in gymnastics, have been associated with an extremely high incidence of isthmic spondylolisthesis.

CLASSIFICATION

Spondylolisthesis is classified into six types (Table 1), as well as by severity of the slip (Table 2).

ASSOCIATED CONDITIONS

Most people with the condition are otherwise physically normal. However, there is an increased risk if one has connective tissue disorder such as Marfan's syndrome or neuromuscular conditions such as athetoid cerebral palsy.

ICD-9-CM

738.4 Isthmic spondylolisthesis
738.4 Degenerative spondylolisthesis

 Diagnosis

SIGNS AND SYMPTOMS

• Back or leg pain
• Gait abnormality
• Abnormal posture (hyperlordotic)
• History of trauma, either acute or mild repetitive, and often sports related

Symptoms can often be insidious; however, they may follow a relatively minor injury. Pain localized to the low back and thigh area may be seen in association with sciatica from an L-5 radiculopathy.

DIFFERENTIAL DIAGNOSIS

The differential diagnosis of spondylolisthesis is extremely important, because the presence of a spondylitic defect is not necessarily the source of a patient's pain. Population studies have shown that the incidence of spondylolisthesis is the same in populations with and without back pain.
A common cause of pain in a patient with a spondylolisthesis is an L4-5 disc herniation. Back pain including tumor, infection, facet arthropathy, stenosis, or degenerative disc disease must be considered.

Table 1. Classification of Spondylolisthesis

Class	Associated Risk Factors
Isthmic	Family history, gymnastics, football lineman
Congenital	Spina bifida occulta
Pathologic	Metastatic cancer or infection
Traumatic	Often associated with spinal cord injury
Degenerative	Seen in sixth and seventh decades of life at L4–5 level
Iatrogenic	Removal of posterior restraints at prior surgery

Table 2. Grade of Spondylolisthesis

Spondylolisthesis Grade	Percentage of Slip
Grade 0	0
Grade I	<25%
Grade II	25% to 50%
Grade III	51% to 75%
Grade IV	76% to 100%
Grade V	Complete displacement

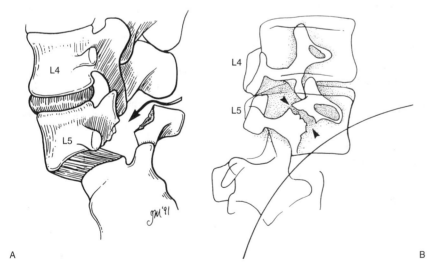

A   B

Fig. 1. Lateral view of spondylolytic spondylolisthesis. Spondylolysis. A 45-degree oblique view of the lumbar space. The *arrow* points to a defect in the pars interarticularis.

Spondylolisthesis

PHYSICAL EXAMINATION

- Watch the patient walk and test the ability to bend forward. Perform a careful neurologic examination, including assessment of rectal sensation and function.
- Patients can present with a hypolordotic posture.
- Patients with a significant slip may show L-5 radiculopathy with extensor hallucis longus weakness and numbness of the lateral calf or dorsum of the foot.
- Perform the limited straight leg raising test. Patients have limited lumbar flexion with significant hamstring tightness.

LABORATORY TESTS

Perform electromyography and nerve conduction velocities to assess L-5 root compression.

PATHOLOGIC FINDINGS

The most common finding is a defect in the pars interarticularis that resembles a fibrous union or pseudoarthrosis. The fibrous mass of the pars defect sometimes pins the L-5 nerve root beneath it.

IMAGING PROCEDURES

- Plain radiographs, including a spot lateral of L-5 to S-1, allow assessment of the presence and degree of spondylolisthesis.
- Oblique views visualize the pars interarticularis (neck of the "Scotty dog") and allow you to see the pars defect.
- Flexion and extension views can assess stability, particularly in degenerative and iatrogenic slips.
- Technetium bone scanning can be used in adolescents, when a clear pars defect is not visualized and early spondylosis is suspected. For this study, a single photon emission computed tomography scan should be ordered.
- Computed tomography myelography allows accurate evaluation of the degree of neural compression in more severe spondylolisthesis. It can also assess both bony and soft tissue compression on the neural elements in degenerative and iatrogenic slips.
- Magnetic resonance imaging can be useful in assessing both the degree of neural compression and the hydration status of the L4-5 disk.
- Use discography or selective blocks to assess whether the L4-5 disc or the pars defect is a patient's pain generator.

Management

GENERAL MEASURES

See the discussion of medical treatment.

SURGICAL TREATMENT

- For high-grade slips and patients in whom nonoperative therapy fails, posterior spinal fusion is indicated.
- For slips that are greater than grade III, fusion should be extended from L-4 to S-1.
- If reduction of the spondylolisthesis is attempted or an L-5 radiculopathy is present, the L-5 nerve root should be widely decompressed.
- The addition of anterior spine surgery may increase the rate of fusion and may prevent postsurgical progression of the spondylolisthesis.

PHYSICAL THERAPY

Therapy to work on hamstring stretching and lumbar lordosis may relieve the discomfort in patients with symptomatic grade 0 or I spondylolisthesis.

MEDICAL TREATMENT

Children and Adolescents

- Patients with asymptomatic grade 0 and I spondylolisthesis require no restrictions.
- Symptomatic patients need activity restriction until they regain painless lumbar flexion and rotation.
- Lumbar bracing in lordosis may be used for up to 6 months to relieve pain.
- Initiate hamstring stretches and abdominal exercises when patient is asymptomatic in a brace.
- Once the patient is asymptomatic, take serial radiographs every 1 to 2 years until skeletal maturity.
- Patients in whom a 12-month regimen of nonsurgical treatment fails or who have symptomatic higher-grade slips require posterolateral fusions.

Adults

- Patients with grade 0 and I slips can be treated as if they had simple mechanical back pain.
- Patients with severe grade II or higher slips require posterior spine fusion and possible nerve route decompression.

- Reduction of high-grade slips, the need for anterior spinal fusion, and the levels to be fused are all controversial topics.
- Medications used should be those typically administered for the relief of back pain: an analgesic with or without a muscle relaxant.

PATIENT EDUCATION

Patients with a high-grade slip must be educated to look for progressive bladder dysfunction. After recovery from a symptomatic episode, new onset of bowel or bladder symptoms may indicate slip progression.

PREVENTION

No preventive measures except long-term brace wear have been found effective in allaying progression of spondylolisthesis. Because of the rarity of significant progression, brace treatment is not commonly recommended for this purpose.

MONITORING

Growing patients should be monitored every 1 to 2 years to rule out progression of the slip.

COMPLICATIONS

- These vary greatly.
- If slip progresses to a high grade, compression of the cauda equina with loss of bowel and bladder function may occasionally occur.
- If reduction of the slip is surgically performed, postoperative L-5 nerve root dysfunction can occur.

PROGNOSIS

Spondylolisthesis predisposes an individual slightly to problems with chronic back pain. Most symptomatic low-grade slips in children and adolescents can be treated nonsurgically and lead to no long-term disability.

RECOMMENDED READING

Grobler LJ, Wiltse LL. Classification, nonoperative and operative treatment of spondylolisthesis. In: Frymoyer JW, ed. *The adult spine.* Philadelphia: Lippincott–Raven, 1997:1865–1921.

Wiesel SW. Spondylosis: degenerative process of the aging spine. In: Kasser JR, ed. *Orthopaedic knowledge update 5.* Rosemont, IL: American Acacemy of Orthopaedic Surgeons, 1996:589–592.

Basics

DESCRIPTION

Sprains refer to damaged ligaments, and they are the result of overstretching of the tissues. Injuries to the ligamentous structures of movable joints are among the most common complaints seen in primary care medicine, as well as in the subspecialty areas of orthopaedic surgery. Sprains can occur in any movable joints. There are no age-related factors, and both sexes are affected equally.

SYNONYMS

- Strain
- Torn ligament

INCIDENCE

Sprains are common.

CAUSES

Abrupt, overstretching of the ligament from an externally applied force or one generated by the periarticular muscles can lead to various degrees of ligamentous injuries.

RISK FACTORS

- "Weekend" athletes
- Running, throwing, or jumping sports
- Inadequate warm-up exercises

CLASSIFICATION

Three grades are recognized:

1. Interstitial injury with no disruption of fiber continuity
2. Partial tear of the ligament with mild laxity but no instability of the involved joint, with preservation of the ligament's continuity
3. Complete tear of the injured ligament

ICD-9-CM

848.9 Sprain/strain, site unspecified

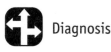

Diagnosis

SIGNS AND SYMPTOMS

- Pain or swelling occurs in minor sprains.
- Patients with incomplete ligament tear may demonstrate mildly increased laxity on stress examination. Ecchymosis over the involved area or gross instability of the joint can be seen in cases of complete disruption of the ligament.

DIFFERENTIAL DIAGNOSIS

- Muscle strain
- Fracture
- Dislocation

PHYSICAL EXAMINATION

- Ecchymosis or tenderness over the area of the ligament strongly suggests the diagnosis.
- Tenderness over the ligament occurs during testing for stability (hence stretching of the ligament).
- Gross instability of the involved joint is diagnostic.

LABORATORY TESTS

There are no laboratory tests to aid in the diagnosis.

PATHOLOGIC FINDINGS

- In grade 1 injuries, the ligament is grossly intact. Microscopically, however, hemorrhages and tearing can be demonstrated in small areas within the ligament.
- Grade 2 injuries can show gross tears and hemorrhages.
- Grade 3 injuries are characterized by complete disruption of the ligament.

IMAGING PROCEDURES

- Stress radiographs may demonstrate grade 2 and 3 injuries.
- Obtain plain films to rule out associated fractures or dislocation.
- Magnetic resonance imaging is best to assess soft tissues injuries, but it is usually not necessary.

Management

GENERAL MEASURES

- Initial treatments consist of rest, ice, compression, and elevation.
- Ice minimizes swelling through local vasoconstrictive effects. It also dulls pain receptors and decreases spasm.
- Compression and elevation further limit soft tissue swelling.

SURGICAL TREATMENT

- Repairs may be done by direct suture with or without autograft, allograft, or synthetic materials reinforcement.
- Most ligament injuries heal without surgical intervention. Rupture of the anterior cruciate ligament frequently requires surgical repair.

PHYSICAL THERAPY

- Ice
- Contrast treatment with hot and cold compresses
- Massage
- Ultrasound
- Pain-free, protected, range-of-motion exercises

MEDICAL TREATMENT

Patients with grade 1 and 2 mild or moderate injuries can be treated with initial immobilization and gradual, pain-free physical therapy to preserve range of motion and to avoid disuse atrophy.

In grade 1 and 2 injuries, normal activity can gradually be resumed once the pain and swelling subsided. Grade 3 injuries require longer immobilization to allow the ligament to heal, especially in nonoperative cases.

PATIENT EDUCATION

- Outline the treatment plan clearly.
- Patient compliance is important in achieving a good outcome.

PREVENTION

Proper warm-up exercise is indicated before a workout or before participating in sports.

MONITORING

Patients are followed at 2- to 3-week intervals to assess range of motion.

COMPLICATIONS

- Joint instability
- Chronic pain
- Stiffness

PROGNOSIS

Prognosis is generally excellent with nonoperative treatment in most patients with ankle and knee collateral ligament injuries.

RECOMMENDED READING

Booher JM, Thibodeau GA. Athletic injury and related skin conditions. In: Booher JM, ed. *Athletic injury assessment,* 2nd ed. Times Mirror/ Mosby, 1989:172.

Brieck JH, Saliba EN. The athletic trainer and rehabilitation. In: Kulund DN, ed. *The injured athlete.* Philadelphia: JB Lippincott, 1988:185.

Sprengel's Deformity

 Basics

DESCRIPTION

Sprengel's deformity is congenital elevation of the scapula (Fig. 1). The scapula is also small and has a restricted range of motion. Other congenital anomalies often coexist.

This condition is present from birth. It may be discovered at birth or after the child starts to use the arms functionally. It is usually diagnosed within the first few years of life, The best ages to perform surgery are between 2 and 8 years, although satisfactory results have been reported as late as 14 years of age. It is more common in girls than in boys, with a ratio of 3:1.

SYNONYMS

- Undescended scapula
- Congenital high scapula

GENETICS

- It is almost always a sporadic condition.
- Only a small number of familial cases have been reported, in which the pattern was autosomal dominant.

INCIDENCE

- Rare
- Incidence less than 1 in 10,000

CAUSES

The normal scapula appears in the fifth week of embryonic life up in the neck, opposite the fifth cervical to first thoracic segments. It then migrates distally to its position in the thoracic region. Therefore, Sprengel's deformity is better termed a failure of descent of the scapula. Its cause is unknown. It may be due to defective formation or later contracture of musculature. A theory has been advanced that abnormally-located "blebs" of cerebrospinal fluid interfere with scapular descent.

RISK FACTORS

- Myelomeningocele
- Congenital cervical fusion

ASSOCIATED CONDITIONS

- Klippel-Feil (cervical fusions) syndrome
- Myelomeningocele
- Congenital scoliosis
- Syringomyelia
- Renal malformations
- Limb malformations may each occur sporadically with this condition, or Sprengel's may occur in isolation.

ICD-9-CM

755.52 Sprengel's deformity

 Diagnosis

SIGNS AND SYMPTOMS

Sprengel's deformity may be bilateral, although most commonly it is unilateral.

The scapula is small and elevated. It is also rotated so the glenoid faces more downward than normal. This places the inferior medial pole closer to the spine and the superior medial pole farther from it. The superomedial pole is prominent in the base of the neck. The angle of the neck may appear more blunted than the opposite side. There is variation in severity, from obvious deformity to one that is barely noticeable. Abduction of the arm is limited, both because the glenoid is turned downward and because the motion of the scapula is decreased. This causes the patient to tilt the trunk when reaching upward; this is often the motion that first brings the diagnosis to light.

DIFFERENTIAL DIAGNOSIS

- Congenital cervicothoracic scoliosis may distort the trunk and ribs, thus giving a similar appearance. Birth palsy of the upper portion of the brachial plexus may cause an inability to abduct the extremity, so use of the arm resembles that of the patient with Sprengel's deformity.
- Injury to the axillary nerve, such as after a shoulder dislocation, produces deltoid muscle weakness.

- Injury to the long thoracic nerve produces winging of the scapula.
- Fascioscapulohumeral dystrophy produces bilateral shoulder weakness.

PHYSICAL EXAMINATION

The prominence of the scapula in the angle of the neck should be noted from both anterior and posterior aspects. The superomedial aspect of the scapula should be palpated to check for a bony connection (omovertebral bar) to the spine. The range of motion should be measured, especially abduction (raising up to side). Neck range of motion should also be checked, and the spine bending test should be performed to look for scoliosis.

If the patient has congenital cervical fusions, hearing should also be tested because there is an incidence of hearing abnormalities.

LABORATORY TESTS

Test results are normal.

PATHOLOGIC FINDINGS

The scapula is smaller than normal. It may be attached at its upper portion to the spinous processes of the lower cervical or upper thoracic spine by a bar of bone or cartilage known as an omovertebral bar. The upper portion of the scapula is abnormally curved forward. The muscles that normally attach the scapula are hypoplastic. Multiple other congenital malformations of other systems may be associated, in random fashion.

IMAGING PROCEDURES

Plain radiography of both scapulae on the same film is needed to confirm the condition and to determine its severity. Further imaging to determine the shape of the scapula or presence of an omovertebral bar is not necessary because it does not affect treatment.

Renal ultrasound should be performed because of the high incidence of associated renal anomalies. Plain radiographs of the spine should be obtained. If there is a sign of associated intraspinal anomaly, it should be investigated with magnetic resonance imaging.

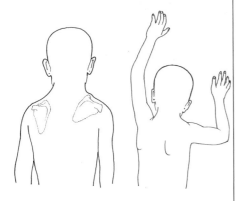

Fig. 1. Sprengel's deformity is an elevated downward-rotated scapula. This produces limitation of abduction (*right*).

Management

GENERAL MEASURES

- Stretching
- Strengthening
- Surgery

SURGICAL TREATMENT

For patients who are unwilling to accept the degree of deformity or limitation of abduction that Sprengel's deformity produces, surgical relocation of the scapula is the only option. There are several techniques to accomplish this; all involve detaching the muscles from their origins or insertions. The procedure results in a noticeable improvement, although it does not restore the appearance or function to normal. The range of abduction is also improved. The incision on the back may tend to spread and become wider than incisions in other areas.

PHYSICAL THERAPY

Physical therapy is useful in nonoperative cases to improve the range of abduction. This consists of active and passive stretching exercises, to be maintained by the parents. The family can assess whether they are satisfied with the results over the first 2 to 4 years of the patient's life.

MEDICAL TREATMENT

Stretching and strengthening are recommended initially, but it is doubtful whether they make any major improvement. During these early years, the patient should be observed to determine the degree of visibility of the deformity and its impact on the function of the arm. Problems in these areas are indications for surgery.

Activity should not be restricted by parents or physician. Often, these children are surprisingly functional.

PATIENT EDUCATION

The parents should be shown the normal and abnormal positions of the clavicle. They should be told that stretching results in slight improvement; surgery results in a good deal more. The length of the surgical incision should be indicated.

MONITORING

The family should bring the child in for several visits, 6 to 12 months apart, when trying to decide about surgery. The best age for surgery is when the patient is 2 to 8 years old, although it has been successfully done on patients both older and younger than this.

COMPLICATIONS

The results of surgery are generally good, but complications include the following:

- Brachial plexus stretch
- Weaknesses of the shoulder muscles
- Incomplete correction
- A wide incision scar

PROGNOSIS

- The deformity is generally static and does not usually improve or worsen with time.
- No evidence indicates that it causes arthritis of the shoulder, although it may be weaker than the other side.

RECOMMENDED READING

Cavendish ME. Congenital elevation of the scapula. *J Bone Joint Surg Br* 1972;54:395–408.

Woodward JW. Congenital elevation of the scapula: correction by release and transplantation of muscle origins. *J Bone Joint Surg Am* 1961;43:219–228.

Stress Fractures

 Basics

DESCRIPTION

A stress fracture occurs when repetitive stresses are applied to a bone faster than it is able to remodel to withstand this challenge. As the stressing force continues, the bone gradually fatigues and eventually breaks. Remodeling occurs in response to the stress but does not happen quickly enough to prevent the break. There are two general types of stress fracture. In the first type, excessive forces are applied to a normal bone such as a metatarsal stress fracture in a military recruit who has just marched 20 miles in boot camp. The second is a fracture occurring with minimal force in a patient with weak bone. An example is a femoral neck stress fracture in an elderly person with severe osteopenia.
Weight-bearing bones of the lower extremity are affected. Most common are the following:

- Metatarsus
- Calcaneus
- Tibia
- Fibula
- Femoral neck

Stress fractures can occur at any age. Typically, people less than 60 years old develop stress fractures after overexertion, whereas persons more than 60 years old develop stress fractures from a smaller stress to an underlying weak bone. Stress fractures occur equally in males and females.

SYNONYMS

- March fracture
- Fatigue fracture

INCIDENCE

- African-Americans are less susceptible to stress fractures than others.
- These are particularly common in runners, military recruits, and athletes.

CAUSES

- Strenuous activity in young people
- Minimal stress in people with weak or osteopenic bone

RISK FACTORS

Two general categories of risk factors are recognized:

- Overuse leading to stress fractures occurs in runners, other athletes, or military recruits.
- Weak bone susceptible to stress fracture is seen in patients with osteopenia, rheumatoid arthritis, or metabolic bone disease.

Patients may also be susceptible to stress fracture after recent foot surgery. This may cause a redistribution of force to the bones of the foot, with considerably more force going to different bones than preoperatively.

CLASSIFICATION

Two classification systems exist for femoral neck stress fractures.

Devas Classification

The Devas system uses the mechanism of injury and age.

- Distraction fractures: transverse fractures occurring in people more than 60 years old
- Compression fractures: occurring in people less than 60 years old

Blickenstaff-Morris Classification

The Blickenstaff and Morris system distinguishes fractures by plain radiograph findings:

Type I.   Endosteal or periosteal callus with no fracture line
Type II. Fracture line present with no displacement
Type III. Displaced stress fracture

ASSOCIATED CONDITIONS

- Osteopenia
- Metabolic bone disease

ICD-9-CM

733.11 Stress fracture

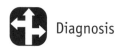 Diagnosis

SIGNS AND SYMPTOMS

The first sign of a stress fracture is point tenderness of a bone. Pain first occurs during activity but subsequently occurs after activity and at night. Often, the patient believes the pain is from a strained muscle and does not seek treatment. The persistence of pain with activity typically brings the patient to a doctor. Femoral neck stress fractures may produce only slight pain in the groin or referred pain to the medial side of the knee. There may be pain on palpation of the greater trochanter. Tibial stress fractures present with pain on palpation of the tibia. There may be thickening of the soft tissues over the bone that may make differentiation from a chronic compartment syndrome difficult.

Stress fractures in the foot present with point tenderness. The most critical factor in diagnosing a stress fracture is clinical suspicion when hearing a history of repetitive stress or weak bone stock.

DIFFERENTIAL DIAGNOSIS

- Infection
- Fracture
- Soft tissue injury
- Acute or chronic compartment syndrome
- Tumor

PHYSICAL EXAMINATION

- Point tenderness is noted in the affected bone.
- Elicit femoral neck tenderness over the greater trochanter.
- The extremes of hip motion cause muscle spasm.
- Antalgic gait may be present.
- Note point tenderness in the tibia and foot.
- Observe swelling and thickening of the soft tissues in the lower leg.

LABORATORY TESTS

There are no serum laboratory tests.

IMAGING PROCEDURES

- Order plain radiographs initially. These will be negative if less than 2 weeks have elapsed from the time of injury.
- Obtain repeat radiographs 2 to 3 weeks after injury to see the stress fracture (Figs. 1 and 2).
- Bone scanning is a sensitive test for stress fractures and shows a fracture 48 hours after injury.
- Magnetic resonance imaging may also be useful in detecting stress fractures.
- These special tests are most useful in the femoral neck, where displacement may cause severe complications and early detection is important.

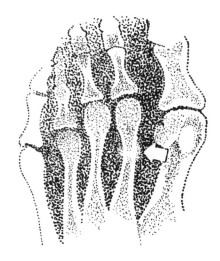

Fig. 1. Stress fracture of the foot most commonly involves the metatarsal shafts. It is signified by sclerosis or a periosteal reaction (*arrow*).

⚡ Management

GENERAL MEASURES

Patients need to decrease the load on injured bone to allow healing to occur. A gentle return to activity is then instituted.

SURGICAL TREATMENT

Femoral neck stress fractures may be treated with cannulated screws (usually three).

PHYSICAL THERAPY

Patients with stress fractures are instructed in partial weight to non–weight-bearing for 6 to 8 weeks.

MEDICAL TREATMENT

Medications

Nonsteroidal antiinflammatory drugs are given for pain.

Femoral Neck Stress Fractures

• Type I fractures should be treated with bed rest. Extremely young patients (less than 7 years) should be immobilized in a hip spica.
• Type II fractures require internal fixation with pins or cannulated screws.
• Type III fractures require a hip compression screw and bone grafting.

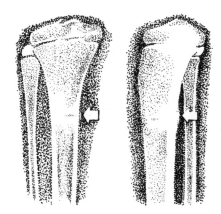

Fig. 2. Stress fracture of the tibia, with sclerosis and periosteal reaction.

Tibia or Fibula Stress Fractures

The patient should be placed on crutches for 6 to 10 weeks.

Foot Stress Fractures

• If the fracture is found within 2 weeks of injury, the patient should rest and should not engage in the offending activity for 2 weeks.
• Repeat radiographs should then be taken.
• If the fracture is found after 2 weeks, the patient should be immobilized with a weight-bearing cast for 4 to 6 weeks.
• If repeat radiographs show the fracture to have healed, the patient may slowly resume activity. Fractures of the fifth metatarsal and fractures that do not heal within 10 weeks require bone grafting.

After initial treatment, activity should be slowly started. Some athletes may require 6 months to increase to their former level of activity gradually.

PATIENT EDUCATION

Military recruits and athletes should be educated to mix their activities and to not overstress their bones.

PREVENTION

• Avoid sudden increases in physical activity levels, especially when involving walking or running.
• Runners should be educated to reduce mileage and to rest when they have acute, new-onset pain with activity.

MONITORING

Radiographs are taken every 6 to 8 weeks to monitor progress to healing.

COMPLICATIONS

Complete displacement is the most common complication of stress fractures. This is rare, however.

PROGNOSIS

• Stress fractures in young people have a good prognosis.
• Older patients or those with metabolic bone disease typically continue to develop fractures in other bones.

RECOMMENDED READING

Blickenstaff LD, Morris JP. Fatigue fractures of the femoral neck. *J Bone Joint Surg Am* 1966;47:1031–1047.

Devas MB. Stress fracture of the femoral neck. *J Bone Joint Surg Br* 1965;47:728–738.

Rockwood CA, Green DP, Bucholz RW, eds. *Rockwood and Green's fractures in adults,* 3rd ed. Philadelphia: JB Lippincott, 1991:1481–1538.

Subtrochanteric Fractures

 Basics

DESCRIPTION

Subtrochanteric hip fractures or simply subtrochanteric fractures by definition extend into the region between the lesser trochanter and a point 5 cm distally. A bimodal age distribution is seen: older patients suffering low-energy trauma and younger patients with normal bone undergoing high-energy trauma. Subtrochanteric fractures account for approximately 10% to 34% of all hip fractures.

CAUSES

• In younger patients with normal bone, the mechanism of injury is high-energy trauma, as occurs in motor vehicle collisions and falls from significant heights. Gunshot wounds constitute approximately 10% of these high energy cases.
• In the older population with weakened bone, low-energy trauma such as a minor fall is more common.
• Less commonly, there is also the pathologic fracture in which weakened bone stock (e.g., secondary to neoplasm or metabolic bone disease) succumbs to the mechanical stresses of normal ambulation or other low-impact activity.
• The mechanical stresses seen in the femur are highest in the subtrochanteric region.

RISK FACTORS

Any condition that generally or focally (such as metastatic disease) weakens the bone may predispose to such an injury with low-energy trauma or even without trauma.

CLASSIFICATION

• Multiple classification systems exist, but it appears that prognostically the most critical factor is fracture stability, based on the degree of comminution of the posteromedial cortex.
• Comminution in this area renders the fracture unstable, whereas bony contact is possible with reduction in stable fractures.

ASSOCIATED CONDITIONS

• When the fracture is associated with high-energy trauma, there should be a high index of suspicion for other injuries both in the ipsilateral extremity and elsewhere such as cranial and vertebral injuries. These injuries can be associated with significant hemorrhage, and as such, the patient should be monitored for hypovolemic shock. In addition, compartment syndrome of the thigh is possible, although rare.
• With any such fracture associated with previous symptoms of pain or a limp or with minimal trauma, neoplasm should be ruled out by appropriate methods including bone biopsy at the time of treatment.

ICD-9-CM

820.32 Subtrochanteric fracture

 Diagnosis

SIGNS AND SYMPTOMS

• The clinical picture is often not subtle and resembles that in any patient with an intertrochanteric or a femoral shaft fracture.
• Pain and deformity are the norm, although nondisplaced fractures are also seen.

DIFFERENTIAL DIAGNOSIS

• Traumatic injury
• Pathologic fracture

PHYSICAL EXAMINATION

Generally, a shortened extremity with a swollen thigh is most evident on examination. A complete neurovascular examination of the extremity should be performed; however, neurologic or vascular injuries are rare unless they are associated with penetrating trauma. An open injury should be ruled out because this requires urgent surgical débridement and irrigation.

LABORATORY TESTS

• A complete blood count to evaluate the hematocrit is advisable in patients with any trauma. Preoperative laboratory tests should be obtained in the event that operative treatment will be necessary.
• Urine and serum electrophoresis may be obtained if possible pathologic fractures are suspected in patients who are more than 45 years of age.

IMAGING PROCEDURES

Anteroposterior and lateral films of the entire femur should be obtained with particular attention to including the femoral neck to rule out concurrent, ipsilateral injury as well to help dictate treatment options.

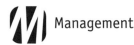 Management

GENERAL MEASURES

• Initial assessment after the trauma includes the Advanced Trauma Life Support protocol when appropriate. Treatment of the associated injuries should be done while traction splinting is in place.
• Skeletal traction should be initiated if the patient is going to be treated nonoperatively or if surgical fixation will be delayed.
• Muscular forces about the fracture tend to flex and abduct the proximal fragment, thus producing a shortened femur with varus deformation. The goals of treatment are to restore femoral length and rotational alignment and to maintain the abductor muscle lever arm by preventing varus deformity.
• Nonoperative treatment may be indicated in some unstable, comminuted subtrochanteric fractures in young, active patients and in patients with open fractures. Skeletal traction or cast bracing may be used, although there is an increased risk of shortening and varus deformity.

SURGICAL TREATMENT

Open reduction and internal fixation comprise the treatment of choice in stable fractures because this approach better achieves near-normal anatomy than do nonoperative procedures and provides for early mobilization. Because this area of the femur undergoes significant compressive and tensile stresses with normal gait, hardware failure is of concern, particularly with unstable fractures. The main operative treatment options include static interlocking nails, cephalomedullary reconstruction nails (with locking screws placed into the femoral head and neck), dynamic compression screws, and external fixators. The optimum choice is determined by the fracture configuration and the patient's age.

PHYSICAL THERAPY

Because the subtrochanteric region of the femur has a high cortical to medullary index, healing occurs more slowly than in fractures of other areas with more cancellous bone at the fractured ends. Accordingly, premature weight bearing may lead to hardware failure and fracture healing delays. Postoperatively, toe-touch weight bearing with crutches or a walker should be initiated within the first 2 to 3 days. Full weight bearing should be achieved gradually over a 3-month period, guided by radiographic healing. No weight bearing should be begun before 3 to 4 months after injury in patients with unstable fractures of the subtrochanteric region (i.e., with a comminuted posteromedial cortex) because the entire stress at the fracture site is borne by the implant alone.

MEDICAL TREATMENT

After the immediate posttraumatic stabilization and workup, medical issues include intravascular volume, antithromboembolic prophylaxis (keeping in mind the timing of definitive surgical management), and treatment of preexisting medical problems.

COMPLICATIONS

The most common complications of treatment of subtrochanteric fractures are nonunion, malunion, shortening, and implant failure. Stable, near-anatomic reduction and internal fixation of these injuries with attention paid to avoiding premature weight bearing help to decrease the incidence of such complications. Avascular necrosis of the femoral head may occur if standard intramedullary nailing is performed through the piriformis fascia.

PROGNOSIS

The prognosis is usually good once the fracture heals.

RECOMMENDED READING

DeLee JC. Fractures and dislocations of the hip. In: Rockwood CA, Green DP, Bucholz RW, et al., eds. *Rockwood and Green's fractures in adults*, 4th ed. Philadelphia: Lippincott–Raven, 1996:1481–1652.

Teitge RA. Subtrochanteric fracture of the femur. *J Bone Joint Surg Am* 1976;58:282.

Subungual Hematoma

 Basics

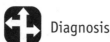 Diagnosis

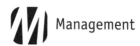 Management

DESCRIPTION

Subungual hematoma is a localized collection of blood between the fingernail and nail bed that results from an injury or laceration of the soft tissue of the nail bed under an intact nail. Pressure of the hematoma against the periosteum of the distal phalanx produces significant pain.

It affects the nails of the finger or toe. Older children and young adults are most commonly affected.

INCIDENCE

• This is one of the most common hand injuries seen in the office or emergency room.
• The long finger is most frequently injured of all of the digits because of its prominence.

CAUSES

• Blunt trauma to the distal phalanx causes this condition.
• Injury in a door is the most common mechanism, followed by smashing between two objects and injury by a saw.

CLASSIFICATION

The injury to the underlying nail bed tissue may be classified as follows:

• Simple laceration
• Stellate laceration
• Crush injury

ASSOCIATED CONDITION

Distal phalanx fracture

ICD-9-CM

No code exists.

SIGNS AND SYMPTOMS

• Typically, in an acute injury, the patient complains of localized pain and gives a history of trauma to the finger.
• Nail deformity is a late sign of a neglected nail bed injury.

DIFFERENTIAL DIAGNOSIS

• Contusion or fracture of the distal phalanx without hematoma formation
• Subungual melanoma, if history of injury is not clear
• Pyogenic granuloma at base of nail, usually caused by perforation with cuticle scissors

PHYSICAL EXAMINATION

• On inspection, the hematoma is visible through the fingernail.
• If there is an underlying fracture of the distal phalanx, one sees diffuse swelling of the fingertip.

IMAGING PROCEDURES

Plain films of the affected finger should be obtained to rule out an associated fracture of the distal phalanx.

GENERAL MEASURES

A painful subungual hematoma, involving more than 50% of the nail bed, is drained by trephining one to three holes in the nail over the affected area with a battery-powered cautery such as an ophthalmic cautery (preferred method), a heated paper clip, or a 16-gauge needle, while the patient presses the pad of the finger firmly against a hard surface. It is not necessary to anesthetize the finger. The nail should be prepared in sterile fashion before the procedure (Fig. 1).

SURGICAL TREATMENT

Surgical repair of a nail bed laceration requires removal of the fingernail. Once adequate regional anesthesia is obtained by a digital nerve block, the distal edge of the nail is grasped with a clamp, and the nail is bluntly dissected from the nail bed and eponychium. After irrigation, the laceration is repaired with fine absorbable suture (e.g., 5-0 or 6-0 polyglactin 910 [Vicryl]). Finally, the eponychial fold must be splinted to prevent formation of adhesions, which can result in deformity of the regrown nail. Either the proximal part of the removed nail or a piece of heavy foil may be used as a

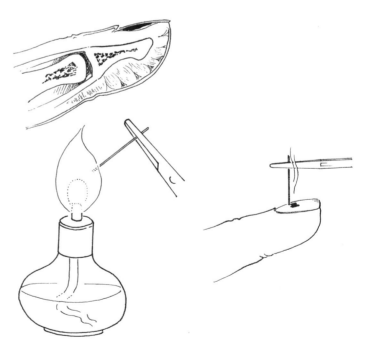

Fig. 1. Subungual hematoma may be decompressed with a cautery or hot needle for pain relief.

splint and should be sutured to the eponychium using 5-0 nylon. The exposed nail bed is covered with petrolatum gauze (Xeroform), and a tubular gauze dressing is applied.

MEDICAL TREATMENT

• Drainage of the hematoma provides prompt relief of pain.
• If fracture is present, splint the distal phalanx as well.
• If the hematoma involves more than 50% of the nail, or if there is an underlying fracture, remove the nail to inspect and repair the underlying nail bed injury.
• If the fracture is nondisplaced, the nail should be replaced as a splint.
• If the fracture is displaced, it should be reduced and fixed.
• The patient may continue activity as tolerated.
• Prescribe nonsteroidal antiinflammatory drugs for pain relief.

PREVENTION

Late deformity of the nail is difficult to reconstruct, and the results are unpredictable. Therefore, guidelines given earlier for inspecting and repairing nail bed injury should be followed to minimize the risk of late deformity.

MONITORING

The patient should be counseled about signs of infection and should be given a follow-up appointment within 1 week if nail bed repair has been performed.

COMPLICATIONS

• Fingernail deformity (i.e., fissured nail) if the eponychial fold is not properly splinted after removal of the nail
• Split or nonadherent nail
• Osteomyelitis, which is a complication of drainage of the hematoma if it is not done in a sterile manner and the wound is not properly dressed

PROGNOSIS

The prognosis is excellent, if proper assessment and treatment are performed.

RECOMMENDED READING

Ashbell TS, Kleinert HE, Putcha SM, et al. The deformed finger nail: a frequent result of failure to repair nail bed injuries. *J Trauma* 1967;7:176–190.

Rosen P, Barkin RM, Danzl DF, et al., eds. *Emergency medicine: concepts and clinical practice.* St. Louis: Mosby–Year Book, 1988:578–579.

Simon RR, Wolgin M. Subungual hematoma: association with occult laceration requiring repair. *Am J Emerg Med* 1987;5:302–304.

Supracondylar Elbow Fracture

 Basics

DESCRIPTION

A supracondylar fracture occurs between the thin bone of the medial and lateral columns of the distal humerus, just proximal to the humeral condyles. The fracture goes through the olecranon fossa of the distal humerus, which is a weak area. These fractures affect the distal humerus of children, with a peak age of occurrence between 5 and 8 years. This fracture is extremely rare in adults. Males are more commonly affected, owing to a generalized increased propensity for fracture.

In adults, the same mechanism (hyperextension) usually causes elbow dislocation. In toddlers, this mechanism usually causes a fracture through the growth plate of the distal humerus.

SYNONYM

Distal humerus fractures

INCIDENCE

This is the most common elbow fracture in children less than 10 years old.

CAUSES

• A fall on an outstretched hand with the elbow hyperextended
• A fall onto a flexed elbow, which is extremely rare

CLASSIFICATION

Classification of Mechanism of Injury

• Hyperextension type
• Flexion type

Classification of Displacement

Type I. Undisplaced
Type II. Displaced, but with an intact cortex; hinge or greenstick
Type III. Completely displaced, with no continuity between fragments; at highest risk for complications

ASSOCIATED CONDITIONS

• Ipsilateral distal forearm fractures
• Ipsilateral midshaft humeral fractures
• Nerve and artery damage (Fig. 1)

ICD-9-CM

812.51 Supracondylar elbow fracture

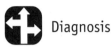 Diagnosis

SIGNS AND SYMPTOMS

• Pain, swelling, and possibly instability occur after an acute traumatic event.
• After a few hours, there is typically ecchymosis in the antecubital region.
• Nerve injuries are common with this fracture, signaled by lack of full active movement.
• Arterial injuries are also possible and produce loss of pulse, color, temperature, and later, movement.

DIFFERENTIAL DIAGNOSIS

• Elbow dislocation
• Bicondylar humeral fracture
• Growth plate fracture (in toddlers)

PHYSICAL EXAMINATION

• Swelling and tenderness are common.
• With type III fractures, an S-shaped deformity at the elbow is common and may be mistaken for a dislocation.
• Perform a thorough neurovascular examination of the involved extremity, because there is a substantial risk of injury.
• Document full active flexion and extension of all digits at both metacarpophalangeal and interphalangeal joints.

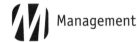

Fig. 1. Supracondylar fracture of the distal humerus may injure the brachial artery or the medial, radial, or ulnar nerve.

• Note significant pain on passive stretch of the fingers, because this may signal compartment syndrome. Check pulse, color, and temperature to assess vascular status.

IMAGING PROCEDURES

• Anteroposterior and lateral radiographs are usually sufficient to diagnose the injury.
• For nondisplaced fractures, a posterior fat pad sign may be the only finding on radiography.
• When ordering a radiograph of a suspected supracondylar fracture, specify the distal humerus as the part to be examined rather than the elbow, because the patient may not be able to straighten the elbow fully.

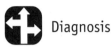 Management

GENERAL MEASURES

Initial treatment should involve immobilization of the injured elbow in 20 to 30 degrees of flexion to prevent further displacement or additional neurovascular damage until the patient can be evaluated by an orthopaedic surgeon.

SURGICAL TREATMENT

• Reduction should be performed with the patient under adequate analgesia or anesthesia for type III fractures and for type II fractures angulated more than 5 to 10 degrees.
• If anatomic reduction cannot be achieved by closed reduction, open reduction should be performed.
• An unstable fracture should be stabilized by pins.

- The elbow is often immobilized in at least 90 degrees of flexion for 3 to 4 weeks. Any activity that encourages use of that arm should be discouraged. After the pins are removed at 4 to 6 weeks, rough play should be prohibited for a month to prevent refracture.
- Compartment syndrome may be prevented by timely recognition of arterial injury. If ischemia time exceeds about 6 hours, fasciotomy of the forearm should probably be included with the rest of the treatment.
- Traction is another option if fixation is not performed.

PHYSICAL THERAPY

- Physical therapy for children is generally not required to regain full elbow motion.
- It is useful in adult fractures. Timing depends on healing and strength of internal fixation. Range of motion is emphasized, followed by strength.

MEDICAL TREATMENT

- Type I injuries: immobilization
- Type II injuries: closed reduction and immobilization or operative intervention
- Type III injuries: operative intervention
- Acetaminophen (Tylenol) or acetaminophen with codeine for pain control

PATIENT EDUCATION

Parents should be informed about the signs of ischemia and compartment syndrome (increasing pain, loss of finger motion, temperature, and color), because these may (rarely) occur in the first few days after reduction, owing to tight dressings or intimal injury to the vessels.

MONITORING

- Patients require radiographs and examinations at 1 to 2 weeks and about 6 weeks after fracture to ensure maintenance of the reduction during fracture healing.
- A small risk of malreduction exists.
- Patients should be seen after bone healing to document good alignment and range of motion.

COMPLICATIONS

- Nerve injuries (5% to 19%): The median nerve is the most common, followed by the radial nerve.
- It may take several months to regain normal function.
- Arterial injuries (5% to 12%): The brachial artery is the most common.
- Compartment syndrome (less than 1%): It may result in Volkmann's ischemic contracture.

- Varus deformity of the elbow: This is a cosmetic deformity, with no functional effect. It may be due to malunion.
- Elbow stiffness: This is uncommon if an anatomic reduction is obtained.

PROGNOSIS

- Prognosis is excellent if anatomic reduction is obtained.
- If malunion occurs, there may be a need for further surgery to correct the deformity.

RECOMMENDED READING

Hotchkiss RN, Green DP. Fractures and dislocations of the elbow. In: Rockwood CA, Green DP, Bucholz RW, eds. *Rockwood and Green's fractures in adults*, vol 1, 4th ed. Philadelphia: JB Lippincott, 1991:929–1024.

Otsuka NY, Kasser JR. Supracondylar fractures of the humerus in children. *J Am Acad Orthop Surg 1997, Jan;5:19–26.*

Wilkins KE. Fractures and dislocation of the elbow 1997, Jan. In: Rockwood CA, Wilkins KE, King RE, eds. *Fractures in children*, 3rd ed. Philadelphia: JB Lippincott, 1991:739–842.

Syndactyly

 Basics

DESCRIPTION

Webbed fingers (or toes) (Fig. 1)
Usually detected at birth
More common in white males

SYNONYM

• Webbed digits

GENETICS

• 10% cases familial
• 90% cases sporadic

INCIDENCE

This occurs in 1 of 2,000 births, with about half of the cases bilaterally symmetric.

CAUSES

Syndactyly is due to a failure of separation of the digits in the sixth to eighth weeks of intrauterine life. The specific cause is unknown. Although syndactyly may be associated in some cases without a positive family history or with a syndrome, in most cases it is an isolated finding.

RISK FACTORS

The presence of other congenital abnormalities constitutes a risk factor for this condition.

CLASSIFICATION

• Classification of internal involvement: simple (skin only) versus complex (bony involvement/ fusion)
• Classification of extent of syndactyly: complete (entire length of digits involved) versus incomplete (joined some part of fingers)

ASSOCIATED CONDITIONS

• Apert's syndrome: acrocephalosyndactyly
• Poland's syndrome: associated with chest wall anomalies and cardiac anomalies
• Congenital constriction band syndrome
• Fenestrated syndactyly (joined at the tips)
• Proteus syndrome
• Neurofibromatosis: slight increase in incidence

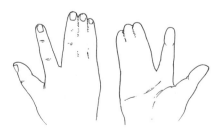

Fig. 1. Syndactyly or webbing of the fingers can be simple or complex.

ICD-9-CM

755.1 Syndactyly

 Diagnosis

SIGNS AND SYMPTOMS

No pain is associated with this condition.

PHYSICAL EXAMINATION

• Observe joined fingers, which can be associated with many anomalies.
• Examine the joints for active and passive range of motion.
• Test the two joined digits at each level to see whether they can move separately; if they can, this indicates no bony or complex syndactyly.
• The amount of excess skin between the digits is a sign of the difficulty of reconstruction.
• Inspect the nails; if they are joined, it is likely that the underlying bones are joined as well.

PATHOLOGIC FINDINGS

• Insufficient amount of skin present
• Abnormal fascial interconnections in excess
• Abnormal interconnection between flexor and extensor tendons
• Various anomalies of bones and joints

IMAGING PROCEDURES

• Plain radiography is indicated to differentiate simple from complex syndactyly.
• Angiography or magnetic resonance angiography may be needed in difficult cases of syndactyly to assess the structure of the underlying vascular supply of the two digits. If it branches distally instead of proximally, this may limit the extent of separation possible.

 Management

GENERAL MEASURES

Release of webbing can improve cosmesis and function, but webs less than a few millimeters distally, or those causing minimum inhibition to spread of the fingers, do not need surgical intervention. Complex syndactyly, especially, with only one branching neurovascular bundle can be difficult to correct surgically. The timing of surgery is controversial, but it is usually recommended after 6 to 12 months of age.

SURGICAL TREATMENT

• Many different techniques of release are available. The exact surgical procedure depends on the degree of syndactyly.
• A large dorsal flap with a wider proximal base than the distal end is a good technique for simple and incomplete syndactyly.
• Skin grafting is necessary depending on the amount of skin defect after release.
• Division of bones is needed in complex syndactyly.
• Postoperative dressing is an important part of treatment. The dressing is extended above the elbow, and a long arm plaster cast can be beneficial. The same dressing is continued until postoperative day 14 to 28.

PHYSICAL THERAPY

This is not needed unless for postoperative motion.

PATIENT EDUCATION

The patient or parents should be educated about the complexity of procedure, which they often underestimate. In particular, the need for obtaining soft tissue coverage and the difficulty of increasing range of motion of an abnormal joint should be explained.

MONITORING

Children should be monitored for partial recurrence of the web, or scar contracture, as they grow.

COMPLICATIONS

• Stiffness
• Scar contracture
• Circulatory deficit, resulting in loss of digit (rare), a complication that can be minimized by operating on only one side of the digit at a time, so a collateral vessel is preserved.

PROGNOSIS

The prognosis is good, although minor differences in width and appearance of the reconstructed digit are common.

RECOMMENDED READING

Dobyns J, Wood V, Bayne LG. Congenital hand anomalies. In: Green DP, ed. *Textbook of hand surgery*. New York: Churchill Livingstone, 1993:251–350.

Hoover GE, Flatt AE, Weiss MW. The hand in Apert's syndrome. *J Bone Joint Surg Am* 1970;52:878–895.

Basics

DESCRIPTION

Two common fractures of the talus, talar neck and body fractures, are presented here. Another common talus fracture, talar dome osteochondral fracture, is covered under ankle osteochondritis dissecans. Because of the tenuous blood supply to the talus, this bone can be categorized with other bones that are predisposed to posttraumatic avascular necrosis, including the femoral head and the scaphoid. The clinician must understand the presenting features of this injury because of the exceedingly high rate of avascular necrosis of the talus associated with these fractures.

Talus fractures are usually due to high-energy trauma, and talar neck fractures are commonly associated with medial malleolar fractures. There are no age- or gender-related associations.

INCIDENCE

This is second in frequency of all tarsal fractures.

CAUSES

The cause is high-energy trauma with forefoot hyperextension.

RISK FACTORS

Motor vehicle accidents are risk factors.

CLASSIFICATION

Hawkins' System

Type I. Nondisplaced vertical fracture of the talar neck
Type II. Displaced fracture of the talar neck with subluxation or dislocation of the subtalar joint; ankle joint is normal
Type III. Displaced fracture of the talar neck, associated with dislocation of the ankle and subtalar joints

Talar Body Fractures

Type I. Coronal or sagittal fractures
Type II. Horizontal fractures

ICD-9-CM

825.21 Talus fracture

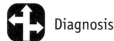 Diagnosis

SIGNS AND SYMPTOMS

- Extreme pain about the talus and hind foot, associated with high-energy trauma
- Ecchymosis
- Deformity

DIFFERENTIAL DIAGNOSIS

- Ankle fractures
- Ankle dislocation
- Talar dislocation
- Calcaneus fracture
- Navicular fracture

PHYSICAL EXAMINATION

Check the ankle and hind foot for the following:

- Focal tenderness
- Deformity
- Ankle and subtalar motion

PATHOLOGIC FINDINGS

Occasionally, fractures occur through cysts or bone tumors.

IMAGING PROCEDURES

- Anteroposterior and lateral radiographs of the ankle and foot are the baseline studies needed.
- An oblique view of the talar neck can be helpful.
- The foot is held in maximal equinus (plantar flexion) and 15 degrees of pronation for this view.
- Computed tomography is usually required to delineate fracture displacement.

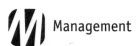 Management

GENERAL MEASURES

Ice, immobilization, and elevation are indicated.

SURGICAL TREATMENT

- Open or closed reduction
- Fluoroscopy, frequently used with fixation performed with Kirschner wires or cannulated screws
- Short leg, non–weight-bearing cast postoperatively

PHYSICAL THERAPY

Range of motion exercises are begun on removal of the cast.

MEDICAL TREATMENT

- Type I talar neck fractures may be treated with a below-knee cast for 12 weeks and non–weight bearing for 6 weeks.
- Type II fractures are an orthopaedic emergency and require immediate reduction either by closed or open (surgical) means. An adequate reduction is a fracture displacement of less than 5 mm and malalignment of less than 5 degrees.
- Type III fractures almost always require surgery to obtain an adequate reduction.
- Talar body fractures have a higher incidence of posttraumatic avascular necrosis.
- Displaced fractures that cannot be reduced and closed require open reduction and internal fixation.

PATIENT EDUCATION

Inform patients of a high incidence of talar osteonecrosis.

MONITORING

Radiographic follow-up is done to monitor talus beaking and Hawkins' sign (absence of subchondral lucency at the talar dome).

COMPLICATIONS

Avascular necrosis of the talus may occur.

PROGNOSIS

The integrity of the talar vascular supply can be confirmed with follow-up radiographs demonstrating Hawkins' sign. This is a subchondral lucency (talar dome subchondral bone osteopenia) that results from bone resorption after a talus fracture with an intact blood supply; therefore, the presence of Hawkins' sign excludes avascular necrosis of the talus.

RECOMMENDED READING

Mizel, M, Lutter LD. *Foot and ankle orthopaedic knowledge update.* Rosemont, IL: American Academy of Orthopaedic Surgeons, 1994.

Tarsal Tunnel Syndrome

 Basics

DESCRIPTION

Tarsal tunnel syndrome is the term used to describe entrapment neuropathy of the posterior tibial nerve (Fig. 1). The neuropathy may involve the nerve itself within the tarsal tunnel or one of its branches after leaving the canal. This condition is analogous to carpal tunnel syndrome, but it occurs much less frequently. Around the ankle, the deep fascia is strengthened posteriorly by the flexor retinaculum, which passes over the posterior tibial nerve, vessels, and tendons from the back of the ankle to the sole of the foot. The tunnel itself is fibroosseous, with the tibia anteriorly and the posterior process of the talus and calcaneus laterally. The posterior tibial nerve, a branch of the sciatic nerve, enters the tunnel proximally and within the tunnel divides into three terminal branches in 93% of cases: medial and lateral plantar and medial calcaneal nerves. The calcaneal branch shows the most variability with respect to whether it branches proximal to, within, or distal to the tarsal tunnel.
Patients are usually middle aged to elderly. Men and women are affected equally.

CAUSES

• A specific cause can be pinpointed in only some patients.
• In general, tarsal tunnel syndrome usually results from specific injury or a space-occupying lesion within the tarsal tunnel, as follows:

—Tendon sheath ganglion
—Lipoma within the tarsal tunnel
—Exostosis or fracture fragment impinging on the nerve
—Medial talocalcaneal bar protruding into the tunnel
—Enlarged venous complex surrounding the posterior tibial nerve within the tunnel
—Severe pronation of the hind foot with resultant stretching of the posterior tibial nerve
—Neurilemoma of the posterior tibial nerve within the canal

ICD-9-CM

355.5 Tarsal tunnel syndrome

 Diagnosis

SIGNS AND SYMPTOMS

• Characteristically, patients find it difficult to describe the pain.
• Complaints usually are burning, tingling, and numbness of toes and plantar aspect of the foot. Symptoms are often aggravated with activity and improve with rest, although some patients feel worse at rest and better while on their feet.
• Approximately 33% of patients have radiation of their pain proximally along the medial aspect of the leg to the level of the midcalf.

DIFFERENTIAL DIAGNOSIS

• Interdigital neuroma
• Intervertebral disc lesion
• Plantar fasciitis
• Peripheral neuritis or neuropathy
• Peripheral vascular disease
• Diabetic neuropathy
• Ganglion
• Fracture
• Valgus hind foot
• Rheumatoid arthritis
• Venous varicosities
• Tenosynovitis
• Tarsal coalition
• Lipoma

PHYSICAL EXAMINATION

• Physical examination and electrodiagnostic studies make up the mainstay of diagnosis. Some experts believe that the diagnosis can be made only with a strong history of tingling and burning, positive findings on examination, and a positive nerve conduction study.
• The nerve may be tender or may demonstrate Tinel's sign (tapping of the nerve with the index or middle finger) with percussion along its course.
• Fusiform or more diffuse swelling of the soft tissues may occasionally be palpated.

• Sensory and motor deficits often are difficult to assess and are not generally present.
• Look at the posture and range of motion of foot to rule out an old injury or arthrosis.
• Obtain nerve conduction studies of the medial and lateral plantar nerve.
• Sensory conduction velocity is believed to be the most accurate study (sensitivity as high as 90%). Obtain conduction velocities of the common peroneal nerve to rule out peripheral neuropathy.

LABORATORY TESTS

Routine laboratory tests can be used to rule out other conditions that may mimic tarsal tunnel syndrome.

PATHOLOGIC FINDINGS

One may find focal swelling or scarring of the nerve at surgical release.

IMAGING PROCEDURES

• Routine radiographs
• Magnetic resonance imaging if a space-occupying lesion is suspected

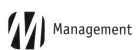 Management

GENERAL MEASURES

These are based on the cause of the condition.

SURGICAL TREATMENT

• This is indicated if conservative measures fail.
• Postoperative management consists of 3 weeks of immobilization and non–weight bearing on the affected lower extremity.
• Good results are generally seen when a well-localized, offending lesion is excised.
• Of patients without an identifiable cause of the disorder, 75% obtain significant relief from tarsal tunnel release; the remainder obtain little or no relief.
• Some reports have noted recurrence, but no report has shown successful results of reoperations on these patients.

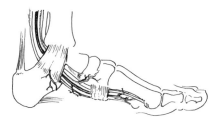

Fig. 1. Tarsal tunnel syndrome is compression of the tibial nerve behind the medial malleolus under the retinacular ligament.

PHYSICAL THERAPY

This may have a role in desensitization.

MEDICAL TREATMENT

- Treatment is based on the cause.
- Space-occupying lesions must be excised.
- Otherwise, nonsurgical treatment is indicated initially.
- Prescribe nonsteroidal antiinflammatory drugs or steroid injection if adjacent tenosynovitis is the cause.
- Treat postural abnormalities with orthotic devices to keep the foot in a neutral position (to prevent pronation). Treat edema with elevation and compression stockings.
- Normal activity can be performed as tolerated.

PATIENT EDUCATION

Patients are shown proper orthopaedic management.

MONITORING

Patients are followed closely to prevent postdecompression swelling.

COMPLICATIONS

Nerve scarring and reflex sympathetic dystrophy may occur in a few cases.

PROGNOSIS

The best results are obtained when specific focal lesions are found at decompression.

RECOMMENDED READING

Crenshaw AH, ed. *Campbell's operative orthopaedics,* 8th ed. St. Louis: CV Mosby, 1992:2777–2781.

Mann RA, Coughlin MJ, eds. *Surgery of the foot and ankle,* 6th ed. St. Louis: CV Mosby, 1993:514.

Tennis Elbow (Lateral Epicondylitis)

 Basics

DESCRIPTION

Lateral epicondylitis is a clinical syndrome that involves pain and tenderness with specific activities, including tennis; hence its common name "tennis elbow." Patients are generally in their fourth or fifth decade and present with pain over the lateral extensor muscles, lateral to the elbow. Males and females are affected equally. Complaints should not include paresthesias that radiate distally; nerve compression syndromes should be suspected when these symptoms are involved.

Tennis elbow commonly affects the origin of the extensor tendons of the forearm at the lateral epicondyle (most commonly, the tendon of the extensor carpi radialis brevis).

CAUSES

- Mechanical overload
- Senescent degeneration of the common extensor tendons
- Owing to overstressing muscles, breakdown and replacement of normal tendon collagen fibers with disorganized healing tissue

RISK FACTORS

- Sporting or work activities causing repetitive overload of the forearm extensors
- Common in carpenters, butchers, and politicians who must grasp hands frequently
- In tennis players, predisposing or contributing factors include small racquet grip, tight strings, or faulty mechanics, factors that should be recognized to help improve symptoms and prevent recurrence

ICD-9-CM

726.32 Tennis elbow

 Diagnosis

SIGNS AND SYMPTOMS

- Aching pain, sometimes described as burning, is felt in the region of the lateral epicondyle of the humerus with radiation into the forearm musculature.
- Symptoms are exacerbated with activity and improve with rest.
- On physical examination, the point of maximal tenderness is over the lateral epicondyle and can extend 1 to 2 cm distally.
- Pain is exacerbated with resisted wrist dorsiflexion and long finger extension, especially with the elbow in full extension.

DIFFERENTIAL DIAGNOSIS

- Radial tunnel compression syndrome (most commonly a compression of posterior interosseous nerve as it enters the supinator muscle). Electromyography may be required to demonstrate the radial tunnel syndrome.
- Lateral elbow instability
- Injury or fracture of radial head or capitellum
- Olecranon bursitis
- Muscular strain or sprain of ulnar collateral ligament
- Medial epicondylitis
- Osteochondritis dissecans

PHYSICAL EXAMINATION

- Note tenderness over the origin of the common wrist extensor tendons at the lateral epicondyle of the elbow.
- Tenderness may extend up to 2 cm distally.
- Reproduce pain with passive flexion of the fingers and wrist with the elbow extended.
- Check for radial tunnel syndrome, in which pain is reproduced with active middle finger extension against resistance (Fig. 1).

PATHOLOGIC FINDINGS

- Microscopic tears within the substance of the extensor carpi radialis brevis
- Replacement of normal tendon collagen fibers with tissue composed of fibroblasts and vascular granulation-like tissue, described as "angioblastic proliferation"

IMAGING PROCEDURES

Routine anteroposterior and lateral radiographs of the elbow are obtained to rule out fractures or other lesions in the elbow.

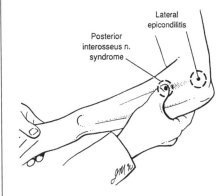

Fig. 1. Areas of palpation to differentiate lateral epicondylitis from posterior interosseous nerve syndrome. The tenderness in tennis elbow is over the bony prominence of the lateral epicondyle; that in the posterior interosseous nerve syndrome is two fingerbreadths distal to this.

 Management

SURGICAL TREATMENT

- Reserved for cases refractory to conservative treatment (less than 5% of cases)
- Consists of débridement and repair of degenerative section of tendon.

PHYSICAL THERAPY

Once symptoms have diminished, a stretching and strengthening program directed at forearm extensors may help to prevent recurrence.

MEDICAL TREATMENT

- Initially, conservative measures of rest, ice, massage over the affected area, and use of nonsteroidal antiinflammatory medications are recommended.
- A counterforce brace (tennis elbow band) may improve symptoms during activities of daily living. Occasionally, injections of cortisone are helpful; however, exercise care, because repetitive injections can increase the risk of extensor tendon rupture.
- Encourage patients to rest the affected extremity as much as possible.
- Patients should wear a tennis elbow band while performing activities of daily living.
- Patients can resume exercise on a graduated basis.

PATIENT EDUCATION

Lateral epicondylitis is typically a result of chronic overload of the wrist extensors. Activity modification is an important element of treatment.

PREVENTION

Use good form while playing tennis (i.e., wrist held stiff and motion at the elbow and shoulder).

MONITORING

Repeat radiographs in 3 months if the pain persists.

COMPLICATIONS

Complications are rare after nonoperative and surgical treatment.

PROGNOSIS

Patients who experience one episode of tennis elbow are at high risk of future episodes.

RECOMMENDED READING

Brashear HF, Raney RB. *Handbook of orthopaedic surgery*, 10th ed. St. Louis: CV Mosby, 1986:477–479.

Clark CR, Bonfiglio M. *Orthopaedics*. New York: Churchill Livingstone, 1994:246–247.

Basics

DESCRIPTION

Tenosynovitis is painful inflammation of a tendon along with the surrounding sheath. It affects any long, synovial-sheathed tendon, most commonly the fingers, wrist, or ankle.
The condition is rare in children and is most common in early to middle adulthood. Females are affected slightly more frequently than males.

SYNONYM

Tendinitis

INCIDENCE

• This is one of the most common musculoskeletal problems affecting the general population.
• Most people experience at least one episode of tenosynovitis.

CAUSES

• Excessive use or constriction of a tendon causes inflammation of the sheath (tenosynovium), which then becomes thickened.
• Activities associated with increased risk include the following:

—Furniture moving
—Mail sorting
—Keyboarding
—Rein flicking (in horseback riding)

• Draping heavy objects over the wrist (e.g., heavy grocery bag) can cause de Quervain's tenosynovitis (inflammation of the extensor tendons of the thumb).
• Women in the 30- to 50-year age group who are engaged in activity involving repetitive motion constitute the majority of noninfectious, nonrheumatologic cases.
• Pregnancy can precipitate tenosynovitis, especially de Quervain's.
• Rheumatoid arthritis and lupus flare-ups, with synovial inflammation, can manifest as tenosynovitis.

RISK FACTOR

Repetitive motion, especially increasing in level, is a risk factor.

CLASSIFICATION

By Duration

• Acute: few days' duration, usually resolves promptly with rest and nonsteroidal antiinflammatory drugs
• Chronic: duration of symptoms greater than 2 to 3 weeks; may have more changes in tendon and its sheath; more difficult to cure

By Location

• Achilles tenosynovitis
• Flexor tenosynovitis
• Biceps tenosynovitis
• De Quervain's tenosynovitis (of the thumb extensor and abductor tendons)

ASSOCIATED CONDITION

Rheumatoid arthritis

ICD-9-CM

727.0 Tenosynovitis

 Diagnosis

SIGNS AND SYMPTOMS

• Pain over the affected tendon, either acute or insidious
• Usually following a period of unusual or new activity
• Worse with continued use
• De Quervain's tenosynovitis: tender on the radial side of the wrist, worse with ulnar deviation
• Trigger finger possible in some long flexor tendons of the fingers, with a snapping or popping feeling during extension

DIFFERENTIAL DIAGNOSIS

Infection of tendon sheath

PHYSICAL EXAMINATION

• Tenderness in a longitudinal distribution, along the course of the involved tendon
• Tenderness mild, moderate or severe
• Possible associated swelling along the tendon sheath

LABORATORY TESTS

• No specific changes are noted.
• Laboratory studies may be useful to rule out infection.

PATHOLOGIC FINDINGS

Localized inflammation and thickening of the tendon sheath are revealed microscopically by the presence of acute inflammatory cells (polymorphonuclear leukocytes).

IMAGING PROCEDURES

Radiographs are needed only if there is a history of penetrating trauma and to assess the presence of arthritis in adjacent joints.

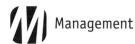 Management

GENERAL MEASURES

• Avoidance of offending activities
• Splinting (to put the tendon at complete rest or to restrict exercise)

SURGICAL TREATMENT

• For patients in whom conservative measures fail
• Release of the tendon sheath around the inflamed area
• Complete release of the abductor pollicis longus, followed by splinting in de Quervain's tenosynovitis

PHYSICAL THERAPY

Occupational therapists manage these problems in the upper extremity, making use of the following:

• Splints
• Strengthening and stretching exercises
• Job and activity modification

MEDICAL TREATMENT

• Have patients rest from the causative activity; this may require 1 to 3 weeks.
• Splinting may help.
• Prescribe nonsteroidal antiinflammatory drugs; sustained-release preparations are now available for patients with compliance problems.
• After symptoms subside, have patients gradually resume activity. Even if the condition is asymptomatic, causative factors in the work environment should be modified, if possible.

PATIENT EDUCATION

• Question patients thoroughly about causes.
• Teach ways to modify these behaviors.

PREVENTION

Avoid repetitive manual activity or a sudden increase in activity.

MONITORING

Patients are followed at 4- to 6-week intervals to check range of motion and healing of the tendon.

COMPLICATIONS

Tendinitis may fail to resolve, usually because of chronic changes in the tendon.

PROGNOSIS

• Most cases resolve with the foregoing measures.
• The posterior tibialis and Achilles tendons are especially prone to disease recurrence.

RECOMMENDED READING

Froimson AI. Tenosynovitis. In: Green DP, ed. *Operative hand surgery*. New York: Churchill Livingstone, 1993:1989–1992.

Platter P, Mann R. Disorders of tendons. In: Mann RA, Coughlin MJ, eds. *Surgery of the foot and ankle,* 6th ed. St. Louis: CV Mosby, 1993:805–836.

Thoracic Outlet Syndrome

 Basics

DESCRIPTION

Thoracic outlet syndrome (TOS) is a group of signs and symptoms that result from compression of the neurovascular supply to the upper limb in the supraclavicular area and shoulder girdle. It presents more commonly in young adults to middle-aged patients and is most typically seen in females, by a ratio of approximately 3.5:1.

SYNONYMS

- Scalene anticus syndrome
- Costoclavicular syndrome
- Hyperabduction syndrome
- Cervical rib syndrome
- Droopy shoulder syndrome

INCIDENCE

- Incidence unknown
- Condition not common

CAUSES

The cause of TOS is frequently multifactorial and may be influenced by trauma, repetitious job activities, anatomic predisposing factors, and some systemic diseases (e.g., diabetes, thyroid disease). TOS refers to compression of the subclavian vessels and brachial plexus at the superior aperture of the thorax.

A job that requires continuous overhead activity (e.g., painting ceilings) may cause signs and symptoms of brachial plexus compression over a short period, as compared with a job requiring one's upper extremities to be in less extreme elevation (e.g., keyboard operator, truck driver), which may contribute to symptoms over a period of years.

RISK FACTORS

- Cervical ribs
- Congenital fibrous bands
- Diabetes mellitus
- Thyroid disease
- Alcoholism
- Aggravating factors include the following:
- Obesity
- Extremely large breasts in women
- Emotional depression, causing patients to adopt a slumping posture

ASSOCIATED CONDITIONS

Complaints of carpal and cubital tunnel syndrome are noted. It is believed that a nerve that has some degree of compression on it in the neck is more susceptible to nerve compression problems at other points along its course, such as at the elbow or the wrist. Thus, patients with TOS are more susceptible to developing cubital and carpal tunnel syndromes, and vice versa. This has been termed the "double crush syndrome."

Patients with arthritis, diabetes mellitus, thyroid disease, and alcoholism have nerves with increased susceptibility to the development of superimposed nerve compression.

ICD-9-CM

353.0 Thoracic outlet syndrome

 Diagnosis

SIGNS AND SYMPTOMS

Neural Compression

- Patients may complain of pain in neck or shoulder, and numbness and tingling involving entire upper limb or forearm and hand. (Fig. 1).
- The ulnar side of the limb and the two ulnar digits are predominantly involved, although the middle finger may also be included.
- Nocturnal pain and paresthesias are common and must be differentiated from symptoms caused by carpal tunnel syndrome, which commonly affects the radial side of the hand.
- Frequently, patients experience difficulty in using the limb in an elevated, overhead position, such as when holding a hair dryer.
- Some patients demonstrate a decline in the strength or dexterity of the hand, even without obvious atrophy.
- Sensory findings are often subtle, are usually on the ulnar aspect of the hand, and may include the medial aspect of the forearm. Pain in the arm, shoulder, neck, and chest and headache may accompany any of these other complaints.

Vascular Compression

- Much less frequent
- Coldness
- Weakness
- Easy fatigability of the arm
- Diffuse pain
- Occasionally, Raynaud's phenomenon
- Venous compression may be intermittent or, less frequently, constant, resulting in swelling of the limb or varying degrees of cyanosis.

DIFFERENTIAL DIAGNOSIS

Lesions of the Cervical Spine

- Herniated intervertebral disc
- Degenerative disc disease
- Osteoarthritis of the spine and spinal cord tumors
- Lesions compressing the brachial plexus
- Tumors of the apex of the lung
- Trauma

Lesions Involving Peripheral Nerves

- Carpal tunnel syndrome (entrapment neuropathy of the median nerve)
- Ulnar nerve compression or dislocation at the elbow
- Compression of the radial or suprascapular nerves
- Neuropathies of alcoholism, heavy metal intoxication, avitaminosis, or diabetes mellitus

Arterial Lesions

- Peripheral or coronary atherosclerosis
- Aneurysm
- Occlusive changes
- Embolism
- Raynaud's disease
- Reflex sympathetic dystrophy
- Causalgia
- Vasculitis
- Differentiate venous complications of thrombophlebitis or mediastinal venous obstruction from intermittent compression or thrombosis of the vein in the thoracic outlet.

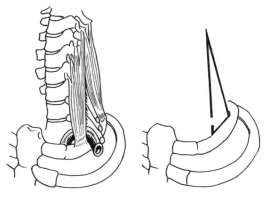

Fig. 1. In thoracic outlet syndrome, the brachial plexus or subclavian artery (L) may be compressed in the scalene triangle (R) or by an extra rib.

PHYSICAL EXAMINATION

- The diagnosis of TOS is a clinical one.
- Assess the neck and supraclavicular fossa on both sides.
- The ipsilateral scapula may be held lower and more anteriorly.
- The clavicle may appear more horizontal than normal.
- There may be tenderness over the brachial plexus.
- Positive Tinel's sign referred to the ulnar aspect of the hand may be present.
- Examine the shoulder girdle for glenohumeral instability, which may produce symptoms similar to those of TOS.
- Perform a complete, bilateral, upper extremity motor and sensory examination.
- Test the intrinsic muscle strength in the hand.
- Document the vasomotor status of the limb as well as the presence or absence of swelling.
- "Stress tests" or provocative maneuvers used in the clinical diagnosis of TOS:

—These must be carefully interpreted. (It is not significant, for example, to be able merely to obliterate the pulse by some position of the arm, because this is possible in many asymptomatic people. A test is not positive unless, without prompting, the patient complains of reproduction of the symptoms when the arm is placed in the provocative position.)
—Conduct Adson's maneuver with the patient's arm at the side, the neck hyperextended, and the head turned toward the affected side.
—Perform Wright's maneuver, with the patient's arm abducted and externally rotated. It has a higher sensitivity, and this may be increased by having the patient take a hold a deep breath. Perform this test with the elbow extended to limit the effects of possible ulnar neuropathy at the elbow (which would be exacerbated by elbow flexion).

PATHOLOGIC FINDINGS

Compression of the neurovascular supply to the upper limb in the region of the suprascapular area and shoulder girdle is noted.

IMAGING PROCEDURES

- Obtain plain anteroposterior and lateral radiographs of the cervical spine to evaluate for discogenic disease, adventitious ribs, or overly long transverse processes.
- Magnetic resonance imaging is useful if there is a strong suspicion of disc disease, but it does not help in the diagnosis of TOS.
- Evaluate the chest radiograph for apical lung tumors, which may be responsible for neurovascular compression, especially in patients with a history of smoking.
- Electrodiagnostic studies may be helpful in identifying associated carpal and cubital tunnel syndromes.

Management

GENERAL MEASURES

From 50% to 90% of patients with TOS can be successfully managed conservatively.

SURGICAL TREATMENT

Scalenectomy, first rib resection, or some combination is most applicable to patients with TOS and is associated with more successful outcomes.

PHYSICAL THERAPY

- The cornerstone of conservative therapy is a carefully regulated program of muscle strengthening and postural reeducation exercises.
- The trapezius, rhomboid, and levator scapulae muscles can be strengthened using elastic bands or free weights with the arms elevated less than 90 degrees and with avoidance of bracing of the scapulae to avoid provocative positions.
- Patients often do not experience symptomatic improvement before 2 months.
- Exercises must be continued until reversal of muscular atrophy and weakness and development of correct posture.
- The preoperative exercise routine can be resumed 1 month postoperatively in surgical patients. Most patients with recurrences can be rehabilitated with a physical therapy program of postural reeducation and muscle strengthening.

MEDICAL TREATMENT

- Conservative therapy is based on a stringent program of exercises to strengthen the muscles of the pectoral girdle.
- The aim is to augment the tone of the suspensory muscles of the acromioclavicular joint so the costoclavicular space can remain wide.
- Patients must continue with the exercises until the muscular atrophy and weakness have been reversed and patients have developed an awareness of correct posture.
- If a carefully supervised exercise and postural program fails, and the patient has intractable pain, surgery may be indicated. Surgery should be presented as an option only for those patients who believe that they cannot continue with the condition as it is and who understand the potential risks and benefits of the proposed procedure.
- Explanation of the pathologic process of TOS helps to alleviate the patient's concerns and makes the patient more receptive when instructed to avoid certain activities and postures. Specific contributory factors should be identified and addressed when possible, such as repetitive elevated positioning of the arms at work.

PATIENT EDUCATION

- Explain the pathogenesis of TOS to patients, because an understanding of the mechanism helps the patient to recognize the need for modifying activities and postures that would narrow the thoracic outlet such as overhead movements, hyperabduction of the arm, use of shoulder straps, and carrying heavy handbags.
- Attempts to alter the ergonomic characteristics of the job should be made, or a new job should be considered.

PREVENTION

- No known fully effective means of prevention is known.
- Diminish the risk by avoiding frequent overhead lifting or hyperabduction of the arm and by weight control.
- Women with extremely large breasts can wear long-line bras.

MONITORING

- Follow the patient's physical therapy progress.
- Postoperative disease recurrence is possible, secondary to scapular muscle weakness and an inability to support the shoulder girdle or secondary to inadequate release of the site of compression.

COMPLICATIONS

- Pneumothorax
- Infection
- Vascular injury
- Injury to brachial plexus
- Shoulder girdle instability

PROGNOSIS

- From 50% to 90% of patients with TOS can be successfully managed conservatively.
- With proper selection of patients for surgery, the majority (75%) should be significantly improved.

RECOMMENDED READING

Leffert RD. Thoracic outlet syndrome. *J Am Acad Orthop Surg* 1994;2:317–325.

Pang D, Wessel HB. Thoracic outlet syndrome. *Neurosurgery* 1988;22:105–121.

Urschel HC Jr, Razzuk MA. Current concepts: management of thoracic-outlet syndrome. *N Engl J Med* 1972;286:1140–1143.

Thumb Arthritis

 Basics

DESCRIPTION

Degenerative joint disease commonly presents in the hand and is associated with pain, swelling, loss of motion, and, later, deformity. Frequently, the thumb is the earliest site of involvement, with the first carpometacarpal joint affected first, especially in osteoarthritis. The carpometacarpal joint is considered the most important single joint of the hand. Thumb arthritis may be unilateral or bilateral, occurring in the nondominant hand as commonly as in the dominant one. It generally affects more women than men.

INCIDENCE

The incidence is highest in the population older than 55 years of age.

CLASSIFICATION

Various forms of arthritis affect the thumb, including the following:

- Osteoarthritis
- Rheumatoid arthritis
- Gout

ICD-9-CM

716.95 Arthritic hand

 Diagnosis

SIGNS AND SYMPTOMS

- Joint pain
- Warmth
- Swelling
- Stiffness
- Crepitus
- Triggering (catching of tendon, with snapping and locking), often localized to the base of the thumb (the carpometacarpal joint) or the metacarpophalangeal joint, most noticeable during activities such as pinching and grabbing

DIFFERENTIAL DIAGNOSIS

- Ligamentous injuries
- Tendon injuries (e.g., de Quervain's disease)
- Scaphoid fractures

PHYSICAL EXAMINATION

- Perform a careful and thorough examination of the hand and thumb, with attention to range of motion of the joints (carpometacarpal, metacarpophalangeal, interphalangeal) and associated swelling, erythema, and soft tissue masses.
- Test for "snuffbox" tenderness and tendinitis (Finkelstein's test).

LABORATORY TESTS

No serum laboratory tests are needed.

PATHOLOGIC FINDINGS

- Rheumatoid arthritis: This is characterized by hypertrophic synovitis that eventually destroys joint cartilage compresses or disrupts tendons, compresses adjacent nerves, and eventually dislocates and erodes the joint itself.
- Osteoarthritis: Loss of articular cartilage is associated with spur formation and loss of motion but not associated with tendon ruptures or triggering as frequently as in rheumatoid arthritis.

IMAGING PROCEDURES

Plain films reveal a loss of joint space, sclerosis, spur formation, and subchondral cysts.

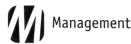 Management

GENERAL MEASURES

- Supportive measures include rest, heat, analgesics, and nonsteroidal antiinflammatory drugs.
- Intraarticular corticosteroid injections may be helpful during flare-ups.

SURGICAL TREATMENT

- Metacarpophalangeal joint: Early surgical treatment may involve synovectomy of the joint and tendon advancement or tendon transfer. If the joint is grossly unstable, or the articular surface is destroyed, arthrodesis (fusion) may be indicated.
- Carpometacarpal joint: This may be treated with arthroplasty, consisting of resection of portions of the bones and inserting a Silastic prosthesis or nonautogenous tendon. Arthrodesis may still be performed later if the prosthesis fails.

PHYSICAL THERAPY AND OCCUPATIONAL THERAPY

This is often helpful after surgery to regain motion, to reduce swelling, and to regain function.

MEDICAL TREATMENT

- Activity limitation or modification
- Nonsteroidal antiinflammatory drugs
- Intraarticular steroid injection
- Rheumatologic or orthopaedic consultation for those with symptoms refractory to attempted trials at conservative management

MONITORING

Patients must be followed at 4- to 12-week intervals for assessment of function and for detecting postoperative wound complications.

COMPLICATIONS

Surgery may be complicated by damaging the radial sensory nerve, or by wound infection, prosthesis failure, chronically subluxating, or an unstable joint.

PROGNOSIS

The prognosis is fairly good. Arthrodesis is the most reliable pain relief procedure, but it results in permanent limited motion. Interpositional tendon arthroplasty is the most common and overall most effective procedure.

RECOMMENDED READING

Green DP, ed. Operative hand surgery, vol 2, 3rd ed. New York: Churchill Livingstone, 1993:1680–1683.

Jupiter J. Flynn's hand surgery, 4th ed. Baltimore: Williams & Wilkins, 1991:407–417.

Milford L. The hand, 3rd ed. St. Louis: CV Mosby, 1988:1–24.

Basics

DESCRIPTION

Thumb extensor/de Quervain's tendinitis is stenosing tenosynovitis of the first dorsal compartment of the wrist, containing the abductor pollicis longus and the extensor pollicis brevis. Patients present with pain and discomfort on the radial aspect of the wrist.

It often occurs in middle-aged women, although men and women of all ages can be affected.

INCIDENCE

This condition is common.

CAUSES

• Repetitive motions of thumb or wrist
• Associated with racquet sports, fly fishing, and golf (often affecting the nondominant hand in golfers); can be associated with rheumatoid arthritis

ASSOCIATED CONDITION

Rheumatoid arthritis

ICD-9-CM

727.04 de Quervain tendinitis

Diagnosis

SIGNS AND SYMPTOMS

• Pain and tenderness on the radial aspect of wrist, often isolated to directly over the first dorsal compartment
• Pain and discomfort exacerbated by extension or abduction of the thumb or radial-ulnar deviation of the wrist
• Repetitive activities particularly painful

DIFFERENTIAL DIAGNOSIS

• Degenerative joint disease of the first (thumb) carpometacarpal joint
• Intersection syndrome (much rarer)

PHYSICAL EXAMINATION

• Note pain, tenderness, swelling, bogginess, and crepitus over the first dorsal compartment of the wrist. This is the radial aspect of the radial styloid.
• Positive Finkelstein's test helps confirm the diagnosis.
• Note exacerbation of the symptoms (pain) with the thumb clenched in the palm and ulnar deviation of the wrist.
• Examine the first carpometacarpal joint, grind test, and range of motion to rule out degenerative joint disease; these entities can coexist. Intersection syndrome is rarer and is often associated with more severe symptoms. On physical examination, the pain localizes 4 cm proximal to the wrist, rather than over the radial styloid as in de Quervain's syndrome.

LABORATORY TESTS

No serum laboratory tests are needed.

PATHOLOGIC FINDINGS

The dorsum of the wrist is anatomically divided into six separate extensor tendon compartments. The first compartment contains the abductor pollicis longus and extensor pollicis brevis, which can become inflamed and irritated as they enter and pass through the rigid fibroosseous tunnel of the first compartment. Intersection syndrome is thought to be an inflammatory condition that exists at the point where the first dorsal compartment and the third dorsal compartment (the extensor carpi radialis longus and brevis) cross. This is approximately 4 cm proximal to the wrist.

IMAGING PROCEDURES

Anteroposterior and lateral views of the wrist and first carpometacarpal views are helpful in ruling out other disorders and in differentiating between degenerative joint disease of the first carpometacarpal and de Quervain's syndrome.

Management

GENERAL MEASURES

With most types of tendinitis, rest and avoidance of aggravating conditions are the mainstays of treatment.

SURGICAL TREATMENT

• A radial incision is made over first dorsal compartment with release of the fibrosseous tunnel and all its septa, as well as the release of the fascial sheaths of each tendon and the compartment.
• Multiple anatomic variations are present.

PHYSICAL THERAPY

Splinting is often helpful to the tendon at rest.

MEDICAL TREATMENT

• The first line of therapy is nonoperative care. This includes the following:

—Immobilization of thumb and wrist, usually in a thumb spica splint
—Steroid injection into the first dorsal compartment
—Success rates in the literature ranging from 55% to 100%

• Recalcitrant or recurrent symptoms often require surgical release of the first dorsal compartment.
• Decrease activity until symptoms resolve.
• Nonsteroidal antiinflammatory drugs and analgesics are given.

PATIENT EDUCATION

Patients are counseled to avoid repetitive activities that worsen their pain. Attention to workplace ergonomics is also important.

MONITORING

Patients are followed at 3-month intervals until their symptoms resolve.

COMPLICATIONS

The most serious complication of surgical intervention is transection of the dorsal sensory radial nerve, which lies in proximity to the first dorsal compartment. This can leave the patient with a small area of anesthesia, or more seriously, with a painful neuroma, which often requires surgical resection.

PROGNOSIS

The prognosis is good.

RECOMMENDED READING

Froimson AI. Tenosynovitis. In: Green DP, ed. *Operative hand surgery*. New York: Churchill Livingstone, 1993:1989–1992.

Thumb Ligament Injuries

 Basics

DESCRIPTION

Thumb ligament injuries most commonly involve an incomplete or complete rupture of the ulnar collateral ligament resulting from a forced radial deviation (abduction). Injuries to the radial collateral ligament can also occur, but they are less common.
These injuries occur in men and women of all ages.

SYNONYMS

- Gamekeeper's thumb
- Skier's thumb

INCIDENCE

These injuries are most common in skiers and ball-handling athletes.

CAUSES

Forced radial deviation (abduction) of the thumb is the cause.

RISK FACTORS

- Skiing accidents involving ski poles or falls
- Athletic activities involving ball handling, such as baseball, football, or basketball

CLASSIFICATION

These injuries are complete or incomplete, based on the integrity of the ligament and its bony insertion.

ASSOCIATED CONDITIONS

- Avulsion fracture of the tendon insertion
- Capsular injuries or Stener's lesions (complete rupture of the ulnar collateral ligament with the adductor aponeurosis interposed between the distally avulsed ligament and its insertion into the base of the proximal phalanx), which are important to recognize and are not always readily apparent

ICD-9-CM

842.10 Thumb ligament sprain

 Diagnosis

SIGNS AND SYMPTOMS

- Pain
- Swelling
- Weakness
- Deformity localized to the ulnar base of the thumb
- Loss of pinch function

DIFFERENTIAL DIAGNOSIS

- First metacarpal or proximal phalanx fractures
- First carpometacarpal joint arthritis

PHYSICAL EXAMINATION

- Ulnar swelling, weakness, or a local palpable mass from a rolled avulsed ligament or bone fragment may be present.
- The examiner can often radially deviate the patient's thumb passively to a marked angle, as compared with the opposite, uninjured thumb.
- Often one needs a digital block to complete a full examination, because of pain and swelling in the acute setting.
- Surgical repair is often necessary with opening of the joint.

PATHOLOGIC FINDINGS

Attenuation or rupture of the ulnar collateral ligament of the thumb is noted.

IMAGING PROCEDURES

Plain films, with stress testing of bilateral thumbs, are often helpful.

 Management

GENERAL MEASURES

- For acute injury: rest, elevation, ice, immobilization in a thumb spica splint, analgesics, and orthopaedic follow-up
- For chronic injury: thumb spica brace, activity modification, or orthopaedic surgery consultation for elective ligament repair

SURGICAL TREATMENT

- This may be performed by suture repair in the acute setting.
- For old injuries, tendon or fascial grafts may be necessary.
- When there is crepitus or pain on a grinding type of manipulation of the joint, arthrodesis (development of arthritis) (fusion) may provide the best result.

PHYSICAL THERAPY

This may be helpful postoperatively to increase range of motion and to assist in resuming various activities.

MEDICAL TREATMENT

- Commonly, proper rest is all that is needed for restoration of function, although pain and swelling may persist for several weeks. A thumb spica splint or cast immobilization may be indicated for a short period, or up to 6 weeks if there is an associated avulsion fracture.
- If the ligament rupture is complete and acute, primary repair should be performed.
- When the diagnosis is delayed for 1 month or longer, fibrosis makes identification and repair of the ligament more difficult.

PATIENT EDUCATION

Patients should limit activities with immobilization to allow for natural, or postsurgical, healing, followed by removable splinting as needed while activities are slowly resumed.

PREVENTION

Prevention involves knowing the mechanism associated with this injury.

MONITORING

Monitoring is done by the orthopaedic surgeon, to assess proper restoration of function and stability. Patients are followed at 4- to 8-week intervals until healing is complete with a full range of motion.

COMPLICATIONS

- Chronic instability
- Nonunion of avulsed fragment
- Degenerative joint disease

PROGNOSIS

Generally, the prognosis is good.

RECOMMENDED READING

Green DP, ed. Operative hand surgery, vol 1, 3rd ed. New York: Churchill Livingstone, 1993:162–163.

Jupiter J. Flynn's hand surgery, 4th ed. Baltimore: Williams & Wilkins, 1991:149–152.

Tibial Plafond Fracture

 Basics

DESCRIPTION

Pilon fractures are a special subset of ankle fractures. They are intraarticular fractures of the distal tibia involving varying degrees of articular and metaphyseal injury (Fig. 1). The word "pilon" comes from the French root meaning "pestle" or "rammer," conveying that the talus actually drives into the tibial articular surface. The distal tibia is also known as the plafond (roof) over the talus, and thus these fractures are also called "plafond fractures." These are often devastating injuries.
The injury itself refers to the trauma of the distal lower extremity, is often associated with marked soft tissue injury, and can be associated with significant neurovascular compromise.
These are high-energy injuries and can be associated with other lower extremity, spinal, pelvic, abdominal, thoracic, or cranial injuries. Tibial plafond fractures are often, although not exclusively, associated with the population at risk for high-level trauma, that is, young males. Practitioners should be even more vigilant of vascular or tissue compromise in elderly or debilitated patients.

SYNONYM

Pilon fracture

INCIDENCE

These are rare injuries, comprising only 1% of all lower extremity fractures and 5% to 10% of all tibial injuries. Anecdotally, the incidence has been increasing with the advent of the automobile air bag.

CAUSES

High-Energy Injuries

• Motor vehicle accident
• Fall from height
• High-energy axial loading: the common denominator

Lower-Energy Injuries

• Skiing injuries

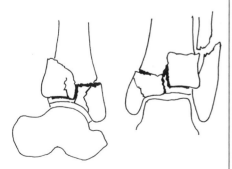

Fig. 1. Tibial plafond fracture.

RISK FACTORS

• Individuals at risk for high-level trauma (e.g., young males, alcohol abuse, drug use)
• Employees who work at heights

CLASSIFICATION

There are multiple classification systems. As with any fracture, it must be determined whether the fracture is open or closed. At this point, identify the specific fracture at hand. The most commonly used classification system is the one proposed Ruedi and Allgower:

• Type I fracture is a nondisplaced or insignificantly (minimally) displaced intraarticular fracture (of the distal tibia).
• Type II is an intraarticular fracture that is displaced.
• Type III is a displaced fracture with marked comminution.

This classification system has marked clinical and prognostic implications. Type I fractures have good prognosis and can be treated with splint or cast immobilization. Type II and III fractures require surgical intervention and are associated with a more guarded prognosis.

ASSOCIATED CONDITIONS

Patients are at high risk of associated pelvic, spinal, abdominal, thoracic, or cranial injuries.

ICD-9-CM

823.8 Tibial plafond fracture

 Diagnosis

SIGNS AND SYMPTOMS

• Severe pain
• Swelling
• Inability to bear weight
• The swelling can encompass the entire foot and much of the distal third of the tibia can be isolated to severe ankle swelling.

DIFFERENTIAL DIAGNOSIS

• Ankle fracture
• Talus fracture
• Calcaneus fracture
• Midfoot fracture
• Forefoot fracture
• Tibial shaft fracture

PHYSICAL EXAMINATION

• Perform a complete assessment of the ABCs (airway, breathing, circulation), head, neck, chest, abdomen, spine, and pelvis, as well as complete an examination of both lower extremities.
• Note marked swelling about the ankle, which can involve the entire foot and much of the distal tibia or can be isolated to severe ankle swelling.
• Pay special attention to the neurovascular and soft tissue status.

LABORATORY TESTS

Order appropriate tests for the level of injury.

• Hematocrit
• Type and crossmatch
• Urine and stool check for blood, as indicated.
• All preoperative laboratory tests necessary for age group, level of injury, and institution

IMAGING PROCEDURES

• Plain radiographs are obtained: anteroposterior, lateral, and mortise views of the ankle; anteroposterior and lateral views of the foot; tibia-fibula films.
• The classification system discussed earlier is based on appearance on the ankle views. If there is no displacement (type I), no other views are necessary. If there is displacement or comminution, a computed tomography scan or conventional tomogram can be helpful for surgical planning.
• Some surgeons find that radiographs of the opposite extremity assist in reconstruction in severe cases.

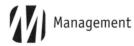 Management

GENERAL MEASURES

Always evaluate the neurovascular and soft tissue status. The soft tissue is often the limiting factor, as well as the major cause for complications. Ice, immobilization, and elevation, initiated as early as possible, regardless of whether the patient is going to surgery or not, are important and beneficial to soft tissue survival. There is a bimodal distribution for the ideal time for surgical intervention, either within the first 12 hours from the time of injury, before soft tissue swelling has occurred, or after 10 to 12 days of ice, immobilization and elevation, when the reactive swelling has subsided.

Tibial Plafond Fracture

SURGICAL TREATMENT

Open Reduction and Internal Fixation

Basic principles of open reduction and internal fixation were laid out in a logical manner in 1969 by Ruedi and Allgower in their classic work.

- Repair the fibula, which is often not comminuted and brings the extremity to length.
- Reconstruct the distal tibia with lag screws.
- Bone graft the tibial metaphyseal defect.
- Plate the medial aspect of the tibia.

External Fixation

The principles of using an external fixator are actually similar:

- Fibula out to length (with or without a plate)
- Tibia articular surface aligned by ligamentous taxis (limited percutaneous fixation if necessary)
- Optional limited exposure for metaphyseal graft

General Considerations

- Better reduction often leads to superior results.
- A skin bridge of at least 7 cm between all incisions has been found to lower the complication rate.

MEDICAL TREATMENT

- Type I: This responds well to closed therapy including a well-padded splint, ice, elevation, and non-weight bearing. The splint can be converted to a cast when swelling begins to subside.

- Type II and III: These injuries require surgical intervention and are associated with poor results and multiple complications. There is currently a debate on whether to perform open reduction with internal fixation or external fixation with or without limited internal fixation. In various clinical series, the reported frequencies of osteomyelitis, amputation, osteoarthrosis, and nonunion are as high as 20%, 6%, 54%, and 18%, respectively.
- The current trend is toward external fixation with limited internal fixation because of its equivalent clinical results and lower complication rate.
- With severe injuries, there is a role for primary arthrodesis, although this is rare, and again, the orthopaedic community appears to be moving away from this management approach.
- Delay weight bearing until the fracture has united, no matter what mode of therapy is used. This is often 3 to 4 months, but it can be shorter in type I fractures, treated nonsurgically.
- Some surgeons progress to light toe-touch before this point.
- Some surgeons also begin motion (nonweight bearing) as early as tolerated in patients who have undergone open reduction and internal fixation.
- Current studies are evaluating hinged external fixators.
- Patients require pain medication in the acute setting and intravenous antibiotics for 24 to 48 hours after surgical intervention.

PATIENT EDUCATION

Patients are counseled on the high risk of posttraumatic arthritis.

MONITORING

Plain radiographs are obtained once a month until union is achieved.

COMPLICATIONS

- Serious injury with conservative estimates of 20% to 50% complication rate, including a 6% chance of amputation
- High likelihood of early ankle degenerative joint disease
- Possible need for revision operations or ankle arthrodesis
- Compartment syndrome
- Soft tissue coverage issues
- Wound dehiscence
- Superficial wound infection
- Pin infection with external fixation
- Deep wound infection
- Osteomyelitis (can necessitate late below the knee amputation)
- Posttraumatic arthrosis

RECOMMENDED READING

Brumback RJ, Mcgarvey WC. Fractures of the tibial plafond: the pilon fracture. Evolving treatment concepts. *Orthop Clin North Am* 1995;26:273–285.

Greind RV, Michelson JD, Bone LB. Fractures of the ankle and the distal part of the tibia. *J Bone Joint Surg Am* 1996;78:1772–1783.

Ruedi TP, Allgower M. Fractures of the lower end of the tibia into the ankle joint. *Injury* 1969;1:92–99.

Wyrsch B, McFerran MA, McAndrew M et al. Operative treatment of fractures of the tibial plafond. *J Bone Joint Surg Am* 1996;78:1646–1657.

Basics

DESCRIPTION

The tibial plateau is the proximal weight-bearing surface of the tibia. It articulates with the femoral condyles to form the knee joint. The tibial plateau can be divided into medial and lateral components. A tibial plateau fracture is any fracture involving the articular surface of the tibia (Fig. 1).

INCIDENCE

• Tibial plateau fractures comprise 1% of all fractures and 8% of fractures in elderly persons.
• Isolated medial plateau fractures comprise about 10% to 23% of these injuries.
• Isolated lateral plateau fractures comprise about 55% to 70% of these injuries.
• Combined medial and lateral plateau fractures comprise about 11% to 31% of these injuries.

AGE

• Bimodal age distribution: peak incidence in men in the fourth decade and peak incidence in women in the seventh decade
• Mechanism of distribution: high-velocity trauma and an osteoporotic population with lesser mechanisms of injury, respectively

CAUSES

• Isolated varus, valgus, or axial forces, or a combination of these forces
• Depending on the study, most of these fractures are the result of motor vehicle accidents, pedestrian versus motor vehicle accidents, and (slightly less) accidental falls from a height
• Less frequently, caused by a fall, twist, or bicycle accident
• Sports injuries representing an estimated 5% to 10% of these injuries

RISK FACTORS

• Those at risk for high-impact trauma (e.g., young age, male gender, alcohol and drug abuse, urban environment)
• The elderly with poor bone quality are at risk for falls

CLASSIFICATION

Schatzker's classification

Type I.   Lateral split fracture
Type II. Lateral split/depression fracture
Type III. Central depression fracture
Type IV. Medial plateau fracture (with or without intercondylar spine involvement)
Type V.   Combined medial and lateral plateau fracture
Type VI. Fracture of the metaphysis separating the articular portion of the fracture from the tibial shaft

• Type I to III: all are lateral plateau fractures. Many clinicians believe that type IV fractures can represent a fracture dislocation, and this injury has the highest concurrence of vascular or neurologic injury.
• These fractures are often the result of high-impact trauma, so associated abdominal, thoracic, pelvic, spinal, skeletal, or cranial injury may be present.
• Neurovascular injury and compartment syndrome may occur.
• Associated injuries to the menisci, the cruciate ligaments, and the lateral collateral ligaments of the knee are possible.

ICD-9-CM

832.00 Tibial plateau fracture

Diagnosis

SIGNS AND SYMPTOMS

• Pain, swelling, and often deformity
• Inability to bear any or full weight
• Inability to move the knee partially or fully

DIFFERENTIAL DIAGNOSIS

• Any other injury about the knee, the distal femur, or the proximal tibia
• Femur fracture
• Supracondylar fracture
• Femoral condylar fracture
• Tibia metaphyseal injury
• High tibial shaft injury
• Soft tissue injuries, such as of the anterior cruciate ligament, posterior cruciate ligament, lateral collateral ligament, medial collateral ligament, meniscus, or any combination

PHYSICAL EXAMINATION

• Because injury is associated with high-impact trauma, the patient usually requires a complete trauma evaluation and always requires a complete physical examination.
• Special care must be taken to evaluate the skin and subcutaneous tissue (open versus closed, tissue quality) and the neurologic and vascular status of the extremity.
• These injuries may be associated with neurovascular compromise (most common in the Schatzker type IV, but can occur with any fracture pattern).
• Perform a careful neurologic examination for nerve injury (most often peroneal and most common with Schatzker type IV) and compartment syndrome (rare, but most common with bicondylar fractures of types V and VI) because both occur with this injury.
• Varus and valgus stability can be gently assessed.

IMAGING PROCEDURES

Radiography

High-quality anteroposterior and lateral radiographs are used to identify the fracture lines and to estimate displacement.

Computed Tomography

• This important adjunctive study to plain radiographs influences decision making.
• Perform scout views to ensure the images obtained are tangent to the articular surface, and cuts of 5 mm or less are recommended.
• Preoperative scans are common practice.

Magnetic Resonance Imaging

MRI is not typically used for displaced tibial plateau fractures. It is useful in identifying intra-articular injury and for the diagnosis of nondisplaced fractures acutely.

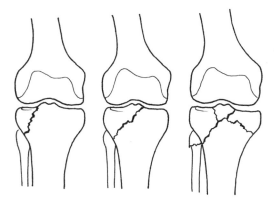

Fig. 1.   Tibial plateau fracture may involve one or both sides of the joint.

Tibial Plateau Fracture

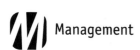 Management

GENERAL MEASURES

Initial Care

Ice, elevation, and immobilization should be initiated as early as possible (even during evaluation of patient). A large, bulky dressing with plaster and splints is used before closed or open treatment to prevent excessive swelling.

Surgical Considerations

If the patient is treated surgically, a postoperative, large, bulky dressing with well-constructed splints, ice, elevation, analgesia, and frequent nursing and clinical assessments for compartment syndrome are indicated.

Closed Treatment

• This is reserved for nondisplaced fractures, knees already affected by severe arthritis, severely compromised soft tissue envelope (i.e., necrotic, already infected), or a severely compromised patient.
• The leg should be placed in a well-padded, well-constructed long leg cast that is completely bivalved.
• Cast immobilization is indicated for 4 to 6 weeks.

Skeletal Traction

• This is used in patients who require surgery but cannot tolerate it.
• Place the leg in balanced suspension.
• Initiate passive range of motion as soon as it can be tolerated (usually 2 to 3 weeks).
• At 4 to 6 weeks, a cast or brace is applied.

Activity

Regardless of treatment, patients should not weight bear until the fracture is healed, usually in 12 weeks.

SURGICAL TREATMENT

Indications

• Open fracture
• Intraarticular step-off of more than 3 to 5 mm or tilt of a condyle (of more than 5 degrees) of the lateral plateau and any step-off or tilt of the medial side as relative indicators (per other studies and advancing understanding of biomechanics and physiology)
• Varus or valgus instability of the knee
• Varus or valgus angulation of the extended knee
• Ligamentous injury
• Floating knee (fracture of the tibia and femur, the knee floats in between)

Timing of Surgery

• Open fractures: emergency
• Closed fractures: dependent on soft tissue envelope. Immediate fixation to up to 2 weeks.

Open Procedure

• Minimally displaced fractures: percutaneous pinning with limited open procedures either arthroscopically or fluoroscopically assisted; may require the creation of a small metaphyseal cortical window to elevate joint depressions and place bone graft (autologous cancellous has been found to be superior)
• Single condyle fractures: some treatable open; require only a screw with a washer, but usually a buttress plate; most surgeons using a long midline incision
• Complex fractures: requiring multiple screws and plates, bone grafting, and other techniques to elevate depressed portions and to stabilize the plateau

Closed Treatment

• Cast brace treatment with early mobilization and delayed weight bearing
• Immobilization possible for 4 to 6 weeks without decreased final range of motion
• Progression to a hinged brace with progressively increasing range of motion
• Weight bearing delayed until evidence of good healing, often as long as 12 weeks
• Patients with severe soft tissue injuries treated with small wire external fixators

Open Treatment

• Cast brace immobilization for 10 to 14 days if fixation is adequate and early range of motion
• Weight bearing delayed usually until fracture is clinically healed
• In knees treated with open reduction and internal fixation, a regimen of more than 2 weeks of immobilization postoperatively associated with decreased range of motion and poorer clinical results
• With adequate stabilization surgically treated knees should start early range of motion.

PHYSICAL THERAPY

Range of motion and quadriceps strengthening exercises are performed until full range of motion is achieved.

MEDICAL TREATMENT

Analgesics are given.

PATIENT EDUCATION

• Patients may develop early arthritis depending on the severity of the initial cartilage injury.
• Compliance with motion and weight-bearing status is essential for a good outcome.

COMPLICATIONS

• Skin compromise
• Infections
• Compartment syndrome
• Loss of fixation
• Malunion
• Nonunion
• Wound and infection complications low with limited procedure
• Large bicondylar repairs associated with higher levels of complications

PROGNOSIS

• These fractures can be devastating injuries. The incidence of post-traumatic arthritis is often related to the amount and location of initial displacement and ultimate reduction of the fracture.
• With careful selection for appropriate therapy, the results can be remarkably good.
• In studies evaluating the use of closed reduction (criteria variable), many patients did well.
• Likewise, in studies of patients with surgical intervention for displaced fractures, as many as 65% to 85% had satisfactory results.
• Cast immobilization for 4 to 6 weeks has not been found to effect posttreatment range of motion adversely. (In contrast, in those knees treated with open reduction and internal fixation, it has been found that a regimen of more than 2 weeks of immobilization postoperatively is associated with decreased range of motion and poorer clinical results. Thus, with adequate stabilization, surgically treated knees should start early range of motion).

RECOMMENDED READING

Hohl M. Fractures of the proximal tibia and fibula. In: Rockwood CA, Green DP, Bucholz RW, et al., eds. *Rockwood and Green's fractures in adults*, 3rd ed. Philadelphia: JB Lippincott, 1991:1725–1761.

Kasser JR, ed. *Orthopedic knowledge update 5*. Rosemont, IL: American Academy of Orthopaedic Surgeons, 1996.

Reid JS. Fractures of the tibial plateau. In: Levine AM, ed. *Orthopaedic knowledge update: trauma*. Rosemont, IL: American Academy of Orthopaedic Surgeons, 1996:159–170.

Schatzker J. Tibial plateau fractures. In: Browner BD, Jupiter JB, Levine AM, et al., eds. *Skeletal trauma*. Philadelphia: WB Saunders, 1992:1745–1769.

Basics

DESCRIPTION

This is a fracture of the tibial shaft.

INCIDENCE

- Most common diaphyseal fracture
- Incidence estimated at 2 per 1,000 yearly
- Can occur in any age group

CAUSES

- Low-energy falls
- Twisting mechanisms
- High-energy crush injuries
- Impaction injuries

RISK FACTORS

- High-impact sports
- Motor vehicle accident

CLASSIFICATION

The Ellis grading system incorporates the soft tissue involvement and helps to define management and prognosis after tibial shaft fracture.

ASSOCIATED CONDITIONS

- Fibular fracture
- Knee ligament injuries
- Femur fractures
- Neurovascular injury
- Compartment syndrome

ICD-9-CM

823-80 Closed for tibia
823-82 Closed for tibia
823-90 Open for tibia

 Diagnosis

SIGNS AND SYMPTOMS

- Instability of the leg at the fracture site
- Swelling
- Ecchymosis
- Pain
- Tenderness

DIFFERENTIAL DIAGNOSIS

- Compartment syndrome
- Fibular fracture

PHYSICAL EXAMINATION

- Evaluate the knee and ankle.
- Perform a skeletal screening examination.
- Scrutinize the wound closely for signs of skin penetration.
- If concerned about compartment syndrome, obtain pressure measurements.

IMAGING PROCEDURES

Anteroposterior and lateral radiographs of the tibia, which include the ankle joint distally and the knee joint proximally, are obtained.

 Management

GENERAL MEASURES

Closed Fractures

Fractures that are less than 50% displaced, are less than 1 cm shortened, and have less than 10% of angulation in any plane may be treated in a long leg cast.

Fractures with Greater Displacement, Angulation, or Comminution

These are treated with reduction and fixation using an intramedullary nail, plate, and screws or an external fixator, depending on the nature of the fracture.

Open Fractures

- These are treated with urgent, and often repetitive, irrigation and débridement.
- Definitive treatment of open fractures involves either external fixation or open reduction with an intramedullary nail, depending on the severity of the fracture, and again is based on the nature of the fracture.

Compartment Syndrome and Neurovascular Injury

- Tibial shaft fractures are often associated with these conditions.
- Closely monitor compartment tension.
- Evaluate the neurovascular status of the limb, immediately on presentation and frequently thereafter.

Activity

Tibial shaft fractures often require 2 to 6 months of non-weight bearing or protected weight bearing on the affected extremity.

SURGICAL TREATMENT

Internal Fixation

This involves either placement of an intramedullary nail starting at the knee and extending to the ankle or placement of a plate and screws.

External Fixation

This involves placement of pins in the proximal and distal portions of the fracture and reduction of the fracture and maintenance of the reduction with the external frame.

PHYSICAL THERAPY

Gait training for non-weight bearing is indicated.

MEDICAL TREATMENT

Analgesics are given.

PATIENT EDUCATION

Patients should be informed that these fractures are occasionally difficult to treat and have a prolonged healing time.

MONITORING

Closely monitor the patient's neurovascular status and look for compartment swelling.

COMPLICATIONS

- Compartment syndrome
- Neurovascular injury
- Malunion, delayed union, or nonunion
- Osteomyelitis

PROGNOSIS

- Low-energy injuries with displacement of less than 50% have a good prognosis.
- The incidence of complications increases and the prognosis worsens with high-energy, comminuted fractures.
- Open fractures have the worst prognosis and the highest incidence of complications.

RECOMMENDED READING

Browner BD, Jupiter JB, Levine AM, et al., eds. *Skeletal trauma.* Philadelphia: WB Saunders, 1992:1771–1869.

Clark CR, Bonfiglio M. *Orthopaedics.* New York: Churchill Livingstone, 1994:194–195.

Tibial Spine Fracture

Basics

DESCRIPTION

This is a fracture of the tibial spine or intercondylar eminence of the proximal tibia (Figs. 1 and 2). These injuries can represent fractures of the anterior tibial spine (part of the insertion of the anterior cruciate ligament [ACL]), the posterior tibial spine, or the entire eminence. In children, these fractures are believed to represent ACL equivalent injuries that have traveled through the incompletely ossified tibial spine.
The following are affected:

• Predominantly isolated knee injury
• Associated ligamentous (collateral ligament) or meniscal injuries about the knee are also common

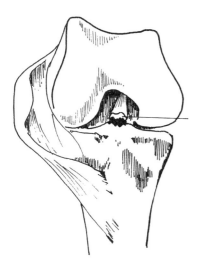

Fig. 1. Tibial spine fracture.

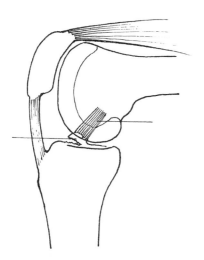

Fig. 2. Tibial spine fracture is best seen on the lateral radiograph and may involve only a small fragment of bone, but it signals ligament injury.

• Roughly 15% of tibial plateau fractures having associated tibial spine or intercondylar eminence fractures

INCIDENCE

• Relatively rare
• In children, reported to be about 3 per 100,000 per year

CAUSES

• Fall from a bicycle (most commonly reported mechanism)
• Twisting or severe stressing of the knee joint (varus or valgus, anterior and posterior, hyperflexion or extension)
• Athletic injury
• Motor vehicle accident

CLASSIFICATION

The Meyers and Mckeever classification is based on the degree of fracture displacement:

Type I. Minimally displaced
Type II. Displacement of the anterior portion of the fragment with a posterior hinge intact
Type IIIA. Complete separation of the fragment but the fragment stays in its native orientation
Type IIIB. Fragment completely avulsed and rotated

ICD-9-CM

823.05 Avulsion for tibial spine

Diagnosis

SIGNS AND SYMPTOMS

• Pain, swelling, and effusion associated with hemarthrosis
• Reluctance to bear weight
• Patient possibly lacking full extension secondary to bony block

DIFFERENTIAL DIAGNOSIS

• Isolated ligamentous injuries
• Coincidental ligamentous injuries (ACL, posterior cruciate ligament, medial collateral ligament, lateral collateral ligament)
• Patella fracture
• Patella tendon rupture
• Tibial tubercle fracture
• Tibial plateau fracture
• Isolated or coincidental meniscal injury

PHYSICAL EXAMINATION

• Note swelling and effusion.
• Rule out block of full extension.
• Gently assess for knee stability (anterior, posterior, varus or valgus).
• Acute hemarthrosis is present, and anterior laxity may be present (often difficult to detect in the acute setting because of guarding).

PATHOLOGIC FINDINGS

• Most often, one sees an avulsion at the insertion of the ACL.
• The ACL fans out and also inserts on the anterior horn of the medial meniscus, which can be pulled into the fracture site and can block reduction.

IMAGING PROCEDURES

• Plain radiographs: Anteroposterior and lateral views of the knee are usually adequate; findings on the lateral radiograph are the foundation of the classification system and help to guide appropriate therapy.
• A tunnel view or a radiograph parallel to the slant of the tibia can be helpful sometimes.

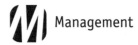

Management

GENERAL MEASURES

Many of these injuries can be treated nonsurgically. Surgery is required if the fragment cannot be reduced or if there is a block to full extension.

Initial Measures

- Ice, elevation and immobilization should be initiated, even during evaluation.
- If the hemarthrosis is causing severe pain, aspirate under sterile conditions.

Type I and II Fractures (and Some Type IIIA Fractures)

- Most can be treated with closed reduction and a long leg cylinder cast.
- Many references cite the need for general anesthesia, but intravenous conscious sedation is adequate for these patients.
- Most commonly, placing the leg in full extension or hyperextension reduces the fragment.
- Positioning for immobilization: Hyperextension has fallen out of favor; anything from full extension to 10 degrees of flexion is appropriate.
- The length of immobilization is 4 to 6 weeks after either closed or open treatment.

Type III Fractures

- Most authors believe that these fractures must be surgically fixed.

- Others believe that only fractures that will not reduce or are blocking full extension require surgical intervention.

SURGICAL TREATMENT

- This can be done with an open procedure or arthroscopically.
- Sometimes it requires the removal of interfracture soft tissue to obtain reduction.
- Fixation can be with a screw or heavy suture. (In children, screws should not cross the physis unless the child is nearing skeletal maturity.)

MONITORING

If the fracture is treated nonoperatively, it should be followed closely to rule out displacement.

COMPLICATIONS

Sometimes, loose bodies become clinical significant after acute treatment.

PROGNOSIS

- Most children have objective evidence of ACL laxity at long-term follow-up, regardless of the treatment method.

- Open reduction does not affect the loss of extension or the anterior laxity.
- Patients are often aware of a difference between the left knee and the right, and some note instability or "giving way."

RECOMMENDED READING

Kasser JR, ed. *Orthopaedic knowledge update 5.* Rosemont, IL: American Academy of Orthopaedic Surgeons, 1996:447.

Richards BS, ed. *Orthopaedic knowledge update: pediatrics.* Rosemont, IL: American Academy of Orthopaedic Surgeons, 1996:262.

Rockwood CA, Green DP, Bucholz RW, et al., eds. *Rockwood and Green's fractures in adults,* vol 2, 3rd ed. Philadelphia: JB Lippincott, 1991:1752–1755.

Willis RB, Blokker C, Stoll TM, et al. Long-term follow-up of anterior tibial eminence fractures. *J Pediatr Orthop* 1993;13:361–364.

Tibial Torsion

Basics

DESCRIPTION

Tibial torsion is a condition in which the tibia, along with the ankle and foot, is rotated either internally or externally (i.e., inward or outward) on its axis (Fig. 1). This rotation is seen in the course of normal development, but on occasion it may represent a developmental abnormality. Abnormal values are usually described as more than two standard deviations from the mean for a given age.

SYNONYMS

- In-toeing (medial torsion or "pigeon toeing")
- Out-toeing (lateral torsion)

GENETICS

- Internal tibial torsion is a combination of genetic factors and intrauterine position.
- A family history is important, because the subdivision into hereditary and nonhereditary forms is of practical significance in the prognosis and treatment.

INCIDENCE

- Abnormal internal or external tibial torsion as an isolated deformity is common.
- It is usually seen in infants and children less than 3 years of age, after walking behavior has developed.
- In general, younger children display more internal than external rotation.
- No particular predilection for males or females has been noted.

CAUSES

This is caused by a combination of genetic factors and intrauterine position. Intrauterine positioning may also be a factor in the hereditary form of tibial torsion.

CLASSIFICATION

- Internal tibial torsion
- External tibial torsion
- Neuromuscular torsion: may be associated with cerebral palsy or spina bifida

ASSOCIATED CONDITIONS

In infants, abnormal medial tibial torsion is often associated with congenital metatarsus varus or developmental genu varum.

ICD-9-CM

736.89 Internal tibial torsion

Diagnosis

SIGNS AND SYMPTOMS

- Because the child seen for rotational concerns is commonly the first born, the parents have not had the opportunity to witness the natural rotational and angular changes that occur as a child grows. A parent who was treated for the same condition with an orthosis may believe that the child will require the same treatment.
- The primary concern is often the appearance of the child's legs while walking or running.
- Tripping and falling may be noticed by the parent.
- Pain is rare. Parents may describe the child as having a limp, but there is no painful component to the gait.

DIFFERENTIAL DIAGNOSIS

- Blount's disease (pathologic genus varum with internal tibial torsion)
- Abnormal femoral anteversion
- Metatarsus adductus
- Cerebral palsy
- Hip dysplasia

PHYSICAL EXAMINATION

Assess the child from the hips to the toes. If the child is ambulatory, visually evaluate the child's gait; this usually demonstrates the problem that concerns the parents.

Look for a Heel-Toe Gait and a Limp

The absence of a heel-toe gait may be the initial sign of an underlying neurologic disorder (e.g., cerebral palsy). A limp may explain the rotational position of the extremity, because the child may be positioning the limb in a more comfortable position to avoid pain while walking.
Unilateral developmental dysplasia of the hip may present as in-toeing associated with a limp.

Foot-Progression Angle

Observe the angular difference between the long axis of the foot and the line of progression the child is moving along. The normal foot-progression angle is slightly externally rotated. In-toeing or out-toeing of more than 5 degrees outside the normal range for a given age is abnormal.

Examine the Patient When He or She is Lying Down

First check the child's hips for stability in the supine position before specific assessment for rotational malalignment. Then place the child prone to evaluate hip rotation and tibial torsion. The pelvis must remain level and stationary during the examination for proper measurement.
Clinical estimates of femoral anteversion and tibial torsion are noted. Femoral anteversion is estimated by the angle between the vertical axis and the long axis of the leg at the position in which the greater trochanter is the most prominent on internal and external rotation. Tibial torsion can be assessed by comparing the bimalleolar axis with the position of the tibial tubercle.

Note the Foot Shape

Metatarsus adductus may be the primary cause of in-toeing, particularly in the infant.

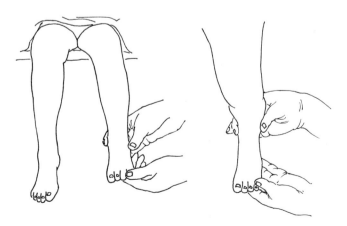

Fig. 1. Internal tibial torsion is characterized by inward rotation of the foot with respect to the knee.

IMAGING PROCEDURES

• Physical examination usually provides the information needed to form a treatment plan, although radiographs are indicated in some instances.

• If there is asymmetric limitation of hip abduction or if hip abduction in the toddler is less than 60 degrees, an anteroposterior radiograph of the pelvis is needed to rule out hip dysplasia.

• Radiographs of the feet may help to confirm clinically suspected metatarsus adductus.

• Radiographs of the tibia are not helpful in assessing tibial torsion.

• Computed tomography is the most widespread imaging technique for evaluating femoral rotation. Ultrasonography can be used to measure the amount of femoral or tibial rotation, and measurements closely approximate those of computed tomography scans. Both tests, however, are often unnecessary, because these conditions can usually be evaluated clinically.

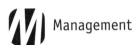 Management

GENERAL MEASURES

• Internal tibial torsion is the most common cause of in-toeing in children less than 3 years of age.

• With increasing age and growth, tibial torsion tends toward a normal tibial position, with the lateral malleolus 20 to 30 degrees posterior to the medial malleolus.

• Virtually all children born with internal tibial torsion have tibial torsion within the normal range by 3 years of age.

• Most nonsurgical treatment consists of a careful explanation to the parents of the course of in-toeing or out-toeing in the examined child, because most rotational concerns normalize with time and growth.

• The use of night splints (i.e., Dennis Browne bars), braces, heel or sole wedges, and orthotics has not been proven to influence derotation of the tibia. Most orthopaedic surgeons do not use these devices.

• In children born with excessive external tibial torsion, particularly if it is asymmetric, spontaneous correction is limited, and rotational osteotomy may be needed later.

• For children with excessive or asymmetric tibial torsion after 5 years of age, derotational tibial osteotomy may be considered if the parents are concerned about the gait.

• Often, the persistence or worsening of in-toeing past 3 or 4 years of age is due to the emergence of abnormal femoral anteversion.

• Children born with "normal" external tibial torsion do not usually undergo further external rotation during the first few years of life, and the final tibial torsion stays within the normal range.

Activity

No particular modification is needed.

SURGICAL TREATMENT

Derotation osteotomy is the only surgical treatment to consider for children with rotational abnormalities; however, surgery should only be considered after an adequate number of years has passed. One must be certain that the expected natural derotation will not sufficiently correct the rotational abnormality. In general, tibial rotational osteotomy is seldom needed in children younger than 5 years of age. In children with cerebral palsy, surgery may be appropriate at an earlier age, particularly if soft tissue surgery is also planned to aid in walking development.

Tibial derotation osteotomy is indicated if the thigh-foot angle remains internally rotated 20 degrees or more or if the external tibial rotation is 35 degrees or more. This is an elective decision, best left up to the family.

Rotational osteotomy is most commonly performed just above the distal tibial growth cartilage and is held with a cast with or without internal fixation. Healing takes 6 to 8 weeks.

PHYSICAL THERAPY

This is not usually indicated or beneficial.

PATIENT EDUCATION

Education of the parents is of paramount importance in managing family concerns. Most patients with tibial torsion improve to a satisfactory degree naturally.

MONITORING

Annual or biannual observation and examination are useful to document the expected rotational changes with growth, particularly if the parents need periodic reassurance.

COMPLICATIONS

• If the young child frequently trips because of tibial torsion, this will usually improve with time as he or she gains coordination.

• Potential surgical complications include growth plate injuries, neurovascular injuries, nonunion, and hardware problems.

PROGNOSIS

• This condition is usually self-limiting and part of natural development.

• If the tibiae of the parents and the adolescent siblings have normal alignment, the probability of spontaneous correction by the age of 7 to 8 years is great.

• If there is a familial incidence of persistent abnormal internal tibial torsion, the prognosis for spontaneous correction is slightly lower.

RECOMMENDED READING

Morrissy RT, Weinstein SL, eds. *Lovell and Winter's pediatric orthopaedics*, vol 2, 4th ed. Philadelphia: Lippincott–Raven, 1996:1047–1053.

Tachdjian MO. *Pediatric orthopaedics*, vol 2, 2nd ed. Philadelphia: WB Saunders, 1990:2810–2817.

Toe Fracture

 Basics

DESCRIPTION

- Fracture through the phalanx of the toes
- Simple or comminuted
- Most common forefoot fracture

CAUSES

This is caused by blunt trauma to the foot or toes.

RISK FACTORS

Walking barefoot is a risk factor.

ICD-9-CM

826.0 Fracture of the phalanx

 Diagnosis

SIGNS AND SYMPTOMS

- Pain
- Acute swelling
- Difficulty in wearing shoes
- Difficulty in ambulating
- Bruising

DIFFERENTIAL DIAGNOSIS

- Contusion
- Joint dislocation

PHYSICAL EXAMINATION

- Erythema
- Swelling
- Tenderness to palpation
- Crepitus
- Subungal hematoma, which may be present if the distal phalanx is involved

IMAGING PROCEDURES

Anteroposterior, lateral, and oblique radiographs of the toe (not foot) identify the fracture and help to dictate the necessary treatment.

Management

GENERAL MEASURES

- Most nondisplaced fractures, even in the presence of comminution, may be treated by buddy-taping the affected toe to the adjacent toes to enhance stability.
- A stiff-soled shoe can be used to assist in ambulation.
- Any patient with a displaced fracture should have the fracture splinted and should be referred to an orthopaedic surgeon for further treatment.

Activity

Buddy-taping and weight bearing with a stiff-soled shoe are recommended as tolerated for 4 to 6 weeks.

SURGICAL TREATMENT

Comminuted fractures, highly angulated fractures, and intraarticular fractures may require open reduction and pin or screw fixation, especially fractures of the first toe.

PHYSICAL THERAPY

This is typically not necessary.

MEDICAL TREATMENT

- Nonsteroidal antiinflammatory drugs
- Analgesics

PATIENT EDUCATION

Pain may persist for weeks after the fracture has healed.

MONITORING

Serial radiographs are obtained.

PREVENTION

Steel-toed shoes should be used in construction-type jobs.

COMPLICATIONS

- Malunion and nonunion of phalangeal fractures of the toes are rare.
- Patients with persistent pain in a malunion or nonunion may ultimately require surgical intervention.

PROGNOSIS

The prognosis is good.

RECOMMENDED READING

Delee J. Fractures and dislocations of the foot. In: Mann RA, Coughlin MJ, eds. *Surgery of the foot and ankle,* 6th ed. St. Louis: CV Mosby, 1993:1465–1471.

Basics

DESCRIPTION

Idiopathic toe walking in toddlers is common. It is most commonly caused by a shortened Achilles tendon. Some of these children eventually adopt normal walking patterns with growth. Persistent and exclusive toe walking beyond 3 years of age should prompt an examination for underlying neuromuscular problems. However, most children have what is termed, by exclusion, idiopathic toe walking.

GENETICS

Up to 50% of patients have a positive family history.

INCIDENCE

- Common
- Usually noted when a child first begins to walk (under 3 years of age)
- Both sexes equally affected

CAUSES

- Habit or patterning
- Shortened Achilles tendon

RISK FACTORS

- Positive family history
- History of premature birth
- Low Apgar score

ICD-9-CM

727.81 Toe walking

Diagnosis

Idiopathic toe walking is diagnosed on the basis of the history and physical examination. It is a diagnosis of exclusion. Neuromuscular abnormality must first be excluded.

DIFFERENTIAL DIAGNOSIS

- Arthrogryposis
- Cerebral palsy
- Muscular dystrophy
- Tethered cord syndrome
- Charcot-Marie-Tooth disease

PHYSICAL EXAMINATION

- Examination should be made with the child in shorts.
- The position of the feet during all phases of walking and standing should be noted.
- Attention should be focused on the neurologic examination to detect a subtle abnormality.
- The range of ankle dorsiflexion should be noted, with the knee both flexed and extended.
- The calf should be palpated for any abnormal masses.
- The hamstrings and adductors should be checked for tightness.
- Passive and active range of motion of the ankles should be documented.

PATHOLOGIC FINDINGS

The child may have a contracted Achilles tendon.

SPECIAL TESTS

- The combination of gait analysis and electromyographic (EMG) studies is sometimes useful in differentiating idiopathic toe walkers from patients with cerebral palsy.
- Computerized gait analysis may differentiate a child with mild cerebral palsy from an idiopathic toe walker.
- Although series comparing the results of EMG studies in idiopathic toe walkers and in toe walking in patients with cerebral palsy have been variable, an out of phase gastrocnemius complex on EMG analysis strongly suggests a neurologic abnormality in a toe walker.

Management

GENERAL MEASURES

Casting

- Increased ankle dorsiflexion can be achieved by stretching and serial casting, placing the foot in maximum dorsiflexion (i.e., at least 10 degrees of ankle dorsiflexion, while allowing the normal heel-toe gait to develop).
- The cast should be changed weekly until the desired ankle range of motion is obtained.

Activity

- Initially, patients should be seen weekly for cast changes.
- Night braces with the ankle in maximal dorsiflexion may be helpful to maintain the dorsiflexion achieved with casting or surgery.

SURGICAL TREATMENT

Z-lengthening of the Achilles tendon can improve ankle dorsiflexion. Surgery, however, should be delayed for several years in a child with idiopathic toe walking to allow maturation of gait and to avoid overlengthening.

PHYSICAL THERAPY

Passive and active range-of-motion exercise of the ankles may be used to treat mild cases.

PATIENT EDUCATION

- Patients and their families may be instructed to perform home heel-cord stretching exercise.
- Some idiopathic toe walkers can assume a heel-toe gait with persistent persuasion.

COMPLICATIONS

- Undiagnosed neurologic abnormality
- Overlengthening of the heel cord
- Recurrence

PROGNOSIS

- Most idiopathic toe walkers develop the normal gait by the age of 3 years.
- Persistent toe strike gait beyond this age requires careful neurologic evaluation.

RECOMMENDED READING

Kalen V, Adler N, Bleck E. Electromyography of idiopathic toe walking. *Pediatr Orthop* 1986;6:31.

Torticollis

Basics

DESCRIPTION

Torticollis is a limitation of motion of the cervical spine that causes the head to be held in a tilted position. It may result from muscular, skeletal, or neurologic abnormalities (Fig. 1).

SYNONYMS

- Skeletal wry neck
- Congenital wry neck
- Cock-robin deformity
- Sandifer's syndrome (torticollis resulting from reflex)

GENETICS

- Multiple congenital causes of torticollis exist, of which a few have a genetic predisposition.
- Skeletal dysplasias are the most common genetic syndromes associated with torticollis.

INCIDENCE

- It is rare.
- Because of the multiple causes, it is difficult to give a specific figure for incidence. It affects an estimated 1 in 1,000 patients.
- The most common cause is rotatory subluxation of the atlantoaxial joint, an acquired condition.
- Congenital muscular torticollis is usually evident in the first 6 to 8 weeks of life.
- Other causes may appear throughout childhood or may become evident well into adulthood.
- Males and females are affected equally.

CAUSES

- Congenital muscular torticollis: caused by contracture of the sternocleidomastoid muscle
- Congenital bony torticollis: may be due to occipitocervical abnormalities

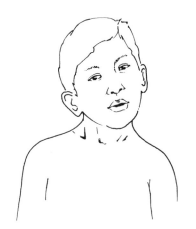

Fig. 1. Torticollis typically produces lateral flexion to one side and rotation to the other.

- Acquired torticollis: may result from neurogenic, traumatic, inflammatory, or idiopathic causes (see Differential Diagnosis)
- Bony abnormalities: atlantooccipital synostosis, basilar impression, odontoid abnormalities, cervical hemivertebrae, or asymmetry of occipital condyles
- Atlantoaxial rotatory subluxation, the most common bony abnormality, characterized by rotatory displacement of C-1 on C-2; may be congenital or secondary to inflammation or trauma

RISK FACTORS

- Local trauma to the infant's neck during delivery, especially during a difficult delivery, is a risk factor.
- Upper respiratory infection, pharyngitis, or trauma are risk factors for atlantoaxial rotatory subluxation.

CLASSIFICATION

- Congenital abnormalities
- Acquired abnormalities

ICD-9-CM

754.1 Congenital
847.0 Traumatic

Diagnosis

SIGNS AND SYMPTOMS

- The hallmark sign is tilting of the head to one side with limitation of range of motion.
- Usually the patient rotates the head away from the neutral (straight) position, but not toward it.
- The chin rotates toward the opposite side that the ear is leaning.
- Patients may present with a neck mass (contracted sternocleidomastoid muscle).
- Neck pain is a common complaint, usually in adults.
- Older patients may also complain of occipital pain, vertigo, or dizziness aggravated by certain movements of the head.
- If torticollis persists beyond infancy, secondary asymmetry of the cranium (plagiocephaly) may remain.

DIFFERENTIAL DIAGNOSIS

Neurogenic Causes

- Spinal cord tumors of the cervical spine
- Cerebellar tumors
- Syringomyelia
- Ocular dysfunction

Traumatic Causes

- Subluxations
- Fractures and dislocations of the occipitocervical junction

Inflammatory Causes

- Cervical adenitis
- Rheumatoid arthritis

Idiopathic Causes

- Atlantoaxial rotatory subluxation or displacement

PHYSICAL EXAMINATION

- The patient's head is tilted with the ear toward the involved side and the chin rotated away, with limitation of range of motion toward the corrected position.
- In some cases of muscular torticollis, there may be a palpable mass on the involved side (contracted sternocleidomastoid muscle).
- Remodeling of the head or face may result from pressure while sleeping.
- A short, broad neck with a low hairline may be seen in patients with bony abnormalities or Klippel-Feil syndrome.

LABORATORY TESTS

There are no specific laboratory tests unless an inflammatory or neoplastic origin is being considered. Ophthalmologic, audiologic, and gastroenterologic evaluations are sometimes needed if no obvious skeletal causes are seen.

PATHOLOGIC FINDINGS

In congenital muscular torticollis, the sternocleidomastoid muscle is fibrotic, replaced by scar tissue in a nonspecific fashion.

IMAGING PROCEDURES

- Anteroposterior and lateral radiographs of the cervical spine should be obtained in any case of torticollis to identify bony abnormalities.
- Computed tomography is used to evaluate rotatory subluxation, dislocation, or fracture.
- Magnetic resonance imaging is used if a neurologic lesion of the brainstem or neck is suspected

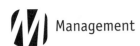 Management

GENERAL MEASURES

Congenital Muscular Torticollis

• This responds to stretching exercises in 90% of patients treated before 1 year of age.
• Positioning of the crib and toys will encourage the child to stretch the involved side.

Atlantoaxial Rotatory Subluxation

• Patients usually recover with physical therapy if the condition is detected within the first week.
• If treatment is delayed, traction or even surgery is required.
• Use of a soft collar and analgesics is appropriate for these cases.
• Patients with recalcitrant cases may require muscle relaxants and a hard collar or brace.

Activity

• Contact sports and vigorous athletics should be restricted until the condition has been treated.
• Specifics depend on the underlying cause.

SURGICAL TREATMENT

• Severe atlantoaxial rotatory subluxation or other severe bony abnormality may require fusion of C-1 and C-2.

• Congenital muscular torticollis that is refractory to stretching may require release of the sternocleidomastoid muscle.

PHYSICAL THERAPY

• Stretching exercises may be beneficial in cases of muscular torticollis or recent-onset rotatory subluxation.
• Specific instructions should be given to the therapist.

MEDICAL TREATMENT

Analgesics (acetaminophen, ibuprofen) are given.

PATIENT EDUCATION

• Once the cause is known, anatomic models may be used to explain the cause of the torticollis to patients and families.
• Patients and families should be made aware of the usual course and the possible need for different methods of therapy.

MONITORING

• Neurologic status should be closely followed.
• Bony abnormalities, such as rotatory subluxation, may require repeated computed tomography scans.

PREVENTION

The condition cannot be prevented, but prompt referral and treatment may preclude the need for surgery.

COMPLICATIONS

• Fixed subluxation
• Plagiocephaly (in late-treated muscular torticollis)

PROGNOSIS

Most cases resolve spontaneously or with treatment.

RECOMMENDED READING

Canale ST, Griffin DW, Hubbard CN. Congenital muscular torticollis: a long-term follow-up. *J Bone Joint Surg Am* 1982;64:810–816.

Phillips WA, Hensinger RN. Management of rotatory atlantoaxial subluxation in children. *J Bone Joint Surg Am* 1989;71:664–670.

Ramenofsky M, Buyse M, Goldberg M, et al. Gastroesophageal reflux and torticollis. *J Bone Joint Surg Am* 1978;60:1140–1141.

Triangular Fibrocartilage Tear

 Basics

DESCRIPTION

The triangular fibrocartilage complex (TFCC) is a complex of ligaments and cartilaginous structures that stabilize the distal radioulnar joint during pronation and supination of the forearm. Injury to the TFCC may result in acute or chronic wrist pain, often on the ulnar side. The TFCC is triangular and extends from the ulnar styloid to the sigmoid notch of the distal radius. The central portion is more cartilaginous and acts as a meniscal homologue, similar to the menisci of the knee joint. A few wrists contain a true meniscus with a free edge that can be seen arthroscopically.

SYNONYMS

- Ulnar impingement syndrome
- Ulnar-sided wrist pain

INCIDENCE

- Uncommon
- Peak incidence: 30 to 60 years of age

CAUSES

- Hyperpronation or dorsiflexion of the wrist may result in a tear of the TFCC, equivalent to a distal dislocation of the ulna (Fig. 1).
- It may be associated with distal radius or ulna fracture (or fractures of both bones).

RISK FACTORS

- Jobs that require repeated, loaded pronation and supination of the wrist
- Jobs that require heavy lifting

ICD-9-CM

842.00 Wrist pain

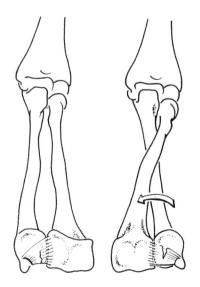

Fig. 1. Triangular fibrocartilage tear may occur with forearm rotation.

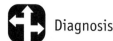 Diagnosis

SIGNS AND SYMPTOMS

- Most common complaint: ulnar-sided wrist pain, especially with repeated pronation and supination
- History of hyperpronation or dorsiflexion injury to the wrist (acute cases)
- History of repeated pronation and supination (chronic cases)

DIFFERENTIAL DIAGNOSIS

- Fracture of the radius, ulna, or any of the carpal bones
- Rupture or tendinitis of the extensor carpi ulnaris, flexor carpi ulnaris, or the carpal ligaments
- Arthritis of the radiocarpal, ulnocarpal, or radiocarpal joints
- Carpal instability, possibly the result of scaphoid or lunate lesions and deformity

PHYSICAL EXAMINATION

- Localize the area of pain carefully (e.g., use tip of the index finger to isolate the area of tenderness more precisely).
- Examine each joint of the wrist and hand for range of motion and to detect crepitation, pain, or snaps.
- Palpate the extensor carpi ulnaris while flexing and extending the wrist to rule out subluxation.
- Assess the neurovascular status of the hand and forearm.

SPECIAL TESTS

Arthrogram of the radiocarpal joint may be indicated:

- A tear of the TFCC allows dye to extrude into the radioulnar joint, which does not normally communicate with the radiocarpal joint.
- Some patients may require later injections of the distal radioulnar or midcarpal joint for full evaluation.

IMAGING PROCEDURES

- Anteroposterior and lateral radiographs of the wrist in neutral pronation and supination are obtained.
- Films of the wrist in pronation and supination may be helpful in assessing radioulnar joint instability.
- Ulnar height should be assessed.
- In the normal wrist, the distal radial and ulnar joint surfaces should be at the same level on the anteroposterior radiograph.
- Variance of the ulna may result from fracture or instability of the distal radioulnar joint.

Management

GENERAL MEASURES

Injury with Fractures

- Reduce and immobilize the fracture.
- The distal radioulnar joint should be assessed for reduction whenever distal forearm or wrist fractures are manipulated.
- When operative care of the fracture is indicated, acute repair of the TFCC should also be performed.

Injuries without Fracture

- Conservative treatment with a short arm cast in neutral rotation and analgesics for 6 weeks should be attempted.
- Gentle range of motion can slowly be reintroduced when the cast is removed.
- Patients with continued pain and instability may require further study and subsequent operative repair.

SURGICAL TREATMENT

- Repair of the ruptured TFCC can be attempted either arthroscopically or with an open procedure if sufficient tissue is present.
- Tears in the central area of the TFCC without instability may require arthroscopic débridement.
- Variance of the ulnar height may need to be addressed though shortening of the ulna or by reconstruction of the distal radioulnar joint with a tendon or band of fascia lata used to stabilize the joint.
- In severe cases, with advanced radioulnar arthritis, fusion of the joint may be considered (Sauve-Kapandji procedure).

PHYSICAL THERAPY

Patients with reduced range of motion after TFCC injury or fracture may benefit from stretching exercises.

MEDICAL TREATMENT

Analgesics are indicated.

COMPLICATIONS

Posttraumatic arthritis can occur, often delayed by years or even decades.

PROGNOSIS

- The prognosis is good.
- Some persistent pain may occur even with adequate repair.

RECOMMENDED READING

Aulicino PL, Siegel L. Acute injuries of the distal radiolulnar joint. *Hand Clin* 1991;7:283–293.

Bowers WH. The distal radioulnar joint. In: Green DP, ed. *Operative hand surgery*, 3rd ed. New York: Churchill Livingstone, 1993:973–1019.

Basics

DESCRIPTION

A "trigger finger" is a manifestation of stenosing tenosynovitis characterized by locking of the metacarpophalangeal or proximal interphalangeal joints with flexion of the digit. As the affected digit is slowly flexed, it snaps or triggers into a flexed position. Once the digit triggers, extension is difficult; occasionally, the digit must be extended manually.

This condition affects digits 2 to 5 in the adult, with the ring and middle fingers most commonly affected, and the thumb in the pediatric patient. Children (congenital type) and middle-aged patients predominate. The adult variety of trigger finger is more common in women than in men.

INCIDENCE

The incidence is unknown.

CAUSES

A nodule usually develops on the flexor tendon, most likely in response to abrasion of the tendon in the tendon sheath. The nodule then impinges on one of the rings of fibrous tissue encircling the flexor tendon sheath known as the A1 pulley, and the result is "triggering" when the digit is extended (Fig. 1). This is a self-perpetuating problem, because the irritation from triggering prevents the swelling from going down.

In the pediatric population (less than 2 years old), a congenital narrowing of the tendon sheath may be present, resulting in congenital trigger digit, most commonly the thumb.

RISK FACTORS

• Rheumatoid arthritis
• Increased age
• Diabetes mellitus

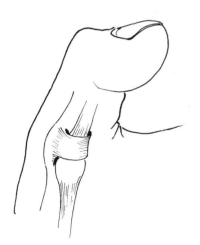

Fig. 1. In trigger finger, a nodule in the tendon sheath prevents it from sliding under the pulley. The finger does not extend.

ASSOCIATED CONDITIONS

• In congenital trigger digit, an association with trisomy 13 exists.
• In the adult patient, other disorders related to tenosynovitis, such as de Quervain's disease and carpal tunnel syndrome, may be present.
• Systemic disorders that cause connective tissue abnormalities, such as diabetes, gout, and rheumatoid arthritis, may also be present.

ICD-9-CM

727.03 Trigger finger Acquired
756.89 Congenital

 Diagnosis

SIGNS AND SYMPTOMS

• Symptoms: painful locking or snapping of the digit into a flexed position with flexion
• Signs: a nodule in the palm of the hand, just distal to the distal palmar crease

DIFFERENTIAL DIAGNOSIS

• Tendon rupture
• Fixed (ankylosed) joints

PHYSICAL EXAMINATION

By gently palpating the flexor tendon sheath of the affected digit in the region of the distal palmar crease and then having the patient flex the digit, the offending nodule may sometimes be palpated. In children less than 2 years old, 30% have bilateral involvement.

LABORATORY TESTS

There are no serum laboratory tests to aid in this diagnosis.

IMAGING PROCEDURES

They are usually not necessary, because trigger finger is a clinical diagnosis.

 Management

GENERAL MEASURES

The triggering often unlocks with rest.

SURGICAL TREATMENT

• A small transverse incision is made in the region of the A1 pulley (just distal to the distal transverse palmar crease) and overlying the affected flexor tendon.

• The A1 pulley is incised.
• After surgical release, the hand is bandaged for several days.
• Activity is gradually resumed.

PHYSICAL THERAPY

None is needed.

MEDICAL TREATMENT

• Age less than 2 years: Many of these patients require surgical intervention.
• In children less than 9 months of age, 30% of these cases will resolve spontaneously.
• In children more than 12 months old, only 10% of these cases will resolve spontaneously.
• In adults, treatment commences with injection of the tendon sheath (but not the tendon) with lidocaine and cortisone in the region of the A1 pulley. A single injection results in a 35% to 84% success rate; the use of more than three injections has a 77% to 88% success rate.
• For those in whom nonoperative therapy fails, surgical incision of the A1 pulley has a 98% cure rate.
• No restrictions are placed on activity after injection.
• After surgical release, the hand is bandaged for several days. Gradual activity is then commenced.

PATIENT EDUCATION

Patients are advised to have surgical release for recurrent symptoms.

MONITORING

None is necessary after surgical release.

COMPLICATIONS

• Errant injections may result in damage to the tendon or digital nerves and vasculature.
• These complications are rare.
• Surgical risks are small (digital nerve laceration, tendon rupture).

PROGNOSIS

The prognosis is good.

RECOMMENDED READING

Green DP, ed. *Operative hand surgery,* 3rd ed. New York: Churchill Livingstone, 1993:1992–1994.

Lister G. *The hand: diagnosis and treatment,* 3rd ed. Edinburgh: Churchill Livingstone, 1993:345–346.

Tumor

 Basics

DESCRIPTION

Bone tumors can be divided into four categories, as follows:

Benign Primary

Benign bone tumors are common. These lesions usually occur in young patients. Osteochondromas, osteoid osteoma, and giant cell tumors are the most common benign bone tumors.

Malignant

• Malignant bone tumors are rare and make up less than 1% of deaths from cancer. Bone sarcomas are malignant neoplasms of connective tissue origin.
• Generally, primary malignant bone tumors occur in the first 3 decades of life.

Metastatic

• Metastatic tumors are the most common destructive tumors encountered in adults.
• Generally, tumors metastatic to bone occur in the fourth through eighth decades of life.

Lesions that Simulate Bone Tumors

Conditions simulating tumors are not common and include a wide variety of lesions. The most common lesions that simulate bone tumors in adults and children include the following:

Children

• Infection
• Eosinophilic granuloma
• Stress fracture

Adults

• Paget's disease
• Hyperparathyroidism
• Myeloma and lymphoma are common lesions that occur in bone but are not of mesenchymal origin.
• Soft tissue tumors are benign or malignant and rarely metastasize to bone.
• Although primary soft tissue sarcomas are twice as common as all bone sarcomas combined, together they constitute slightly more than 1% of all cancer deaths.

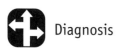 Diagnosis

SIGNS AND SYMPTOMS

• Pain

—Most patients with bone tumors present with musculoskeletal pain.
—Typically, it is described as dull, deep, aching pain.
—It often becomes constant and occurs at night.

• Swelling occurs.
• Loss of function at the involved site is noted.
• Weight loss occurs.
• Acute symptoms of a pathologic fracture are noted (in up to 10% of patients, pathologic fracture is the first evidence of the underlying disease).
• Soft tissue tumors

—These are more common.
—Patients may present with a small lump or a large mass.
—The lesion is often enlarging and may be painful or painless.

PHYSICAL EXAMINATION

• Patients with suspected bone tumors should be carefully examined.
• Perform a complete musculoskeletal examination.
• Inspect the affected site for soft tissue masses, overlying skin changes, and adenopathy.
• When metastatic disease is suspected, examine the thyroid gland, lungs, abdomen, prostate, and breasts.

IMAGING PROCEDURES

Radiography of the Lesion

• Plain radiographs in two planes are the first imaging examinations indicated.
• Reviewing radiographs of a lesion

—Determine the matrix characteristics (bone, cartilage, or amorphous).
—Determine the anatomic location within the bone (epiphyseal, metaphyseal, diaphyseal).
—Determine the number of lesions.
—Determine the effect of the lesion on bone.
—Determine the response of the bone to the lesion.

Technetium Bone Scanning

This is indicated if there is clinical suspicion of malignancy and the plain radiographs are normal.

Skeletal Survey (More Sensitive)

• This is indicated in patients with myeloma, in whom the bone scan may be negative.
• The skeletal survey includes the following:

—Anteroposterior and lateral views of the cervical spine, thoracic spine, and lumbosacral spine
—Anteroposterior views of the pelvis, femora, tibiae, fibulae, humeri, radii, and ulnae.

Magnetic Resonance Imaging

This is the preferred modality for screening the spine for occult metastases, myeloma, or lymphoma.

Chest Radiography

This should also be obtained when malignancy is suspected.

Soft Tissue Tumors

• Initial radiographic evaluation begins with plain radiographs in two planes.
• Magnetic resonance imaging is then the best imaging modality to define the anatomy and to depict the lesion more precisely.

DIFFERENTIAL DIAGNOSIS

This is based on clinical and radiographic findings. The patient's age helps to select diseases that are common in the given age group.

Young (10 to 25 years) Patients

Benign

• Infection
• Eosinophilic granuloma
• Enchondromatosis

Malignant

• Osteosarcoma
• Ewing's sarcoma
• Leukemia or lymphoma

Older Adults

Benign

• Paget's disease
• Hyperparathyroidism

Malignant

• Metastatic bone disease
• Multiple myeloma
• Lymphoma
• Primary mesenchymal tumors
• Chondrosarcoma
• Malignant fibrous histiocytoma

Matrix Characteristics

• Cartilage calcification may appear stippled with apparent rings, whereas bone may be cloudlike and may show trabeculae.
• Cartilage-forming tumors include enchondroma, osteochondroma, chondromyxoid fibroma, chondroblastoma, and chondrosarcoma.
• Bone-forming tumors include osteoid osteoma, osteoblastoma, osteochondroma, osteosarcoma, and blastic metastases.

Number of Bone Lesions

• This indicates whether the process is monostotic or polyostotic.
• Multiple destructive lesions in patients older than 40 are most likely metastatic bone disease, multiple myeloma, or lymphoma.

• In younger adults, multiple lytic lesions are most likely a vascular tumor, multiple enchondromatosis, or Langerhans' cell granulomatosis (eosinophilic granuloma).

• In children younger than 5 years of age, multiple destructive lesions may represent metastatic neuroblastoma or Wilms' tumor or Langerhans' cell granulomatosis (histiocytosis X).

Anatomic Location of the Lesion

• Chondroblastoma and giant cell tumors most commonly occur in the epiphysis of long bones.

• Ewing's tumor often involves the diaphysis.

• Osteosarcoma is most commonly seen at the metaphysis of the distal femur and the proximal tibia.

Effect of the Lesion

• A lytic lesion is less dense (radiolucent).

• An osteoblastic lesion is more dense (radiopaque).

High-Grade Malignant Lesions

• These usually spread rapidly through the medullary canal.

• Cortical bone is destroyed early, and tumor may spread to the soft tissues.

• Often, the host has little ability to contain the process, and it may appear diffuse or permeative.

Low-Grade Malignant Lesions

• These tend to spread slowly.

• Host bone often can contain the lesion with a thickened cortex or rim of periosteal bone, to give a well-circumscribed appearance.

• Reactive new bone formation with periosteal elevation into an "onion skin" pattern may suggest Ewing's sarcoma, osteosarcoma, or osteomyelitis.

LABORATORY STUDIES

These are often nonspecific, but routine studies should be obtained in any patient with suspected tumor.

Patients 5 to 30 Years of Age

• Complete blood count with differential
• Peripheral blood smear
• Erythrocyte sedimentation rate

Patients More Than 40 Years of Age

• Complete blood count with differential
• Peripheral blood smear
• Erythrocyte sedimentation rate

• Serum calcium and phosphate
• Serum or urine protein electrophoresis
• Urinalysis

Biopsy

• This is key to diagnosis.

• It is beneficial to the pathologist and the surgeon to have a narrow working diagnosis at the time of the biopsy.

• The biopsy should be done at the center where the treatment is to be given.

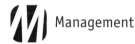 Management

GENERAL MEASURES

Immediately after Diagnosis

• Referral should be made to a musculoskeletal oncologist for proper staging, biopsy, and treatment as appropriate.

• An improperly placed biopsy needle or biopsy incision can have a significantly adverse affect on the patient's clinical course, and thus patients should be referred only to orthopaedists who specialize in tumor management.

• A team approach to treatment includes an orthopaedic tumor surgeon, pathologist, medical or pediatric oncologist, radiation oncologist, social worker, and physical therapist.

• For diagnosis of a malignant primary sarcoma, a pulmonary computed tomography scan is performed to evaluate for metastases; this helps to complete the staging and to determine the treatment plan and prognosis.

Determining Treatment

• The diagnosis, histologic grade, and the size of the tumor are essential for determining treatment and prognosis.

• This helps to determine whether adjunctive treatment (chemotherapy or radiation therapy) is to be given before to surgical treatment.

Treatment Options

Neoadjuvant (Preoperative) Chemotherapy

This has a significant impact on both the efficacy of limb salvage and disease-free survival for patients with osteosarcoma and Ewing's tumor.

External-Beam Irradiation

• It is used for local control of Ewing's tumor, lymphoma, myeloma, and metastatic bone disease.

• It is also used as an adjunct, in combination with surgery, for the treatment of soft tissue sarcomas.

• The ionizing irradiation can be delivered preoperatively, perioperatively with brachytherapy afterloading tubes, or postoperatively.

Radiation Therapy

• This is used to destroy any cells that may have escaped surgical treatment.

• In some cases, it is used to shrink the tumor preoperatively in locations where it is difficult to determine tumor margins clearly.

PATIENT EDUCATION

Patients are appraised of the staging strategy and the treatment based on the diagnosis.

MONITORING

The pulmonary system is monitored closely after treatment of primary sarcomas, as follows:

• First 2 years: every 3 to 4 months
• From 2 to 5 years: every 4 to 6 months
• From 5 to 10 years: every 6 months

COMPLICATIONS

• Cauda equina syndrome

—True orthopaedic emergency: 0.2% of lumbar discs and often in metastatic tumors
—Massive, central lumbar disc herniation with saddle anesthesia (S2-4)
—Bowel and bladder paralysis (unable to void, rectal incontinence)
—Emergency magnetic resonance imaging and discectomy or decompression needed

PROGNOSIS

Prognosis depends on the specific lesions, as follows:

• In general: 5-year survival
• Low grade: 80% to 90%
• High grade: 40% to 60%

RECOMMENDED READING

Bonfiglio M, Buckwalter JB. Musculoskeletal tumors. In: Clark CR, Bonfiglio M, eds. *Orthopaedics: essentials of diagnosis and treatment.* New York: Churchill Livingstone, 1994:351–372.

Frassica FJ, McCarthy EF. Orthopaedic pathology. In: Miller MD, ed. *Review of orthopaedics,* 2nd ed. Philadelphia: WB Saunders, 1996:292–335.

Unicameral Bone Cyst

 Basics

DESCRIPTION

Unicameral bone cyst is a benign membrane-lined, fluid-filled lesion of bone that develops in childhood and fills in by maturity. It usually occurs in the proximal humerus and proximal femur 80% of the time, in order, at the proximal tibia, distal tibia, distal femur, calcaneus, distal humerus, radius, fibula, ilium, ulna, and rib. Typically, the lesion is centrally located either adjacent to the physeal plate or in the metaphyseal or diaphyseal region. Rarely, it crosses the physis into the epiphysis. It may also occur in flat bones. It is rarely seen in adults.

SYNONYMS

- Simple bone cyst
- Solitary bone cyst

GENETICS

No known relationship exists.

INCIDENCE

- It is most common in children 4 to 10 years old.
- All lesions are diagnosed in patients less than 20 years old.
- The age of diagnosis has ranged from 1.5 to 18 years.
- There is a 2 to 1 ratio in boys versus girls.

CAUSES

The origin is unknown, but suggested causes include the lesion arising from an intraosseous hematoma, a necrotic lipoma, lymphatic or venous obstruction, or an intraosseous synovial rest.

CLASSIFICATION

Active

This is usually seen in children younger than 10 years. A lytic area abuts the physis and may fill the entire metaphyseal region. Typically, it has a thinner cortical wall, which makes the lesion more prone to fracture and recurrence (approximately 50%).

Inactive

This is usually seen in children older than 12 years. A lytic area is separated from the physeal plate by normal cancellous bone. Typically, it has a thicker cortical wall, which makes it less prone to fracture and recurrence (approximately 10% to 15%).

ASSOCIATED CONDITIONS

None are known.

ICD-9-CM

733.21 Unicameral bone cyst

 Diagnosis

SIGNS AND SYMPTOMS

- The patient is usually asymptomatic unless fracture occurs as a result of a thinned-out cortex.
- Most cysts are discovered as a result of a fracture, which typically occurs with minimal trauma such as throwing a ball.
- The remaining lesions are either found incidentally on an unrelated radiograph or not at all.
- If symptomatic, the patient presents with localized pain and swelling or stiffness of the adjacent joint.

DIFFERENTIAL DIAGNOSIS

- Aneurysmal bone cyst
- Fibrous dysplasia
- Enchondroma
- Giant cell tumor
- Eosinophilic granuloma

PHYSICAL EXAMINATION

Usually, nothing is detectable on examination unless the patient is symptomatic, as mentioned earlier. With respect to recurrent fractures resulting from a unicameral bone cyst, patients must be examined for angular deformities resulting from malunion and for limb length discrepancies secondary to growth arrest.

PATHOLOGIC FINDINGS

Gross

Examination reveals a cystic cavity with a membrane lining of variable thickness (2 to 10 mm) usually containing yellowish fluid that may be blood-tinged or frankly bloody if it has been recently fractured or previously aspirated and injected. Septa may be present with loculations of fluid particularly if a fracture has previously occurred.

Microscopic

A membrane containing fibrous tissue and occasional spicules of bone are seen along with occasional osteoclasts, chronic inflammatory cells, and giant cells.

IMAGING PROCEDURES

Radiography

The typical appearance is a centrally located, expansile, radiolucent lesion with a well-marginated border located in the metaphyseal region causing thinning of the adjacent cortex. The "fallen fragment" or "fallen leaf" sign indicates the presence of a fracture with movement of a cortical piece of bone to a dependent portion of the fluid-filled cyst and suggests the presence of a cavity instead of a solid tumor. The cyst moves away from the epiphysis as the lesion becomes inactive.

Magnetic Resonance Imaging

This may be performed if there is a question of a solid lesion. A bright uniform signal in the T_2-weighted image is consistent with a high water content suggesting a cyst.

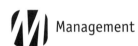 Management

GENERAL MEASURES

If found incidentally, a unicameral bone cyst may be treated with observation or with dual-needle aspiration of the cyst followed by injection of methylprednisolone, bone marrow, or other substance. If it is discovered as a result of a pathologic fracture, the bone may be allowed to heal. About 10% of fractures are followed by spontaneous healing of the cyst. The rest of these patients are usually offered injections. If a simple bone cyst is persistent, surgical curettage and bone grafting may be required.

SURGICAL TREATMENT

Needle aspiration may be performed by inserting two needles with stylets into the lesion under fluoroscopic guidance. Removal of the stylets and attempted aspiration will prove whether the lesion is fluid filled. Placement of the needles in the proper position may be confirmed with radiographic dye. If the dye is unable to be injected or there is no fluid on aspiration, then an open biopsy should be performed, assuming the possibility of a solid lesion. If the lesion is fluid filled, 40 to 200 mg of methylprednisolone may be injected into the cyst and, if necessary, injection may be repeated at 2-month intervals up to three times. Newer protocols include injecting other substances into the cyst, such as marrow or bone paste. Approximately 75% of patients require multiple injections. Treatment by this method is thought to occur by stimulating the cyst to heal.

Persistent or recurrent cysts may require open curettage and bone grafting. Various graft sources have been used such as autograft (cortical, cancellous, and bone marrow aspirate), allograft (cortical and cancellous), and injectable demineralized bone matrix. The rate of recurrence is approximately 50% with active cysts and 10% to 15% with inactive cysts. In critical, high-stress regions such as the base of the femoral neck, internal fixation with a plate may be indicated.

PATIENT EDUCATION

Patients must be advised that the persistence rate is approximately 85% in cysts treated with observation after a fracture. If treated with injections or bone grafting, an active cyst recurs in 50% and an inactive cyst recurs in 10% to 15%. The risk of refracture remains as long as the cyst is present. Activity modification may greatly reduce the risk of refracture, but this may not be practical for this specific age group, depending on the patient.

COMPLICATIONS

- Growth arrest may occur, giving rise to limb length discrepancies along with malunions that cause angular deformities.
- Avascular necrosis may occur as a result of fracture through proximal femoral lesions.

PROGNOSIS

- The unicameral bone cyst eventually heals spontaneously and fills in with bone, but it may involve recurrent fractures, injections, or curettage and bone grafting before resolution.
- Results of treatment vary with the location or size of a cyst and the age of the patient.
- The rate of recurrence is higher when the cyst occurs in the proximal humerus versus the femur or tibia.
- When a cyst is present in flat bones, recurrence is rare. Smaller cysts have a lower rate of recurrence than larger cysts.
- Younger patients tend to have a higher recurrence rate than older patients.
- Malignant degeneration of the unicameral bone cyst is nonexistent.

RECOMMENDED READING

Dahlin DC, ed. *Bone tumors,* 3rd ed. Springfield, IL: Charles C Thomas, 1978:385–387.

McCarthy EF, Frassica FJ, eds. *Pathology of bone and joint disorders with clinical and radiographic correlation.* Philadelphia: WB Saunders, 1998:277–279.

Morrissy RT, Weinstein SL, eds. *Lovell and Winter's pediatric orthopedics,* 4th ed. Philadelphia: JB Lippincott, 1996:448–450.

Spjut HJ, Dorfman HD, eds. *Tumors of bone and cartilage,* 2nd series. Washington, DC: Armed Forces Institute of Pathology, 1970:347–353.

Vertebral Osteomyelitis

 Basics

DESCRIPTION

Vertebral osteomyelitis is an infection of vertebral bodies.

SYNONYM

Back infection

INCIDENCE

This condition is rare.

CAUSES

- Most infections are from the hematogenous route, commonly pelvic inflammatory disease and cystitis.
- It occurs in adults, in men more than in women, and in the lumbar spine more than the thoracic and the thoracic more than the cervical.
- Organisms include *Staphylococcus aureus*, gram-negative bacteria (*Escherichia coli, Proteus, Klebsiella, Pseudomonas*), and *Mycobacterium tuberculosis*.
- Most infections are in the vertebral body rather than in the posterior elements.

CLASSIFICATION

- Acute: less than 3 months' duration
- Chronic: greater than 3 months' duration

RISK FACTORS

- Diabetes (both type 1 and type 2)
- Alcoholism
- Intravenous drug abuse

ASSOCIATED CONDITIONS

This occurs in immunocompromised patients:

- Cancer
- Human immunodeficiency virus infection

ICD-9-CM

730.8 Osteomyelitis, spine

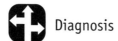 Diagnosis

SIGNS AND SYMPTOMS

- Possible extreme illness
- Backache increasing in intensity, becoming constant
- Night pain
- Insidious onset: 8- to 10-week delayed diagnosis common because of lack of radiographic changes
- Fever
- Malaise
- Pain with spinal motion
- Possible late epidural abscess development
- Straight leg raising restricted

DIFFERENTIAL DIAGNOSIS

- Tumor
- Fracture
- Disc herniation

PHYSICAL EXAMINATION

Common findings include the following:

- Severe pain with percussion of the spinal cord
- Paravertebral muscle spasm
- Painful straight leg raising

LABORATORY TESTS

- Elevated white blood cell count with a left shift in 50% of patients
- Erythrocyte sedimentation rate consistently elevated; used to monitor disease course
- Blood cultures positive in 50%

IMAGING PROCEDURES

- Plain radiographs: Changes lag 4 weeks behind the clinical course.

—Early: Findings include localized rarefaction of vertebral end plates, rapid adjacent vertebral involvement and disc space narrowing, fuzziness of cortical end plate, and "divot" out of the anterosuperior or anteroinferior vertebral body.

—Later: Destructive erosion of contiguous vertebral bodies, most extensive anteriorly, sclerosis and reactive bone, and a soft tissue mass are noted.

- Bone scan or gallium scan detects disease early.
- Magnetic resonance imaging is also good for early detection.
- Infection versus tumor

—In infection, the disc space is usually destroyed first.

—With tumor, the disc space is spared, whereas tumor deposits in the vertebral body.

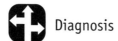 Management

GENERAL MEASURES

For diagnosis, obtain blood cultures, source cultures (urine or sputum), and percutaneous or open biopsy before starting antibiotics.

- Biopsy mandatory for diagnosis
- Needle biopsy, 71% positive
- Unsafe in cervical or thoracic region unless guided by computed tomography
- Open biopsy, the most accurate method; can débride also

SURGICAL TREATMENT

Surgery is indicated with the following:

- Failure of medical management
- Formation of large abscess
- Progressive neurologic deficit
- Biomechanical instability
- Failure to obtain adequate needle biopsy for diagnosis
- Epidural abscess, a surgical emergency that may cause a progressive neurologic deficit

PHYSICAL THERAPY

Physical therapy generally worsens the pain and should alert the clinician to the possible presence of infection and neoplasm.

MEDICAL TREATMENT

- Early in disease evolution: intravenous antibiotics to culture sensitivities, bracing, bed rest
- Late in disease evolution: surgery, failure to respond to intravenous treatment, abscess formation
- Continued treatment until normal erythrocyte sedimentation rate, resolution of pain and fever, evidence of fusion
- Bracing for 3 months
- Radiography every 6 weeks

MONITORING

- Radiography every 4 to 8 weeks
- New magnetic resonance imaging if fever or increase in pain

COMPLICATIONS

- Abscess
- Neurologic compromise
- Cauda equina syndrome
- Destabilization of spine with bone destruction

PROGNOSIS

Most patients can be cured with appropriate antibiotics and surgical debridement as necessary.

Basics

DESCRIPTION

Congenital vertical talus is an uncommon disorder, a rigid flatfoot that requires early identification and aggressive treatment. Its essence is a dislocation of the talonavicular joint.

It may be unilateral or bilateral. More than half of affected patients have other neurologic, genetic, or connective tissue disorders. The deformity occurs *in utero,* but it may be first identified any time from infancy to adulthood.

SYNONYMS

- Congenital convex pes planus
- Congenital rigid rocker-bottom foot

GENETICS

- This is unknown, but it is probably variable.
- In some cases, vertical transmission as an autosomal dominant trait with incomplete penetrance has been described.

INCIDENCE

The condition is rare, but it has a high association with other disorders and anomalies. Ten percent of children with myelodysplasia have congenital vertical talus; it also can be associated with trisomy 13, 15, and 18 and with arthrogryposis. In 20% to 40% of cases, congenital vertical talus occurs as an isolated anomaly. It affects males and females equally.

CAUSES

Muscle imbalance between the dorsiflexor muscles of the forefoot and plantar flexor muscle of the hind foot cause disruption in the middle of the foot (talonavicular joint). Ligamentous laxity and *in utero* malposition may be causative factors in some cases.

RISK FACTORS

- Myelodysplasia
- Ligamentous laxity
- Arthrogryposis multiplex

CLASSIFICATION

- Isolated
- Syndrome-related

ASSOCIATED CONDITIONS

- Arthrogryposis
- Larsen's syndrome
- Myelomeningocele
- Trisomy 13, 15, 18

ICD-9-CM

754.69 Congenital vertical talus

Diagnosis

SIGNS AND SYMPTOMS

- Signs: Moderate reversal of the arch and a crease on the dorsum of the foot near the sinus torsi
- Symptoms: Lack of push-off strength; painful callus under the head of the talus possible if untreated

DIFFERENTIAL DIAGNOSIS

- Calcaneovalgus foot
- Flexible flatfoot

PHYSICAL EXAMINATION

- The other extremities, as well as the spine, should be checked for anomalies.
- Measure strength in both lower extremities.
- Observe the foot in stance and gait if child is walking.
- It is easily distinguishable from the more common calcaneus and flexible flatfoot.
- The foot is convex, has a rocker bottom, and is rigid.
- The heel is in a fixed equinus with a tight Achilles tendon.
- The head of the talus is prominent and palpable medially in the sole of the foot.
- The hind foot is in valgus.
- The forefoot is abducted and in dorsiflexion at the midtarsal joint (Fig. 1).
- As the patient becomes older, the appearance of the foot becomes more distinctive.

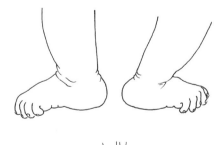

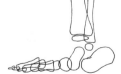

Fig. 1. Vertical talus produces a dorsal crease and a plantar prominence.

PATHOLOGIC FINDINGS

- The calcaneus is in equinus and laterally displaced.
- The talus is hypoplastic, angled medially, and plantar flexed.
- Fixed dorsal dislocation of the navicular is noted.
- Contracture of the Achilles tendon (posteriorly) is evident.
- Contracture of the toe extensor and the tibialis anterior (anteriorly) is seen.
- Specially positioned plantar flexion lateral radiograph is helpful (see later).

IMAGING PROCEDURES

- Order radiographs.
- The talus is plantar flexed (on the lateral radiographs) and is angled medially (on the anteroposterior films).
- The navicular is dorsally dislocated and is perched on the neck of the talus.
- The forefoot is dorsally displaced and abducted.
- The calcaneus is in a fixed equinus.
- Only the most posterior aspect of the talus articulates with the tibia, and, in extreme cases, the talus is parallel to the tibia. In extreme plantar flexed views, the navicular will not reduce, and the line through the talar axis will pass plantar to the metatarsal axis. Normal is dorsal to the cuboid and in line with the metatarsal axis. However, the navicular does not ossify until about age 3 years, in either the normal foot or congenital vertical talus. The position of the navicular may be inferred from the orientation of the first metatarsal.

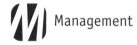

Management

GENERAL MEASURES

- Stretching
- Surgery

SURGICAL TREATMENT

- The essential features are open reduction and pinning of the talonavicular joint. The associated contracted tendons should also be lengthened (Achilles and anterior tibialis). The medial joint capsules may be stabilized, or, in older children, the talonavicular joint may be fused. The oldest children may require triple arthrodesis.

Vertical Talus

- Postoperative percutaneous pins of the talon-avicular joint are usually removed at 6 weeks.
- The foot is usually casted for 6 to 12 weeks.
- When early surgical intervention is pursued (before age 2 years), an extensive soft tissue release or reconstruction is performed. This is combined with a reduction and pinning of the navicular. Late treatment in the 2- to 6-year-old child requires subtalar fusion. In adolescents and adults, salvage is performed by triple arthrodesis and often requires removal of a large portion of the talus. Recurrent deformity in the 2- to 6-year-old child is treated with soft tissue reconstruction and subtalar fusion.

MEDICAL TREATMENT

- If the condition is recognized, surgical intervention is preferred before the patient is 2 years old.
- Casting and manipulation alone are not usually effective, although they can be used preoperatively to stretch soft tissue.

PATIENT EDUCATION

Patients should be informed of the chances of inheritance in future children. The natural history of this condition, if left untreated, which is severe callus formation, skin breakdown, and poor push-off, should also be discussed. The risk of hip dysplasia should be mentioned and excluded. The possible need for further surgery should be mentioned.

MONITORING

Even after surgery, the patient should be followed periodically to verify normal growth.

COMPLICATIONS

- Complications of nontreatment: callus, skin breakdown, poor push-off
- Complications of treatment: stiffness, residual varus or valgus, need for further surgery

PROGNOSIS

The condition is progressive if it is untreated.

RECOMMENDED READING

Ogata K, Schoenecker PL. Congenital vertical talus and its familial occurrence. *Clin Orthop* 1979;139:1–28.

Seimon LP. Surgical correction of vertical talus under the age of 2 years. *J Pediatr Orthop* 1987;7:405.

Sullivan JA. The child's foot. In: Morrissy RT, Weinstein SL, eds. *Lovell and Winter's pediatric orthopaedics,* 4th ed. Philadelphia: Lippincott–Raven, 1996:1089.

Basics

DESCRIPTION

Wrist pain is a common symptom. It may be caused by different conditions including trauma, overuse, and infection. It is important to obtain a detailed history to make the correct diagnosis and to provide appropriate treatment. The history should include onset, duration, frequency, and location of the pain. Information regarding swelling, erythema, abnormal clicks, aggravating activities, range of motion, sensory changes, motor strength, and general health conditions is essential.

CLASSIFICATION

- Traumatic
- Inflammatory
- Degenerative
- Infectious
- Neurologic

ASSOCIATED CONDITIONS

- Rheumatoid arthritis
- History of trauma

ICD-9-CM

719.43 Pain in joint

 Diagnosis

SIGNS AND SYMPTOMS

The location of wrist pain is indicative of the cause. Patients may present with swelling and pain localized as radial wrist pain, dorsal wrist pain, ulnar wrist pain, palmar wrist pain, and general wrist pain.

DIFFERENTIAL DIAGNOSIS

By location of pain, the differential diagnosis is as follows:

Radial Wrist Pain

- De Quervain's tenosynovitis
- Scaphoid fracture or nonunion

Dorsal Wrist Pain

- Tenosynovitis of extensor tendons
- Ganglion cyst

Ulnar Wrist Pain

- Distal radioulnar joint instability
- Flexor carpi ulnaris tendinitis
- Fracture of the hook of the hamate

Palmar Wrist Pain

- Flexor tenosynovitis
- Carpal tunnel syndrome

General Wrist Pain

- Arthritis
- Infection

PHYSICAL EXAMINATION

Radial Wrist Pain

De Quervain's Tenosynovitis

- This is caused by inflammation of the first dorsal compartment (extensor brevis and abductor longus).
- The patient may provide a history of repetitive activities of the wrist.
- Finkelstein's test (with thumb flexed into palm, pain is reproduced by ulnar deviation of the wrist) is usually positive

Scaphoid Fracture

Patients usually have a history of trauma, most often a fall on an outstretched arm.

Dorsal Wrist Pain

Tenosynovitis of Extensor Tendons

- The patient usually presents with a complaint of pain in the dorsum of the wrist that may radiate proximally and distally.
- Usually, the patient has a history of repetitive activities and overuse.
- Pain occurs on flexion and extension.
- Sometimes, a sharply demarcated scalloped edge of the extensor synovial sheath can be palpated with wrist motion.

Ganglion Cyst

- This is the most common mass on the dorsal surface of the wrist.
- Most arise from the scapholunate ligament.
- Generally, they are movable and transilluminate light.
- The size of a cyst may vary with time.
- Generally, only large cysts cause pain.

Ulnar Wrist Pain

Distal Radioulnar Joint Instability

- Most patients have a history of trauma to the wrist.
- Pain is located at the distal radioulnar joint, especially with pronation and supination.
- Instability can be palpated or visualized with stress loading.
- Radiographs may show increased space between distal radius and ulna; if radiography is inconclusive, computed tomography may be helpful.

Flexor Carpi Ulnaris Tendinitis

Pain on the flexor carpi ulnaris is usually detected on resisted wrist flexion and ulnar deviation.

Fracture of the Hook of the Hamate

- Patients have a history of direct impact to the ulnar palm, especially in golf and tennis players.
- Pain occurs on palpation of hamate and resisted flexion of the fourth and fifth fingers.
- Radiographs of the wrist in the carpal tunnel view show the fracture.

Palmar Wrist Pain

Flexor Tenosynovitis

- This is similar to extensor tenosynovitis.
- The patient usually presents with a history of overuse of the wrist.
- Pain is located on the volar aspect of the wrist and is aggravated with wrist motion; it may radiate proximally or distally.

Carpal Tunnel Syndrome

- This is the most common compression neuropathy in the upper extremity.
- Patients frequently complain of pain around wrist, numbness and tingling sensation to the radial three digits, clumsiness, and weakness.
- Patients frequently wake up at night with numbness in the fingers.
- Tinel's test of the carpal tunnel and Phalen's test may be positive.
- Decreased sensibility in median nerve distribution and thenar atrophy are late signs of this condition.

General Wrist Pain

Arthritis

- Inflammatory arthritis and osteoarthritis involving the radiocarpal, intercarpal, and carpometacarpal joints will present with pain in the wrist.
- Patients with osteoarthritis may have a history of trauma in the past.
- Swelling, stiffness, and decreased range of motion are usually present.
- Patients with inflammatory arthritis, especially rheumatoid arthritis, have swelling of tendon sheaths and thickening of synovium.
- Deformity of joints is a sign of advanced disease.
- Radiographs of patients with osteoarthritis generally show narrowing of joint space, subchondral sclerosis, and osteophytes.
- Radiographs in inflammatory arthritis show narrowing of joint space, osteopenia, bone erosion, and deformity.

Wrist Pain

—Wrist Infection

- Immunocompromised patients or those with a history of intravenous drug use are at higher risk of infection.
- Pain, swelling, erythema, decreased range of motion, and other cardinal signs of infection may be present.
- Elevated leukocyte count, erythrocyte sedimentation rate, and C-reactive protein are signs of infection. Joint fluid analysis shoes that a finding of more than 80,000 white blood cell and more than 75% polymorphs strongly suggests a septic joint (the absolute white blood cell count may vary and may overlap with other conditions).

LABORATORY TESTS

White blood cell count, erythrocyte sedimentation rate, and C-reactive protein are indicated to assess for infection.

IMAGING PROCEDURES

Radiography

- Plain anteroposterior and lateral radiographs are obtained to look for fracture, with a carpal tunnel view for fracture of the hook of the hamate and carpal tunnel syndrome.
- A scaphoid view is used to assess scaphoid fracture.

Magnetic Resonance Imaging

This may be useful in the diagnosis of triangular fibrocartilage complex tear.

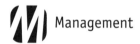 Management

GENERAL MEASURES

- Tendinitis and tenosynovitis can be treated with rest, modification of activity, ice, immobilization, nonsteroidal antiinflammatory drugs, and local injection of steroid if warranted.
- Nondisplaced fractures should be treated with immobilization and nonsteroidal antiinflammatory drugs.
- Rheumatoid arthritis of the wrist should be treated by a rheumatologist as a component of general systemic condition.
- Ganglion cysts may be aspirated or excised.
- Patients with mild to moderate carpal tunnel syndrome symptoms can be managed conservatively. Conservative treatment (oral antiinflammatory medicine, wrist splint, and modifi-

cation of activity) is unlikely to cure the condition, but it may alleviate the symptoms enough to obviate the need for surgical intervention. Injection of cortisone to the carpal tunnel may be indicated for persistent carpal tunnel syndrome.
- Patients with wrist infections should be admitted to a hospital. After joint fluid is sent for culture and sensitivity, intravenous antibiotics should be started as soon as possible. Open irrigation is usually indicated; however, both serial aspiration of the joint and open irrigation of the joint are acceptable means of treatment. After hospital discharge, antibiotics are usually continued for several weeks. Early range of motion is paramount in preserving long-term joint function.

SURGICAL TREATMENT

De Quervain's Tenosynovitis

A few patients require surgical release of the first dorsal compartment.

Displaced Scaphoid Fracture

Internal fixation by Kirschner wire is done using a palmar approach.

Distal Radioulnar Joint Instability

If the triangular fibrocartilage complex is involved, treatment is controversial. Patients who cannot be treated by immobilization may require arthroscopy and open repair of the triangular fibrocartilage complex tear. If distal radioulnar joint instability is accompanied by intraarticular and extraarticular fracture of the distal radius or ulna, fixation of fracture and Kirschner wire pinning of the distal radioulnar joint instability are indicated.

Fracture of Hook of the Hamate

This fracture tends to be displaced, and the incidence of nonunion is greater. If the fragment is small, surgical excision of the fractured fragment is recommended. If the fracture is at the base of the hook, open reduction and internal fixation are recommended.

Flexor Tenosynovitis

Surgical tenolysis is indicated for chronic recalcitrant tendinitis.

Carpal Tunnel Syndrome

Surgical release is considered definitive treatment and is indicated when conservative treatment has failed or when signs of advanced carpal tunnel syndrome including decreased sensibility, muscle atrophy, and significant nerve conduction study and electromyographic changes exist.

Arthritis

Surgical intervention (e.g., resection, fusion) is reserved for patients with severe symptoms in whom conservative treatment has failed.

MEDICAL TREATMENT

- Nonsteroidal antiinflammatory drugs
- Local steroid injection for tenosynovitis and tendinitis in persistent case
- Intravenous antibiotics in case of wrist infection

PATIENT EDUCATION

Patients with work-related carpal tunnel syndrome may alleviate the condition by job modification.

PROGNOSIS

Most cases can be largely alleviated by one of the foregoing methods.

RECOMMENDED READING

Anlicino PL, Siegel JL. Acute injuries of the distal radioulnar joint. *Hand Clin* 1991;7:283–293.

Cooney WP, ed. *The wrist: diagnosis and operative treatment.* St. Louis: CV Mosby, 1998.

Donatto KC. Orthopaedic management of septic arthritis. *Rheum Dis Clin North Am* 1998;24:275–286.

Gelberman RH, Rydevik BL, Press GM, et al. Carpal tunnel syndrome: a scientific basis for clinical care. *Orthop Clin North Am* 1988;19:115–124.

Gelberman RH, Wolock BS, Siegel DB. Fractures and non-union of the carpal scaphoid. *J Bone Joint Surg Am* 1989;71:1560–1565.

Harvey FJ, Harvey PM, Horsley MW. De Quervain's disease: surgical or nonsurgical treatment. *J Hand Surg Am* 1990;15:83–87.

Basics

DESCRIPTION

A wrist sprain is an injury to the bones and ligaments of the wrist that results in pain from an incomplete ligament tear. No long-term disability is associated with it. Because many serious injuries are easily confused with wrist sprains, the patient with significant swelling or persistent pain should be suspected of having a more serious injury.

Wrist sprain occurs most commonly in adults; it is rare in children. Suspect an injury to the growth plate if swelling and tenderness are seen. Elderly persons are more likely to suffer a fracture. Males and females are equally affected.

INCIDENCE

This is a common injury, because the wrist is part of our first reflexive defense against injury.

CAUSES

- This injury usually occurs from a fall on an outstretched hand.
- It may also occur from a twisting injury as the hand is grasping an object.

RISK FACTORS

- Frequent falls
- Overuse

CLASSIFICATION

Grade I. No ligament damage (stretch of the ligament without tearing)
Grade II. Partial tear
Grade III. Complete tear

ASSOCIATED CONDITIONS

When people fall on an outstretched hand, there is a continuum of injury from stretching and mild tearing of the ligament to fracture of the bones and dislocation of the articulation such as the following:

- Scaphoid fracture
- Radial styloid fracture
- Perilunate dislocation

ICD-9-CM

842.00 Wrist sprain

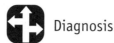 Diagnosis

SIGNS AND SYMPTOMS

Signs

- Swelling over the wrist joint

Symptoms

- Pain on range of motion
- Stiffness
- Decreased grip strength
- Little pain on axial loading

DIFFERENTIAL DIAGNOSIS

The diagnosis of a wrist sprain is clinical, and it is primarily made by palpation over the ligaments and exclusion of more serious injuries.

Navicular or Scaphoid Fracture

This is a serious injury, which may go on to a painful nonunion if it is not immobilized. It is signaled by pain in the "snuffbox" area of the hand, between the extensor and abductor tendons to the thumb. A scaphoid view on the radiograph usually demonstrates it. If not, a bone scan may be ordered, or the wrist may be immobilized in a thumb spica cast for 2 weeks and then rechecked.

Scapholunate Interosseous Ligament Injury

This is a tear of the ligament between the lunate and scaphoid bones, which joins these two important carpal bones. It may result in late wrist instability and clicking, if torn. The signs are a gap of greater than 3 mm between the scaphoid and lunate on plain radiograph or an angle of greater than 60 degrees between these bones on the lateral radiograph.

Avulsion or "Chip" Fracture of the Lunate or Triquetrum

This injury may also simulate a sprain. This is best seen on coned or detailed lateral films of the wrist. Longer immobilization is required.

de Quervain's Tenosynovitis

This is an overuse injury of the extensor-abductor tendons of the thumb that results in aching on the radial side of the wrist and a positive Finkelstein's test.

Triangular Fibrocartilage Tear

This involves the distal radioulnocarpal joint.

Distal Radioulnar Joint Subluxation

This is noted by a dorsal prominence over the distal ulna, especially in pronation.

Subluxation of the Extensor Carpi Ulnaris Tendon

This injury usually occurs with pronation and supination of the wrist.

Lunate Dislocations

These are serious injuries and occur following falls and high-energy trauma to the wrist. The lunate is completely dislocated, and this injury is frequently overlooked on plain radiographs.

PHYSICAL EXAMINATION

- Inspect the wrist for amount of swelling.
- Carefully perform range of motion; it should be possible to achieve a complete range if done slowly. Check pronation and supination of the wrist.
- Palpate the structures on the dorsum of the wrist individually for tenderness and to focus on the subsequent radiographic examination.
- Palpate the volar part of the wrist; if tender, the likelihood of a serious injury increases.
- Inspect the snuffbox for tenderness.
- Palpate the wrist extensor tendons, both over and away from the wrist.

LABORATORY TESTS

There are no serum tests.

PATHOLOGIC FINDINGS

- A sprain of the wrist involves partial stretching or disruption of the ligaments holding the radius and the carpal bones in alignment.
- No major interosseous ligament injury or fracture should be seen.

IMAGING PROCEDURES

- Obtain anteroposterior, lateral, and oblique films of the wrist. The oblique film is also termed the navicular view and is most useful to rule out an occult injury to this bone.
- Order a clenched-fist view if scapholunate instability is suspected. A positive view shows more than 3 mm of space between the scaphoid and lunate.
- Coned (specially focused) lateral view of the wrist may be needed to rule out avulsion fractures of the triquetrum of the lunate.
- Magnetic resonance imaging or fluoroscopy may be used by the orthopaedist or hand surgeon specialist in cases of an unclear diagnosis or to search for an occult injury.
- Bone scan may be done to rule out occult fracture in the presence of normal plain films.

Wrist Sprain

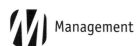 Management

GENERAL MEASURES

- Immobilization for comfort
- Counseling to return to activity when symptoms subside
- Specialist referral if symptoms persist
- If a navicular fracture is suspected, the wrist should be immobilized in a thumb-spica cast and reexamined in 2 weeks
- If carpal instability is suspected, refer patient to a specialist.

SURGICAL TREATMENT

Surgery is not indicated for simple wrist sprains. Major ligament tears that result in instability often necessitate surgical repair, either ligament reconstruction or wrist fusion.

PHYSICAL THERAPY

The patient may perform therapy at home with an exercise program or directly under the supervision of a therapist. The goals of rehabilitation are range of motion, strength, and dexterity.

MEDICAL TREATMENT

- If a sprain is suspected, ice, immobilization, and analgesics are appropriate.
- Nonsteroidal antiinflammatory agents are useful for patients with severe pain.
- A wrist splint may be made of padded plaster or fiberglass or may be ready made for easy removal and reapplication.
- Remove the wrist splint when the pain subsides, usually in 5 days, at the most.
- If pain persists beyond 5 days and is not improving, referral to a specialist may be indicated.

ACTIVITY

- When pain subsides, early return to activity should be encouraged.
- If clicking or pain develops, then, the wrist should be reevaluated.

PATIENT EDUCATION

Instruct the patient when to remove the splint in 5 days and to begin range of motion and activities of daily living.

MONITORING

The patient should be seen 7 to 14 days after the injury. If the pain has resolved, no further evaluation is necessary. If significant pain is still present, radiographs and consultation with an orthopaedic or hand surgeon should be performed.

PREVENTION

If feasible, patients should avoid falling on the outstretched hand.

COMPLICATIONS

- Reflex sympathetic dystrophy: a syndrome of sympathetically maintained pain resulting in exaggeration of the injury response
- Anklyosis

PROGNOSIS

- Full recovery is expected after a wrist sprain.
- If it is not achieved, evaluate the patient for other conditions.

RECOMMENDED READING

Green DP, ed. *Operative hand surgery,* 3rd ed. New York: Churchill Livingstone, 1993:7, 627, 799, 861.

Index

Index

Index

Index

Index

Index

Index